HIGH ANGLE
RESCUE TECHNIQUES

HIGH ANGLE
RESCUE TECHNIQUES

Third Edition

Tom Vines
Training Officer
Carbon County Sheriff's Search and Rescue
Red Lodge, Montana

Steve Hudson
President, Pigeon Mountain Industries, Inc.
Deputy Director, Walker County Emergency Management
Lafayette, Georgia

With 627 illustrations

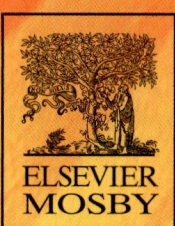

ELSEVIER
MOSBY

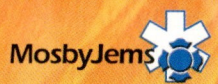

ELSEVIER
MOSBY

11830 Westline Industrial Drive
St. Louis, Missouri 63146

HIGH ANGLE RESCUE TECHNIQUES   ISBN 0-323-01914-5
Copyright © 2004, Mosby, Inc. All rights reserved.

Previous editions copyrighted 1992, 1999

International Standard Book Number 0-323-01914-5

Acquisitions Editor: Linda Honeycutt
Developmental Editor: Laura Bayless
Publishing Services Manager: Linda McKinley
Project Manager: Rich Barber
Design Manager: Bill Drone

Printed in China

Last digit is the print number: 9   8   7   6   5   4   3   2   1

No one person can develop knowledge of rope rescue in isolation. Any sense of the right approach to rope rescue, and how to do it safely, comes though association with other people in the field of rope rescue. That is why we dedicate this book to those people with whom we have associated in training and discussions, and those we never met, who have provided us with a knowledge of rope rescue and how to approach the challenge of rescue.

We also dedicate this volume to all those people in rescue who devote their time in training to do rescue well, who stand ready for the rescue call, and give their energy and skill to the rescue of people in need.

Tom Vines
Steve Hudson

Contributors

Michael V. Callahan MD, MSPH, DTM&H
Medical Director, Rescue Medicine
CIMIT/Massachusetts General Hospital
Boston, Massachusetts

Jim Kovach
Rescue Instructor
Cuyahoga Valley Career Center
Brecksville, Ohio
Bowling Green State Fire School
Bowling Green, Ohio

Loui McCurley
Technical Specialist
Alpine Rescue Team, Colorado
VP Technical Marketing
Pigeon Mountain Industries
Lafayette, Georgia

Ken Phillips
Chief of Emergency Services,
National Park Service
Grand Canyon National Park, Arizona

Introduction

About two decades have passed since we first began work on the first volume of *High Angle Rescue Techniques.* But it seems like light years in rescue history. Those past years have seen a great revolution in all aspects of the high angle environment, particularly in rope rescue. There have been great changes in equipment (rope and hardware) and in techniques (how equipment is used). Much of the equipment and many of the techniques, formerly accepted, have been questioned.

One important change has been the increased number of disciplines involved in rope rescue. Some time ago, it was primarily cave and mountain rescuers who were involved in rope rescue. Now, those rescuers have been joined by other communities. These other rescue disciplines include the fire service, industry, construction, and others.

Rope rescue concepts have leapt borders. During the past decade, the cross border unions from various parts of the world have contributed greatly to the advances in rope rescue. Perhaps most importantly, rope rescue itself has developed a sense of community. Knowledge is being developed and shared among the many professionals who practice in the field. No one ever stops learning. Each time we work with someone new, teach a class, work a rescue, or just discuss ropework with others, we learn more about the high angle environment. The greatest benefit for all of us in the rescue community is our working together to share this common knowledge. This sense of community and teamwork is vital to the advancement in rescue technology.

The world of rope rescue is too complex and changing to be dominated by any one authority or expert. None of the authors involved with *High Angle Rescue Techniques* considers himself or herself to be the expert in the field. We all feel, however, that we have been in the fortunate position of having access to a great deal of information from many different sources in the Americas and Europe. Our feeling is that the best service we can make to the people in this field is to provide them with the best possible information available, collected from many reliable resources; this is what *High Angle Rescue Techniques* is all about.

New Topics with the Third Edition

This edition of *High Angle Rescue Techniques* includes new and expanded information for rescuers. The success of a rescue often depends on how well it is organized, so this edition includes an expanded section on organizing and managing the rescue. Rescues often involve injuries or medical emergencies, so the third edition contains an expanded section on medical considerations in rescue. Litters are an important tool in rescue, so we have expanded and updated material on litters and set aside a special chapter for them. The number of communications and electrical towers is increasing, so this new edition contains a new chapter on rescue considerations for towers. Many rescuers are interested in using highlines in their operations, so there is a new chapter on highlines. At some point in many rescues, helicopters become involved, so the text contains a thorough review of their use in rescue. Rescuers have become increasingly sophisticated with equipment testing, so the third edition includes a special chapter on testing of rescue systems and equipment.

How to Use This Book

High Angle Rescue Techniques has evolved over the years. Many people have commented and made suggestions on the first two editions. Where possible, we have implemented that feedback into the third edition. We realize that this book's usefulness and popularity have been due to its simplicity. Consequently, this text will remain a manual for basic and team rope rescue. Remember that this book is designed as a training manual to be used under the guidance of a qualified instructor. High angle ropework is a dangerous activity. To be both safe and effective, you must have tools specifically designed for rope rescue and the knowledge to use them. For these reasons, this is not intended to be a self-instructional text.

High Angle Rescue Techniques is divided into two sections. The first 10 chapters are concerned with personal rope skills basic to becoming a high angle rope technician. The second half of the book focuses on rescue skills that every rescue team must have.

High Angle Rescue Techniques is also a step-by-step manual, creating a series of building blocks in high angle training. Therefore, the most critical skills, such as knowledge of rope and equipment, are covered initially. These are followed by skills such as belaying and rappelling. Finally, everything is put together in the last chapters, which focus on team rescue skills.

Here is a list of some of the special features used in each chapter of this book:

Warning Boxes

Warning boxes notify readers of an operational procedure, practice, or condition that may result in injury or death if they do not carefully follow the warning. These warnings are one of the most important features of this manual. Always remember that the high angle environment is a dangerous one. When you find one of these warnings in the text, stop and carefully read the warning. Make certain you understand it before proceeding.

Caution Boxes

Caution boxes notify readers of an operational procedure, practice, or condition that may result in damage to the equipment if not carefully observed. Although the caution boxes are not as vital as the warning boxes, paying attention to these boxes will help you preserve equipment and prevent certain dangerous situations.

Suggestion Boxes

In many aspects of the high angle environment, there are small hints, often learned through years of experience, which may make the job easier. Throughout this text, these are listed in the suggestion boxes.

Objectives

Each chapter lists a number of objectives that relate to knowledge or skills you should be able to display after completing that chapter. Mastery of this information or these skills indicates you have taken steps toward competency as a high angle rope technician. Proper instruction is critical in mastering the objectives. You cannot assume you have mastered a concept or skill without a qualified evaluation.

Key Terms

A command of the language of the high angle environment is essential for good communication in that environment. Terminology for high angle rope work comes from several different languages and from diverse activities such as mountaineering, caving, sailing, fire fighting, and textile manufacturing. It is important to know that some of these terms may have a unique or expanded meaning in high angle rescue terminology.

At the beginning of each chapter you will find lists of new words introduced in that particular chapter. All these words, in addition to some other terms of interest, are reproduced together in the glossary at the end of the text. And all of the key terms and glossary terms are boldfaced and italicized when they first appear in the text.

Evaluation Exercises

To help you in the learning process, the end of each chapter has cognitive and affective exercises that focus on the major elements in that chapter. Use these questions to see if you have grasped the important concepts in the chapter and check to see if your answers are correct in the answer key at the end of the book.

In most chapters, there are also psychomotor exercises that are designed to help you review specific physical skills related to the high angle environment.

Advantages and Disadvantages

High angle rescue is a discipline in which some inflexible rules are necessary for safety. However, in some cases there are safe choices for both equipment and technique. In this manual, we have tried to provide all viable options. Our philosophy is that the ideal high angle rope technician is one who is well trained and has the ability to adapt to any kind of situation. A better-informed rescuer can make intelligent decisions, whatever the situation.

Prerequisites

Beginning with Chapter 9, Rappelling, prerequisites are listed before each chapter. It is very important that you not move on to more advanced skills without first thoroughly mastering the prerequisite skills. If this progression is not followed, you will have problems executing the skills, which could result in unsafe conditions for yourself and others. This list of prerequisites can also serve as ready guidelines for reviewing important basics.

Acknowledgments

As with most projects the size of *High Angle Rescue Techniques*, this text, in all three editions represents the work of many more people than just the authors. We would like to thank all those individuals and organizations who helped with the evolution of this project. It is impossible to list all of the individuals who have taught us techniques, made suggestions, listened to ideas, told us of mistakes (ours and theirs), introduced us to others with special skills, and all the other things that have helped shape our own knowledge. Many of these people were providing such help years before we started working on the new edition of this book. We are taking this opportunity to say, "Thank you!"

This expanded version of *High Angle Rescue Techniques* was largely made possible by the efforts of contributing authors: Michael Callahan, MD, Jim Kovach, Loui McCurley, and Ken Phillips.

Several individuals and organizations also deserve special acknowledgment for their direct contributions to our efforts over the years. We would like to acknowledge the fine work of photography by David Scott Smith and Jonathan Hollada. Photographic resources, equipment and models, and other critical assistance were provided by Carbon County Montana Sheriff's Search and Rescue; Walker County Georgia Emergency Services; Pigeon Mountain Industries, Inc.; Karen Padgett; Diane Cousineau; Kris Green; and Jeremiah Tapp. Thanks also to Scott Carmine, Shane Catlett, and the City of Dalton Fire Department.

We also acknowledge Steve Dewell, Rob Spears, Russ Salo, Robert Golubski, and David Gilbert. All of these people could not have donated their time unless their spouses, families, and employers were also willing to spare a little of their time. Once again, thank you all.

Publisher Acknowledgments

The editors would like to thank the following people for lending their expert advice on the third edition of *High Angle Rescue Techniques:*

Peter Connick

Captain
Chatham Fire Rescue
Chatham, Massachusetts
Adjunct Faculty
Cape Cod Community College
West Barnstable, Massachusetts

Attila J. Hertelendy, BHsc., CCEMT-P, NREMT-P

Associate Instructor
University of Nevada, Reno
Fire Science Academy
Reno, Nevada

Ronald H Jones

Safety Officer
Aurora Fire Department
Treasurer
Cayuga County High Angle Rescue Team
Aurora, New York

Barbara Klingensmith, MS, FF/EMT-P

Florida State Fire College
University of Florida
Ocala, Florida

Jack Reall

City of Columbus Fire Division
Sunbury, Ohio

Contents

1 The High Angle Environment 1
- **The High Angle Environment. 2**
  - Mountaineering 2
  - Climbing 2
  - Vertical Caving 3
- **High Angle Rescue. 3**
  - Rope Rescue 3
  - Fire Service Rescue 3
  - Tactical Operations 3
  - Industrial Rescue 3
  - Rope Access 3
  - Tower Rescue 4
  - Other Ropework Users 4
- **The High Angle Rope Technician. 4**
  - Training 4
  - Continued Skills Maintenance 4
  - Comfort in the High Angle Environment 4
  - Safety 4
  - Think Systems 5
  - Characteristics of an Effective Rescuer 5
  - Use of Low-Risk Methods First 5
  - Preparation for Self-Rescue 6
  - Backup of Other Rescuers 6
  - Care of Equipment 6
  - Attention to Detail 6
  - Team Concepts 6
  - Warning Call 7
- **Rope Rescue Technician Skills 7**

2 Personal Equipment and Protection, 9
- **Clothing, Fitness and Health, and Personal**
  - **Equipment 10**
  - Headgear 10
  - Hydration 11
  - Protection from Heat and Cold 11
  - Clothing 12
  - Footwear 12
  - Gloves 12
  - Seat Harnesses 13
  - Harness Suspension Pathology 13

- Foot Supports 14
- Seat Harness Qualities 14
- Differences Between Climbing and Rescue
  - Harnesses 14
- Rescue Harnesses 14
- Full Body Harnesses 15
- Seat/Chest Harnesses 15
- Chest Harnesses 15
- Organizational Standards 15
- Securing Hardware in the High Angle
  - Environment 16
- Shoulder Slings 16
- Light Sources 16
- Knives in the High Angle Environment 17

3 Rope and Related Equipment 19
- **Determining the Right Rope for the Task. . . . 20**
  - Ropes for Technical Climbing and
    - Mountaineering 20
  - Ropes for Rappelling and Ascending 21
  - Ropes for Rescue Use 21
- **The Role of the Fall Factor. 22**
  - The Role of Fall Factors with Short Ropes . . 22
- **Fibers Used to Make Rope 23**
  - Natural Fibers 23
  - Synthetic Fiber Ropes 23
- **Rope Construction 24**
  - Laid 25
  - Plaited 25
  - Braided 25
  - Double Braid 25
  - Kernmantle 26
- **Choosing a Rope 27**
  - Dynamic versus Static Ropes 27
  - Size and Strength 27
  - Determining the System Safety Factor 27
  - Breaking Strength of Rope 29
- **Rope Colors 29**
  - Process for Coloring Ropes 29
- **Accessory Cord 29**

Webbing 29
  Webbing Materials 29
  Webbing Construction 30
  Webbing Size 30
  Webbing Strength 30

4 Care and Use of Rescue Rope and Related Equipment 33
Care of Ropes 34
  Keeping a Rope History Log 34
  Tagging Ropes 34
  Storing Ropes 34
  Bagging Ropes 35
How Ropes are Damaged 36
  Harmful Substances 36
  Overloading a Rope 36
  Damage from Falling Objects 37
  Abrasion 37
  Heat Fusion 39
  Rope Damage through "Flash" Rappels 39
  Rotation of Ropes Used in Rappel
      Training 39
  Strength Loss through Knots 39
Inspecting a Rope 40
  Establishing Responsibility for Life Safety Ropes
      40
  Retiring a Rope 40
Washing Rope 40
  Rope Washing Devices 42
  Cleaning Ropes with a Washing Machine . . . 42
  Fabric Softeners 42
  Special Cleaning Problems 43
Dressing Rope Ends 43
Care of Webbing 43
Hints for Rope Handlers 43
  Preventing Tangles 43
  Throwing and Dropping Rope 45

5 Basic High Angle Hardware 47
Hardware for the High Angle System 48
  Carabiners 48
  Descenders 56
  Rope Grabs 59
  Hardware for Anchoring 61
  Belaying 62
  Pulleys 64
  Edge Rollers 65

6 Knots 67
Knots in the High Angle Environment 68
  The Qualities of a Good Knot 68
  How Knots Affect Ropes 68
  Backing up Knots 69
  Dressing Knots 69

Specific Knots for the High Angle
  Environment 69
  Overhand Knot (For Rope and Webbing) . . . 69
  The Figure 8 Family 69
  Ring Bend (Water Knot) 74
  Double Overhand Knot (for Rope) 74
  Clove Hitch (for Rope and Webbing) 75
  Bowline on a Coil (for Rope) 75
  Interlocking Long-Tail Bowline (for Rope) . . 75

7 Anchoring 79
Anchors and the High Angle System 80
  Anchor Points 80
  Natural Anchors 80
  Anchors on Structures 80
  Less Obvious Anchors 81
  Artificial Anchors 81
  Placement of Anchors 81
  Positioning of Anchors 81
  Directionals 82
  Backing Up Anchors 83
  Materials for Anchors 84
  Keeping Anchors in Place 87
  Anchor Plates 87
  What to Do When No Anchors Appear to Be
      Available 88
  Multipoint Anchors 89

8 Belaying of One-Person Loads . . . 97
Belaying 98
  Belaying Is a Serious Commitment 98
  One-Person versus Rescue Belay 98
  The Belay System 98
  Belay Failure: The Human Element 99
  Belay Practice System 100
  Belaying Signals 101
Belaying Techniques 102
  The Münter Hitch 102
  Using a Free Running Belay Device 106
  Belaying with the ATC 106
  Belay Plates in Figure 8 Descenders 109
  Assisted Catch Belay Devices 109
Additional Cautions for Belayers 112
  Arranging the Belay Direction 112
  Maintaining Proper Slack in the Belay
      Rope 113
  Securing the Belayer 113
  Bottom Belay (for Rappelling Only) 113
  Body Belays 114

9 Rappelling 115
Rappelling 116
  Importance of Control 116
  How Rappelling Works 116
  Rappels Using Body Friction 117

Mechanical Rappel Devices 118
Rappel Stance 128
Getting Over the Edge 128
Emergency Descent Systems 138
Self-Belay Techniques 138
Protecting the Rappel Rope Below You . . . 139
Extricating Jammed Rappel Devices 139
Preventing a Rappel Off the End of a
    Rope 140

10 Basic Ascending Techniques 143
  The Purpose of Ascending. 144
  How Ascending is Accomplished. 144
    Types of Ascenders 144
  The Basics: A Prusik Hitch 145
    Selecting Rope for a Prusik Hitch 145
    Creating a Prusik Loop 145
    Attaching a Prusik Loop to a Rope 145
    Other Uses for the Prusik Loop 145
  Greater Holding Power: The Three-Wrap
    Prusik 147
  Mechanical Ascenders for Personal Use . . . 148
    Parts of the Light-Use Ascender 148
    Right-Handed and Left-Handed
      Ascenders 148
    Ascender Slings 148
    Using a Light-Use Ascender 149
  Creating an Ascending System. 151
    Tying Off Short 152
    Chicken Loops 154
    Examples of Ascending Systems 154
    Ascending Over an Edge 157
    Changing Over 158
    Extricating an Obstruction from a Jammed
      Rappel Device 160

**11 Rescue Preplanning and
    Response: Rescuer Safety and
    Situational Awareness 165**
  **Organization and Management: The
    Crucial Elements in Rescue Success or
    Failure. 166**
    Preplan 166
    Incident Command System 169
    Notification 172
    Response 172
    Investigation 172
    Critical Incident Stress Management 173
    Leadership 173
    Goals and Direction 173
    Strategy and Allocation of Resources and
      Time 173
    Communications 173
  **Key Points for Maintaining an Organized
    Rescue. 175**

  Important Safety Reminders 175
    After-Action Review: Hot Debrief 176
    Incident Review 177
    Situational Awareness 177
    Communicating for Safety 177
  Incident Risk Management Process. 177

**12 Medical Considerations in High
    Angle Rescue 181**
  **Medical Care during a High Angle Rescue
    Operation 182**
    Medical Preplanning 182
    Medical Personnel 182
    Medical Skill Level 183
    Medical Control 183
    Financial Resources 184
    Medical Equipment 184
    Litter Medical Kit 185
    Preparation and Training 187
  Assessment and Interventions 187
    Airway and Breathing 187
    Circulation 188
    Head and Spine Considerations 189
    Nonmedical Patients 189
    Medical (Trauma) Patients 189
  **Rescue and Medicine: Putting It
    Together. 190**

13 Rescue Belaying 191
  Rescue Belays. 192
    Brake Belays 192
    Tandem Prusik Belay System 192
    Load-Releasing Hitches 193
    540° Rescue Belay Device 198

14 Pickoff Rescue Techniques 203
  Using the Pickoff Rescue 204
    Pickoff Rescue Situations 204
    Teamwork and Communication 204
    Skills and Equipment Required for a
      Pickoff Rescue 204
    The Belay Question 205
    Medical Considerations 205
    Rescue of a Subject Wearing a Seat
      Harness 205
    Rescue of a Subject Not Wearing a Seat
      Harness 209
    Alternative Approach: Lowering/Raising
      Pickoff 211
    Rescue of an Unconscious Subject 212

**15 Use of Litters in High Angle
    Rescue 213**
  Litters in Rescue Operations 214
    Litter Functions 214

Types of Litters.......................... 214
  Metal Basket Litters 214
  Plastic Basket Litters 215
  Break-Apart Litters 216
  Choosing a Litter for Rescue Operations ..216
  Flexible Litters 216
Packaging the Subject in the Litter 217
  Protecting the Subject in the Litter 217
Packaging the Subject for Rope Rescue.... 221
  Packaging the Subject in the Litter 221
  Litter Subject Tie-Ins 221
Carrying the Litter 225
  Litter Slings 225
  Litter Wheels 226

16 Low Angle Evacuation 229
The Need for Low Angle Evacuation...... 230
  Examples of Low Angle (Slope)
    Evacuation 230
  Elements of Low Angle Evacuation 230
  Standard Requirements for Slope
    Evacuation 232
  Litter Rigging for Low Angle Evacuation ..232
  Litter Team for Low Angle Evacuation 234
  Packaging the Subject for Low Angle
    Evacuation 234
  Optional Personnel in Low Angle
    Evacuation 234
  Litter Tender Body Positions in Low Angle
    Evacuation 234
  Litter Tender Strategy for Low Angle
    Evacuation 235
  Litter Tender Tie-Ins 235
  Brake and Anchor Systems for Low Angle
    Lowering 236
  Braking Systems for Low Angle
    Evacuation 236
  Rope Management in Low Angle
    Evacuation 237
  The Belay Question 237
  Communications 237
  A Typical Low Angle Lowering 238
  Hauling 240
  Safe Movement of Personnel in Low Angle
    Evacuation 246

17 High Angle Lowering 249
The High Angle Lowering System........ 250
  Lowering System 251
  Braking Systems for Lowering 252
  Belays for Lowering 252
  Communication in Rescue Lowering 252
  Principles of Rescue Lowering 253
Little Lowering Systems................ 261
  Single Line versus Double Line Lowering ..261

  Procedure for Lowering a Litter (Single
    Line with Belay) 266
  Rigging the Litter for Single Line
    Lowering 267
  Medical Considerations for Rescue Subjects
    in High Angle Lowering 269
  Double Line Lowering Systems 270
  Passing Knots 274

18 Hauling Systems 277
Rescue Hauling Systems 278
  Purposes of Hauling Systems 278
  How Hauling Systems Work 279
  Calculating Mechanical Advantage 280
  Multiplying the Mechanical Advantage 280
  Calculating Mechanical Advantage and
    System Efficiencies 283
  Elements of Hauling Systems 284
  Preventing Edge Friction in Hauling
    Systems 287
  Role of the Haul Team 288
  Tag Lines 288
  Getting Over the Edge 288
  Communications 288
  Rigging and Using Hauling Systems in
    Rescue Operations 288
  1:1 TMA Hauling System 288
  Hauling from a Confined Space 290
  2:1 Hauling System without the
    Diminishing V 291
  Setting Up a 2:1 System 291
  3:1 (Z-Rig) Hauling System 291
  4:1 (Piggyback) Hauling System 292
  General Considerations for Rescue Hauling
    Systems 293

19 Tower Rescue 295
Tower Rescues: a Growing Need......... 296
Hazards in Tower Rescues.............. 296
Personal Rescue Equipment 296
Rescue Gear 297
Tower Climbing 297
  Free Climbing 297
  Built-In Fall Protection 297
  Lead Climbing 297
  Lanyard Systems 298
Rescuer Safety 299
  Climber Exhaustion 299
  Other Factors 300
Tower Rescue Size Up 301
Completing the Rescue 301
Preplanning 301
  Contacts and Resources 301
  Equipment and Personnel 302
Training 302

20 Highlines **303**
  Highlines in Rescue 304
    Use of Highlines 304
    Problems with Highlines 305
    Elements of a Highline 305
    Highline Loads 306
    Determining the Amount of Sag in the
      Highline 310
    Steps in Rigging a Highline 312
    Anchor Materials 312
    High Directionals 312
    Rigging a Highline 312
    More Complex Systems 315
    Helpful Hints .315
    English Reeve System 315

21 Helicopter Rescue Operations . . **317**
  Helicopters in Rescue Operations 320
    Decision Making and Situational
      Awareness .320
    When to Use a Helicopter 320
    Weather and Nighttime Limitations 321
    Mission Planning and Preplanning 321
    Outside Helicopter Rescue Assets 322
    Mission Management 323
    Landing Zones 324
    Load Calculation 324
    Helicopter Rescue Crews 326
  **Helicopter Flight Characteristics and
    Limitations** **328**
    Helicopter Aerodynamics 328
    Autorotation .329
    Translational Lift 330
  Types of Helicopter Landings **330**
    One-Skid Landings 330
    Toe-In Landings 331
  Helicopter Performance **332**
    Density Altitude 332
    Hover Ceiling 332
    Center of Gravity 332
    Maximum Gross Weight 332
  Basic Helicopter Safety **332**
    Preboarding 332

    Safety During Helicopter Operations 333
  Personnel Protective Equipment **333**
  Applicable U.S. Federal Regulations **335**
    In-Flight Emergency: Survival Plan
      Checklist 335
    Water Ditching Survival Training 336
    Rescue Subject Care and Transport
      Considerations 336
    Additional Rescue Subject Care
      Considerations 337
  Helicopter Rescue Techniques. **337**
    Helicopter Hoist Rescue 338
    Helicopter Rappel 340
    Helicopter Short Haul Operations 341
    Rescuer Let-Down/Lowering (Dynamic Short
      Haul) 343
    Cargo Let-Down 343

**22 Testing of Systems and
    Equipment** **347**
  Reasons for Testing Rescue Equipment . . . 348
  Component Testing 348
    Carabiners: an Example of Component
      Testing 348
    Performing Your Own Tests 350
  Systems Testing 350
  Backyard Testing 350
    Planning the Test Project 350
  Crunching the Test Results. **356**

**Appendix A Standards Setting
Organizations and Further
Reading** **359**

**Appendix B Checklists for Rescuer
Skills** **361**

Answer Key **373**

Glossary **381**

Illustration Credits **390**

1

The High Angle Environment

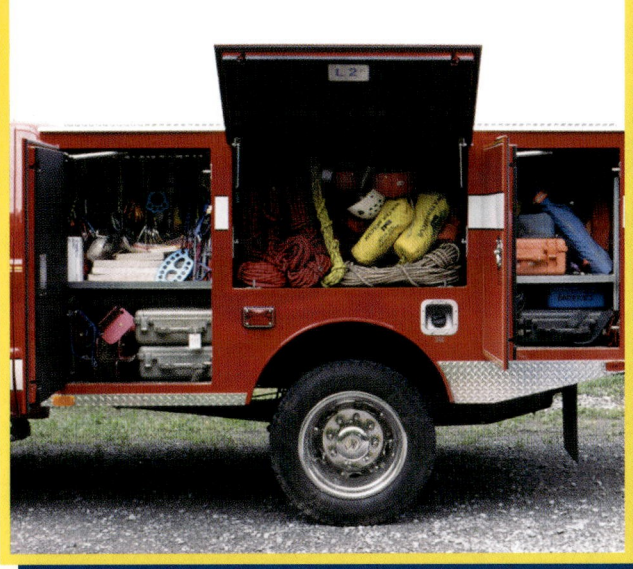

The material in this chapter conforms to guidelines published by the National Fire Protection Association (NFPA), specifically standard 1983-01, *Standard for Life Safety Rope and System Components* (2001). NFPA standards are revised regularly, and readers are advised to review the latest version of this standard.

International System of Units (SI)

This book was written in the United States, where the "English system" of measurement (e.g., pounds, quarts) is commonly used. To make the information more accessible to readers outside the United States, equivalent measurements in the International System of Units (SI) have been included. In some cases, the SI units are approximate conversions from the English system.

Objectives

On completion of this chapter, you should be able to:

1. Identify the environments in which high angle rope techniques and equipment are used for access and rescue and identify the major differences in those applications.
2. Define the primary difference between climbing and the single rope technique (SRT).
3. Describe a situation that has the potential for self-rescue.
4. List some of the equipment necessary for self-rescue situations.
5. Discuss the importance of practicing skills correctly every time and of the use of evaluation tools.
6. State the universal warning call for falling or rolling objects.

Key Terms

Ascending Climbing directly on the rope using mechanical cams or specialized knots.

Belayer The person who controls a safety rope connected to another person or persons to keep them from falling.

Carabiner Metal snap links used to connect elements of a high angle system.

High Angle A very steep environment in which a person is primarily supported by the rope system. One or more ropes are necessary to prevent the involved persons from falling.

Low Angle An environment, such as a flat or mildly sloping area, in which a person is primarily supported by the surface and not by the rope system. One or more ropes may be used for safety or for lowering.

Mountaineering The use of combined skills, such as climbing and snow and ice travel, to ascend a mountain.

Rappelling Using the friction of rope against one's body or through a descender to descend a rope under control.

Rock Climbing Ascending while making direct contact with the rock. Rope and other equipment may be used for safety in the event of a fall.

Rope Access The commercial use of mountaineering and caving rope techniques to access work sites. To ensure safe operation, the systems usually involve at least main and belay (safety) lines.

Rope Rescue Rescue in high angle and steep slope environments where the use of rope and related equipment is necessary.

Single Rope Technique (SRT) Ascending and descending directly on the rope without direct aid from contact with the rock, walls, or structures.

System The combination of components used in the high angle environment to construct a functioning unit. Two examples would be a lowering system and an anchor system.

Vertical Caving Traveling through caves with vertical or near vertical sections that require the use of rope and ascending and descending equipment.

The High Angle Environment

Throughout history, humans have been able to conquer much of the world around them by devising means to operate comfortably in environments such as the ocean, which nature had originally created hostile to them. One of the last environments conquered by humans is the high angle environment. Here, gravity is the great adversary. Although humans have not vanquished gravity, they have been able to create ways to temporarily overcome it and in some cases to use it to their advantage.

There are actually a number of different ways of operating in the high angle environment, depending on your needs.

Mountaineering

People have engaged in the vertical sport of mountaineering for hundreds of years. **Mountaineering** combines a number of skills, including climbing, camping, snow and ice travel, and often the test of will to survive against the very worst of natural forces. The most obvious goal may be reaching the top of a mountain, but often there are less obvious goals, including surviving the worst conditions in nature: cold, high wind, and high altitude illness.

Since World War II, tremendous advances have been made in mountaineering equipment. Among the most significant is the development of ropes using synthetic fibers.

Climbing

Climbing is a more specialized activity than mountaineering and is sometimes further defined as **rock climbing**. It may not involve any change in altitude more than walking from the parking lot. Or it often may involve the ascent of a short piece of rock so challenging that the climber may spend weeks working out the right "moves" so that he or she can make the climb efficiently. Climbing can also involve "big walls" that take several days to ascend and can include ice, snow, or mixed terrain.

Climbers often practice by *top roping*. In top roping, one end of the rope is dropped from the top of the climb to the bottom and tied to the climber. A safety person, or **belayer**, controls the other end of the rope, which can be threaded through a carabiner at the top and controlled by the belayer either on the ground or at the top.

In *lead climbing*, the first climber starts at the bottom of a climb with the rope attached to his or her harness and running back to a belayer. While ascending, the climber attaches the rope to intermediate anchors created by placing special pieces of climbing hardware, called *protection*, into the rock. This protection could be permanent bolts set into the rock or items temporarily placed, such as cams, chocks, and pitons. **Carabiners** are clipped into the protection, and the rope is run through them. These intermediate pieces of protection reduce the potential falling distance of the lead climber as that person progresses up the route to the next belay station. Often the belayer follows the lead climber once the next belay station has been reached. The former lead climber acts as belayer in a top rope–type climb for the former belayer.

In *free solo climbing*, a climber ascends alone and without safety gear such as rope. Free solo climbing is in vogue among a very few climbers, but most climbing is still done with the climber roped *(free climbing)*. The essential elements of free climbing are (1) a rope with a great deal of stretch so that it can catch the falling climber and also absorb the shock created by the fall, and (2) protection or anchoring hardware so that the rope can be attached to the rock and "protect" the climber.

In recent years climbing has diverged into several specialties. A relatively new development is climbing on artificial climbing walls in indoor "climbing gyms." This is often done by top roping, but some of the more sophisticated gyms have walls with prebolted protection and lead routes on which climbers can place their own protection for lead climbing.

Vertical Caving

Vertical caving is one of the youngest of the vertical sports, beginning only in the 1950s. It also differs significantly from climbing. Instead of the vertical caver climbing the rock itself, he or she descends and ascends on the rope and usually does not intend to use the rope for protection in case of a fall from the rock. This method of climbing is known as **single rope technique (SRT)** (see Chapter 3). Vertical caving uses two primary ropework skills, rappelling and ascending.

A common technique used in vertical caving technique is the controlled descent on a rope. Vertical caving puts more emphasis on the skill of rappelling than does climbing. This is because vertical cavers often have to rappel long distances, sometimes several hundred feet, and in adverse conditions such as dark and wetness. The other vertical caving skill, **ascending**, is climbing directly on the rope using mechanical cams or specialized knots.

Vertical caving is not a widely followed sport, but it has had a significant influence on the equipment and techniques used in other vertical activities, particularly high angle rescue and industrial rope access. One of the most important of these effects has been the development of a rope that is very durable and that stretches very little *(static rope)*.

High Angle Rescue
Rope Rescue

Depending on the environment and the rescuers involved, **rope rescue** may also be called *vertical rescue* or in some cases *technical rescue*. In these situations a rope and other associated gear are necessary so that the subject of the rescue can be moved from hazard, kept stabilized and safe, and protected from falling.

Originally, most of the equipment and techniques used in rope rescue were the same as those used in mountaineering. However, in recent decades a major shift has occurred away from these types of equipment and techniques toward ones more specialized for rescue. A significant example is rescue rope, which has shifted from a stretchy line, as is used in mountaineering, to a line with very little stretch and more durable construction, similar to that used in vertical caving.

Fire Service Rescue

The use of life support rope and associated equipment in the fire service has undergone tremendous change during recent decades. This is partly because of well-publicized tragedies, such as the one that occurred in June 1980 in New York City, in which a rope failed during a rescue attempt and two firefighters fell to their deaths. Further impetus for these changes has come from fire service organizations such as the National Fire

Protection Association (NFPA), the International Association of Fire Fighters (IAFF), and the International Society of Fire Service Instructors (ISFSI).

Perhaps the most significant of these changes has been the recognition that the use of natural fiber rope for life safety is a dangerous and irresponsible practice, a realization that resulted in a massive changeover by fire departments to synthetic fiber ropes.

Tactical Operations

The increase in terrorist incidents and other forms of violence has prompted greater preparation by law enforcement and the military in the use of high angle operations. Many of these innovations have taken place in operational procedures, such as the use of helicopters. However, tactical practitioners have contributed to the high angle technology used by many other disciplines. An important example of this is the *figure 8 with ears descender* (also called a *rescue 8*). An early form of the device was developed by the Special Air Services (SAS) in England, and it was later adapted initially in North America through the joint efforts of California Law Enforcement personnel and mountaineer and inventor Russ Anderson. (See p. 57 for a discussion of the advantages of the figure 8 with ears over the conventional figure 8).

Industrial Rescue

Industrial rescue incidents can occur in high angle and confined areas, such as refineries, chemical plants, and open pit and underground mining sites, that pose the risk of falls, entrapment, medical emergencies, and exposure to dangerous materials. The principles of high angle rescue are the same in industrial and natural environments, but environmental circumstances may either help or hinder industrial rescuers. In industrial rescue situations, abundant structural anchors usually are available, and the response time generally is short. The rescue teams may be either on-site or predesignated response units, such as fire departments.

A very specialized type of industrial operation is the *confined space rescue*. Confined spaces often contain hazardous materials and dangerous machinery. Most significant are the hazardous atmospheres that require rescuers to safeguard themselves with protective clothing and a breathing apparatus. In addition, the presence of hazardous materials can require rescuers to use specialized equipment rope constructed from fibers resistant to corrosive substances.

As a result of the high death rate among those attempting rescues in confined spaces, the U.S. Occupational Safety and Health Administration (OSHA) has established regulations specific to rescuers in confined spaces.

Rope Access

An approach rapidly growing in popularity is the commercial use of mountaineering and caving rope techniques to access work sites. Using **rope access** to get to hard-to-reach work sites may be quicker and simpler than using traditional structural installations such as scaffolding and platforms. Rope access has a wide range of uses, including window cleaning, bridge painting, and engineering inspection of building exteriors and ocean oil platforms. In most rope access techniques used on a work site, the worker has two ropes, or lines: a working line and a back-up safety line, with a harness as the primary means of attachment. As the use of rope access at work sites increases, rope rescue teams increasingly will be called upon to extract these workers from accidents that on-scene teams can't handle.

The Society of Professional Rope Access Technicians (SPRAT) develops consensus safety standards for vertical rope access work. SPRAT has developed the standard *Requirements for Rope Access Work,* which applies to the four job positions in rope access work: Rope Access Supervisor, Technician, Worker, and Attendant (see Appendix A).

Tower Rescue

Other industrial situations may require rope access procedures to allow workers to do their jobs. An example would be a worker climbing up a structural tower.

Other Ropework Users

The highly sophisticated entertainment environments currently in use require lighting technicians, stagehands, and special effects workers to climb into rigging high above the stage. Increasingly, these workers are using ropework techniques to access the rigging.

The High Angle Rope Technician

There has been a tradition in the high angle environment of specializing in a particular discipline, such as rock climbing. However, many people are borrowing techniques and equipment from all disciplines in the high angle environment and putting them to use for their own particular needs. Some of these individuals might be described as *high angle rope technicians,* people competent in a number of high angle skills who can use them for particular needs, such as rope rescue.

High angle rope technicians are trained and experienced in the skills needed in the high angle environment. They use the technology of the high angle environment to conquer gravity and to move about with ease in any direction needed. They also may use the technology of rope rescue to carefully move subjects away from dangerous situations and into safe areas, where any injuries can be treated.

High angle rope technicians follow some basic principles so as to be both safe and successful in their work.

Training

High angle rope skills cannot be learned simply by reading a book. This book is designed as a training manual to be used under the guidance of a qualified instructor experienced in the field of high angle techniques. Such instructors can be found in established training organizations, such as government organizations and fire training centers or independent schools with a long

history of training in high angle techniques. You should choose an instructor or training school with experience in the environment in which you will be working, and the instructor should be knowledgeable about the relevant standards and regulations. For example, if you expect to be working in an area that could involve confined spaces, the instructor must understand the government regulations that apply to confined space entry and confined space hazards. An instructor in fire service rescue must be knowledgeable about the relevant NFPA standards. You should avoid individuals who have taken only one class in high angle techniques, yet have anointed themselves instructors in those procedures.

Continued Skills Maintenance

Instruction in high angle techniques is only the first step. High angle skills deteriorate quickly without constant practice and regular training. A training schedule should be an indispensable part of every high angle technician's routine. The difference between a competent high angle rope technician and one who can only talk about doing it is that the competent technician really has the skills for the job. It is essential not only that a person understand the skills, but also that he or she use them instinctively. In sudden emergencies, people react with actions that are instinctive. The only way to make high angle skills instinctive is *practice.*

An instructor should use an evaluation sheet to help show that every student has performed the skills satisfactorily (an example of an evaluation sheet is shown in Appendix B). This checklist has a space for the instructor to indicate that the student has performed the skills satisfactorily and a space for the student to confirm that he or she has performed the skills. This method helps double-check the training system and may protect the instructor at a later date should the student fail to perform the skill correctly and claim that the failure was the result of a training lapse.

Comfort in the High Angle Environment

A fear of heights is natural to human beings, and a degree of it is necessary for survival. Individuals without any fear or respect for the hazards involved in high angle work are a danger to themselves and to others. However, until a person feels at ease operating in the high angle environment, that discomfort will prevent the person from being effective in these activities. As with any unaccustomed environment, the approach to movement, to using equipment, and to working alongside others is completely new. You should be able to work at the highest building or cliff face in your response area. The only way to become accustomed to working hundreds of feet in the air and to become effective doing it is to spend time there. In other words, *practice.*

Safety

Beyond doubt, the primary objective of high angle activity is doing it safely. This primary objective is achieved through mental and physical concepts and through team organization.

Personal Red Flags

An individual should be aware of a number of "red flags," or danger signs, when working in the high angle environment, including the following:

- Tunnel vision (an obsession with a detail or unexpected problem that causes the rescuer to lose situation awareness).
- Physical fatigue.
- Mental or physical impairment caused by environmental factors such as heat or cold.
- Impairment caused by alcohol or drugs.
- Fear of speaking out when a dangerous situation is noted.
- Overconfidence, leading to lack of attention to the task at hand.
- Inability to concentrate because of outside concerns, such as family or personal problems.
- Overexcitement ("adrenaline rush"): Feel your pulse; if it is racing well beyond your normal rate, sit down and cool off.
- Failure to ask for help or assistance. People sometimes have a dangerous tendency to fail to admit they are in over their heads, because doing so would make them look bad. If you feel you are getting in over your head, ask for help (a belay, if appropriate) or back off. If you are at all uncertain about how to tie a knot or use a piece of equipment, ask for advice or get some feedback.

Physical Safety Concepts

The following are some physical safety rules that should be observed at all times:

- Establish safety lines; everyone at the edge must be tied in.
- When appropriate, use redundant systems (e.g., more than one anchor).
- Wear a helmet and other appropriate personal protection equipment (this applies to all on site).
- Check equipment constantly to make sure it is in safe condition.

Think Systems

This book examines the necessary elements of the high angle system and the ways in which their strengths and weaknesses determine the effectiveness of the system and, ultimately, the outcome of the operation.

One ideal that should be kept in mind by anyone working in the high angle environment is think *systems*. Although some elements are essential and important, activities in the high angle environment are rarely completed with only one rope, only one piece of hardware, or only one person.

The high angle environment system consists of many elements, such as rope, hardware, anchors, and other elements, which cannot be viewed in isolation. For the elements to operate safely and properly, they must be viewed together as a system.

Just as a chain is only as strong as its weakest link, the high angle system is only as effective as its weakest element. For example, if your equipment system uses a rope that has a tensile test strength of 9,000 lbf (40 kN) but it is attached to an anchor that pulls out at 500 lbf (2.2 kN), the strength of the entire

| Box 1-1 | **Weight versus Mass: Units of Measure** |

Precise measurement requires a distinction between *weight* and *mass*. Pounds and kilograms are measurements of weight. An accurate measurement of force is expressed in newtons. A newton (N) is the unit of force required to accelerate a mass of 1 kilogram 1 meter per second. The impact loads on rope and the breaking strength of equipment are usually expressed in kilonewtons (kN); in the English system, this is expressed in pounds/force (lbf). Major organizations that set standards for high angle rescue use the International System of Units (SI). Equivalents are as follows:

1 newton = 0.225 lbf
1 kN (1,000 newtons) = 225 lbf

system is only 500 lbf (2.2 kN). (See Box 1-1 for information regarding pounds/force [lbf] and kilonewtons [kN].)

Study this book carefully to learn the strengths of your component pieces of equipment. As you come to understand the various rigging systems, you will learn that each system component can be rigged in ways for maximum strength and often in ways that will weaken the overall system as well. Learn to engineer the systems you use and build them in a way that yields maximum strength as a total system.

Characteristics of an Effective Rescuer

Although it is difficult to define exactly all the characteristics of an effective rescuer, certain traits stand out. One of the most significant is the rescuer's concern for the subject, the person being rescued. The rescuers must realize that the rescue subject is the reason for everyone's involvement. This is a human being in distress, a person in physical and perhaps emotional pain. A rescuer may contribute to that distress by regarding the rescue subject more as an object than as a person. Rescuers must continually communicate with the rescue subject in their care, even when the subject is unconscious. Hearing is the last sense to go in an unconscious person, and many people will recall conversations that took place around them while they were unconscious.

Use of Low-Risk Methods First

The approach to the rescue subject should be the one that involves the least amount of danger both to the subject and to the rescuers. Some examples of this lower risk approach include the following:

- Always evaluate the situation before approaching it. Depending on the specific environment, dangers to rescuers could include hazardous atmospheres, energized wires, falling rocks, or hostile individuals.
- Don't rush. Rushing causes mistakes that endanger both the rescuers and the subject. Move carefully and meticulously. Don't crowd other rescuers.
- Choose the least dangerous route to the subject.
- Use the simplest rescue system that works effectively and safely. In rope rescue, the simplest way of doing the job is

usually the most effective way. The more complicated the rescue system, the greater the chance of something going wrong.

- Instead of setting up operations directly above the subject, where rocks or hardware might fall on the person (and other rescuers), move slightly off to one side. Keep all non-essential personnel away from the area, because they might dislodge rocks and other objects.
- Appoint a team safety officer to oversee equipment use, anchoring, rigging belays, personal rappelling and ascending, and seat harness tie-ins. The safety officer should be among the most experienced of the team members and must be able to oversee all aspects of the operation.
- Ensure that all rescuers wear protective gear, such as helmets, to prevent head injury from falling objects and to reduce injury if the rescuer takes a fall. All personnel qualified for high angle operations should wear their seat harnesses so that they are ready for any immediate needs.
- Before rescue operations begin, set up safety lines. Anyone near the edge must clip into one of them. If continued access up and down a steep slope is needed, a securely anchored safety line should be set from top to bottom off to the side, slightly away from the rescue site.

Preparation for Self-Rescue

Whatever the activity, a person who works in the high angle environment must always keep in mind that anything can go wrong, and someday it probably will. Therefore you should be ready for something to go wrong and be ready to extricate yourself. Prepare and train yourself for an emergency. Keep on yourself the gear necessary to perform self-rescue, including a small assortment of carabiners, a couple of slings made from webbing or rope, and either a set of Prusik loops or a pair of ascenders (see Chapter 10 for an explanation of the specific purpose of this gear).

Backup of Other Rescuers

In the same way, each rescuer should be ready at any time to extricate any other rescuer who gets into difficulty. Whenever any team member is not at work performing a task, all attention should be focused on the activity at hand. Everyone, no matter how intelligent and experienced, has an occasional lapse. All team members should be alert to the development of any unsafe condition and be ready to make appropriate corrections.

Care of Equipment

One sign of good mechanics or carpenters is their meticulous care of the tools of their trade. The same is true of a high angle rope technician, who must care for rope and hardware. However, in the case of high angle gear, good care is critical, because lives depend on these tools. Considerations for avoiding loss and damage to rescue gear include the following:

- Do not lay unsecured equipment at the edge of a drop. It can easily be kicked or knocked over the edge and be damaged or lost. Even worse, the object could injure those working below.
- When using equipment on a vertical face, keep all gear secured. It should be either attached to the system or secured to the equipment sling that many harnesses have.
- Do not lay equipment on the ground or floor. Hardware is easily lost in debris or dirt, and grit damages hardware. Prepare for this when you first arrive on the site. Either lay out an equipment tarp or hang a sling on a tree or other beam. All hardware not in use should be placed on the tarp or clipped into the sling.
- Inspect all gear after each operation. The time to discover that gear is defective is during inspection, not during a rescue.
- Ropes need special care (see Chapter 4). A traditional rule is never step on a rope. Many experienced vertical rope-workers are fanatical about never stepping on a rope. Stepping on a rope grinds grit into the core, where it can damage the load-supporting fibers. More than that, however, to many people a person who steps on a rope shows contempt for the well-being of the person who uses the rope.
- Take all defective gear out of service immediately.
- Belay all lowering and raising of rescue subjects. Any rescuers who request them must be provided with belays.

Attention to Detail

Attention to detail in the high angle environment is necessary for rescuers to work effectively and to prevent injury to themselves and others. This environment is unforgiving, and a lapse that might go unnoticed on level ground could result in severe injury or death in the high angle environment.

There is, of course, a need for balance. You must not be so obsessed that you are unable to complete a task. However, only a focused mind can examine a system quickly and immediately determine if all the necessary details are in place, and this only comes with practice.

Although attention to detail is an essential trait for the high angle rope technician, the nature of high angle operations requires that a person have the ability to improvise. Every high angle situation is different, with varying circumstances in terms of weather and terrain. Therefore a well-trained individual with good judgment is preferable to one who is well trained to perform in only one way.

Team Concepts

Many accidents or near misses occur because of organizational and management failures. Rescuers can help avoid this by training together often so that individual skills are combined into one working unit. Another form of insurance is the use of a safety officer. The *safety officer* is an individual who makes sure that safe procedures are followed during training and real rescues. The safety officer should be someone other than the team leader, because the leader often is too busy to check all safety systems (Chapter 11 presents more information about the safety officer).

Warning Call

One of the most common dangers in the high angle environment is falling objects, either hardware dropped by others or dislodged rocks. Whenever a hard object begins to fall, even if no one is thought to be below, the universal warning is to yell *very loudly*, "Rock!" Do not say, "Look out," "Heads up," or anything other than "Rock."

Rope Rescue Technician Skills

To summarize, a rope rescue technician is one who is trained in the necessary skills for rope rescue, has shown that he or she is competent in those skills, and continually trains to maintain them. He or she should be able to do the following:

- Demonstrate the proper use and care of rope.
- Demonstrate the proper use and care of other equipment needed in the high angle environment.
- Demonstrate the ability to tie correctly and without hesitation the 10 knots described in Chapter 6, plus the Münter hitch and the Prusik hitch.
- Demonstrate the ability to rig safe and secure anchors.
- Demonstrate the ability to safely and confidently belay another person.
- Demonstrate the ability to rappel safely, confidently, and under control; the ability to tie off a rappel device to operate safely with hands free of the rope and then return to a safe and controlled rappel; and the ability to operate on the rope with the body in any position, including the inverted position.
- Demonstrate the ability to ascend safely; the ability to tie correctly and without hesitation a friction hitch, as well as how to use it; the uses and limitations of mechanical ascenders; and the ability to safely ascend a fixed rope using both friction hitches and mechanical ascenders.
- Demonstrate the ability while on rope to confidently and safely change over from rappelling to ascending and from ascending to rappelling; also the ability to extricate himself or herself from a jammed rappel device (or similar problem) without using a knife.

In addition to personal vertical skills, the rope rescue technician must train and qualify in other areas before qualifying in the area of rescue. Among these skills are:

- *Emergency medical skills.* Team members should be trained at least to a level of DOT first responder (see the section on Medical Considerations for Patients in High Angle Rescue in Chapter 12).
- *Team skills.* Some examples are litter-handling techniques and lowering and hauling systems.
- *Communication skills.* These include not only the ability to communicate electronically but also the standard voice communications required in specialized team operations such as rescuer lowering and hauling systems.
- Other skills, depending on the environment, such as land navigation, snow and ice travel, or survival.

Evaluation Exercises

Cognitive and Affective Exercises

1. Identify the five environments, both recreational and work related, in which high angle rope techniques and equipment are used for access and rescue; also identify the major differences in those applications.

2. Single rope technique implies which of the following:

   A. The climber is using the rope to ascend or descend.
   B. The climber is using the rope to "safety" himself or herself.
   C. The climber is without a belay.
   D. The climber is climbing one rope length.

3. Free climbing implies that:

   A. The climber is climbing the rope to go upward.
   B. The climber is ascending, making direct contact with the surface he or she is on, while using rope and other equipment to provide safety in the event of a fall.
   C. The climber is rock or ice climbing.
   D. The climber is using a rope to make forward progress during a difficult vertical event.

4. Which of the following might be considered a self-rescue situation:

   A. While traversing a glacier, one of the rescue party falls into a crevasse.
   B. While a rescuer is rappelling, his or her shirt gets caught in the figure 8 device.
   C. The rescuer slips while climbing but is caught by the rope and is hanging upside down below an overhang.
   D. All of the above.

5. Of the following, what would be considered minimal equipment for self-rescue preparedness:

   A. In your pack: Several locking carabiners, a figure 8 descender, several slings, and some Prusik loops.
   B. In your pack: Several pieces of protection, ascenders, and Prusik loops or slings.
   C. On your person: A small assortment of carabiners, a couple of slings made from webbing or rope, and either a set of Prusik loops or a pair of ascenders.
   D. On your person: Extra carabiners, a sling, and a rappel device.

6. While performing a rescue operation, you notice something falling from above your position. You should:

   A. Yell, "Rock!"
   B. Yell, "Falling!"
   C. Shout in a loud voice, "Something is falling toward you!"
   D. Shout, "Look out!"

7. It is important that personnel learn the correct way from the beginning because:

   A. Under stressful situations in real incidents, people will revert to the way they did it the first time.
   B. People frequently cannot understand things until the fourth time.
   C. Participants must make mistakes before they can learn.
   D. It is not important; incorrect procedure can be remedied at any time.

2

Personal Equipment and Protection

The material in this chapter conforms to guidelines published by the National Fire Protection Association (NFPA), specifically standard 1983-01, *Standard for Life Safety Rope and System Components* (2001). NFPA standards are revised regularly, and readers are advised to review the latest version of this standard.

Objectives

On completion of this chapter, you should be able to:

1. List four points to consider when selecting a helmet for use in the rope rescue environment.
2. List several considerations for the "shell" and "insulated" layers of clothing for rope rescue personnel.
3. List several considerations for hand and foot protection in rope rescue.
4. List several considerations for a secure and comfortable seat harness.
5. Cite an example of the safety standards that apply to safety equipment in the rope rescue environment.
6. Describe the considerations for selection of personal equipment for use in the rope rescue environment.
7. List federal, private, and international organizations that set standards for rescue equipment.
8. Describe a scenario that would result in a catastrophic failure if a knife is used improperly in the rope rescue environment.

Key Terms

ASTM (formerly known as the American Society for Testing and Materials) An international organization that develops standards through a "full consensus" method. ASTM standards that apply to the rope rescue environment include those relating to search and rescue, recreational climbing equipment, and arboriculture equipment.

CEN (European Committee for Standardization) The standards-setting authority for the European Union. CE standards cover a wide range of products, including those used for recreational climbing, protection from industrial falls, and rope access.

Chest Harness A type of harness worn around the chest for upper body support. In the high angle environment, it should never be used as the only source of support; it should always be used in conjunction with a seat harness.

Emergency Seat Harness A temporary tied harness that is used when a manufactured, sewn seat harness is not available.

Escape Belt A device that fastens around the waist like a belt that is intended for use by the wearer only as an emergency self-rescue device. It should never be used as the sole means of suspension.

Full Body Harness A type of harness that offers pelvic and upper body support as one unit.

Harness Suspension Pathology A potentially fatal condition that can occur when a person hangs motionless in a seat harness for a long period. The position in the harness, along with harness strap compression, reduces venous blood flow from the extremities (particularly the legs) to the right side of the heart, with subsequent reduction in cardiac output. This can result in unconsciousness and possibly death in minutes.

Helmet A head covering that protects against head injury both from falling objects and from head impact. When used in this book, the term helmet denotes head protection specifically designed for high angle work.

Ladder Belt A device that fastens around the waist and is intended for use as a positioning device for a person on a ladder. It should never be used as the sole means of suspension.

NFPA (National Fire Protection Association) A U.S. national organization that sets safety standards including life safety equipment training, and professional qualification standards for rope rescue teams.

Seat Harness A system of nylon or polyester webbing that wraps and supports the pelvic region to attach the wearer to the rope or other protection in the high angle environment. There are three classes of NFPA harnesses:
- Class I: A light duty seat harness meant for emergency escape and light duty work by one person.
- Class II: A seat harness meant for heavy duty work by one person or in rescue situations in which another person's weight may be added in the course of the rescue.
- Class III: A full body harness meant for fall protection and rescue where inversion might occur.

UIAA (Union of International Alpine Associations) An organization that sets performance standards for ropes, harnesses, ice axes, helmets, and carabiners to be used by climbers and mountaineers.

Clothing, Fitness and Health, and Personal Equipment

Making the correct choice of clothing and personal equipment to use in the high angle environment can give you, as a high angle rope technician and rescuer, a greater margin of safety, add to your comfort, and enable you to perform your job more effectively and efficiently.

Headgear

A critical piece of personal protective equipment is the *helmet*. A helmet can protect the wearer from injury or can reduce the severity of injury from falling objects such as rocks or climbing hardware. It also can reduce the severity of brain injury should you fall and hit your head.

You should buy only helmets specifically designed for high angle activities. Other types of helmets may provide only an illusion of protection and can actually be dangerous to the wearer. *Construction-type or motorcycle helmets are not suitable for high angle work.* They are not designed to offer protection from the forces that may be applied to the head in the high angle environment. Many construction helmets offer at best only minimum protection, and they tend to slip off the head when protection is needed most.

Many types of helmets may be uncomfortable or inconvenient to wear in the high angle environment. For example, motorcycle helmets tend to be very uncomfortable during hot weather and can diminish hearing. Rescue operations often take a long time, and rescuers are in hazard zones for many hours. A comfortable, well-fitting helmet is essential in such situations, because the helmet must be worn for long periods.

It is very important that helmets have a secure chin strap. Helmets with elastic chin straps are not suitable for high angle work. As the elastic chin strap stretches, the helmet may flip off the head and leave the wearer without head protection. This often occurs when the helmet is stressed, such as when the wearer falls or is hit by falling objects.

Any helmet used in high angle work should also have a *three-point suspension*. This means that in addition to support points on both sides of the helmet, a third one is positioned at the rear. The third suspension point helps prevent the helmet from falling forward over the eyes. The chin straps on many construction-type helmets are designed to release easily when the helmet snags on something. A good high angle helmet should have a chin strap that requires much greater force to cause release; this helps keep the helmet on the user's head in a tumbling fall.

The shells of helmets used in high angle rescue are constructed of materials such as plastic, fiberglass, composites of fiberglass, and composites of Kevlar in various plastics. The shell should have the rigidity to resist impact to the helmet and penetration by sharp objects. At the same time, it should have enough give to absorb some of the blow that otherwise would be directly transmitted to the skull and spine. The design of the helmet should protect the head against objects falling from above and hitting from the side.

The inside suspension of the helmet should hold the shell away from the skull during a blow to the helmet and should provide air circulation and comfort, particularly during hot weather.

A slight brim helps prevent rainwater or spray from dripping into your face. However, your helmet should have a narrow enough profile to allow you a good upward field of vision and to ensure that the back of the helmet does not catch on a pack when you raise your head.

Helmets that have earned climbing helmet certification to the **Union of International Alpine Associations (UIAA)** or the **European Committee for Standardization (CEN)** of the European Union usually are adequate for high angle work. Helmets certified to the **National Fire Protection Association (NFPA)** have good impact resistance, but many fire helmets are inadequate for high angle rope work. Those with extended rear brims are cumbersome in the high angle environment. Also, their bulkiness tends to obstruct vision, making it difficult to maneuver in the sometimes cluttered and confined high angle environment, and they can be very uncomfortable in hot weather. A more recent NFPA helmet standard (NFPA 1951) has been established for helmets used in urban search and rescue (USAR). This guideline is part of the NFPA *Standard on Protective Ensemble for USAR Operations.*

The cardinal rule is: *Don't buy a cheap helmet for high angle work.* Spending a few extra dollars on a helmet with good suspension and impact absorption is cheap compared with the cost of ending up brain dead.

Hydration

By composition, the human body usually is about two thirds water. For the body to operate efficiently, little variation from this norm can be tolerated. Water is involved in every function of the body. Body fluid transports nutrients and oxygen to muscles and the brain. It also is responsible for lubrication and temperature control. Studies have shown that most people performing physical labor in extreme temperatures become dehydrated.

The following are some of the ways in which dehydration can affect you:

- Keeping warm becomes more difficult.
- You cannot think at full efficiency. Even moderate dehydration greatly affects your ability to do complex problem solving.
- Your energy reserves are diminished.

- Electrolyte shifts affect your fine motor skills.
- Disabling headaches and muscle cramps occur.

Dehydration diminishes body functions and can cause a dangerous loss of judgment. This is a very insidious process, because most people drink fluids only when thirsty, and thirst is a poor indicator of the need for hydration. A more reliable indicator is urine output. Clear or light-colored urine usually indicates adequate hydration.

Dehydration is not a problem confined to hot environments. It also is common in cold environments, because people are less motivated to drink fluid. *The important thing is to drink fluids constantly, even when you are not thirsty, so that you have clear or light-colored urine.*

Urination, particularly in social situations such as a rescue, may seem inconvenient and embarrassing. However, if you are not urinating regularly, you are not hydrated. Keep at least 2 quarts (2 L) of water in your pack, particularly if no group water sources are available. The best fluid to drink for hydration is plain water.

Protection from Heat and Cold

Humans are physically weak and vulnerable compared with many other creatures on earth. It is our brain that has enabled us to survive and prevail. If brain function is threatened, then survival is at risk.

One of the greatest weaknesses of the human body is that it was designed to survive only in a narrow temperature range. Existence outside this range for a prolonged period, whether in temperatures that are too hot or too cold, progressively inhibits the body from functioning; it causes dangerous mental confusion and eventually death.

We lack the natural defenses of animals (e.g., having fur to stay warm and panting to lose heat), therefore we must create artificial defenses to protect ourselves from temperature extremes.

The human body loses or gains heat in four ways: conduction, convection, radiation, and respiration.

1. Conduction (direct contact with cold or hot object)
   - Example of heat loss through conduction: Sitting or lying on a cold metal structure
   - Example of heat gain through conduction: Sitting or lying on hot concrete or rock slabs
2. Convection (air currents rob body heat or overload it)
   - Example of heat loss through convection: Standing on a tower where a cold wind is blowing
   - Example of heat gain through convection: Working in a containment vessel on a hot day
3. Radiation (radiant heat robs the body of heat or adds heat)
   - Example of heat gain through radiation: Working in the sunshine on a hot day
   - Example of heat loss through radiation: Working with the head uncovered in a cold environment
4. Respiration (the body is cooled or heated through the respiratory system):
   - Example of heat loss through respiration: Inhalation of cool air, which is warmed by the respiratory system before being exhaled
   - Example of heat gain through respiration: Increase in body temperature caused by hot ambient air

One secret to maintaining temperature equilibrium is being adaptable to changes in temperature and weather. This means being able to add or remove clothing and other protection regardless of the heat or cold challenge.

Clothing

The principle of clothing protection is to maintain warmth when needed but also to allow the body to lose warmth before becoming overheated. The principle of insulation is the retention of air in the fibers of the garment. The great danger to insulation is wetness, either from the outside (rain, snow) or the inside (perspiration). Wetness quickly saps body heat.

One important piece of clothing that protects from outside wetness is a "shell," which is a jacket or a parka made of water-proof material such as coated nylon or Gore-Tex. A shell can protect against both precipitation and the cooling effects of wind. However, during intense physical activity, lack of air circulation under the shell can result in the production of large amounts of perspiration. As a result, the interior of the shell may become as saturated with sweat as the outside is with precipi-tation. The shell, therefore, must have a means of venting heat away from the body before perspiration begins. Unzipping a zipper down the front of the garment can serve this purpose. Some outdoor clothing also has zippers along the side or under the armpits to help release body heat before it produces perspiration.

Several types of fabric are available, in addition to Gore-Tex, that are designed to allow body perspiration to escape while protecting the wearer from precipitation. How well this concept works, however, still depends on specific climate conditions and use by the wearer. Some users have found that in incessant, heavy rain, the fabric allows wetness to soak through. Also, production of large amounts of perspiration can overwhelm the fabric system and inhibit its function. Whatever the specific type of rainwear you use, if you can stand for half an hour under a shower and still not get soaked through, it will probably protect you in the outdoor rope rescue environment.

An insulating layer of clothing should be worn under the shell. This provides warmth, but it must also protect the wearer against chilling even when wet, either from precipitation or perspiration. The key for insulation value is the ability to retain air in the fibers and not get wet from outside or inside the garment.

Cotton is the least desirable fabric in wet and cold envi-ronments because it tends to lose its insulating qualities when wet. The traditional choice for a fabric that retains warmth when wet is wool. A more recent development, and a fabric that is more comfortable next to the skin, is polyester pile. However, both fabrics (particularly pile) offer little shielding from the wind, therefore they need to be worn with an outer windbreaker shell.

For the outdoors, underwear made of synthetic materials such as polypropylene has become common. It dries quickly and tends to draw moisture away from the skin, which prevent it from having a cooling effect on the body.

Clothing should protect the rope rescue technician against adverse environmental conditions and provide maximum comfort for any activity. Shirts and pants must be sized so that

⚠ Warning

Underwear made of materials that can melt, shrink, or stick to skin when exposed to heat and flame may not be appropriate for individuals working in helicopters or in other situations in which flash fire is a possibility. Under intense heat, such as that produced by a flash fire, the synthetic material may melt into the skin, complicating the burn injury.

they do not bind when the arms are extended above the head or when the legs are raised.

Footwear

Among the requirements for footwear are comfort, protection, and adhesion. Although boots increasingly are partly or completely fabricated of materials such as Gore-Tex or plastic, leather is still the material with the qualities most needed in a multipurpose boot for rope rescue.

Boots should provide support to the ankles and protect the feet from scrapes, cuts, and bruises, yet they should be pliable enough to be comfortable after hours of standing or walking. The soles should not be "slick," like the soles of street shoes, but rather should have adhesion to help the wearer maintain balance against the surfaces found in the rope rescue environment. Rubber boots, such as those commonly used in the fire service, are not appropriate for rope rescue operations. They do not have the needed foot protection, and they impede foot and leg movement.

Lug soles, particularly those made from Vibram, have been very much in fashion, but they may not be required as long as the boot sole provides adhesion. Furthermore, in some cases a lug sole may actually be a disadvantage. Some types of lug soles may become dangerously slick when wet or caked with mud.

For specialized rock climbing, technical climbing boots may be used, which have soles constructed of special rubber compounds that may adhere to the rock better. Many of these climbing boots have little or no welt, therefore they may be better for certain climbing techniques, such as "edging" along the rock. However, because they are specifically made for climbing, they are not comfortable for walking or standing for long periods.

A good choice of socks is important for warmth, comfort, and prevention of injury such as blisters. A two-sock combination can reduce friction on the skin that causes blisters. An inner sock made of a synthetic, such as polypropylene, wicks moisture away from the foot so that it stays dry. A thick outer sock, made of a material such as wool, increases warmth and provides some protection for the foot.

Gloves

Gloves are worn in the rope rescue environment to protect the hands against the weather and, more important, against burns and abrasions from a running rope. Gloves shield the hands and prevent discomfort that might cause the rope rescue technician to lose control of the rope.

While providing protection, gloves must allow the hands to retain a sense of feeling so that the fingers can manipulate equipment. Therefore gloves constructed of soft leather, such as deerskin or goatskin, offer the best compromise. Heavily insulated gloves, such as those sometimes worn by firefighters, should not be used in ropework. They tend to prevent a proper feel of the rope in rappelling or rope handling.

Commercial versions of rope handling gloves are available that have added protection across the palm but thinner material on the fingers so that the hands retain a sense of feeling. Gloves with extra heat protection for what is called fast rope handling are sometimes used in tactical operations. However, if you need gloves with such extra heat protection (more than a few layers of leather), you are rappelling too fast for rescue ropework.

Seat Harnesses

A **seat harness** is among the most important pieces of equipment for rope rescue activities. It is essential that you choose a harness for safety, security, and comfort.

Rope rescue seat harnesses are constructed of nylon or polyester webbing. The webbing wraps the pelvic region to support it and attaches the rescuer to the rope or other protection. Figure 2-1 shows an example of a sewn, manufactured seat harness.

An unsuitable seat harness or one that is badly fitted can result in such severe discomfort that it can prevent the wearer from performing a task. Even worse, it can be dangerous to the wearer. The most secure and comfortable seat harnesses are presewn and manufactured.

Although a tied **emergency seat harness** may be used in a pinch, it is no substitute for a well-designed, sewn, manufactured harness. It is extremely difficult to make a tied seat harness that is as secure and comfortable as a well-designed and carefully manufactured product. One reason for this is it takes a great deal of skill to tie secure knots in a tied seat harness. Another

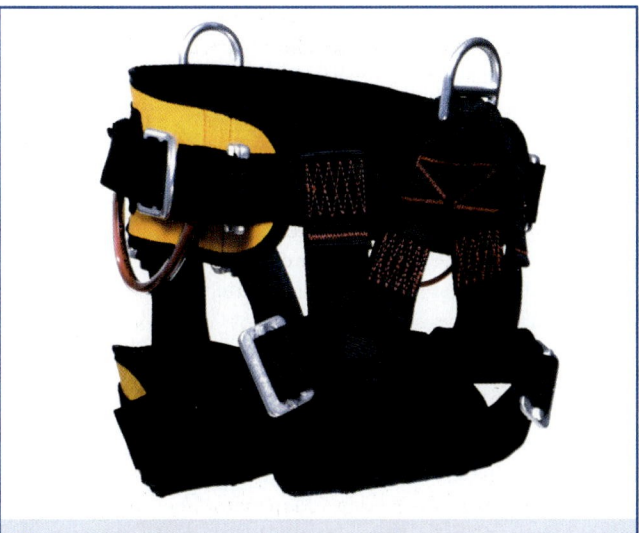

Figure 2-1 Manufactured sewn seat harness.

Warning

Life belts, *ladder belts*, pompier belts, and similar safety belts with support only around the waist must not be used as the single point of support in high angle activities. These types of equipment are designed only as a safety element to help prevent falls from ladders or other elevated positions.

When a person hangs free in them, the belts can constrict the waist and rib cage, impairing breathing and possibly damaging internal organs. They also can slip up under the armpits, causing permanent damage to nerves and resulting in permanent paralysis of the arms. Their use, in place of a seat harness, as the single support can result in injury, permanent disability, or death.

reason is that the narrow webbing usually used in tied harnesses does not give the support of the wider material used in manufactured harnesses. The narrow material, along with the knots, constricts blood circulation and causes severe discomfort to body parts.

Even more critical is a well-engineered harness design. The harness should support your pelvic girdle so that your weight does not create pressure points on the nerves and arteries in the groin and back. In a high angle rescue situation, a person may have to be hanging in the harness for a relatively long period. Twenty minutes is not an unusual time, and periods longer than an hour are a possibility. Although no harness is totally comfortable in these conditions, the tied seat harness tends to cause greater discomfort and possible circulatory problems.

While hanging in an inadequate seat harness, the wearer's discomfort begins as the narrow webbing or rope compresses the kidneys and thighs. This becomes even more painful as circulation to the legs is constricted. After only a few minutes, leg muscles are deprived of perfusion and become useless. Ultimately, the person may be threatened by dangerous blood pressure changes and buildup of blood toxins.

Harness Suspension Pathology

One other condition that everyone in high angle rescue should be aware of is **harness suspension pathology**, a potentially fatal condition that can occur when a person hangs motionless in a seat harness for a long period. The condition results when the individual's position in the harness, along with harness strap compression, reduces venous blood flow from the extremities (particularly the legs) to the right side of the heart, with subsequent reduction in cardiac output. This can result in unconsciousness and possibly death in minutes. Most at risk are individuals who are unconscious, hypothermic, dehydrated, or fatigued. Anyone who appears to be in danger of harness suspension pathology should be gotten down and unclipped from the harness as quickly and safely possible. There are reports of victims of harness suspension pathology dying suddenly after being brought to the ground and released from the harness, therefore affected individuals must be handled carefully and monitored closely.

A potential medical consequence of harness suspension pathology is crush syndrome, which can lead to renal failure and other life-threatening conditions. Medical responders should consider the potential for crush syndrome in their treatment, closely monitor vitals signs, and have the individual examined by a physician.

Rescuers who must hang in a harness for long periods can reduce the potential for harness suspension pathology by repositioning and moving about in the harness to facilitate blood flow. Individuals involved in high angle rescue should consult their medical control officer about treatment of the condition and conduct their own research into this condition.

Foot Supports

In situations in which a rescuer may be suspended in a seat harness for long periods, especially in a free drop (i.e., not in contact with a wall), even the best harness becomes uncomfortable. Using foot loops, stirrups, or an etrier (a short ladder made of webbing) to stand in for a few moments provides relief by restoring circulation. Of course, this helps only if the person is conscious and able to stand or wiggle around. Wiggling around in the seat harness can also enhance circulation.

You can attach the foot supports with a Prusik hitch or ascender on the rope above your rappel device or rope attachment point (see Chapter 10, Basic Ascending Techniques, for information on Prusiks and ascenders). You can also attach them directly to your seat harness main attachment points.

Seat Harness Qualities

The requirements for and qualities of a secure, comfortable seat harness include the following:
- The webbing should be wide (at least 2 inches or 50 mm) for comfort at critical points such as the waist and thighs. Padding can make the webbing even more comfortable.
- Stitching should be securely and evenly sewn and of contrasting color so that abrasion and wear can be detected.
- The harness should have leg and thigh supports, such as leg loops. These add comfort and support by spreading your body weight, or the force of a fall, over other portions of the body, such as the thighs and buttocks.
- The harness should allow you freedom of movement both when you are hanging in it and when you wear it on the ground.
- The harness should be easy to put on and to adjust.
- The harness should not slip down when you walk around.
- When you fall and are caught by the harness, it should allow you to easily return yourself upright.
- The harness must not allow you to fall out when you are upside down.
- The harness should have a front tie-in point designed so that you maintain a correct center of gravity whatever activity you are performing.
- The stress points, such as the tie-in, should be faced with extra webbing and/or use heavy metal connectors.

- Depending on how it is to be used, the harness should be certified by appropriate standards, such as those established by the UIAA, NFPA, CEN, *ASTM* (formerly the American Society for Testing and Materials), or American National Standards Institute (**ANSI**).

Because anatomy varies from person to person and because the rope rescue environment requires different kinds of activity, no one seat harness design is suitable for everyone. Before selecting a particular seat harness and investing the money, you should try several different designs to see which one is best for you.

Differences Between Climbing and Rescue Harnesses

Most climbing harnesses are made to be lighter weight, are often cut for ease of movement, and are made for recovering from leader falls. Harnesses specifically designed for rescue usually are heavier and bulkier because they have wider webbing and padding for comfort for sitting for long periods. They are not designed for lead climbing. Rescue harnesses generally have a metal attachment point into which carabiners are clipped directly. Climbing harnesses have a reinforced webbing loop to directly attach the belay rope. The rope usually is attached directly to the harness with a loop created from a figure 8 follow-through (Flemish bend).

> ### ▤ Warning
>
> A seat harness by itself should not be used as the only tie-in point for swift water operations. If you are attached only to a seat harness in swift water, the force of the current can easily force your upper body back over into the water, making it impossible for you to right yourself—and you will drown. Swift water technicians usually use a tie-in point higher on the body, such as a chest harness. Obtain instructions on this procedure from a qualified swift water technician.

Climbing and rescue harnesses are also designed to meet test standards for different organizations. Climbing harnesses generally are designed to meet the UIAA, CEN, and ASTM (F08) standards. Rescue harnesses are designed to meet standards developed by the NFPA and ANSI. The CEN has also set a rescue/industrial standard.

Rescue Harnesses

Rescue harnesses are specifically designed for rescue use. Rescue harnesses often feature wider webbing and optional padding for greater comfort. They usually are heavier and bulkier than climbing harnesses. Many rescue harnesses also have a large D ring for a front attachment point.

Full Body Harnesses

In certain circumstances, a combination of a seat harness with a chest harness (Figure 2-2) or a **full body harness** (Figure 2-3) may be preferable to only a seat harness. Such situations may include the following:

- When a person is involved in a dangerous activity that requires that he or she constantly be held upright. For example, a rescuer might be entering a confined space and is equipped with a harness attached to a retrieval line.
- When equipment is worn that makes a person top heavy, such as a breathing apparatus. The chest portion of the harness helps distribute the extra weight of the apparatus on the body.
- When a person is of greater than average weight. The higher tie-in point helps the person stay upright.
- During certain climbing or mountaineering activities when it is necessary to be held upright should a fall occur; for example, while wearing a heavy pack that would make it difficult to right oneself.
- For placement on a subject in certain rescue situations (see Chapter 13, Pickoff Rescue Techniques).

In these situations, a full body harness or a combination seat/chest harness may provide needed security, but in some circumstances a full body harness may be a disadvantage. In certain rescue situations some individuals may find the full body harness too constraining, preventing the range of motion needed for rescue activities.

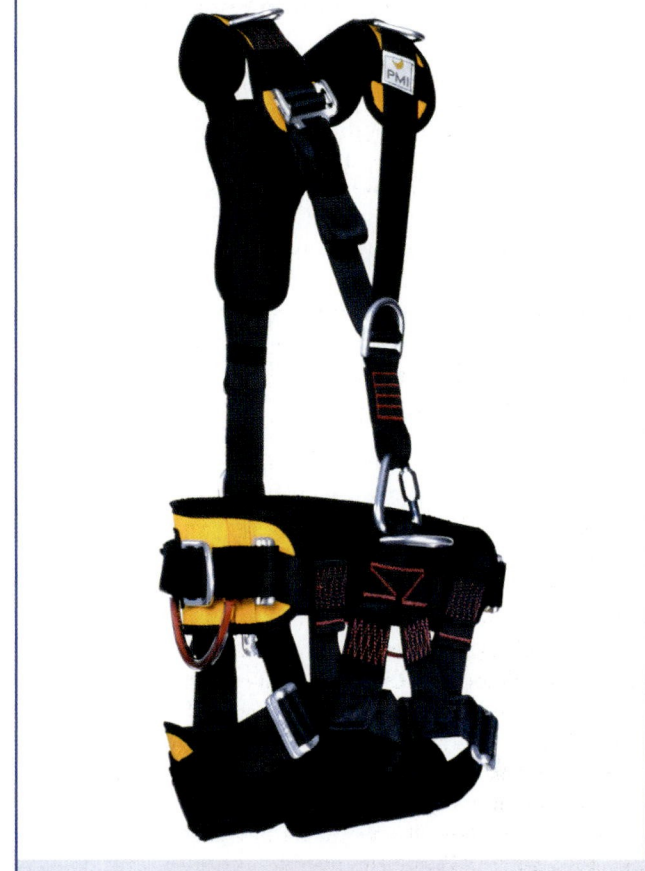

Figure 2-3 Full body harness.

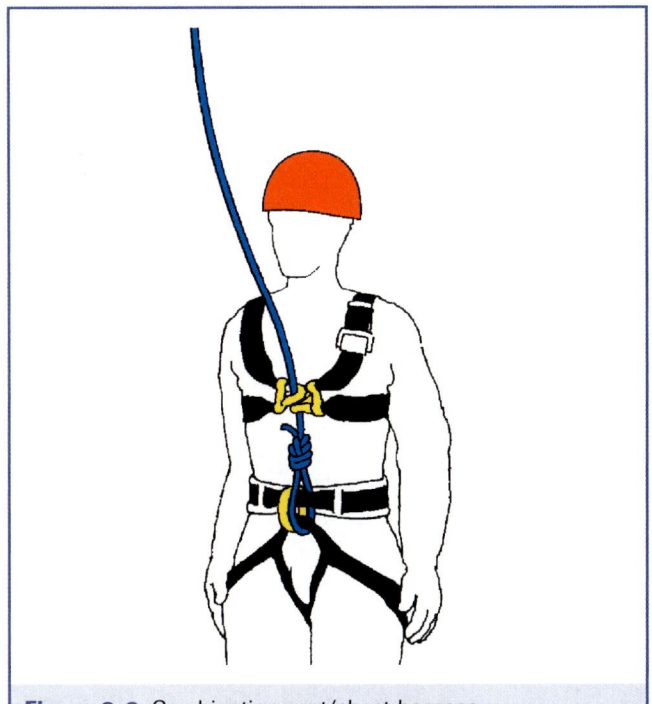

Figure 2-2 Combination seat/chest harness.

Seat/Chest Harnesses

The seat/chest harness combination may be preferable for some rescuers because it allows the wearer to choose options based on the specific conditions. A chest harness, worn with a seat harness, can be quickly connected or disconnected to the system, depending on the needs of the user. Should the wearer need to be held upright without using upper body strength, he or she can quickly connect it. If it is too constraining, the wearer can unclip it but continue wearing it. An added advantage to a rescuer's carrying a chest harness is that it can be used to hold a rescue subject upright in certain types of operations.

Chest Harnesses

A **chest harness** is comfortable, easily adjusted, easily combined with a seat harness, and easy to put on and take off. A chest harness should *never* be used alone for high angle activities; it must always be used in combination with a seat harness.

Organizational Standards

Standards established by the ANSI, ASTM (F08), NFPA, CEN, and UIAA apply to the construction and use of some harnesses. Each of these standards applies to a specific group of users; *no one standard applies to everyone who uses high angle equipment.* For example, ANSI standards apply to certain workplace activities, whereas NFPA standards apply to firefighters.

The NFPA's *Standard on Fire Service Life Safety Rope and System Components* classifies harnesses into three groups:

- *Class I:* A light duty seat harness meant for emergency escape and light duty work by one person.
- *Class II:* A seat harness meant for heavy duty work by one person or in rescue situations in which another person's weight may be added in the course of the rescue.
- *Class III:* A full body harness meant for fall protection from falls and for use in rescues in which inversion might occur.

ASTM (F08), UIAA, and some CEN standards apply to mountaineers.

For specific information on any standard, the responsible organization should be contacted. Appendix A provides additional information on standard-setting organizations.

Securing Hardware in the High Angle Environment

Pieces of high angle hardware, such as carabiners, are easily lost during rescue work in the high angle environment. Even worse, hardware can easily be dropped and can injure a person who happens to be in the path of its fall. When rescuers are working in the high angle environment, all equipment should be kept attached to something secure. A convenient place is the equipment loops that many harnesses have (Figure 2-4).

If equipment slings or loops are not manufactured into the harness, they can easily be created with utility cord.

Shoulder Slings

Some prefer to use shoulder slings for equipment. These may work well, particularly if the equipment is not bulky and does not interfere with high angle activities. However, some strangulation deaths have occurred when climbers have fallen and the shoulder sling became snagged.

Light Sources

High angle operations, particularly in rescue, often take place at night or in enclosed areas with no light. Consequently, all personnel should have with them a reliable source of light. You will need to have both hands free during high angle operations; therefore these light sources should be in the form of headlamps (Figure 2-5). A headlamp follows the movement of your head, usually placing the light where you are looking.

Choose a headlamp that is easily adjustable and field serviceable. Always carry extra batteries and a spare bulb. Many headlamps have battery packs to the rear of the head, which helps balance the weight on your helmet. If you choose this kind of headlamp, you must be sure that it will remain stable on your head and not fall off easily.

Some traditional headlamps have a belt battery pack attached by a cord to the headlamp. Although this may provide a sufficient source of light, high angle technicians sometimes find that the cord snags and becomes entangled or breaks. This is particularly a problem in confined spaces. A possible solution is to wear the cord inside the clothing; however, should the wire short, the wearer may discover a whole new meaning to the term *hot wired!*

The lamp should have an adjustable beam and a secure switch so that the light cannot be turned on accidentally when in storage.

The battery type that has the longest shelf life and is resistant to the effects of cold is the lithium cell. However, it is also the most expensive and has been known to cause explosions by venting gas. After the lithium cell, the alkaline battery is the next most desirable in terms of long life and operating temperature, and it is not as expensive as the lithium battery.

A halogen bulb gives a brighter light than a standard bulb but also drains batteries much more quickly. Some rescuers carry both types of bulbs. They use the standard bulb normally to save the batteries and switch to the halogen bulb when they need extra light.

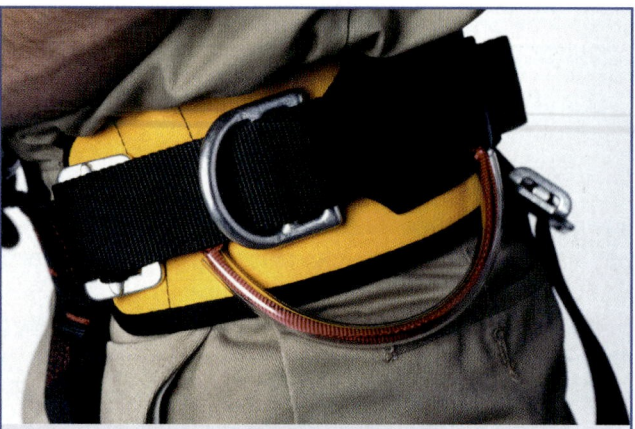

Figure 2-4 Seat harness equipment loops.

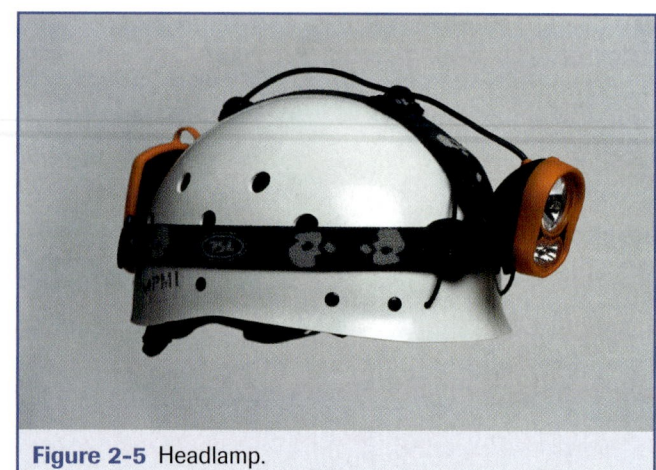

Figure 2-5 Headlamp.

A recent innovation is the use of light-emitting diode (LED) technology. LED lights are not actually filament light bulbs, but rather solid-state diodes that give off light when charged with a current. The new high-intensity models make for extremely lightweight headlamps with incredibly long burn times. Unfortunately for rescuers, most LED lights do not yet have enough brightness to provide a useful light more than short distance. An LED light can be used for close-up work, but it doesn't project enough light to see down a long vertical face, for example. One advantage of an LED lamp is its compactness; it can be slipped into a coat as an emergency or back-up light. An LED/conventional bulb combination headlamp provides the best of long-duration light from the LED and a strong beam when brightness is needed for distance.

Individuals entering potentially explosive atmospheres must use light sources that are intrinsically safe for the particular conditions. This means that the design of the lighting equipment safeguards it against ignition in a hazardous atmosphere. There are several levels or classes of hazards, and lamps that are certified for one level might not be safe in others.

Knives in the High Angle Environment

Carrying knives in the high angle environment has become almost a custom for some. However, careless use of knives can have terrible consequences. In addition to presenting the real danger of personal injury, knives in the high angle environment are a threat to life because of the ease with which they destroy life-supporting equipment.

An exposed knife blade is particularly dangerous to ropes loaded with the weight of one or more people. When stretched, as they are when supporting weight, rope yarns are very susceptible to being cut by any sharp object.

Typically, a person might reach for a knife when his or her T-shirt or hair has gotten drawn into the rappel device and the person is stranded. However, in such a situation the person is likely to be under stress and possibly in pain and may have limited freedom of movement. It would be very difficult to cut his or her way out without touching the knife edge to the rope.

One alternative to a knife is the tool used by emergency services personnel to cut seat belts. This instrument has a recessed blade so that it does not accidentally cut a lifeline as easily as a naked knife blade.

Even better than cutting is the use of advanced skills and optional equipment to extricate oneself from a jammed rappel device and similar situations. One alternative for a ropeworker is to use a Prusik knot or an ascender to take the weight off the rappel device and then extricate himself or herself from such a predicament. (The skills and equipment required for this procedure are described in Chapter 10.)

Evaluation Exercises

Cognitive and Affective Exercises

1. A helmet worn in the high angle environment does all of the following except:

   A. Decreases the risk of significant skull fracture
   B. Decreases the risk of severe brain injury
   C. Decreases the risk of accidents
   D. Protects from falling objects

2. A helmet for the high angle rescue environment should include which of the following:

   A. Chin strap
   B. Certification from an appropriate agency
   C. Three-point suspension system
   D. All of the above

3. All of the following are appropriate footwear for high angle ropework except:

   A. Heavy mountaineering boots
   B. Rubber fire service boots
   C. Vibram-soled, lightweight hiking boots with good ankle protection
   D. Heavyweight leather hiking boots

4. Footwear worn by the high angle technician should have which of the following characteristics:

   A. Comfort
   B. Good sole-to-terrain adhesion
   C. Good ankle protection
   D. All of the above

5. Wearing gloves helps a person maintain control of the rope in the high angle environment because gloves:

   A. Protect the wearer from dirt and grime
   B. Limit feeling the heat of the rope
   C. Protect against burns and abrasions
   D. Improve the grip on materials

6. Which of the following may cause life-threatening complications if used as a single-point of suspension in the high angle environment:

   A. Life belts
   B. Ladder belts
   C. Pompier belts
   D. Escape belts
   E. All of the above

7. A person who is hanging for a long period in an unsuitable seat harness in the high angle environment might experience all of the following except:

   A. Euphoria
   B. Syncope (fainting)
   C. Pain
   D. Hypotension

8. An international organization involved in setting standards for seat harnesses is:

   A. UNICEF
   B. AMGA
   C. UIAA
   D. OSHA

9. A U.S. organization involved in setting standards for rope rescue equipment is:

   A. USIA
   B. NFPA
   C. IODA
   D. USDOT

10. The best strategy for relieving pressure on your lower body while hanging for long periods in a seat harness would be:

    A. Prusik a foot loop to the rope above the harness
    B. Hand hang
    C. Put weight on to the belay line
    D. Add foot loops to the harness

11. All the following situations would require a rope to your seat harness except:

    A. Rappelling
    B. Attending a litter in high angle terrain
    C. Entering the water during a swift water rescue
    D. Having a belay or safety line close to a cliff edge

12. A convenient place to store rigging hardware while rigging a rescue is:

    A. On your seat harness utility loops
    B. On the litter
    C. In your pack
    D. On the ground at the site

13. Which of the following represents a situation in which the use of a knife might lead to disaster:

    A. Catching a T-shirt in a rappel device
    B. Freeing the working rope of a fused Prusik
    C. Cutting brush away from the edge during a rope operation
    D. All of the above

3

Rope and Related Equipment

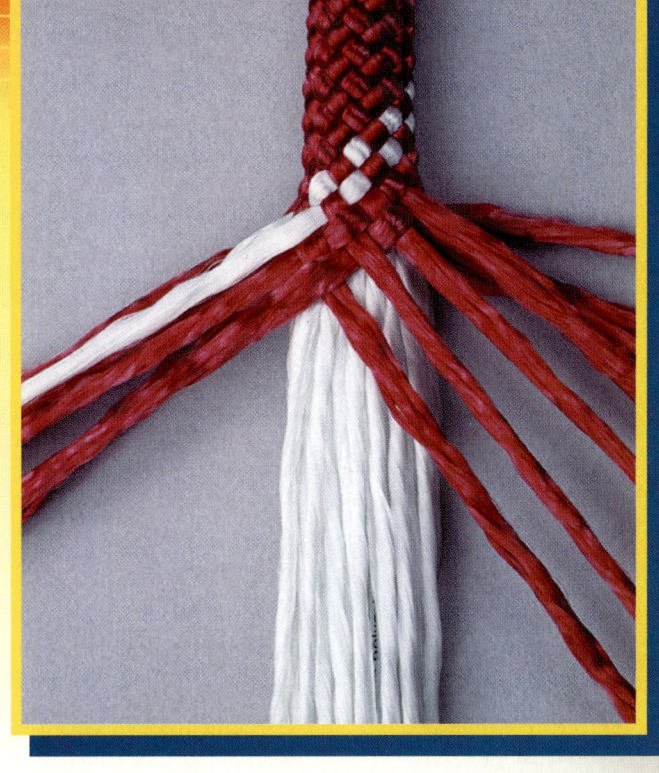

The material in this chapter conforms to guidelines published by the National Fire Protection Association (NFPA), specifically standard 1983-01, *Standard for Life Safety Rope and System Components* (2001). NFPA standards are revised regularly, and readers are advised to review the latest version of this standard.

Objectives

On completion of this chapter, you should be able to:

1. Describe the type of rope used in climbing compared with that used in rescue situations.
2. List the considerations for rope construction needed to create static, low-stretch, and dynamic types of life safety ropes.
3. Identify the design, weakness, and limitations of the rope currently used by your organization or group.
4. Explain the difference between component load ratio, system load ratio, and system safety factors.
5. Given a system and problem, determine the system safety factor.
6. Given a scenario, determine the fall factor for a rescuer.

Key Terms

Abrasion The damaging wear on rope and other equipment caused by rubbing against abrasive material.

Dynamic Rope A type of rope designed for high stretch to reduce the shock on the climber and anchor system. This type of rope usually is used in rock climbing and mountaineering and is certified by the Union of International Alpine Associations (UIAA) or the European Committee for Standardization (CEN) as such.

Fall Factor The distance fallen in relationship to the amount of rope used to catch the fall. The fall factor calculation is used to estimate the impact force on a rope when it is subjected to stopping a falling mass.

Kernmantle A rope design consisting of two elements: an interior core (kern), which usually supports the major portion of the load on the rope, and an outer sheath (mantle), which serves primarily to protect the core but also may support a minor portion of the load.

Kevlar Trade name for a type of Aramid fiber, manufactured by the DuPont Corp., that has high tensile strength, low elongation, and high resistance to heat.

Laid Rope Rope made by twisting three or more strands together with the twist direction opposite that of the strands. Plain, or hawser, laid ropes have three strands, whereas shroud laid ropes have four strands.

Load Ratio The ratio of the component's minimum breaking strength to the anticipated load.

Low-Stretch A quality of a type of rope designed to be used in applications such as rescue, rappelling, and ascending in which high stretch would be a disadvantage and no falls, or only very short falls, are expected before the climber is caught by the rope. The term low-stretch rope can refer to ropes with slightly more elongation than the traditional static ropes or to both types of ropes (see Static Rope, right column).*

Nylon 6 A type of nylon used in rope manufacturing. Because of its shock-absorbing qualities, nylon type 6 is found in most climbing ropes. One trade name for this type of nylon is Perlon.

Nylon 6,6 A type of nylon used in rope manufacturing. With its resistance to wear and reduced elongation under load, most static ropes are constructed of type 6,6. In North America it is manufactured by DuPont and the Monsanto Corporation.

Perlon A trade name for a version of nylon type 6.

Polyester A type of fiber used in some rope manufacturing. Also known by the trade name Dacron.

Polyolefins A group of fiber types (e.g., polypropylene, polyethylene) used in the manufacture of ropes often used in water applications.

Spectra Trade name for a high-modulus polyethylene fiber with high tensile strength.

Static Rope A type of rope designed to be used in applications such as rescue, rappelling, and ascending in which high stretch would be a disadvantage and in which no falls, or only very short falls, are expected before the climber is caught by the rope. Static ropes have slightly less elongation than low-stretch ropes built to the same standard. Less elongation prevents loss of system efficiency from rope stretching (see Low-Stretch Rope).*

System Safety Factor The ratio between the maximum load expected on a high angle system and its breaking strength. The larger the ratio, the greater the safety factor.

Tensile Strength A measurement of the greatest lengthwise stress under slow pull conditions that a rope can resist without failing.

*The Cordage Institute's *Standard on Low Stretch and Static Kernmantle Life Safety Ropes* has attempted to divide what were once known in the United States as *static ropes* into two categories. One type is now known as *static kernmantle* and the other type is known as *low-stretch kernmantle*. Low-stretch ropes built to the Cordage Institute's standard have slightly more elongation than static ropes built to the same standard. More elongation means lower impact forces when the rope is used to arrest sudden load. In this text, the terms *static* and *low stretch*, as well as the associated rope applications, can be used interchangeably.

Determining the Right Rope for the Task

Rope is the universal link in high angle activities and rope rescue. During the past few years, great strides have been made in the technology and manufacture of rope. However, rope is only as good as the use to which it is put, and it performs only as well as the care you give it.

Many different kinds of rope are used for high angle activities. Each kind has a specific design and fiber that determine how it reacts to natural and human forces. Before choosing a rope, you must decide whether it will be used for rappelling or ascending, for rescue, for swift water, for climbing rock or ice, or for another specialized activity. The incorrect use of a rope can result in severe problems for the user and sometimes in tragedy.

Ropes for Technical Climbing and Mountaineering

Ropes for climbers and mountaineers are designed to catch the user if the person falls while climbing. Ropes for lead climbing must have stretch to absorb the energy of the fall without harming the climber. Besides protecting the climber, a good climbing rope helps reduce the force that is transmitted to anchors and "protection," causing them to fail. This kind of rope is called *dynamic,* a term that relates to the use of force in motion. **Dynamic ropes** are also called *high-stretch ropes.* Most of a dynamic rope's ability to stretch is built into it during manufacture and is achieved through various designs that elongate under load, much as with a spring (Figure 3-1).

Two other characteristics of dynamic ropes for climbing and mountaineering are softness and pliability. The feel of a rope is called *hand,* which can be stiff or soft. In a good dynamic rope, the hand is soft enough to run through gear, yet the rope is stiff enough to wear well. These qualities are necessary in climbing because the rope is constantly being moved, knotted and unknotted, and run through hardware. In a climbing rope, these qualities are achieved partly by the manufacture of rope with a sheath, or outer surface, that is loose and thin. Standards for climbing ropes have been established by the UIAA, CEN, and ASTM (formerly the American Society for Testing and Materials) (see Appendix A, Standards-Setting Organizations).

Ropes for Rappelling and Ascending

Rope used for rappelling or ascending does not usually act as a safety for the person on the rope but as a means of travel. This is known as *single-rope technique (SRT)* or, more recently, *rope access.* The user actually travels down the rope using a rappel device or up the rope using ascenders. One example of SRT is vertical caving. In SRT the stretch of a dynamic rope would be a disadvantage, and its thin sheath would be susceptible to **abrasion.**

For SRT activities, many prefer to use a **static rope,** which has very little stretch. In static ropes the interior fiber bundles are constructed nearly parallel to one another so that most of the stretch is through the inherent stretch in the nylon (Figure 3-2). Static ropes typically stretch only about 18% to 20% before breaking.

In addition, static ropes characteristically have a thicker, tighter sheath, which affords greater protection to the core. Because of this type of construction, static ropes do not have the ease of handling of dynamic ropes and may be slightly more difficult for tying knots.

Ropes for Rescue Use

Ropes designed for rescues share some characteristics with ropes designed for SRT: low stretch and high resistance to damage from abrasion. In rescue work the quality of **low stretch** means greater control of the rope for the rescuers, such as in

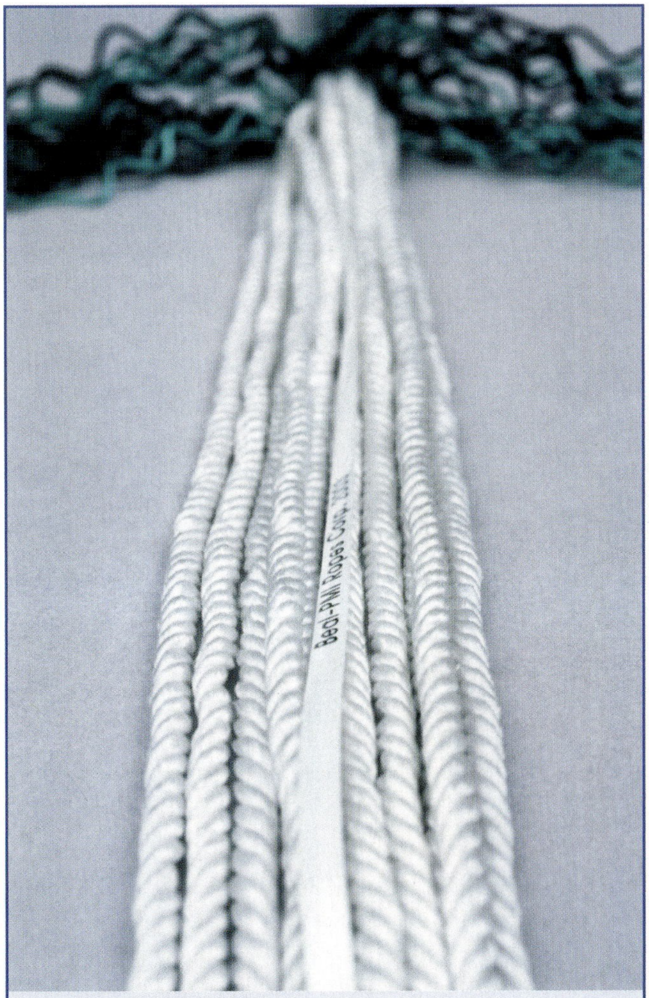

Figure 3-1 Typical dynamic rope core.

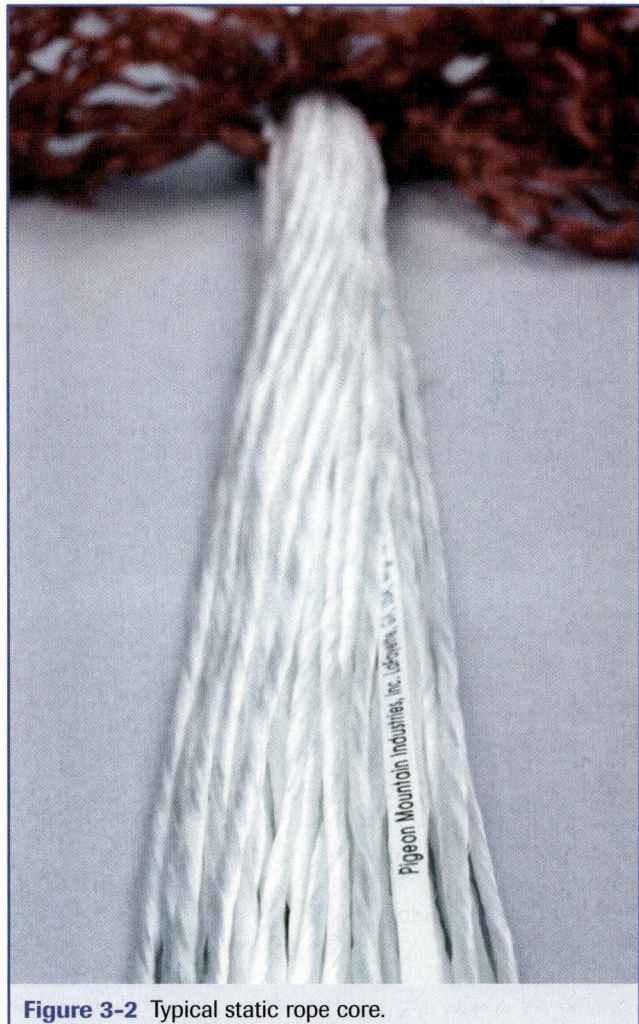

Figure 3-2 Typical static rope core.

lowering a litter. As the litter is eased over the edge of a vertical face, a greater load suddenly comes onto the rope. If a dynamic rope were being used, the result would be a great deal of stretch and a significant drop in the litter. A static rope has less stretch and therefore offers more control.

In addition, a system using a static rope does not have much creep. When a rope is first weighted, the initial stretch occurs. However, additional stretch, known as *creep,* slowly comes into the rope over a period of time as it remains loaded. Creep tends to be greater in a dynamic rope. In a rescue situation, creep would be a disadvantage. For example, it would make it more difficult for a dynamic rope to hold a litter in a constant position on a vertical face while a patient is loaded into the stretcher.

The Role of the Fall Factor

One important method of estimating the forces at work on a rope is to compute the **fall factor** (Figure 3-3). As shown in Figure 3-3, a climber is attached to a rope that will catch the person in a fall and keep the person from hitting the ground. The other end of the rope is directly attached to a point of "protection" that will not come loose. The fall factor (FF) is calculated by dividing the distance the climber on the rope falls by the length of the rope between the person and the point of protection.

$$\text{Fall factor} = \frac{\text{Distance person falls}}{\text{Length of rope}}$$

Consider that the length of rope is 100 feet (30 m) (see Figure 3-3, *A*). If the person were climbing up from below, slipped just before reaching the point of protection, and fell exactly 100 feet (30 m), the calculation would be:

$$\text{Fall factor} = \frac{100 \text{ feet } (30 \text{ m})}{100 \text{ feet } (30 \text{ m})} = 1$$

If the person were climbing up from below and fell before reaching the point of protection, the fall would be less than a factor 1 fall (see Figure 3-3, *B*). For example, if the fall were only 50 feet (15 m), the calculation would be:

$$\text{Fall factor} = \frac{50 \text{ feet } (15 \text{ m})}{100 \text{ feet } (30 \text{ m})} = 0.5$$

Now, note Figure 3-3, *C*. The individual has climbed above the point of protection by a full rope length. If the person were to fall now, the calculation would be:

$$\text{Fall factor} = \frac{200 \text{ feet } (60 \text{ m})}{100 \text{ feet } (30 \text{ m})} = 2$$

Any fall from above the point of protection would be more than a factor 1 fall (see Figure 3-3, *D*). If, for example, the climber fell from 50 feet above the point of protection, the calculation would be:

$$\text{Fall factor} = \frac{150 \text{ feet } (45 \text{ m})}{100 \text{ feet } (30 \text{ m})} = 1.5$$

As the fall factor increases, the severity becomes much worse. Note that it is not just the length of the fall that matters, but the length of the fall in relation both to the amount of rope and to the point of protection.

The Role of Fall Factors with Short Ropes

Recent tests have shown that the fall factor formula for dynamic ropes does not necessarily translate to static ropes, especially

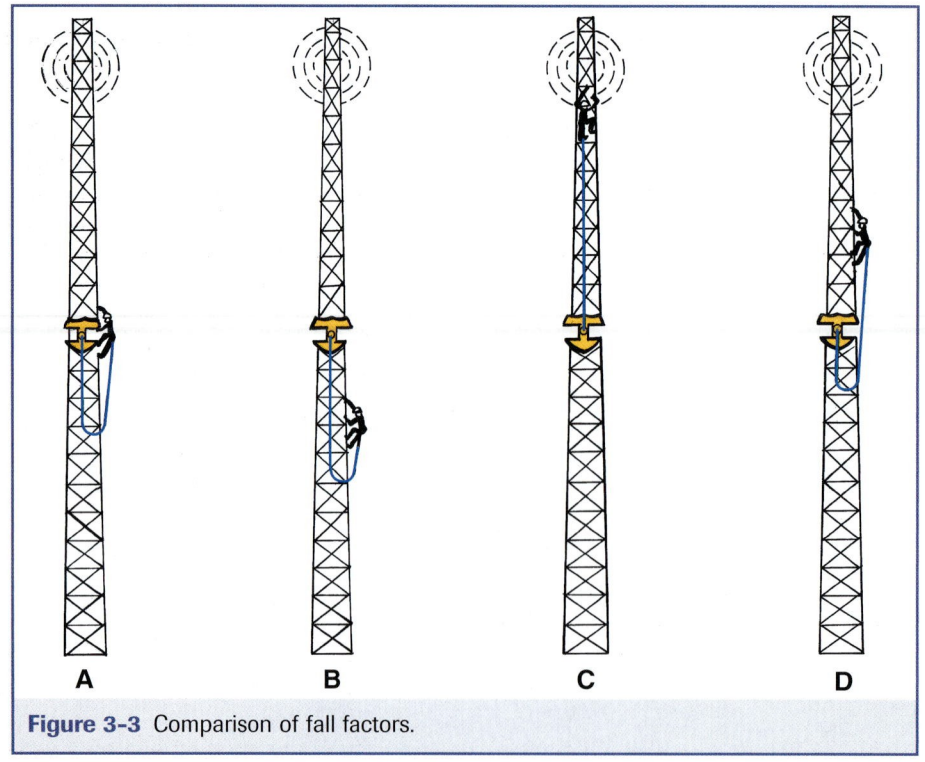

Figure 3-3 Comparison of fall factors.

Warning

Although calculating the fall factor is useful for obtaining general estimates of the forces on a rope in a fall, the situations shown in Figure 3-3 are ideal ones. Other factors often enter into the situation to alter the results, including the following:

❑ The rope may be running through intermediate points of protection or it may be rubbing against rock or other surfaces. This creates drag that may slow the rope's ability to stretch. This in turn effectively shortens the length of rope available to absorb the energy of the fall. The net result would be a much higher fall factor and greater impact forces on the person and on parts of the system, such as the anchors.

❑ In most climbing situations, a fall does not occur completely in free air. The fall factor is of little importance if the person slams into the ground or is bashed against the wall on the way down.

when very short or very long lengths of static rope are involved. In the case of very short static ropes, the forces are slightly less than would be predicted using the fall factor formula. When the formula is applied to very long ropes or to loads greater than single body weight, it tends to underestimate the force. For example, a 0.25 FF on a 5-foot (1.5 m) static rope has a much higher impact force than a 0.25 FF on a 2-foot (0.6 m) section of the same rope. Everything else being the same, there is much less difference in impact forces when different lengths of dynamic ropes are used in the same FF falls.

What may seem to be a short fall can produce high-impact forces on the system and the persons on rope. For example, a rescuer at the edge of a cliff who is helping to move a loaded litter over the edge might be clipped in to a 3-foot safety rope that anchored near his feet. If he should fall, he easily could fall twice the length of the rope with which he is tethered, yielding a severe fall factor of 2, even though he may have traveled only 6 feet (1.8 m) in the fall. The choice of a safety rope with some extra stretch versus one made from a very-low-stretch material can make the difference between a major injury and a minor scare. The choice of fibers and the construction of the rope are important considerations in rope selection.

Fibers Used to Make Rope
Natural Fibers

For many years, ropes made of natural fibers, such as sisal, hemp, and manila, were standard. About the time of World War II, mass production of rope made of synthetic fibers, such as nylon or **polyester**, began.

Currently, synthetic fiber ropes are considered standard for situations in which the safety of a person is "on the line." In vertical sport activities, such as climbing or vertical caving, synthetic fiber ropes have long since replaced those made of natural fibers. Synthetic fiber ropes are also considered the standard for rescue ropes. National organizations such as the International

Association of Fire Fighters (IAFF), the International Society of Fire Service Instructors (ISFI), and the National Fire Protection Association (NFPA) have all condemned the use of natural fiber rope in life safety applications because natural fiber ropes:

- Show low resistance to abrasion
- Have a limited ability to absorb shock loading
- Degrade in strength even with the best care
- Can rot without outward visible signs
- Have lower breaking strengths than ropes of the same diameter made of synthetic fibers such as nylon or polyester
- Do not have strands that are continuous along the rope's entire length because natural fibers are never more than a few feet long

Synthetic Fiber Ropes

Synthetic fiber ropes have several important advantages over natural fiber ropes. For example, synthetic fiber ropes:

- Do not rot
- Do not age as quickly
- Can be made into more advanced rope designs than natural fibers

Several different synthetic fibers are used to make ropes. Each fiber has distinct characteristics that make it suitable for certain uses and unsuitable for others.

Polyolefins (Polypropylene and Polyethylene)
Advantages

- Do not absorb water
- Float (specific gravity of 0.91); consequently, are useful in activities on the water
- Good chemical resistance (pH 2 to 12)

Disadvantages

- Relatively low tensile strength (6 to 6.5 grams per denier [gpd] breaking tenacity)
- Poor abrasion resistance
- Low melting points (150° to 200° F [65° to 93° C]).
- Poor shock absorbing (shock loading) capability
- Poor resistance to damage from sunlight

Polypropylene or polyethylene ropes are often found in water activities. However, because of their low tensile strength, low abrasion resistance, and low melting point, they should not be used for direct loading in life support operations. For example, polyolefin ropes are unsuitable for rappelling and rescue lowering and hauling systems.

Denier

Denier is a weight-per-unit-length measure of any linear material such as yarn. The measurement is a numeric representation of the weight in grams (g) of 9,000 meters of the material. The smaller the number, the finer the yarn. The tensile strengths of yarns are often rated as grams per denier (gpd).

HMPE (Extended Chain, High-Modulus Polyethylene)

Advantages

- High tensile strength (30 to 35 gpd breaking tenacity)
- Float (0.97 specific gravity)

Disadvantages

- Low melting point (about 150° to 200° F [65° to 93° C])
- Poor shock absorbing capability (2.7% to 3.5% elongation at break)
- Very slippery, therefore special knots may be required to hold when tied

HMPE is a polyethylene yarn, and the one best known in the United States is **Spectra.** HMPE products are found in climbers' slings and runners. These are very slippery and do not hold knots very well. Because of HMPE's poor shock absorbing qualities, slings and runners made of this material should be used with dynamic rope or other energy absorbers in the rope system to absorb impact loads.

Aramids

An aramid is a manufactured fiber in which the fiber-forming material is a long-chain synthetic polyamide having at least 85% of its amide linkages attached directly to two aromatic rings.

Advantages

- Resistant to high temperatures (350° F [176° C] working limit)
- High tensile strength (18 to 26.5 gpd breaking tenacity)

Disadvantages

- Easily damaged by abrasion
- Easily damaged by continued small radius flexing (as in knotting)
- Poor shock loading capability (1.5% to 3.6% elongation at break)

Kevlar (an Aramid Fiber)

As with any newer material, the best use of **Kevlar** rope has been the subject of considerable controversy. The consensus seems to be that it may have uses in applications in which it is not subject to continued small radius bending. For example, rock climbers have used Kevlar cord successfully as protection sling material, in which it remains continually knotted, and with dynamic rope or other shock absorbers. However, most seem to agree that current designs of Kevlar rope should not be used in situations in which the rope will be subjected to abrasion and continued small radius flexing, such as in repeated knotting and un-knotting. Kevlar generally is considered unsuitable for activities such as rappelling, ascending, belaying, and rescue lowering and hauling systems.

Recently, some personal escape "ropes" have been produced from Kevlar webbing. These products may work well for their designed use, but it should be noted that because of Kevlar's poor abrasion resistance, such escape lines are designed for limited or one-time use.

Polyester

Advantages

- High tensile strength even when wet (7 to 10 gpd breaking tenacity)
- Good abrasion resistance
- Melting point of about 480° F (250° C) (high temperature working limit of 275° F [135° C])
- Resistant to damage from acids (pH of 3.5 to 7.5)

Disadvantages

- Cannot handle shock loading as well as nylon (12% to 15% elongation at break)
- Susceptible to damage from alkalis
- Does not float (specific gravity of 1.38)

Polyester fibers are found in a number of life safety applications. However, because polyester does not handle shock loading as well as nylon, it generally is not found in climbing ropes. An example of polyester is Dacron, the DuPont trade name for a type of polyester.

Nylon

Nylon actually is produced in several different types. The two most commonly used in life safety ropes are **nylon 6** (also known by its European trade name, **Perlon**) and **nylon 6,6.** Nylon 6 (Perlon) has better elongation qualities than nylon 6,6 and therefore has better shock absorbing qualities. Consequently, nylon 6 is found in most types of climbing ropes. Nylon 6,6 has a slightly higher melting point and a slightly higher breaking point than nylon 6. In addition, nylon 6,6 shows slightly better resistance to wear and less elongation under load. For these reasons, most static ropes are constructed of nylon 6,6. Whether these differences in the nylon actually appear in the rope depend in large part on the individual rope design. Nylon 6,6 is found in some ropes manufactured in North America. The DuPont and Monsanto corporations manufacture nylon 6,6 yarn.

Advantages

- About 10% stronger than polyester in ropes of comparable diameter when dry (7.8 to 10.4 gpd breaking tenacity)
- Good shock loading capability (15% to 28% elongation at break)
- Melting point of about 480° F (250° C) (nylon 6,6); high temperature working limit of 250° F (121° C)
- Good chemical resistance to alkalis (pH 6.5 to 10.5)

Disadvantages

- May lose 10% to 15% of its strength when wet (regains the deficiency when dry)
- Susceptible to certain strong acids, such as those used in storage batteries

Ropes made of nylon yarn are commonly used in life support applications, including climbing, vertical caving, rescue, and tactical operations.

Rope Construction

The choice of a rope for a specific job depends not only on the fiber from which the rope is made but also on the manner in which the rope is constructed.

Laid

Laid construction, also known as *twisted* or *hawser lay,* means that small fiber bundles of material are twisted and then combined in larger bundles, usually in groups of three, which are twisted around one another in the opposite direction (Figure 3-4). **Laid rope** construction resembles the designs of older types of rope made of natural fibers.

Characteristics

- When loaded the fibers tend to untwist slightly, causing spin and kinking. To limit this problem, many modern laid ropes are designed with a "balanced" construction. Even so, this type of rope has a good bit of inherent twist. Even if the rope itself doesn't spin, the laid design adds a great amount of spin during a rappel as the rappel device spirals down the twist of the strands.
- Because each fiber may appear at the surface of the rope somewhere along its length, the load-bearing fibers are more susceptible to damage by abrasion.
- Laid rope tends to be very stretchy.
- This type of rope tends to kink unless handled carefully.

Individuals who still use laid rope in life support operations usually use the tighter lay, or *mountain lay,* design. The *marine lay* design is looser and more susceptible to damage by abrasion. However, the mountain lay design is more difficult to find than the marine lay.

Ropes of laid construction have been displaced in most high angle work by other designs.

Plaited

Plaited rope usually consists of bundles of fibers plaited together (Figure 3-5).

Advantage

- Plaited ropes tend to be soft and pliable.

Disadvantage

- This type of rope is prone to picking (snagging and pulling out of fiber bundles).

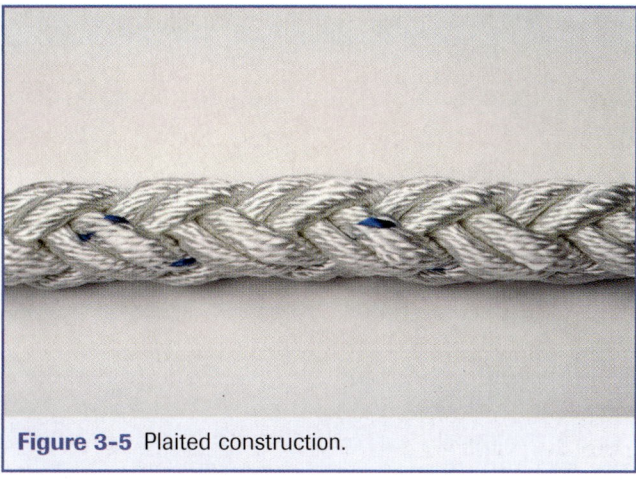

Figure 3-5 Plaited construction.

Braided

The two types of braid used in the construction of braided rope are the solid, or single, braid and the hollow braid.

In a *solid (single) braid* rope (Figure 3-6), the rope is constructed entirely of a single weave of three or more fiber bundles. The design is sometimes called *clothesline braid.* Because the load-supporting fiber bundles in single braid construction are vulnerable to destruction when the rope is being used, single braid ropes have limited use in high angle operations.

A hollow braid rope is essentially a very thick sheath. It sometimes has a filler, such as scrap yarn or filament plastic. It typically is found in inexpensive hardware store–type rope, not in life safety line.

Double Braid

A double braid rope (Figure 3-7) is essentially a rope constructed of a solid braid covered with a hollow braid. One braid acts as the rope core; the second braid is constructed around it to act as a sheath and to help protect the inner braid.

Advantage

- Double braid rope is soft and flexible.

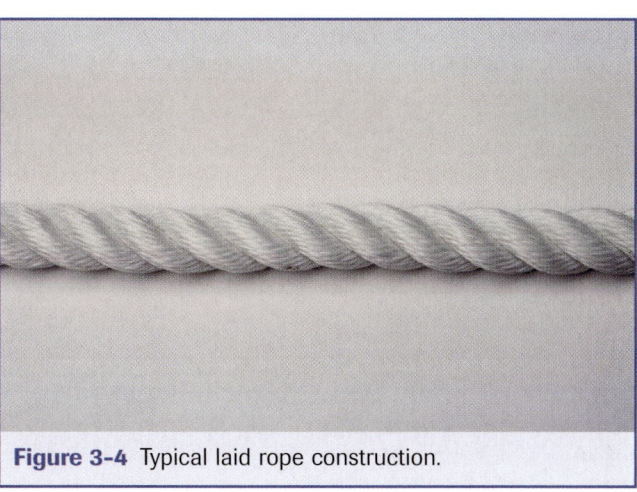

Figure 3-4 Typical laid rope construction.

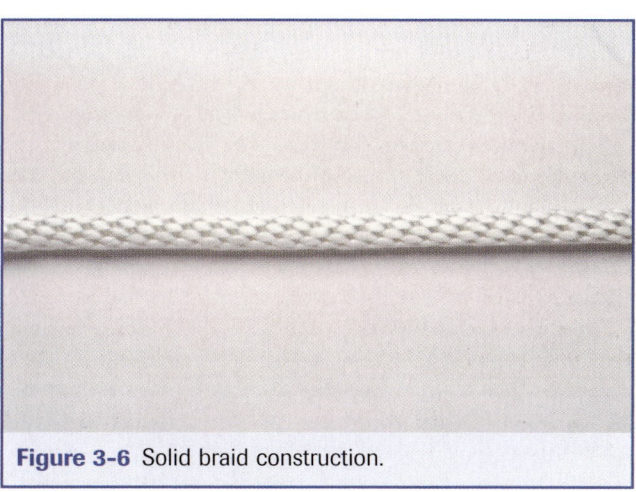

Figure 3-6 Solid braid construction.

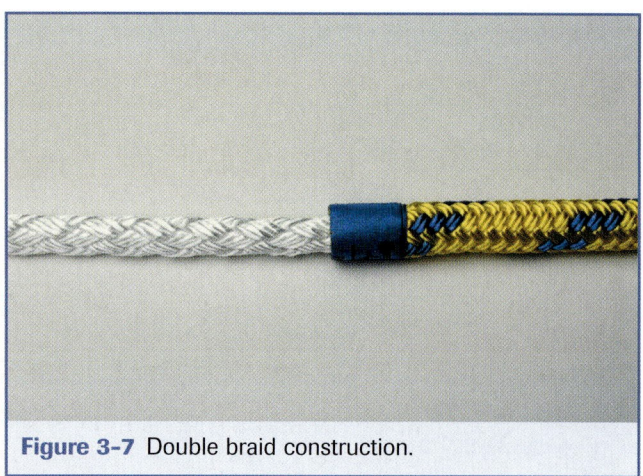

Figure 3-7 Double braid construction.

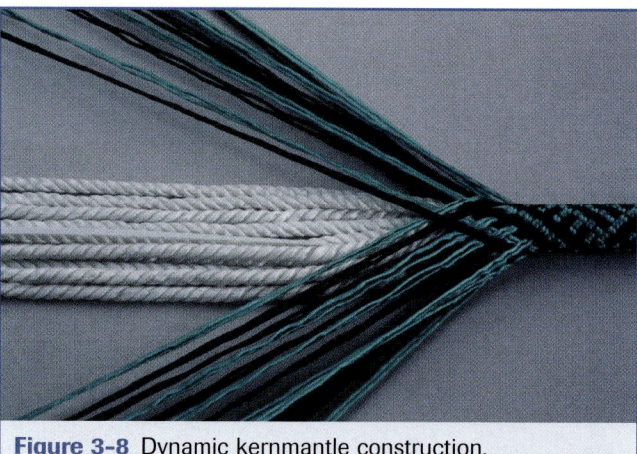

Figure 3-8 Dynamic kernmantle construction.

Disadvantages

- Double braid rope is susceptible to contamination of the core by grit and dirt.
- This type of rope is susceptible to picking.
- Double braid rope is susceptible to abrasion.
- When the rope is cut around its diameter, the sheath tends to slip down on core.

Kernmantle

The term *kernmantle* comes from a compound German word, *kern* (meaning core) and *mantle* (meaning sheath or cover). The kernmantle rope design consists of a central core of fibers that supports the major portion of the load on the rope. This core is covered by a woven sheath, which supports a lesser portion of the load. The tight weave of the mantle protects the core from abrasion, dirt, and environmental effects, such as sunlight. Kernmantle construction produces a rope that is strong and resists damage but easy to handle. Also, kernmantle rope does not have the drawback of severe twisting that affects other rope designs (e.g., laid). The two basic types of kernmantle ropes are *dynamic kernmantle* and *static kernmantle*.

Dynamic Kernmantle

When applied to rope, the term *dynamic* means a rope with high stretch. This stretch is meant to act as a sort of shock absorber when a falling climber is caught by the rope. Some dynamic kernmantle ropes stretch by as much as 60% before breaking.

The stretch is created with a rope core that mechanically lets out under load, much as a spring does. The design of the core varies slightly from one manufacturer to another. Figure 3-8 shows one design of dynamic kernmantle construction. Most dynamic rope cores are constructed of a group of twisted bundles. A small percentage of dynamic ropes have braided cores.

Compared with static kernmantle rope, the sheath, or mantle, of dynamic kernmantle rope tends to be relatively thin but has more fiber bundles over the same area. This means that the sheath covers the core better when the rope is stretched or bent.

Advantages

- The elasticity of dynamic kernmantle rope is an advantage for climbing situations in which long falls are possible.
- This type of rope is very easy to handle and to tie in knots.

Disadvantages

- The thin sheath makes these ropes susceptible to damage from abrasion and to contamination from dirt and grit.
- The elasticity of dynamic kernmantle ropes makes them less suitable for activities such as rappelling and ascending and for many rescue operations.

Static Kernmantle

Static kernmantle ropes are also known as *low-stretch* kernmantle ropes. When applied to rope, the term *static* means a type of rope with very low stretch (no more than 20% of its length at break). A rope core of fiber bundles that are nearly parallel to one another creates this low stretch (Figure 3-9). Some static ropes have so little stretch that what there is results largely from the inherent stretch of the nylon.

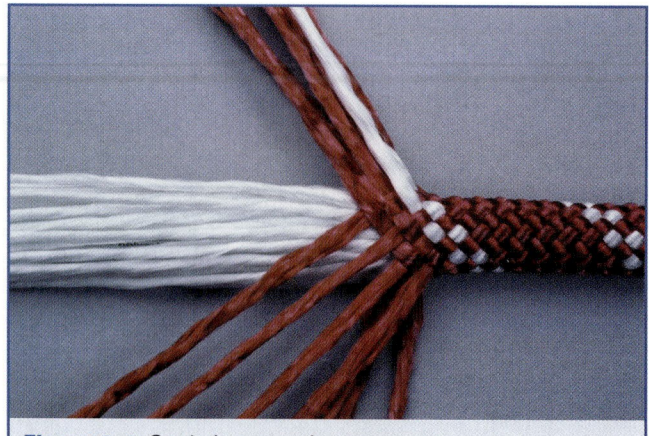

Figure 3-9 Static kernmantle construction.

Because static ropes have so little stretch, they cause a more abrupt stop when catching a fall. This sudden stop subjects the climber's body, the equipment in the system, and the anchors to greater impact loading than would a dynamic rope.

Most static kernmantle ropes also have a thicker, tighter sheath than do dynamic kernmantle ropes. This thicker sheath helps protect the core from damage by abrasion and helps prevent dirt and grit from entering the core and damaging the inner fibers. However, the tighter sheath results in a rope that is stiffer than and not as easy to handle as a dynamic kernmantle rope, with its thinner sheath.

Choosing a Rope

A rope is the one essential element in the high angle system. It is in essence a tool, and as with all tools, the correct rope should be chosen to fit the job.

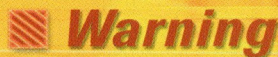

Warning

All references in this book to *dynamic rope* or *static rope* relate to very specific types of rope construction. A dynamic rope is one specifically built for climbing or mountaineering and is not just a stretchy rope. A static rope is either a *rescue static rope* made especially for rope rescue, or a *sport static rope* made for personal ascending or rappelling.

These special ropes are not normally found at the average hardware store. They should be purchased only from reputable dealers and manufacturers who sell their products for these specific uses.

Dynamic versus Static Ropes

If you are going to be doing only recreational rock climbing or mountaineering, your choice should be a dynamic rope. Many types of dynamic rope can be used, depending on the climbing environment and the style of climbing. To choose the correct rope, you should consult an instructional manual on climbing or any of several catalogs from companies that specialize in climbing equipment.

Also, if the rope is going to be used as a belay for falls that result in severe shock loading, a dynamic rope is more appropriate. The point at which a fall becomes severe enough to require a dynamic rope is the subject of considerable debate. Much depends on local conditions, such as the climbing environment, the equipment used, and the experience of the people involved. However, certainly if a fall approaching the severity of FF 0.25 is expected, a dynamic rope should be used. This is not so much for the sake of the rope as to reduce the impact loads on the person attached to the rope and on the anchors.

If your activities are going to be restricted to rappelling and ascending, particularly under harsh conditions, a static rope probably would be preferable. Most rescue workers now use static rope in their operations.

Size and Strength

If you have chosen a static rope and have decided on the type of fiber and construction, you must now decide how strong a rope is needed, or on the **tensile strength.** The tensile strength of a rope depends very much on its cross section of material, or the amount of yarn used per foot of length.

The temptation may arise to choose the largest diameter rope available, usually ⅝ inch (16 mm) for a synthetic fiber, life support rope. However, this could be a serious mistake and could actually hinder activity with the rope. There is also a tendency to pick the strongest possible rope for a particular diameter. Although strength is important, higher strength often is achieved by using materials that do not stretch hardly at all. This lack of stretch means poor energy absorption if an unexpected force is suddenly applied to the system. Special care must be taken when rigging with a very-low-stretch rope. Another way to increase strength in a kernmantle rope of a given diameter is to put less yarn in the sheath and more yarn in the core. Although this makes a rope with a soft hand, it can also make a rope with little sheath to protect the core from cuts, dirt, chemicals, and abrasions.

Most rescue teams select ⁷⁄₁₆-inch (11 mm) or ½-inch (12.5 mm) static kernmantle ropes for their main rescue lines. However, each team should make its own decision based on such factors as rescue needs, environment, and the nature of their team.

Problems with Large-Diameter Ropes

The use of large-diameter ropes poses several problems, including the following:

- Higher cost, because more material is used in the rope.
- Greater weight, because the larger the diameter of a rope, the more it weighs. This can mean difficulty carrying the rope to where it is needed (usually uphill or up flights of stairs).
- Handling problems, because when the rope is hanging vertically, the greater weight means more difficulty in rappelling and handling the rope.
- Incompatibility with other equipment, because many types of high angle equipment are not made for use with ropes over ½-inch (12.5 mm) in diameter.

The one obvious advantage to very-large-diameter ropes is their overall strength. However, in normal field use, larger diameter ropes have only slightly better abrasion and cut resistance than ⁷⁄₁₆-inch (11 mm) and ½-inch (12.5 mm) ropes.

Determining the System Safety Factor

The most realistic way to determine the needed tensile strength of the rope (and therefore its diameter) is to calculate the **load ratio** in the context of the system safety factor. The **system safety factor** estimates conditions expected to be encountered in the local high angle environment plus a realistic margin of safety.

To determine the safety factor for a particular system, you first must analyze the elements of the system; that is, the breaking strengths of the various components, the ways they affect one another, the load, and how the load will be applied. You then add a margin to cover what you don't know or couldn't anticipate.

First, you need to know the breaking strengths of all the individual components of the system. Breaking strengths are advertised in several ways, but most technical rescue equipment manufacturers now provide a *minimum breaking strength (MBS)*, which is determined by calculating three standard deviations below the mean of several laboratory tests. The rope technician should know the approximate MBS of all the equipment in any system she is rigging. It is important to note that some items have several MBS numbers based on the way they are placed in a system.

It is easy to use the MBS to calculate what may appear to be the safety factor of a component by comparing the estimated breaking strength of an item against a specific static load. However, this figure reflects only the *load ratio* of that component, or more specifically, the *component load ratio (CLR)*. The component load ratio is the estimated breaking strength of a given item in relation to a specific static load.

Even more important is the effect of the load on the system as a whole. To find the real safety factor, you need to know the ratio of the expected maximum load on the system to the expected failure point of the weakest point in the system. This takes into consideration all the components and the way they are rigged. This ratio is more accurately known as the *system load ratio (SLR)*. It is important to know the load ratios of each component in your system and also the system load ratio, because these values help you determine the system safety factor.

For example, a 9,000-lbf (40 kN) general purpose rescue rope that you expect will be loaded with a 300-lbf (1.33 kN) rescuer would yield a 30:1 load ratio on the rope itself: 9,000:300 lbf (40:1.33 kN). Because this is the load ratio only of the rope component and nothing else, this is the component load ratio. Bear in mind that if the expected load changes, so does the ratio, even if the same rope is used.

To calculate the system load ratio, you would need to know the strength of the anchor to which the rope is attached, as well as the ways in which anything else might affect the strength of the various components.

Let's say the rope is anchored to a tested 5,100-lbf (22.5 kN) anchor bolt. The system load ratio would be 17:1, because the 9,000-lbf (40 kN) rope is attached to a 5,100-lbf (22.5 kN) anchor, and the 300-lb (1.33 kN) rescuer on that 5,100-lbf (22.5 kN) anchor is a 17:1 load ratio: 5,100:300 lbf (22.5:1.33 kN). However, you also need to think about the way you fastened the rope to the bolt. This usually is done with a knot. Most common knots reduce the rope's strength only by 15% to 30%, therefore our 9,000-lbf (40 kN) rope would still have 6,300-lbf (28 kN) strength with a 70% efficient knot, yielding a 21:1 load ratio, which is higher than the anchor's load ratio.

Knots and anchors are just two of many things that can affect the system load ratio. What happens in any of the above examples if you put two people on the system? In each case, the ratio would be cut in half. In the case of the single anchor point, you would now have an 8.5:1 system load ratio: 5,100:600-lbf (22.5:2.66 kN). Another consideration is the edge over which the rope runs. If it is a very sharp radius edge, it will reduce the strength of the rope even more than the knot does unless the edge is padded somehow.

Another consideration is shock loading, or shock absorption. Will the load likely stay relatively static or take a big bounce?

What if our 600-lbf (2.66 kN) load jumped from a window with a few inches of slack in the rope? That could easily double the load on the system and cut the 8.5:1 static system load ratio to less than 4.25:1.

Once you have determined the reasonable system load ratio based on the above process, you can determine the system safety factor. What ratio is safe? In theory, anything greater than a 1:1 system load ratio will probably hold. However, how "safe" it ultimately will be depends on several things, including how accurately you estimated the maximum load, how accurately you pinpointed the weakest link, and what the consequences might be in the event of a failure. To provide a margin of safety and to determine the safety factor, apply a multiplier of the load to make up for inaccuracies and unknowns in your system analysis.

The margin of safety used is up to the technician and the policy of the rescue group. Start the design of your system by calculating the anticipated load on the system. To add a safety factor to the system load ratio, you must multiply the anticipated static load by at least 4 or 5 and possibly even 10. The greater the chance for a large, unplanned load, such as a dynamic loading, and the more uncertain you are about the lowest component load ratio, the larger your safety factor needs to be. The greater the ratio, the safer the system. However, bear in mind that it is possible to make a system so "safe" that it is also impractical or inefficient (or both) to the point of being dangerous to both the rescuers and the subject.

The goal is to achieve the highest system safety factor that is *reasonable* to rig in the given conditions with time and equipment constraints often beyond your control. True rope technicians know the minimum breaking strengths of the various components they are using, the ways those minimum strengths can be affected by the rigging methods, the quality of anchors, and the force multipliers both in and on the system. They can evaluate the system and build it to provide the highest reasonable safety factor.

Some mountain and wilderness rescue groups accept a safety factor of 10:1, for several reasons. First, they may have to carry rope and equipment for long distances, therefore weight is an important factor. However, mountain rescuers also feel that they have better control of their equipment and are very knowledgeable about its history. They also may be skilled enough to assess equipment limitations, such as potential overloading and other damaging factors. For these reasons, they feel they do not need a safety factor greater than 10:1.

Some rescue disciplines feel they need a higher safety factor. For example, a component safety factor for rescue rope that is commonly used in the fire service is 15:1. Therefore, if 600 lbf (267 daN) is the expected maximum load, with a safety factor of 10:1, the rope should have a minimum breaking strength of 6,000 lbf (26.7 kN.) If a component safety factor of 15:1 is used, the minimum breaking strength should be 9,000 lbf (40 kN.) It is important to note that this 15:1 ratio is a component safety factor and does not mean that the finished system should automatically be expected to have a safety factor this high.

The NFPA has set guidelines for life safety rope and rates them as escape, light use, or general use. The organization's *Standard for Life Safety Rope and System Components* (NFPA 1983-2001) requires a minimum breaking strength of 3,034 lbf (13.5 kN) for an escape rope, 4,496 lbf (20 kN) for a light use life safety rope, and 8,992 lbf (40 kN) for a general use life safety rope. These are the component minimum breaking strengths that can be used to help determine the system load ratio.

Breaking Strength of Rope

The breaking strength of a rope is measured as *tensile strength at break*. On the face of it, this may seem like a very simple idea. However, the many different ways of conducting tests produce different test results on the same piece of rope. Among the different factors that affect the outcome of a tensile test include:

- *The speed of the pull.* A rope pulled apart slowly registers a higher breaking strength than one pulled apart more quickly. (Results may be different in dynamic drop tests, depending on rope materials and construction.)
- *The diameter of the object to which the rope is attached when it is pulled.* A rope pulled to failure by a small-diameter object breaks at a lower tensile strength than a rope pulled with a larger diameter object. Similarly, a rope pulled with a knot in it breaks at a lower strength than one without a knot, because whenever a rope is placed under load in a sharp bend, some strength is lost (see Chapter 4).

Rope Tensile Test Standards

The Cordage Institute's CI 1801, *Low Stretch and Static Kernmantle Life Safety Rope* (1998) can be used for comparisons by rope manufacturers who choose to do so. This standard specifies guidelines such as what the rope is tied to during the test and the rate of pull, along with other criteria.

Certain NFPA standards also apply to rope that is used by those who adhere to that organization's standards. The NFPA should be contacted for specific information on these standards. (See Appendix C for addresses of standards-setting organizations.)

Rope Colors

Although many people choose a rope color for aesthetic reasons, color also can serve a functional purpose. For example, if several ropes are used together, the different colors can help distinguish one line from another so that the user immediately knows which rope to haul or lower.

Another way to use color is to buy a different colored rope for each year, so as to be able to tell quickly the age of the ropes. Also, varying colors can be used for different sizes of rope.

Process for Coloring Ropes

When manufactured, nylon is off-white, therefore any color for a rope must be added at some point during its manufacture. Adding color to the rope material somewhat affects the rope's strength, and in some cases it affects the rope's resistance to damage by sunlight. How much these properties are affected depends on the method used to add the dye to the rope material and, in some cases, on the dye itself.

The two basic methods of adding color to a rope are *solution dying* and *surface-applied dying*. In solution dying, the color is added to the raw material as the yarn is being manufactured. In surface-applied dying, the color is added to the synthetic yarn after it has been manufactured, or it is added to the rope after it has been braided.

Solution dying usually causes slightly more loss of strength in the rope than surface-applied dying. Also, loss of strength varies among colors because of chemical differences in the dyes.

One advantage of kernmantle ropes is that the sheath yarns don't carry much of the load; the dye yarns, therefore, have little effect on the overall strength of the rope. However, the dye could shorten the life of the sheath by weakening its resistance to abrasion.

Accessory Cord

Accessory cord is smaller diameter rope used for a variety of tasks for which the regular rope would be too bulky. Most accessory cord is soft and more flexible, resembling a miniature climbing rope. This makes it easier to knot, and it grips well when used in friction knots such as Prusik hitches. Because it has a soft sheath, you should regularly inspect it for wear and damage. Accessory cord usually is found in sizes up to 9 mm.

⚠ Warning

Climbers' accessory cord does not use the same high-stretch core yarns as dynamic climbing rope and should never be used in place of those ropes for impact load situations.

Webbing

Because of its special characteristics, webbing may be preferable to rope in certain situations. For example, webbing is more comfortable than rope against the body for seat harnesses. Also, webbing commonly is used for anchoring because it is less expensive than rope. In addition, because of its wide, flat surface, webbing may be more abrasion resistant in some rigging applications.

One drawback to webbing is that it does not absorb shock loading as well as many ropes. When webbing is used for anchors, therefore, it tends to transmit more shock loading to the anchor points. This is one reason some people prefer rope to webbing in anchoring.

There are fewer secure knots for webbing than for rope. Because webbing has a slick surface, knots can pull out if they are not carefully tied, safetied, and monitored. Consequently, you may prefer webbing anchor loops that are presewn at the factory.

Webbing Materials

Most webbing is made of nylon or polyester, materials that have the same characteristics as those used to manufacture rope. Some webbing is made from Spectra, which has high tensile strength but does not absorb shock loading as well as nylon or polyester. For this reason, webbing made of Spectra should be used with dynamic rope or other energy absorbers in the rope system to absorb impact loads.

Webbing Construction
Flat Webbing

Flat webbing is constructed of a single layer of material, the same as seat belt webbing. It is less expensive but stiffer and more difficult to work with than tubular webbing.

Tubular Webbing

Because *tubular webbing* is more supple and easier to work with, it is more often used in the high angle environment. The tubular shape is obvious if you look at the webbing from one end and squeeze the two edges together. The two types of tubular webbing are shuttle loom and needle loom.

Shuttle loom tubular webbing has a continuous spiral of the filler along the webbing's warp fibers (Figure 3-10). If you inspect shuttle loom webbing along the edge, it will not have a seam and will appear to have the same construction on the edges as flat webbing.

Needle loom webbing is formed by folding flat webbing lengthwise and stitching the two edges together (Figure 3-11). Because webbing is susceptible to abrasion along its edges, some types of edge-stitched webbing may become unstitched when the thread is broken. The better designed edge-stitched webbing locks the stitches under one another so that they are not as prone to coming unstitched.

Because of the economics of the manufacturing process, shuttle loom webbing is becoming more difficult to find. Older needle loom webbing did not always have an extra lock stitch and could easily unravel if cut. Modern needle loom webbing incorporates a lock stitch that prevents unraveling.

Unfortunately, a few sources of the original needle loom webbing without a lock stitch may still be available. The best way

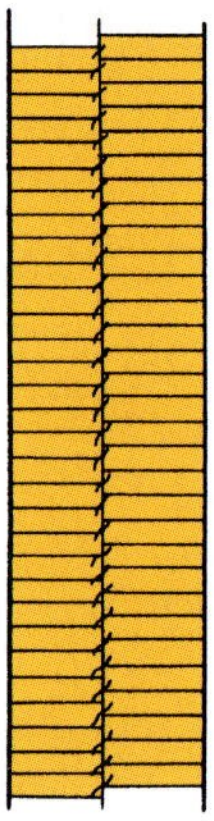

Figure 3-11 Edge-stitched (needle loom) webbing.

to shop for tubular webbing is to be certain of the source, making sure that the seller understands the differences. You can test for the lock stitch by cutting the joined edge and making sure the yarns lock rather than unraveling from the cut spot.

There are hundreds of sizes and types of webbing, and many types are unsuitable for high angle operations. You should buy webbing for life support applications only from quality suppliers who publish tensile strengths and specifications. Be particularly cautious about the use of surplus webbing, which usually has no information about tensile strength, material, specifications, date of manufacture, or history of use. In determining the safety factor for webbing, use the same procedure as for rope and other equipment.

Webbing Size

Webbing ranges in width from ½ inch (12.5 mm) up to 6 inches (150 mm). In high angle work, widths from 1 to 2 inches (25 to 50 mm) are most often used. For seat harnesses, the larger widths are more comfortable.

Webbing Strength

The most common types of webbing sold by suppliers of high angle equipment include the following:

- 1-inch (25 mm) tubular nylon: Most common is Mil-W-5625, which has a tensile strength of about 4,000 lb.
- 2-inch (50 mm) tubular nylon: Tensile strength of about 8,000 lb.
- 1-inch (25 mm) solid nylon: Most common is Mil-W-4088, type 18, which has a tensile strength of about 6,000 lb.
- 1¹⁵⁄₁₆-inch (49 mm) or 2-inch (50 mm) solid seat belt–type webbing, nylon or polyester: Tensile strength of 4,500 to 6,000 lb, depending on the material and type.
- 1²³⁄₃₂-inch (44 mm) flat nylon webbing (Mil-W-4088): Tensile strength of about 9,500 lb.

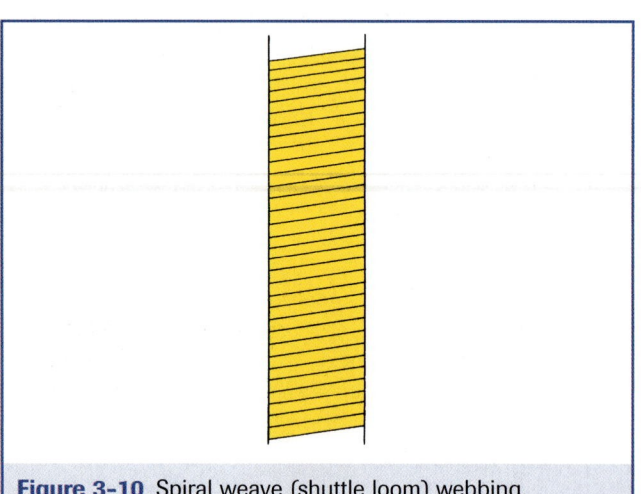

Figure 3-10 Spiral weave (shuttle loom) webbing.

Evaluation Exercises

Cognitive and Affective Exercises

1. Dynamic ropes are designed to stretch because:

    A. Stretch is required for knots.
    B. It allows energy to be absorbed during shock loading.
    C. It allows for a "weak" link.
    D. It allows systems to bend.

2. Static ropes are designed not to stretch because this type of construction:

    A. Reduces stretch in mechanical advantage, rappelling, and ascending situations.
    B. Allows for energy absorption.
    C. Allows the climber to absorb the kinetic energy.
    D. Permits easier knot placement.

3. A climber is connected to a secure point of protection at the top of a 1,200-foot (366 m) cliff with a 6½-foot (2 m) length of rope. While at this point of protection, he falls the full length of the rope. The fall factor is:

    A. 1.5
    B. 2
    C. 1
    D. 0.5

4. A rescuer is connected 200 feet (60 m) up a 650-foot (200 m) tower with a 100-foot (30 m) length of rope to a secure point of protection. She climbs up past the point of protection by 50 feet (15 m) and falls past the point of protection the full length of the rope before being caught by the rope. This is a fall factor of:

    A. 0.5
    B. 1
    C. 1.5
    D. 2

5. A rescuer is climbing a 300-foot (90 m) wall and is being belayed on a 200-foot (60 m) dynamic rope. The belay point is 200 feet (60 m) up the cliff. The climber starts climbing again at the belay point and has climbed 100 feet (30 m) up from the belay point when he falls. He falls free and is caught by the belay. This would be a fall factor of:

    A. 0.5
    B. 1
    C. 1.5
    D. 2

6. The advantages of synthetic fiber rope for high angle activities include all of the following except:

    A. They have higher temperature resistance.
    B. Each fiber runs the entire length of the rope.
    C. They have low resistance to abrasion.
    D. They do not rot.

7. The types of nylon commonly used in rope for high angle activities include:

    A. Polyester and nylon 6
    B. Nylon 6,6 and nylon 6
    C. Perlon and Kevlar
    D. Nylon 6,6 and polyolefins

8. The advantage(s) of plaited rope is/are:

    A. Softness and pliability
    B. Picking
    C. Abrasion resistance
    D. Stiffness

9. Single-braid rope generally is not adequate for high angle operations because:

    A. It is constructed of three fiber bundles.
    B. It is braided as a "clothesline braid."
    C. It is vulnerable to destruction.
    D. All of the above.

10. The term kernmantle refers to:

    A. The core and sheath construction
    B. The solid braid over a single braid
    C. The eight bundles of fibers plaited together
    D. The three fiber bundles twisted together

11. You are about to make a traverse to a subject who is trapped on a ledge approximately 100 feet (30 m) away. The subject is approximately 200 feet (60 m) above the ground, and you are on the same elevation as the subject. Which of the following ropes would you choose for protection during your traverse?

    A. Plaited rope
    B. Dynamic kernmantle
    C. Single braid
    D. Static kernmantle

12. You have reached the subject in the above situation, and you want to set a rope to the bottom for other rescuers to ascend. You would choose which of the following ropes for the ascent rope?

    A. Plaited rope
    B. Single braid
    C. Static kernmantle
    D. Dynamic kernmantle

13. The component load ratio of a rescue rope with a rated minimum breaking strength of 4,500 lbf (20 kN) and with a 600 lbf (2.66 kN) load would be:

    A. 15:1
    B. 7.5
    C. 12.5:1
    D. 10:1

14. Assuming a load ratio of 15:1, the minimum tensile strength rope to be used when the expected load will be 600 lb (2.66 kN) would be:

    A. 4,500 lb (20 kN)
    B. 6,000 lb (28.9 kN)
    C. 7,500 lb (33.4 kN)
    D. 9,000 lb (40 kN)

15. The typical breaking strength of 1-inch tubular webbing is:

    A. 2,500 lb (11.2 kN)
    B. 4,000 lb (17.8 kN)
    C. 5,000 lb (22.2 kN)
    D. 6,000 lb (28.9 kN)

4

Care and Use of Rescue Rope and Related Equipment

The material in this chapter conforms to guidelines published by the National Fire Protection Association (NFPA), specifically standard 1983, *Standard for Life Safety Rope and System Components* (2001). NFPA standards are revised regularly, and readers are advised to review the latest version of this standard.

Objectives

On completion of this chapter, you should be able to:

1. List the elements of a rope log.
2. Identify the storage situations that could harm a rope.
3. List the advantages of bagging a rope for storage and transport.
4. List the situations or substances that may damage a working rope.
5. Cite several methods for protecting a working rope.
6. Define the 4:1 rule.
7. List the steps for inspecting a rope.
8. List the reasons for retiring a rope.
9. List several strategies for preventing tangling of a working rope.
10. Describe the process for throwing or dropping a rope down a face or wall.

Key Terms

Edge Rollers In-line, free-turning rollers that are anchored at an edge of a wall or cliff face to reduce rope friction.

Rope History Log A document that tracks the history of a particular rope. The log contains entries that indicate the manufacturer, diameter, design, tensile strength, date of purchase, when the rope was used, how it was used, and any abuse that could affect its performance or safety.

Rope Tag Identification placed on a rope that distinguishes it from other ropes.

Care of Ropes

The modern high angle rescue rope is a marvel of design and engineering. However, a rope's performance, how long it lasts, and its safety still depend on how well it is cared for. The condition of a rope ultimately depends on its history: the age of the rope, the conditions to which it has been subjected, and the care it has received.

If a rope is owned and used by only one person, that person probably knows the history of the rope. However, if more than one person is using the rope, there has to be a system for tracking the rope's history. The common way of tracking a rope's history is to keep a *rope history log*. Each rope should have its own log.

Keeping a Rope History Log

Each rope must have its own log card with pertinent information on the manufacturer, diameter, design, tensile strength, date of purchase, and critical data. The log card should have enough space to allow rope technicians to note each time the rope was used and for what activity. Specific entries must be made whenever the rope was subjected to abuse that could affect its performance or safety. An example of a rope history log is shown in Figure 4-1.

It is essential that entries for each rope be made every time ropes are returned to storage after use. Every user must follow this discipline; otherwise, the rope history is incomplete.

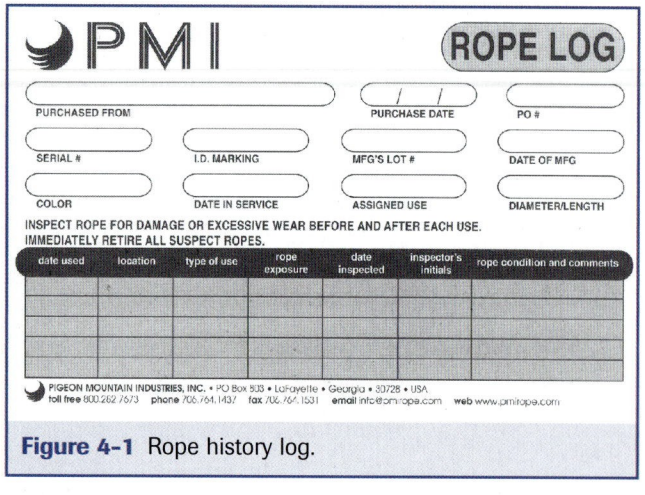

Figure 4-1 Rope history log.

Tagging Ropes

Because most groups with high angle rescue gear have ropes of similar color, length, and diameter, a means of distinguishing each individual rope must be found so that its history can be kept. Each rope should have some distinct identification, such as a number or letter, that corresponds to its card. This identifying mark, known as a *rope tag*, must be placed on the rope so that it is unmistakable and cannot be eradicated or lost. Some examples of rope tagging include the following (Figure 4-2):

- Hot stamping the end of the rope
- Marking the circumference at the end of the rope and protecting the mark with clear plastic tape, clear heat shrink tubing, or a protective coating such as Whip End Dip

Storing Ropes

In short, a life support rope must be stored in a place of its own where it is protected from harm. You can damage your rope if you do the following:

- Leave it in sunlight (all fibers used in life safety ropes, including nylon and polyester, degrade with prolonged exposure to sunlight)
- Expose it to vehicle exhaust systems or to fumes or residues from storage batteries (both of these vehicle components produce substances damaging to rope)
- Leave it on the floor (concrete floors are alkaline, but they may contain damaging substances from materials used in sealants and from acids used in cleaning; stepping on rope grinds in dirt and grit; also, damaging substances can be dropped onto the rope)

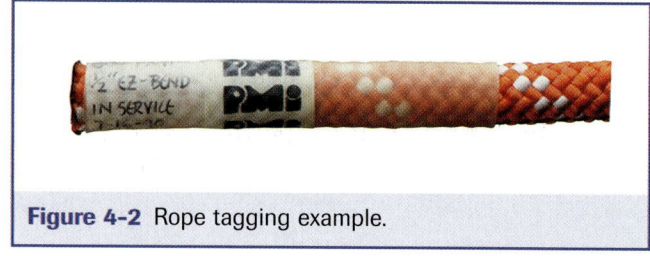

Figure 4-2 Rope tagging example.

- Store it in wet or damp areas (this promotes the growth of mold or mildew on the rope)
- Store it in areas of high temperature (prolonged exposure to temperatures higher than humans can tolerate promotes rope degradation)
- Contaminate it with dirt and grit (dirt and grit work into the core and damage the yarn; avoid needlessly dragging a rope on the ground; never step on a rope)

Bagging Ropes

One of the most convenient ways of storing, transporting, and protecting a rope is called bagging (Figure 4-3).

Some of the advantages of bagging include the following:

- The bag helps protect the rope from damage while keeping it clean.
- You can usually flake rope into a bag quicker than you can coil it. Figure 4-3 shows a fast technique for bagging a rope.
- A bag with a shoulder strap or pack straps is a convenient way to carry the rope.

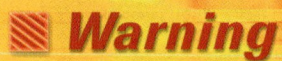

Warning

To avoid damage to the rope, use common sense in dropping bagged rope. For example, do not drop a bag with 600 feet (183 m) of rope down 100 feet (30 m). The 500 feet (152 m) remaining in the bag when the bag hits bottom may be damaged by the impact. Match the amount of rope to the distance of the drop.

- A bagged rope is easy to deploy. Simply secure the upper end of the rope and drop the bag over the edge. In most cases the rope flakes out of the bag without tangles. Secure the bottom end of the rope to the bottom of the bag so that the bag is not lost when you drop it.

Techniques for Bagging Rope

The following are techniques for bagging a rope:

1. If you are wearing a seat harness, clip a carabiner into the harness and run the end of the rope through the carabiner and into the bag. If you are not wearing a harness, begin with the next step.
2. Grasp the top edge of the bag and hold the bag open and upright with your nondominant hand (e.g., *left hand for right-handed individuals*).
3. Lightly trap the rope between your thumb and index finger as it enters the bag.
4. With your dominant hand *(right hand for right-handed individuals)* below the other hand, grasp the rope and pull it into the bottom of the bag.
5. Slide the dominant hand back up to the other hand, take another length of rope, and pull it down into the bag.
6. Continue with these short strokes until the rope is bagged.

Coiling

Before bagging became common practice, coiling commonly was used for storing and transporting ropes. The specific type of coil depends on the circumstances or environment in which the rope is to be used. Some basic types of coils (i.e., mountaineer coil, caver's coil, and butterfly coil) are shown in Figure 4-4.

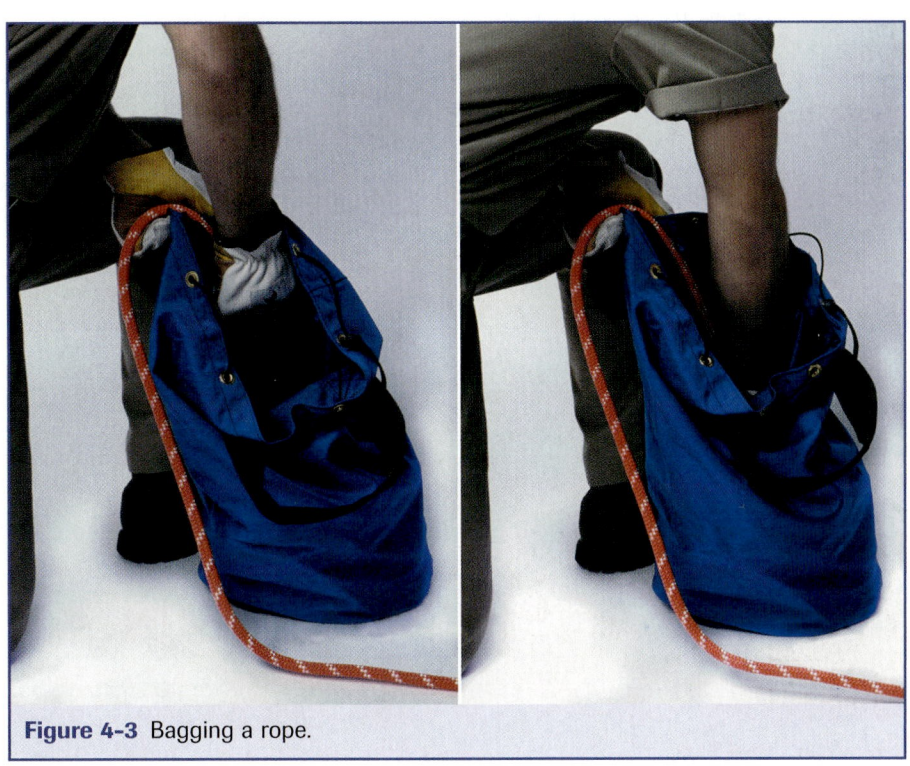

Figure 4-3 Bagging a rope.

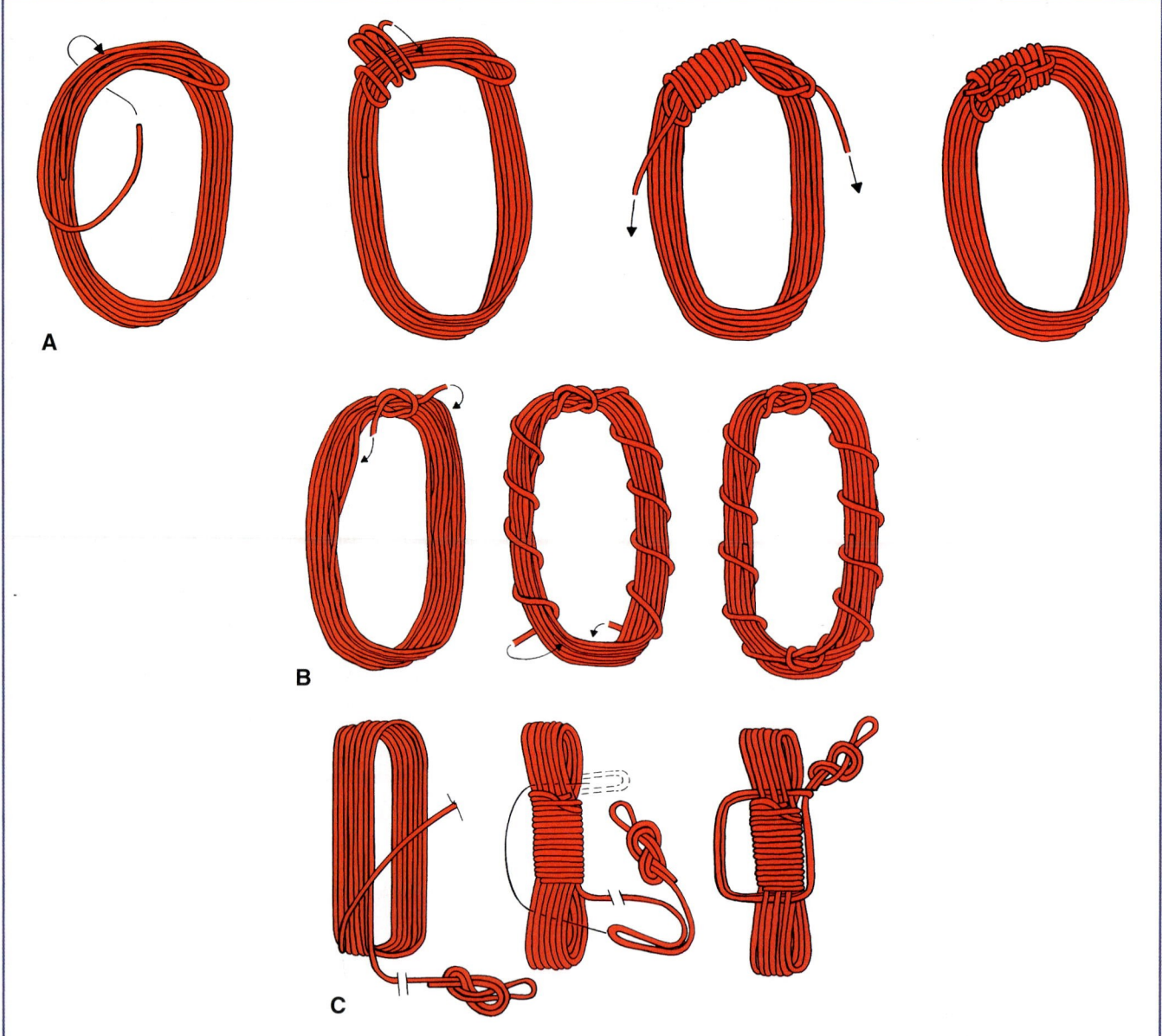

Figure 4-4 A, Mountaineer coil, a traditional climber's coil, can be made quickly. **B,** Caver's coil is designed to be carried through caves without snagging. **C,** Butterfly coil is useful for paying out rope, such as dropping down a face. Also, the ends can be secured so that the coil can be carried on a person like a backpack.

How Ropes are Damaged
Harmful Substances

The following list includes some of the common substances that can destroy or cause deterioration in certain kinds of rope.

Damaging to Nylon

- Acids, particularly those found in storage batteries
- Bleaches

Damaging to Polyester

- Alkali (such as is found in soot)

Damaging to Nylon and Polyester

- Many other strong chemicals (avoid any contact with a chemical unless you know for sure it is harmless to rope fiber)

Overloading a Rope

Overloading a rope causes internal damage that could endanger those using the rope in the future. Damage from overloading usually occurs when a rope is used in activities for which it was not intended and when the load greatly exceeds the rope's safe working load. Some examples of overloading a rope include towing vehicles and lifting heavy objects.

A separate set of ropes, for utility use only, must be used for activities such as these two examples. Utility lines must be stored separately from life support ropes and distinctly marked, for example, *"Utility line—not for life support operations."*

Damage from Falling Objects

Objects such as rocks or tools that fall on the rope, particularly when it is under load, can do serious damage. Anytime you see heavy or sharp objects fall on a rope or when the rope has been used in a rock fall zone, you should inspect the rope for damage.

Abrasion

One of the most common means of destroying a rope or shortening its life is abrasion. This kind of damage usually is avoidable. Damage from abrasion commonly occurs when the rope is under tension and is lowered and raised across a rock or over the edge of a building. Abrasion often happens when a person is doing "bouncy" rappels or ascending, causing the rope to "saw" back and forth across a rock or hard object.

Techniques for Preventing Abrasion

There are numerous ways to avoid abrasion on rope, many of them using simple and inexpensive equipment. Every person and every team that owns a rope should carry equipment for preventing edge abrasion.

Rope Pads

Rope pads are among the simplest and least expensive means of protecting rope from abrasion. They work best for fixed ropes, such as rappel lines. Among the commonly used types of pads are canvas pads (heavy duty canvas can easily be made into protective pads). For greater protection and durability, a square of heavy duty canvas can be folded twice, stitched around the edge to prevent fraying, and then cross-stitched (Figure 4-5). For added convenience, large grommets can be set into two corners. The grommets can be used to attach the pad so that it does not slide away as the rope is moving. A complete edge protection kit should include a variety of pads, ranging from approximately 2 × 3 feet (0.6 m × 0.9 m) to 2 × 6 feet (0.6 × 1.8 m) or larger. Several commercially made canvas rope pads are also available.

Fire Hose Sections of discarded fire hose can also be converted to effective rope pads. To avoid having to feed the rope through the hose, modify the hose in the following manner:

1. Split the hose down the center.
2. To prevent the rope from slipping out, secure the edges of the hose with a closure such as snaps or Velcro (Figure 4-6).
3. Set a hole or grommet in each end of the fire hose so that it can be anchored to prevent it from slipping down the rope.

Improvised Techniques If no premade edge protection is available, other materials may be pressed into service to protect the rope from abrasion. Some examples of improvised rope pads are:

- Packs
- Turnout coats

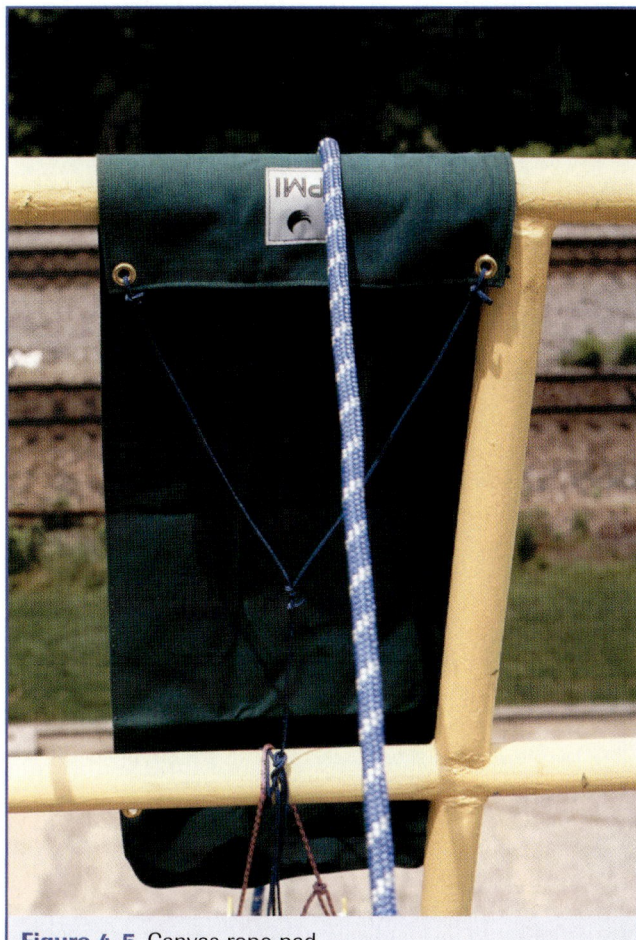

Figure 4-5 Canvas rope pad.

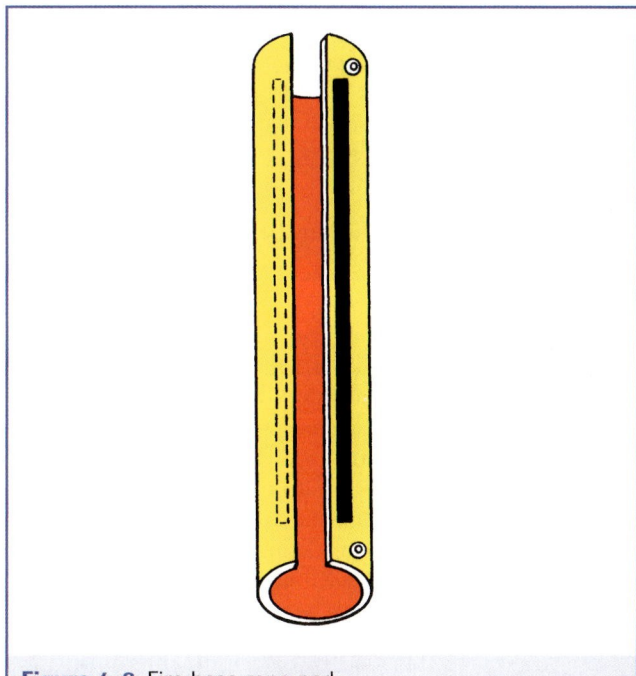

Figure 4-6 Fire hose rope pad.

- Clothing
- Blankets
- Carpet squares

Note that wool carpet squares are preferable because synthetic material may melt under heat fusion with the rope.

Commercial Rope Protectors

A number of rope protection devices are available.

Metal Devices Some metal devices have rollers, others have only skid bars. Metal devices are often used in lowering or hauling operations.

ADVANTAGES
- Afford greater protection
- Reduce friction, particularly in hauling

DISADVANTAGES
- More expensive
- Heavier
- Some models may be prone to tipping over unless anchored carefully.

Soft Protection Soft protection is constructed of canvas and other fabrics. It often is used when the rope is not moving, such as with a rappel rope.

ADVANTAGES
- Less expensive than metal devices
- Weighs less than metal protection

DISADVANTAGES
- May not give as much protection
- Does not reduce friction as much as metal devices

Other types of commercial edge protection may be similar to canvas edge pads or fire hose pads. Some of the fabrics used for these pads are canvas and polyvinyl chloride (PVC)-coated nylon (Figure 4-7). Some are made with closures so that the pad stays wrapped around the rope. One type of edge protector is constructed of a slick, heat-resistant plastic and has grooves to guide the rope.

Mechanical Rope Protection Devices

Edge Rollers ***Edge rollers*** are one of the most effective means of protecting ropes from abrasion. They usually are more expensive than soft edge protection, but they have the added advantage of greatly reducing the friction of rope over an edge. This is particularly important in hauling systems, in which edge friction makes raising more difficult and puts great stress on equipment. Some edge rollers may tip over if they are not anchored carefully.

Three main types of edge rollers are available: single unit rollers, roof rollers, and roll modules.

Two rollers are set into a frame (Figure 4-8). Two or more of these units usually are needed to provide adequate edge protection. They generally must be stabilized by anchoring them with their attachment points. When they are stabilized, these units perform well on irregular surfaces, such as cliffs and other natural conformations.

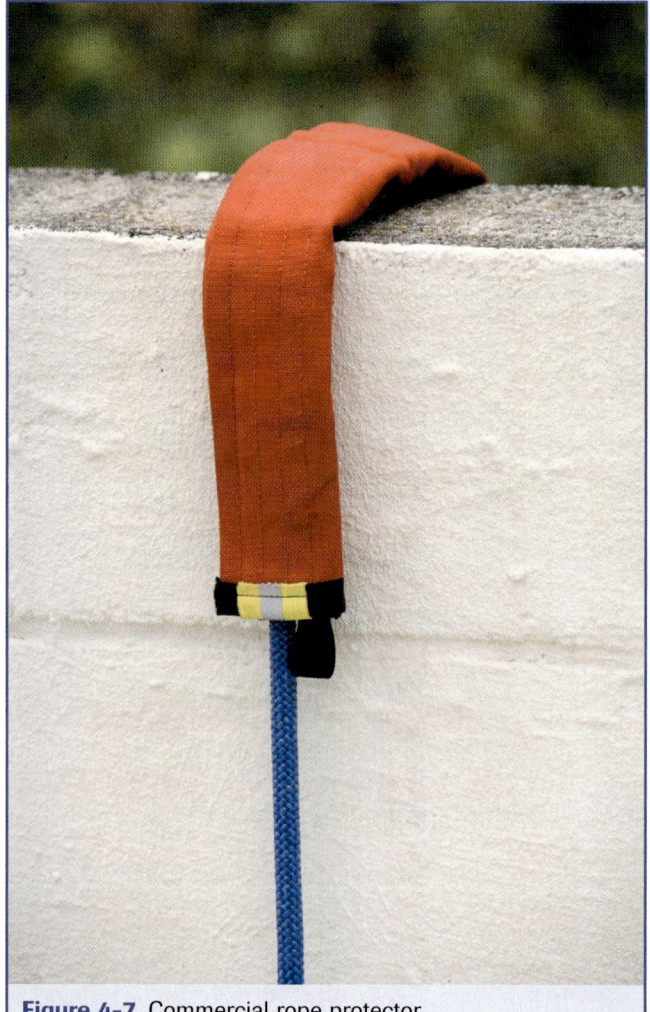

Figure 4-7 Commercial rope protector.

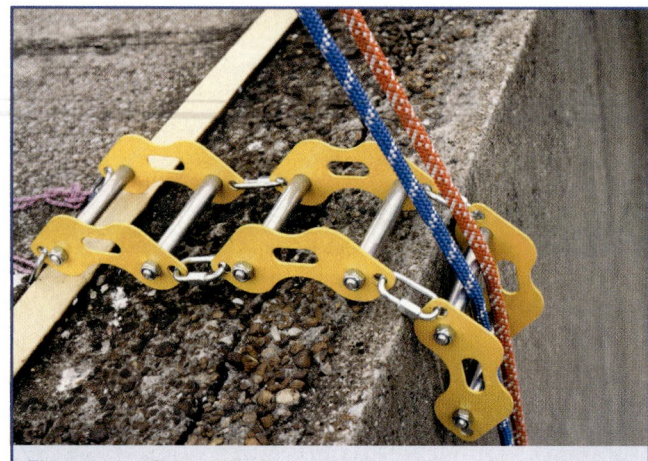

Figure 4-8 Edge roller.

A *roof roller* consists of a unit of two rollers set in a 90-degree frame (Figure 4-9). They are designed for edge protection on buildings and other structures where 90-degree angles are present.

A *roll module* has rollers on the side as well as the bottom, so that if the module tips over, it still offers protection. The four modules are linked with screw links and can conform to a variety of surfaces.

Other Mechanical Edge Protection Another type of mechanical edge protection device has metal units that can be clipped together. One example is the Edge Roller, which is composed of three linked units consisting of hard aluminum side plates with two roller bars each. It can be used linked together with the furnished screw links at sharp edges or separated for long, gradual breakovers.

Heat Fusion

Heat fusion results when two pieces of synthetic material rub together. This is very destructive to rope and can cut a line as surely as a knife. Heat fusion usually occurs when one rope runs across another rope or across webbing, or when one line moves quickly across one spot in a second line that remains stationary. Heat fusion occurs in the following situations:

- Two ropes under tension with one remaining stationary while the other, being lowered, runs across the first
- A loaded rope running across an anchor rope or webbing also under load
- A rappeller holding a rope against the seat harness webbing while performing a rapid rappel

Damage to ropes by heat fusion can happen quickly, without warning, and can be catastrophic. Everyone working in the high angle environment must constantly be on the alert for heat fusion and take steps to avoid it.

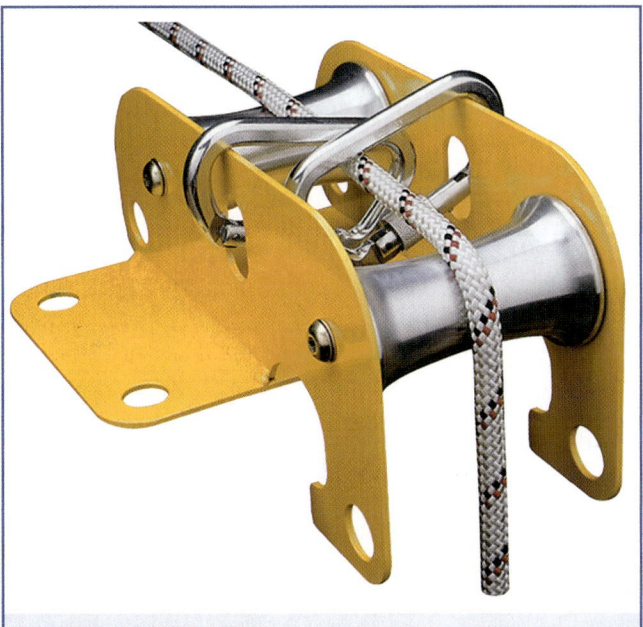

Figure 4-9 Roof roller.

Some ways to prevent heat fusion from rope cross include:

- Rigging ropes so that they do not make contact and create heat fusion
- Holding ropes away from each other with pulleys or edge rollers
- Padding a stationary rope where another rope runs across it
- Making sure never to place a moving rope and a stationary rope in the same edge protection device, such as edge rollers (separate rollers or devices are used)

Note that heat fusion occurs when one rope is stationary and the other moves across it *in one spot* so that heat builds up. If both ropes are moving constantly so that one spot is not subjected to heat buildup, destructive heat fusion is not likely to occur. For example, in a Münter hitch (see p. 102) the rope is running across itself, but all surfaces are moving. Therefore when correctly used, the Münter hitch is not likely to cause heat fusion.

> ### ▨ *Caution*
>
> Whenever you use more than one rope on edge protection devices, be on guard for heat fusion (see left column). Never use both a stationary and a moving rope on the same edge protection device; this can cause the moving rope to cut through the stationary rope—which can happen quickly and without warning.

Rope Damage through "Flash" Rappels

All rappel devices operate through friction of the rope across the device; this results in heat buildup that increases with the speed of the rappel. Fast rappels must be avoided because they can damage rope through heat buildup. Such "flash" rappels also indicate poor technique or lack of control (or both) on the part of the rappeller.

Rotation of Ropes Used in Rappel Training

In ropes in constant use for rappel training that are always anchored on the same end, the handling characteristics eventually change because of sheath bunching at the lower end. When a rope is used for many rappels, the ends of the rope should be alternated as anchors to help prevent a change in handling characteristics.

Strength Loss through Knots

All knots reduce the overall strength of a rope, but some knots cause a greater loss than others. The general rule is this: knots with tight bends, such as bowlines, cause greater strength loss than knots with more open bends, such as the figure 8 family of knots.

Effects of Bending a Rope

Whenever a rope is placed under load in a sharp bend, some strength is lost (Figure 4-10). The rope fibers on the outside of the bend receive a greater share of the load, and those on the inside of the bend receive very little of the load or none at all.

Common situations in which ropes undergo this kind of stress include ropes that have knots or kinks when they run over a sharp bend, such as in a carabiner or small-diameter pulley.

The 4:1 Rule

Rope users have long estimated rope strength loss with what is known as the 4:1 rule: that is, strength loss in rope does not become significant until the rope has a bend less than four times the diameter of the rope. The 4:1 rule applies more to natural fiber and to a few synthetics than it does to nylon rope, for which loss may not be significant until it drops below a 2:1 ratio.

Many users of nylon rope use the 4:1 ratio as a guideline, partly because it provides a safety margin. The 4:1 rule is used when choosing mechanical devices, such as pulleys, to ensure minimal strength loss when these devices are used.

Another reason to use the 4:1 ratio as a guide involves efficiency. Very small pulleys mean low efficiencies as the rope turns around them. Using the 4:1 guide means fewer problems with efficiency.

To choose a pulley using the 4:1 rule, compare the diameter of the rope with the diameter of the pulley sheave. If the diameter of the rope is ½ inch (12.5 mm), the diameter of the pulley sheave should be at least 2 inches (5 cm).

Inspecting a Rope

Rope inspection is an ongoing process that is performed before, during, and after rope use. Rope is inspected in two ways: by look and by feel. After each use, inspect your rope thoroughly by *looking and feeling* along every inch of its length.

When visually inspecting the rope, look for the following:

- *Discoloration:* This includes any obvious change from the rope's original color. Discoloration, particularly brown, gray, black, or green, could indicate chemical damage.

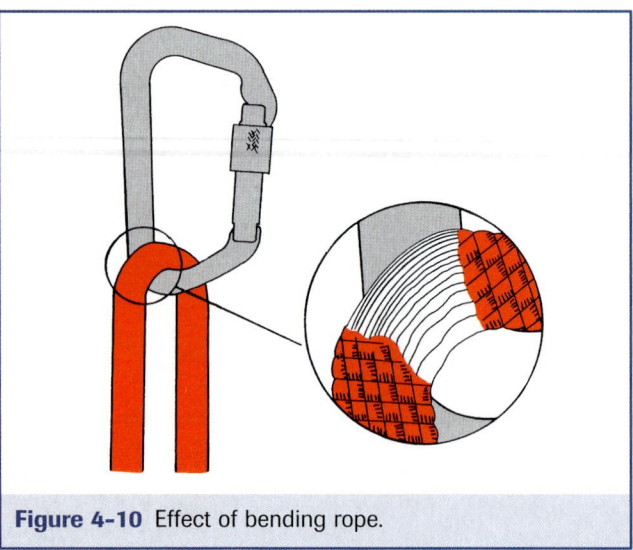

Figure 4-10 Effect of bending rope.

- *Glossy marks:* These could indicate heat fusion damage.
- *Exposed core fibers (white in most static rope):* Exposure of core fibers indicates damage to the sheath.
- *Lack of uniformity in diameter and size:* These characteristics may indicate broken sheath bundles.
- *Inconsistency in texture and stiffness (hold the rope in a loop and check to see whether it has a uniform radius around the entire bend):* An inconsistency in the bend may be the result of a soft spot that indicates core damage (Figure 4-11).

For the touch inspection, run the rope slowly through your bare hands and feel for the following:

- Stiffened fibers
- Obvious changes in diameter
- Soft or hollow spots
- Contamination with dirt and grit

If enough strands are broken, you will feel a localized change in the diameter of the rope, usually a depression or hourglass shape. Some types of damage result in *puffs*, or the protrusion of core fibers from the sheath. If the rope is contaminated with dirt, it should be washed.

Establishing Responsibility for Life Safety Ropes

As with other life safety devices, such as breathing apparatus, ropes used by a team must be assigned a *chain of responsibility*. Someone must be responsible for knowing where they are, how they have been used, who has used them, and what condition they are in. Someone must be responsible for inspecting them after each use, for keeping a log for each rope, and, when appropriate, for removing them from service.

Retiring a Rope

Unfortunately, the only tests currently available for reliably measuring rope strength destroy the rope. Therefore it is essential to be able to determine if a rope should be retired. That ability is the result of education in rope use and construction combined with experience and good judgment (Box 4-1).

Compared with many other types of equipment, rope is an inexpensive tool. The cost of replacing a rope is certainly less than that of a severe injury or loss of life.

Washing Rope

Ropes tend to become dirty with use. Using a rope when it is dirty shortens its life, therefore one element of a rope inspection program is deciding when the rope needs a bath. However, washing for the sake of washing is not a good idea. A rope should be washed only if it shows dirt. Overwashing can cause the rope to stiffen or shrink, or both.

Soiling obviously affects the appearance of the rope, but the most serious effect is hidden. Particles of grit and dirt eventually work their way into the core of the rope and damage the load-supporting yarn as it stretches and flexes. (Stepping on a rope forces more of this damaging material into the rope core.) Furthermore, dirt on the surface of a rope accelerates wear on hardware such as rappel devices, much as sandpaper would.

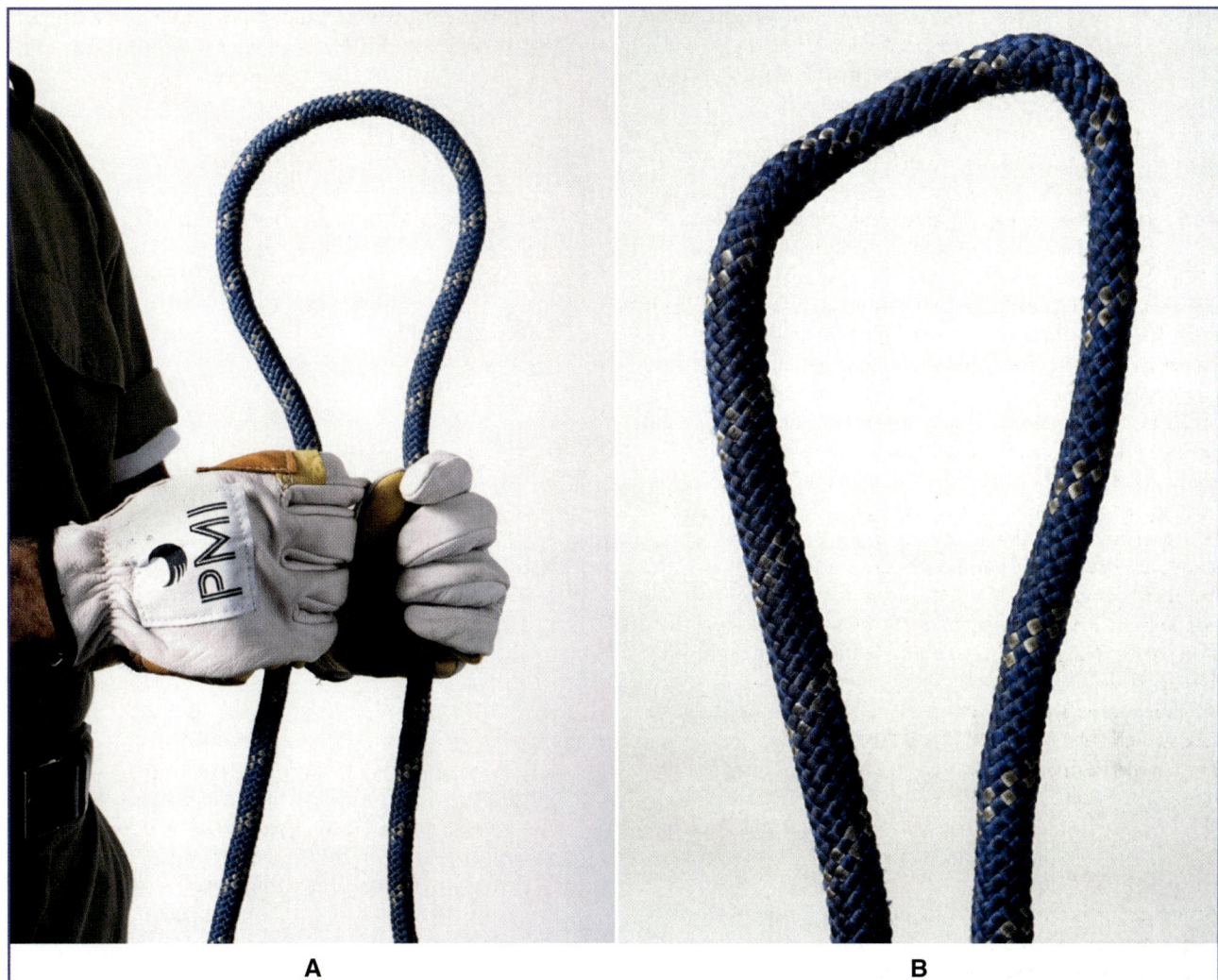

Figure 4-11 Inspection of normal and damaged rope. **A,** Hold the rope in a loop and see if it is a uniform radius around the entire bend. **B,** An inconsistency in the bend may signify a soft spot, indicating core damage.

Box 4-1 | Guidelines for Retiring a Rope

The following general guidelines can help the rope technician decide when to retire a rope.

Sheath Wear

More than half of the outer sheath yarns are broken.

Shock Loading

The rope has been subjected to severe shock loading.

Overloading

The rope has been subjected to an overload for which it was not designed. Examples of overloading for life support rope would include towing a vehicle or hauling heavy equipment or materials.

Chemical Contamination

Unless you know specifically that a chemical is harmless, consider it a contaminant.

Lack of Uniformity in Texture

The rope has soft, mushy places or hard spots.

Age

The rope is simply "worn out" from use.

Lack of Uniform Diameter

The rope necks down to a smaller diameter, resembling an hourglass shape.

Loss of Faith

The rope has been used by individuals you suspect may not have taken proper care of it.
The bottom line is this: When in doubt, throw it out.

Aluminum particles also are damaging to rope. The metal particles are forced into the rope as it runs through metal hardware such as rappel devices. Correct washing of your rope can also remove many of these damaging particles.

Rope Washing Devices

Commercial devices specifically designed for washing ropes are available. Some operate very much like the hose-washing devices used by fire departments. As water jets spray into the center of the device, the rope is pulled slowly through it. One model has a built-in brush to help scrub away the surface dirt (Figure 4-12). It adjusts to various rope diameters up to ¾ inch (19 mm).

Rope-washing devices are most effective against larger particles of dirt; however, they may not get the surface of the rope completely clean. This can be done only with further steps.

Cleaning Ropes with a Washing Machine

Washing machines can thoroughly and effectively clean rope. However, to prevent damage to the rope, the machines must be used carefully, and certain specific precautions must be taken. Washers also can damage the rope through tangling. The following guidelines can be used in washing ropes:

- Coil the rope to prevent tangling. A commonly used coil for washing is the chain coil (Figure 4-13).
- To prevent tangling or abrasion on the agitator, place the rope in a mesh bag. Such bags are used to wash delicate fabrics in washing machines; a scuba equipment mesh bag also can be used. Close the bag securely before placing the bagged rope in the machine.
- Use gentle soaps and follow package directions for their use. Soaps that indicate they are "safe for all synthetics" most likely are safe for rope cleaning. Still, to make sure, some rope owners use only the gentlest cleaners such as Woolite or Ivory Flakes laundry soaps (not dishwashing liquid detergent).
- Some ropes have had an additional chemical "dry" treatment to prevent the rope from picking up water. This is particularly useful in areas where wet ropes might freeze.

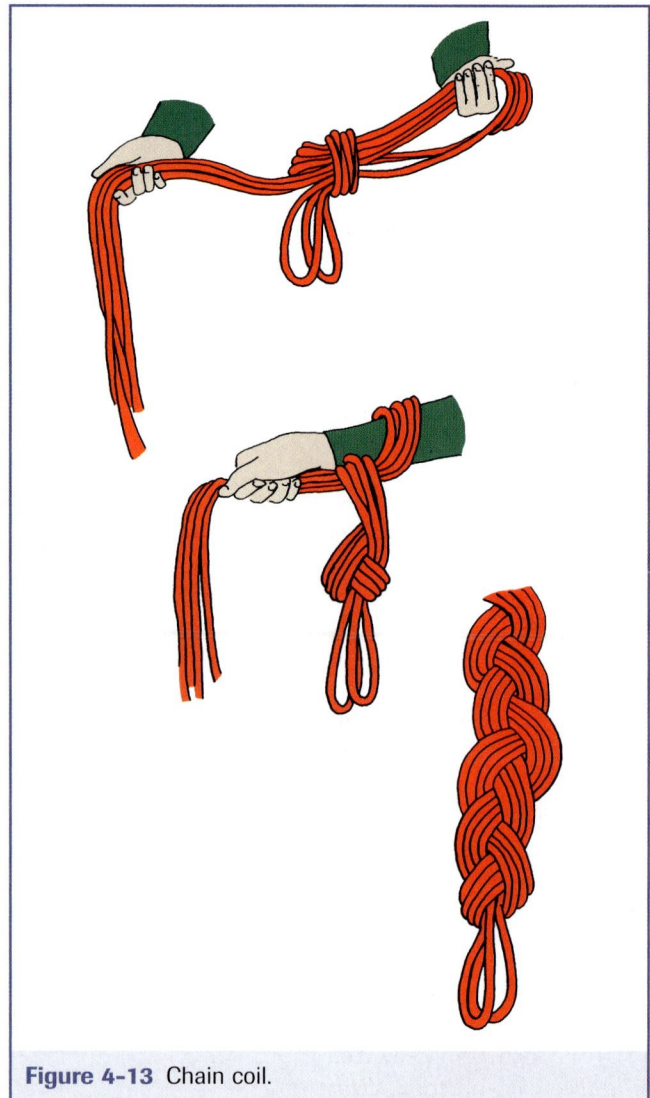

Figure 4-13 Chain coil.

Some of these treatments are easily removed with soapy water, and such ropes should be cleaned only with plain water.

- Do not use bleaches or bleach substitutes.
- Use the "cold water" setting.
- Rinse thoroughly to remove all traces of soap.
- Carefully dry the rope without heat. Hang the rope loosely out of direct sunlight and allow it to air dry.

Fabric Softeners

Some people use fabric softeners to give the rope sheath a soft feel. Ropes rinsed with a fabric softener solution that is mixed according to the fabric softener manufacturer's directions actually should perform better than ropes washed only with soap and water. Fabric softeners can make it easier to tie knots by delaying the rope stiffness that comes with age. The lubricants in fabric softeners can help replace the lubricants originally furnished on the yarns by the manufacturer, which are removed by repeated washing of the rope. Replacing the lubricants helps

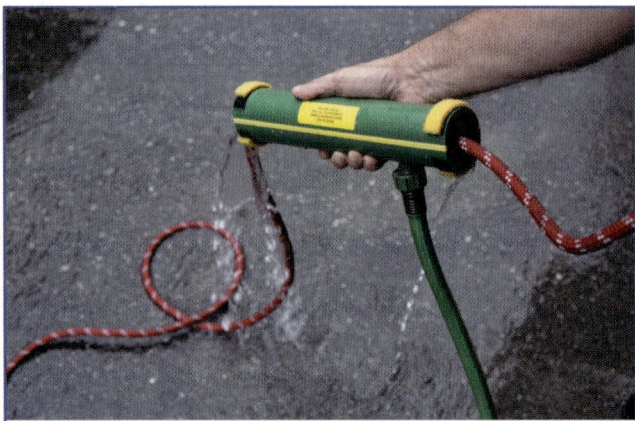

Figure 4-12 Rope washer.

the yarns load more evenly, which might raise the tensile strength slightly in older, well-washed ropes.

Special Cleaning Problems

Despite careful handling, ropes may become spotted with oil, grease, or mildew. There is no indication that any of these substances alone destroys rope fiber. However, they are unsightly and may stain clothing or high angle gear. Petroleum substances may cause other contaminants to stick to the rope.

These substances often can be removed by soaking the rope in cool, soapy water and scrubbing the affected areas with a fingernail brush. Do not use strong, solvent-based cleaners. Many solvents that loosen grease and grime also dissolve nylon. Contact the rope's manufacturer for specific types of cleaning problems.

Dressing Rope Ends

Cut rope ends should always be carefully dressed. Frayed ends have a sloppy, unprofessional appearance, become snagged, and eventually grow in size. This is particularly true with laid rope.

The most effective method of cutting synthetic fiber rope is to use an electric hot cutter (Figure 4-14). Before the rope is cut, the spot where it is to be severed should be firmly taped.

If you do not have a hot cutter, the following steps should be taken:

1. Firmly tape the spot to be cut to prevent fraying.
2. Cut down through the center of the tape.

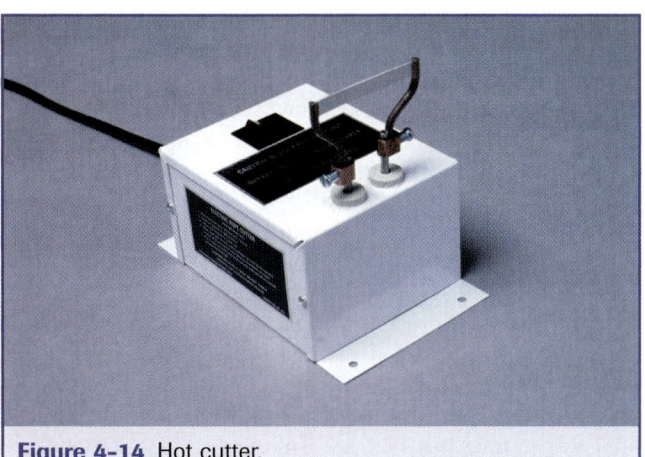

Figure 4-14 Hot cutter.

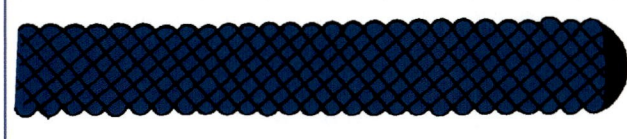

Figure 4-15 Shape of melted rope end.

3. Immediately fuse the cut ends with heat, such as with a lighter or other small flame. Taper the shape of the melt slightly (Figure 4-15). It should not be the shape of a mushroom, because the rope end could get snagged when pulled through hardware or rock.

Care of Webbing

In general, webbing should receive the same care as rope: (1) protect it from abrasion and damaging substances and (2) inspect it after each use.

Note that webbing is more susceptible than rope to damage from shock loading. As with rope, webbing should be protected from friction heat damage.

Hints for Rope Handlers
Preventing Tangles

Rope does not usually come out of a coil without tangling. To ensure that the line runs smoothly in the operation, it should first be *stacked*. This simply means taking the rope off the coil and laying it on the ground on top of itself with the end to be used first on the top (Figure 4-16). The stack should be completed out of the way of the operation but located so that the rope runs off to where it is needed without entangling debris, other rope, or people. Rope stacked in this manner usually slides off the pile smoothly. However, it is a good idea to assign a rope handler to feed the rope to the person using it to ensure that no tangles or kinks develop.

Bagged rope is less likely to tangle. However, friction devices, such as figure 8 descenders, twist the rope, creating tangles between the 8 and the bag. This twisting increases as more rope is fed through the descender. Therefore, when using devices that twist the rope, such as figure 8 descenders, pull the rope out of the bag and stack it on the ground. Some friction devices, such as the brake bar rack, twist the rope very little, therefore the rope usually can be left in the bag when racks are used.

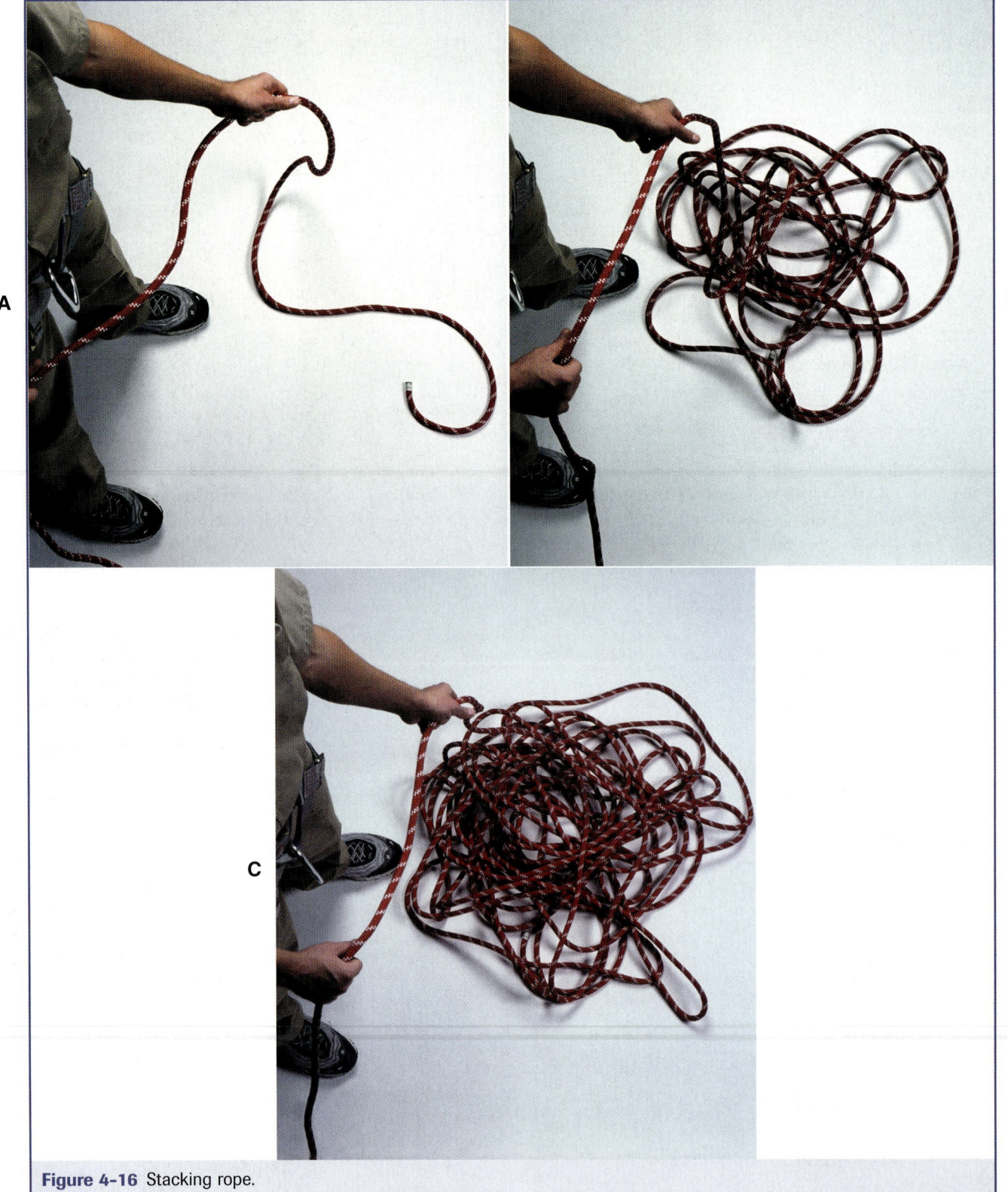

Figure 4-16 Stacking rope.

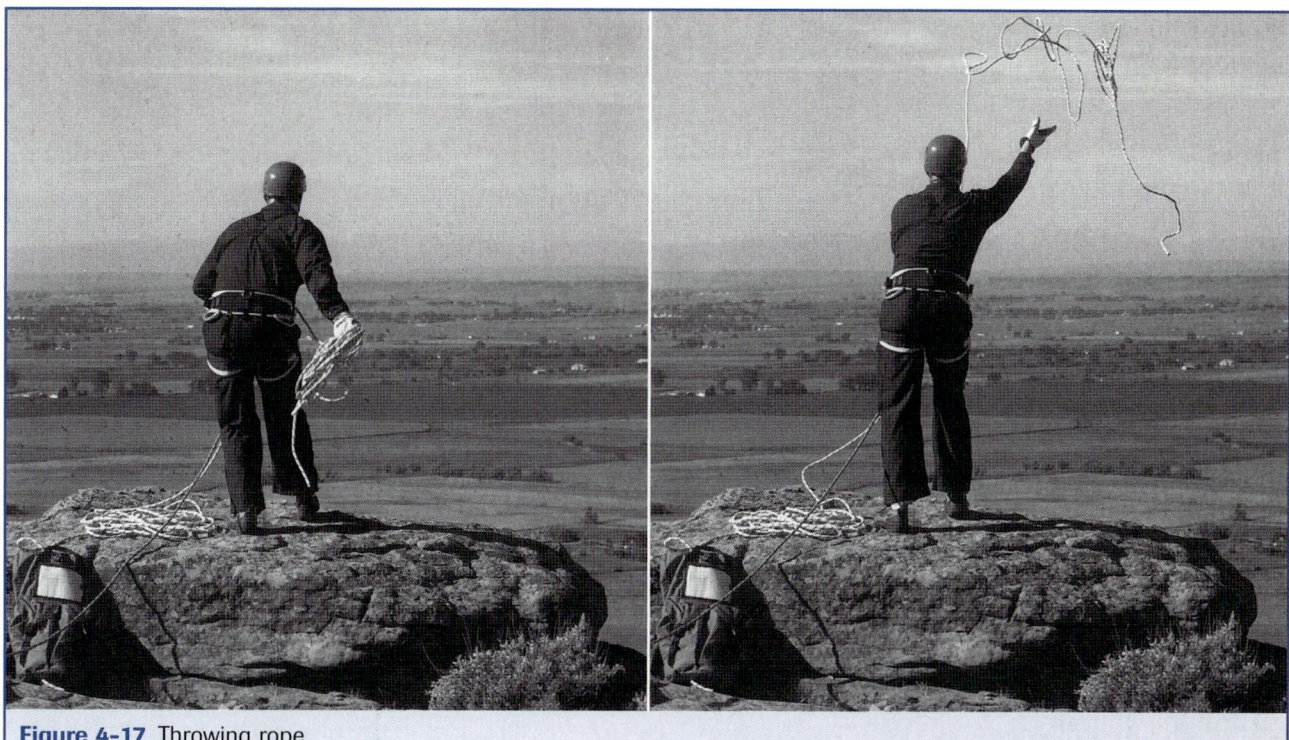

Figure 4-17 Throwing rope.

Throwing and Dropping Rope

In many situations, it is not easy to get rope from the top of a drop to the bottom. As mentioned previously, large bags of rope should not be dropped because of the potential for damage to the rope. In many cases the face of the drop is not completely vertical, but broken. Also, you may not have the rope in a bag but rather in a coil.

Most coils do not automatically feed out when the rope is dropped over the edge. To get a rope over the edge without tangles, proceed as follows:

1. Stack the rope as described earlier. Be sure the top end (at the bottom of the stack) is secured so that it does not slip over the edge.
2. Tie a bulky knot, such as a figure 8, on a bight in the bottom end of the rope; this helps prevent rappelling off the end. This is a particular concern in the dark or when you cannot see the end of the rope.

3. At the bottom end of the rope (the top of the stack), take several loose coils in your throwing hand (Figure 4-17).
4. Add three or four loose coils in the opposite hand. The remainder of the rope should be coming off the top of the stack.
5. Loudly shout "Rope!" so that anyone below is warned of falling rope.
6. With a side arm motion, pitch the loose coils in your throwing hand out horizontally. Note that if the wind is blowing, it may blow the rope off target or back up the cliff. You may have to throw the rope in a downward motion.
7. Allow the momentum of the falling rope to take the coils from your other hand. The rope should now pay out as it is pulled down by its own weight. Be sure to control the rope's speed through your *gloved* hand or, on very long drops, through a descender or belay device.

Evaluation Exercises

Cognitive and Affective Exercises

1. Which of the following are conditions in which rope should not be stored:

   A. Near vehicle batteries
   B. In direct sunlight
   C. In contact with a concrete floor
   D. All of the above

2. The advantages of bagging rope rather than coiling it include all of the following except:

   A. Bagging can be accomplished quicker than coiling.
   B. Bagged rope is more convenient to carry.
   C. Bagged rope is easier to deploy.
   D. Bagging protects the rope from heat damage.

3. An 11 mm static rope can be damaged by any of the following except:

   A. Using it to lower a 600-pound (270 kg) rescue load
   B. Pulling all of the stretch out of the rope during highline operations
   C. Lifting heavy objects
   D. Towing a vehicle

4. Techniques for reducing rope damage from abrasion include:

   A. Using canvas pads
   B. Using a fire hose
   C. Using edge rollers
   D. All of the above

5. A trainee is rappelling down the group's rope but is going very fast. You explain to the trainee that this practice must be discontinued because of the risk of:

   A. Heat fission
   B. Heat fusion
   C. Kinking
   D. Piling

6. All the following are examples of dangerous heat fusion situations except:

   A. A rappeller moving very fast with the rope against the seat harness webbing
   B. A loaded rope running over the anchor rope
   C. A belay using a Münter hitch
   D. Two ropes running under tension, with one stationary and the other running over it

7. All the following are ways to prevent heat fusion except:

   A. Holding a rope away from another rope, using webbing to pull the moving rope
   B. Rigging ropes so that they do not make contact
   C. Holding ropes away from one another with pulleys or edge rollers
   D. Padding stationary ropes at points where another runs over it

8. Using the 4:1 rule, what is the smallest bend that can occur in a ½-inch (12.5 mm) rope before it begins to reduce the strength of the rope:

   A. 2 inches (50.8 mm)
   B. 1.5 inches (38.1 mm)
   C. 1 inch (25.4 mm)
   D. 0.5 inch (12.5 mm)

9. Which of the following are guidelines for determining when a rope should be retired:

   A. Chemical contamination
   B. Overloading
   C. Sheath wear
   D. All of the above

10. Precautions that should be taken when cleaning a rope in a washing machine include all the following except:

    A. Using a front-loading machine
    B. Using any manufactured soap
    C. Chain coiling the rope
    D. Using cool water

Psychomotor Exercises

11. Using a 10.5 or 10.6 mm × 50 m dynamic climbing rope, coil the rope in each of the following methods:

    A. Mountaineer coil
    B. Caver's coil
    C. Butterfly coil

12. Place a 10-foot (3 m) piece of rope over a sturdy table edge and hold moderate pressure on both ends. Using various edge protection devices, place the devices under the rope to protect it and practice securing them in place to compensate for rope movement, both vertical and horizontal.

13. Acquire four 10-foot (3 m) sections of 11 mm and ½-inch rope; two sections with various damage and two new sections. Use these to allow all group members to practice rope inspection.

14. Using a 330-foot (100 m) static rope, practice stacking or flaking the rope out to prevent tangling.

15. Using a 330-foot (100 m) static rope, practice dropping and throwing the rope down a face. Make sure that all personnel are secured to the top with anchor and harness attachments.

5
Basic High Angle Hardware

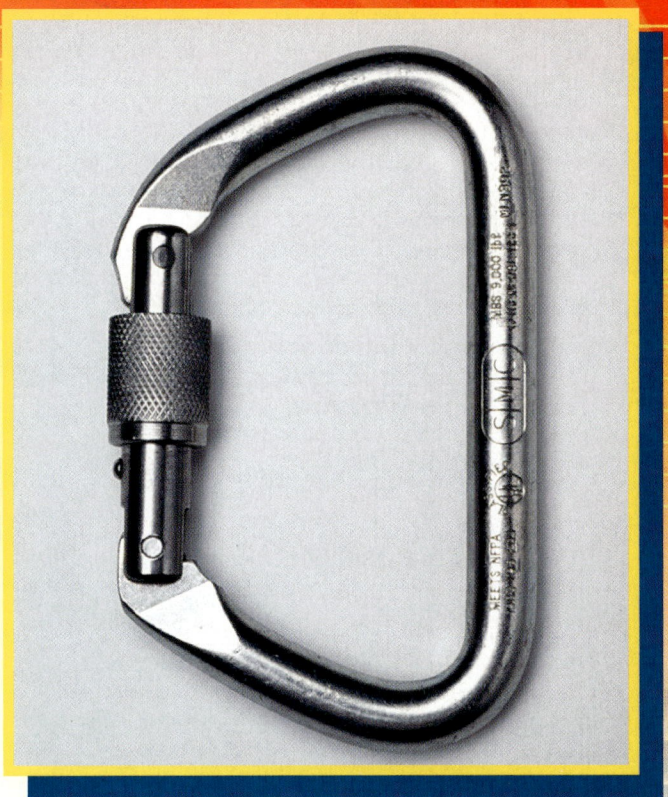

The material in this chapter conforms to guidelines published by the National Fire Protection Association (NFPA), specifically standard 1983-01, *Standard for Life Safety Rope and System Components* (2001). NFPA standards are revised regularly, and readers are advised to review the latest version of this standard.

Objectives

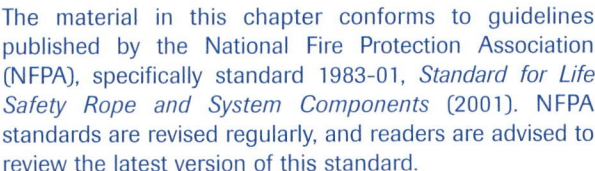

On completion of this chapter, you should be able to:

1. Describe how a carabiner's design can influence its strength.
2. Given a diagram, identify the parts of a carabiner.
3. Given a scenario, identify the appropriate carabiner to use.
4. Given a scenario, identify the appropriate descender device to use.
5. Identify the different types of ascenders and the important considerations in their selection.
6. Describe a scenario using ascenders that may result in a catastrophic failure.
7. Describe the purpose and situations in which the following rock protection would be used:
   - Natural anchors
   - Stoppers
   - Active and passive cams
   - Pitons
   - Bolts
8. Define belaying.
9. Describe the disadvantages of body belaying.
10. Identify the basic types of belay devices.
11. Describe the use of the Münter hitch (Italian hitch).
12. List the uses for pulleys in the high angle environment.
13. Given a scenario, select the best pulley to use.
14. List two main functions of edge rollers.

Key Terms

Ascenders Rope grab devices used by individuals to ascend a fixed rope or, with specific types of ascenders, to devise hauling systems. The two basic categories of ascenders are *light-use ascenders,* which normally are used for no more than one person's body weight, and *general-use ascenders,* which are used as personal ascenders and in hauling systems for progress capture devices and as rope grabs.

Bolts Metal devices used to create semipermanent anchors on a rock surface. A hole is drilled into the rock, and the device is set in the hole. Most bolts have a mechanical means of expanding to jam themselves in the drilled hole. A hanger usually is attached to the bolt so that the bolt can be used as an anchor point.

Brake Bar Rack A descending device (also known as a rappel rack) that consists of a U-shaped metal bar to which are attached several metal bars, which create friction on the rope. Some racks are limited to use in personal rappelling, whereas others may also be used to lower rescue loads.

Cams Devices used in climbing for protection or anchoring that lodge in a rock crack. *Active cams* with springs adjust to the width of the crack. *Passive cams* (nuts, stoppers, and chocks) wedge to fit the crack.

Descenders Metal devices that create friction on the rope to exert a braking action, resulting in a controlled rappel or lowering.

Figure 8 Descender A device used for rappelling and in some cases for lowering. The descender has the general shape of the numeral 8, with a large ring to create friction on the rope and a smaller ring to attach to a seat harness.

Locking Carabiner A carabiner with a locking sleeve on the gate side that secures the gate shut.

Manner of Function The method in which a particular piece of equipment was designed to be used.

Nonlocking Carabiner A carabiner without a means to secure the gate shut.

Piton A slender metal wedge, with an eye for attachment, that is driven into a rock crack for climbing protection or anchoring.

Prusik A soft rope grab that is constructed with rope of a smaller diameter than that of the rope it grabs.

Pulley A device with a free-turning, grooved metal wheel (sheave) used to reduce rope friction; it also has side plates to which a carabiner may be attached.

Rappel Rack See Brake Bar Rack.

Rope Grab A device that grips the rope. The two types are mechanical rope grabs, which usually are made of metal and which grip the rope with a camming action, and rope or webbing rope grabs, which use a hitch to grip the rope.

Hardware for the High Angle System

Rope, webbing, and other software are critical to the high angle system. However, another vital link in the system is the category of equipment known as *hardware.* Hardware includes a variety of gear, usually constructed of metal, that performs specific functions in the high angle environment.

Carabiners

Carabiners are metal connectors that link the elements of the high angle system. They are also sometimes called *biners, snap links,* or *krabs.* (In Europe, the United Kingdom, and some parts of Canada, carabiner is spelled *karabiner.*) The basic parts of a carabiner are the spine, hinge, gate, nose, and latch (Figure 5-1).

Depending on the manufacturer, carabiner latches are designed in a variety of ways. However, there are three basic types. One style of carabiner latch consists of a pin in the top of the gate that slips into a slot in the nose (Figure 5-2, *A*). When the carabiner is loaded, the pin is trapped in the slot. This adds overall strength to the loaded carabiner.

Another basic type of latch consists of a claw on the gate that slips into a slot on the nose (Figure 5-2, *B*). In some versions of this design, the locking mechanism does not completely engage, and the carabiner can fail at very low loads.

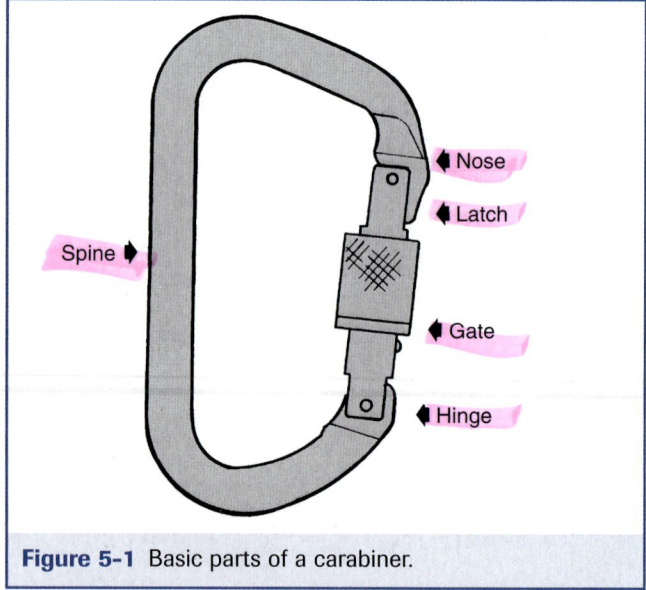

Figure 5-1 Basic parts of a carabiner.

The third type of latch consists of a keyhole-shaped slot in the top of the gate that slips into a matching key-shaped area of the nose (Figure 5-2, *C*). When loaded, the keylock latch engages firmly, which contributes to the carabiner's strength. One advantage of the keylock carabiner over other carabiner designs

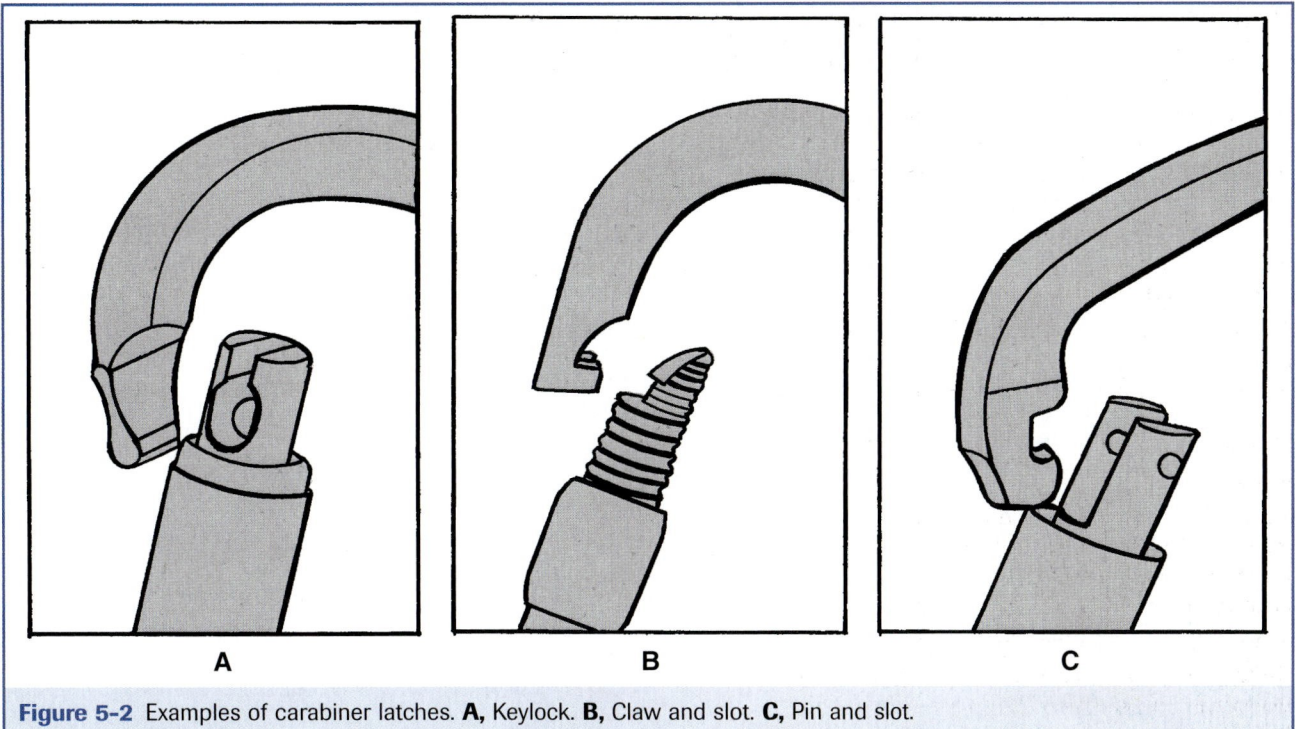

Figure 5-2 Examples of carabiner latches. **A,** Keylock. **B,** Claw and slot. **C,** Pin and slot.

is that the notch does not snag as easily on soft material, such as rope and webbing.

Basic Carabiner Shapes

Carabiners are manufactured in a wide variety of shapes and usually are designed for specific uses. They originally were designed as a simple oval shape (Figure 5-3, *A*). When an oval carabiner is placed under load, the stress is the same on both sides, equally on the spine and the gate. The problem is that in any carabiner, the weakest side is the one with the gate.

The design that takes greatest advantage of the strength of the spine is the D-shaped carabiner (Figure 5-3, *B*). Note that the spine side of the carabiner is longer than the gate side, with the top and bottom of the carabiner flaring toward the spine. The purpose of this design is that when under load, materials such as a rope clipped into the carabiner will slip into position on the

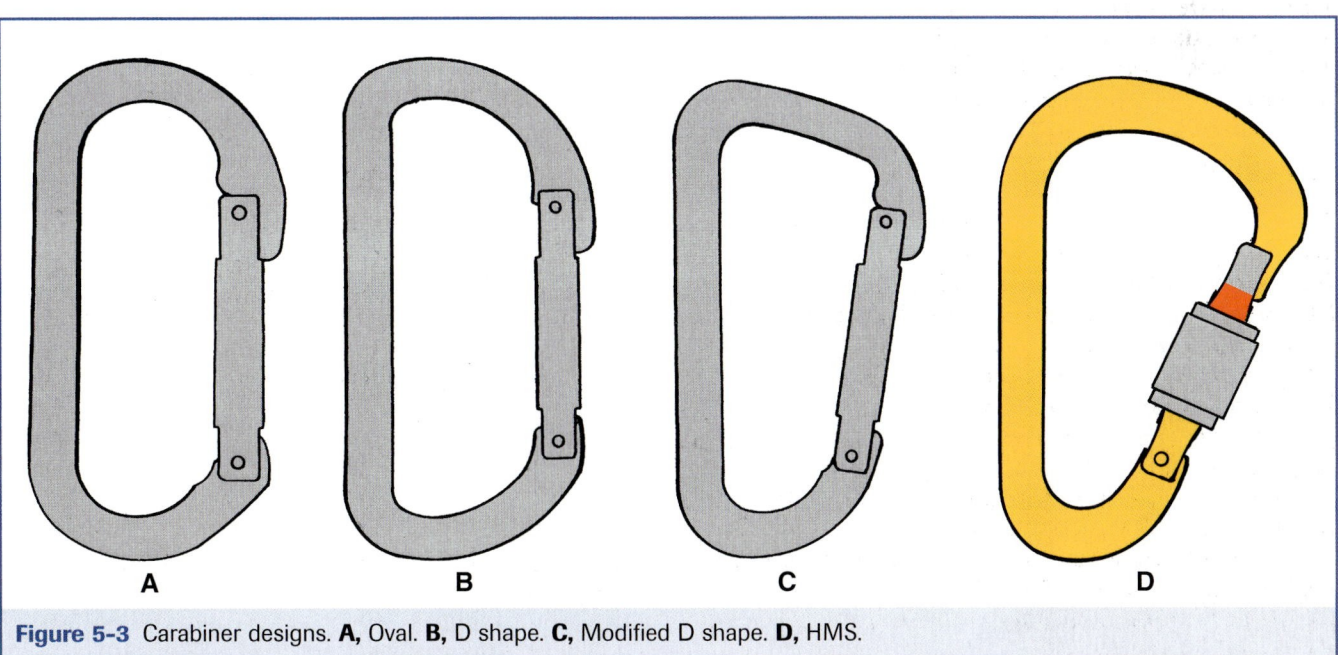

Figure 5-3 Carabiner designs. **A,** Oval. **B,** D shape. **C,** Modified D shape. **D,** HMS.

spine side. The result is greater stress on the stronger side of the carabiner.

Since the development of the D carabiner, other designs have been produced, such as the modified D shape (Figure 5-3, *C*). The HMS (an acronym for the German word *Halbmastwurfsicherung*) is a pear-shaped carabiner designed for use with the Münter hitch (Figure 5-3, *D*) (see Chapter 8).

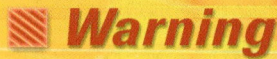

Warning

Strength ratings for carabiners usually represent the ideal situation; in a D carabiner, for example, when material pulls only on a small area of the carabiner next to the spine. If material pulls across a wide area of the carabiner top or bottom (such as wide webbing does), greater stress could be placed on the gate side of the carabiner. Consequently, the carabiner may fail at a load lower than its rated strength.

Carabiner Sizes and Strengths

Because climbers must carry their equipment with them, weight is a primary concern. Consequently, carabiners made primarily for rock climbers tend to be lightweight. Some are constructed of hollow aluminum and have low strength ratings.

For more demanding use and when more than one person's body weight may be involved, such as in a rescue, carabiners need higher strength ratings. Carabiners of this type are made of solid aluminum or steel.

Carabiners also differ in size. Again, because climbers place a premium on weight and bulk, their carabiners tend to be relatively small. In situations such as rescue activities, however, when large amounts of material must be connected inside the carabiner, carabiners need to be larger.

Carabiner Gate Opening

Along with differences in the size and weight of carabiners, there also are differences in the widths of gate openings. For some activities, the carabiner gate opening must be larger. In rescue activities, for example, a carabiner may have to be clipped over a litter rail, which can be as large as 1 inch (25.4 mm) in diameter.

Accidental Gate Opening

The main job of a carabiner is to maintain its link with the other elements of the high angle system. To do this, the carabiner gate must remain securely closed. If it does not remain closed, the connecting elements can come unlinked and the system will fail.

Carabiner gates can come open accidentally in several ways. Among the most common are:

- The carabiner is pressed against the edge of a wall or rock, forcing the gate open (Figure 5-4).
- A rope or piece of webbing is pulled across the carabiner gate, forcing it open (Figure 5-5).

If any chance exists that a carabiner gate may come open and only **nonlocking carabiners** are available, two carabiners should be set together reversed and opposed. That is, the pair of carabiners should be set with their gates reversed to one another and their tops and bottoms opposed to one another (Figure 5-6).

Locking Carabiners

Although two reversed and opposed carabiners usually are very secure, using a single **locking carabiner** (Figure 5-7) often is quicker and more convenient. Although specific designs vary with the manufacturer, locking carabiners usually fall into the following categories:

- A locking sleeve moves on screw threads over the nose of the carabiner to ensure closure.
- A sleeve turns around a pin on the gate to move up and close over the nose.
- A spring-loaded sleeve *(Autolock)* requires a quarter turn to unlock. (This is a very convenient carabiner; however, it

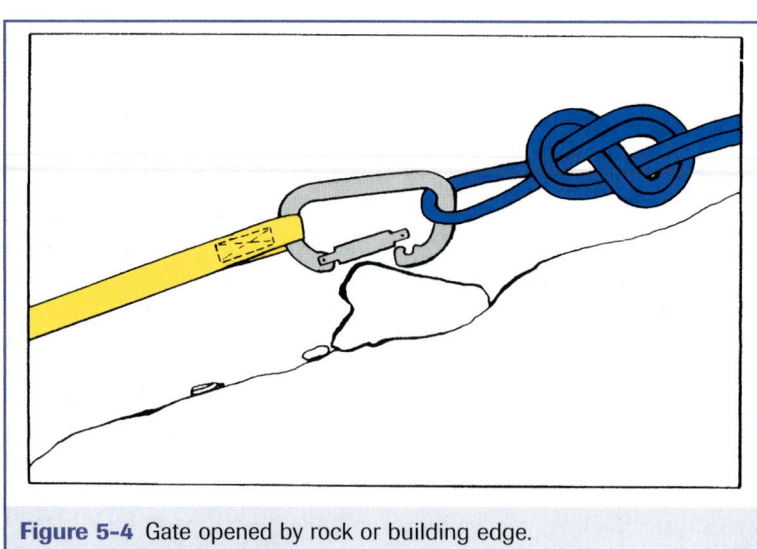

Figure 5-4 Gate opened by rock or building edge.

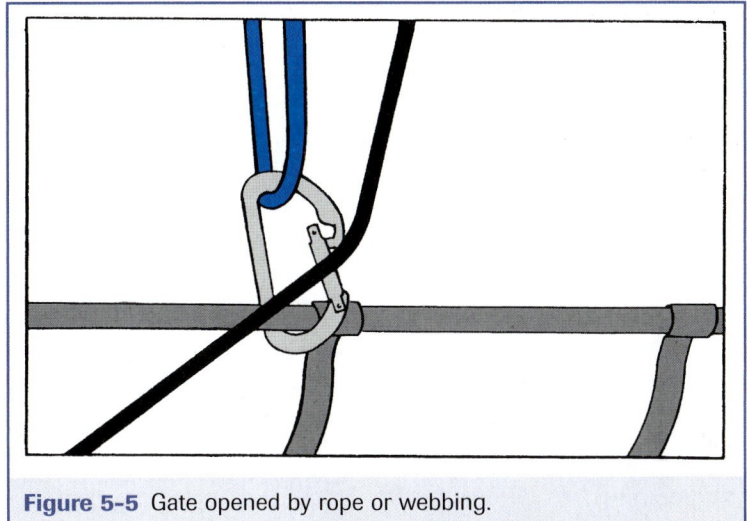

Figure 5-5 Gate opened by rope or webbing.

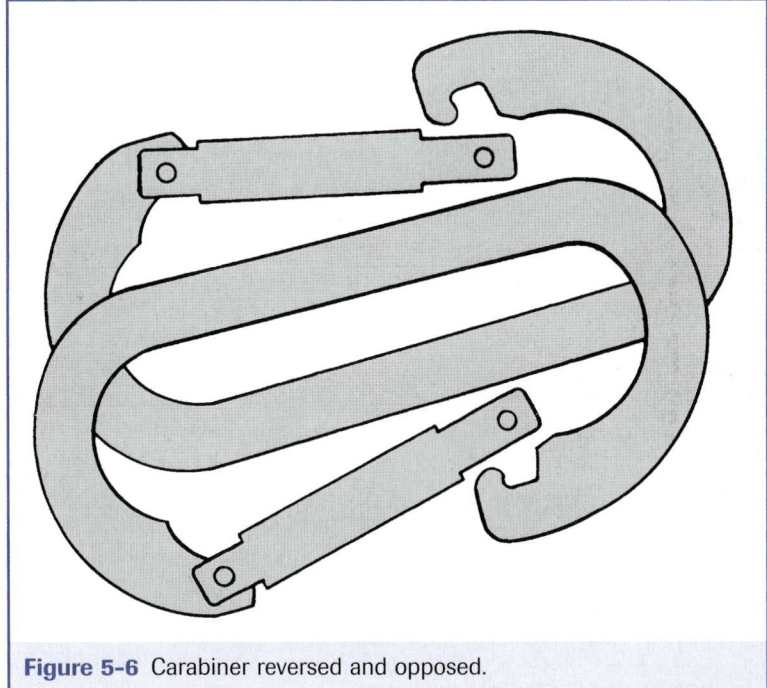

Figure 5-6 Carabiner reversed and opposed.

should be used with caution because some versions come open very easily. Some manufacturers incorporate various safety features into these carabiners, such as having to move the sleeve up or having to press a lock button before turning the sleeve.)

- A sleeve moves downward over the hinge to hold the gate locked. (These hinge-locking carabiners now are rarely seen.)

Carabiner Strength

Not all carabiners are as strong with the locking knob in the unlocked position as they are with the knob in the locked position. With some carabiner designs, the locking knob must hold the claw-type latch together in the locked position for the carabiner to have its full-rated strength. Tests have shown that some of these types of carabiners can fail at a much lower rating than their advertised strength if the gate is unlocked.

In addition to the long-axis locked strength of a carabiner, you should know its long-axis unlocked strength, long-axis gate open strength, and short-axis (gate cross-loaded) strength.

Whatever type of carabiner is used, those using it are responsible for constantly making certain that the carabiner gate stays closed.

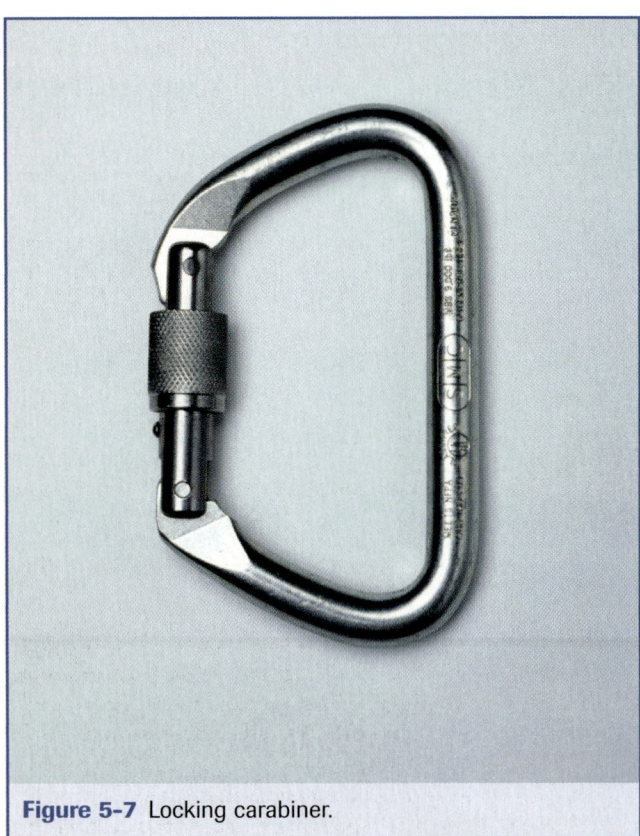

Figure 5-7 Locking carabiner.

⧄ Warning

Locking carabiners can and do come open after being locked. The following are common ways this can happen, along with possible countermeasures.
- ❏ The carabiner gate unlocks by rubbing against a wall or cliff face.
  Countermeasure: Turn carabiner away from the face.
- ❏ With some carabiner designs, vibration can cause the locking sleeve to unscrew.
  Countermeasure: Position the carabiner such that the gate is at the bottom and gravity keeps the locking screw closed. (This may not be an ultimate solution in high vibration environments, such as helicopters.)
- ❏ The gate is opened by rope or webbing running across it.
  Countermeasure: Move the carabiner out of contact with the line or place padding between it and the rope or webbing.

Additional Concerns for Locking Carabiners

If a carabiner chronically becomes unlocked without apparent cause, it should be retired from service. Older design carabiners could become jammed if the locking knob is overtightened, because the locking sleeve ramps up hard against the frame when tightened. If the sleeve is turned slightly while the carabiner is loaded, the spring in the frame jams the sleeve when weight is released. This makes it difficult or impossible to turn the sleeve without reweighting the carabiner. Newer designs leave a gap between the sleeve on the gate and the nose of the frame when the sleeve is screwed completely closed. To check to see if a carabiner is a newer design type, screw it all the way closed; a slight amount of play should remain in the gate.

If an older design carabiner locking mechanism becomes "frozen" through overtightening, the following procedures may release it:

1. If the carabiner is not already on a seat harness, attach it to one. Have the wearer move to a secure position, away from the edge of any drop.
2. Attach the carabiner by a sling to a convenient anchor.
3. Reload the carabiner by sitting down with it attached to the anchor point.
4. Often, the locking nut then can be loosened easily.
5. If it still cannot be loosened, tightly wrap a short piece of webbing around the locking nut to gain leverage.
6. If the previous step does not work, the only option may be careful use of a pair of pliers.

Aluminum versus Steel Carabiners

For the most part, carabiners are made of one of two metals, aluminum alloy or steel.

Aluminum Alloy

Advantages
- Significantly lighter weight
- Does not rust (but can undergo some forms of corrosion)
- Less expensive than steel

Disadvantages
- The locking mechanism on some aluminum designs eventually may wear out.
- Severe shock loading may cause permanent damage.
- Some aluminum carabiners are not as strong as comparable steel designs.

Steel

Advantages
- The locking mechanism on some steel carabiners may hold up better than the locking mechanism on aluminum carabiners.
- Steel carabiners may hold up better under severe shock loading.

Disadvantages
- Steel is heavier than aluminum (an important concern when more than a few carabiners must be carried for any distance).
- Steel carabiners are more expensive than aluminum types.
- Unless plated, steel will rust (consequently, most steel carabiners require more maintenance than the aluminum type).

Some steel carabiners are plated to resist rusting. If you plan to buy plated carabiners, make sure they have stainless steel hinge springs. Unless they are stainless steel, the springs could rust and break. Consequently, the gates would not swing closed automatically, making the carabiner dangerous to use.

If you work in high angle environments exposed to salt spray, such as near the ocean, choose carabiners constructed of all stainless steel (such as those manufactured in the United States by SMC).

Carabiner Standard Labeling

Currently two labeling systems are used for carabiners sold in the United States, and a third is being developed. The two systems now in use are the European Committee for Standardization and the Union of International Alpine Associations (CEN/UIAA) system and the National Fire Protection Association (NFPA) system.

- *CEN/UIAA system:* Carabiners that pass standards established by the CEN and UIAA are labeled with specific markings. These carabiners are stamped with major axis, minor axis, and gate opening strengths, which are shown in kilonewtons (kN) (Figure 5-8). (A newton is a unit of force measurement; 1 N equals about 0.225 lbf, and 1 kN, or 1,000 N, equals about 225 lbf.)

- *NFPA system:* Carabiners that meet the NFPA's **1983 Standard for Fire Service Life Safety Rope and System Components** (2001) also carry special markings (Figure 5-9). These carabiners are marked, "Meets NFPA 1983, 2001 ED." They carry the name or logo of the manufacturer, along with the label of the third party that certifies that the product meets the standard.

NFPA-certified carabiners also have either an *L* or a *G* stamped into the frame. The letter *L* indicates that the carabiner is for *light use* and designed for one-person loads, with a major axis minimum breaking strength, with gate closed, of 27 kN (6,069 lbf). The letter *G* indicates that the carabiner is for *general rescue use,* with a minimum major axis breaking strength, with gate closed, of 40 kN (8,992 lbf).

Other Labeling

Another carabiner standard has been established by the ASTM F32 (Search and Rescue) Committee. The ASTM F32 standard, which covers specifications for carabiners for search and rescue operations, includes test methods and marking requirements.

General Points on Buying Carabiners

Some carabiners carry no labeling and may not be tested to any standard. If the carabiner does not carry NFPA or CE/UIAA labeling, you may not be able to be sure about factors such as open gate strength, the strength of minor and major axes, and other qualities. (There is no ASTM mark for carabiners; many meet ASTM labeling requirements but are not marked as such.)

It is up to you, *the user,* to get the information from the carabiner's manufacturer.

Using Carabiners in Their Manner of Function

A carabiner's manner of function is to be loaded along its long axis, or lengthwise (Figure 5-10). As mentioned earlier, the weakest point of a carabiner is the gate. Consequently, side loading stresses the gate and puts an unnatural force on the carabiner, severely reducing its strength, which may cause it to fail.

Hard Linking

Another possible cause of carabiner failure is hard linking. Hard linking occurs when a carabiner is rigged so that it cannot rotate with the forces placed on it. This twisting force can cause the carabiner to break. Some examples of hard linking include the following:

- The carabiner is clipped into eyebolts on a wall.
- The carabiner is clipped into a second carabiner that cannot rotate.
- The carabiner is clipped directly into a vehicle tow hook.

To avoid hard linking, rig a soft link, such as a section of webbing or rope, between the hard links.

Carabiner Brake Bars

To avoid cross loading, you should avoid using carabiner brake bar systems (Figure 5-11). Brake bars are solid bars of metal with

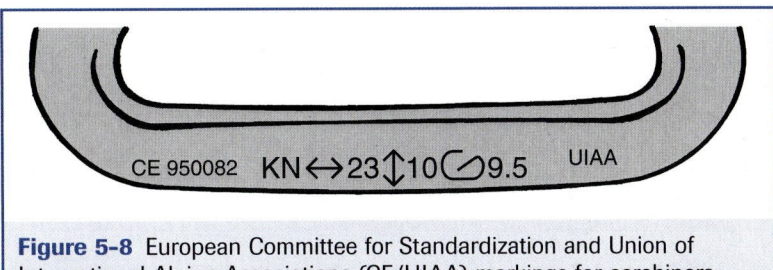

Figure 5-8 European Committee for Standardization and Union of International Alpine Associations (CE/UIAA) markings for carabiners.

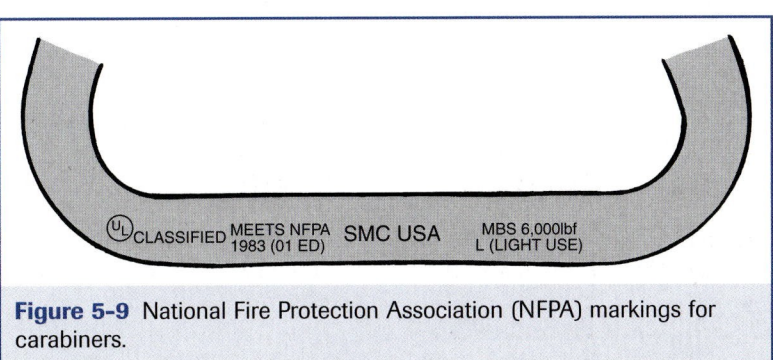

Figure 5-9 National Fire Protection Association (NFPA) markings for carabiners.

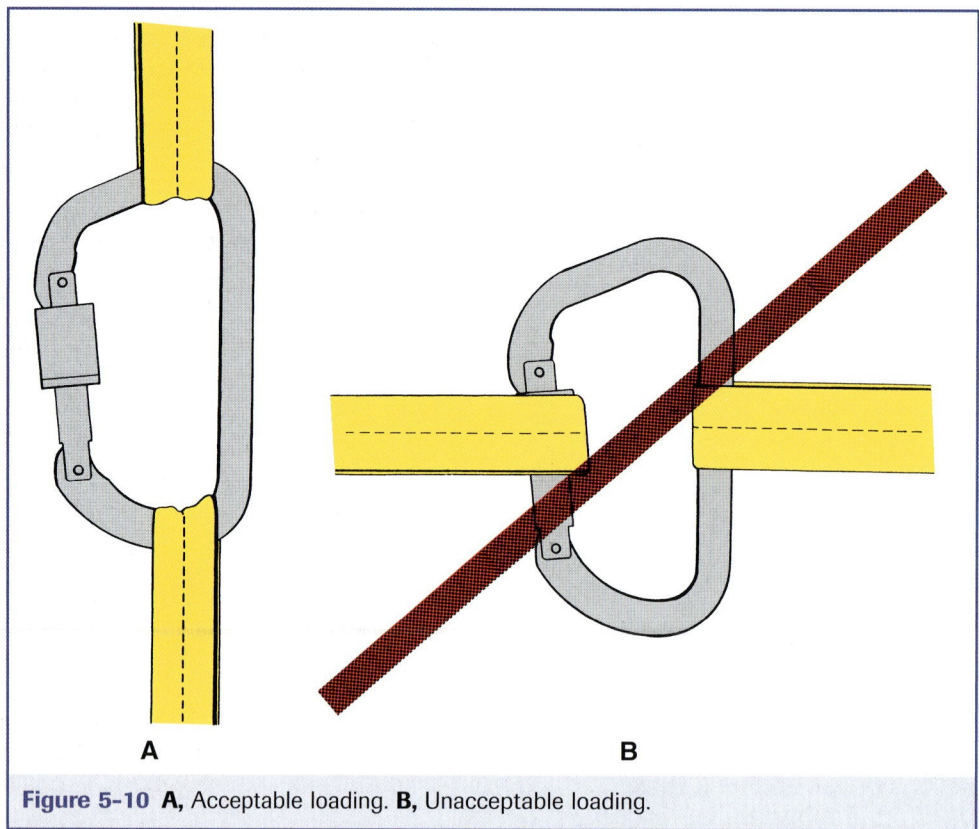

Figure 5-10 A, Acceptable loading. **B,** Unacceptable loading.

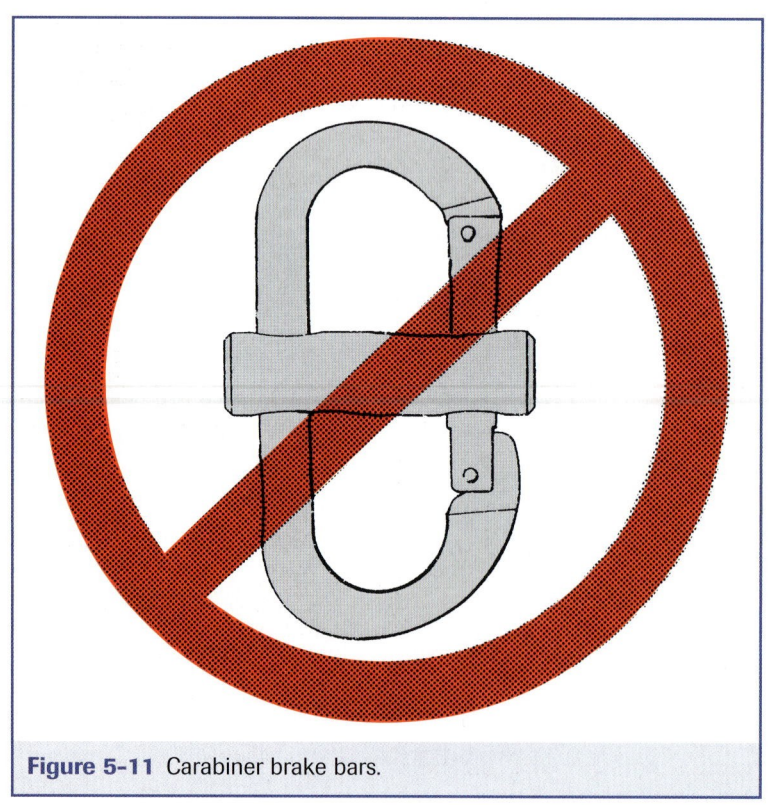

Figure 5-11 Carabiner brake bars.

a hole drilled in one end and a slot cut in the other end. They sometimes were fitted to oval carabiners to create rappel systems and occasionally lowering systems. Because they subject carabiners to forces for which they were not designed, carabiner brake bar systems should be avoided. Carabiner brake bar systems are not as common as they once were but are still used by some in the high angle environment. Brake bars are used on brake bar racks (see p. 57), for which they were designed, and they do not put unnatural stress on these racks.

⬚ *Warning*

All equipment used in the high angle environment is designed to be used in a specific *manner of function*. This is particularly true of carabiners. Any equipment, such as carabiners, that is not used in the designed manner of function may result in failure of the equipment and severe injury or death.

Three-Way Loading

As mentioned before, carabiners are designed for loading along the long axis. However, some seat harness designs have tie-in points consisting of right and left attachments. When a carabiner is clipped into these attachments and then loaded through a rope to a descender or other point, the carabiner becomes loaded from three directions. This can place potentially dangerous side-loading forces on the gate (Box 5-1).

Screw Links

Triangular or semicircular screw links increasingly are being used in place of carabiners when three-way loading is necessary. Instead of the swing-open gate found on carabiners, screw

Box 5-1	Possible Solutions to Three-Way Loading

Use a large, pear-shaped carabiner for the seat harness. Place the two harness attachment points in the large end of the carabiner and the third point, such as the descender, in the small end. You must still be careful that the carabiner does not rotate out of this configuration and turn sideways so that it loads the gate. Use a triangular or semicircular screw link in place of the seat harness carabiner. These devices are designed for loading from any direction.

links have a screw locking sleeve that closes the opening (Figure 5-12). When the screw link is screwed closed completely, it has the same strength regardless of the direction or directions of loading. Screw links have both advantages and disadvantages.

Advantages

- Strength regardless of direction of load
- Inexpensive

Disadvantage

- Must be screwed all the way closed for strength; because of the number of turns required to close the locking sleeve, they can take time to open and close

Care and Inspection of Carabiners

You must inspect each carabiner after use. Check the gate for signs of excessive side loading, such as rough pivoting action and bent parts. Pay particular attention to hinge pins and latches. Make sure that what may look like a scratch is not actually a crack. A deep-gouge scratch in a carabiner can reduce the cross-sectional area needed for strength. Scratches also can provide an entry point for corrosion. Corrosion is particularly critical in hinge pins, latches, springs, and locking knobs.

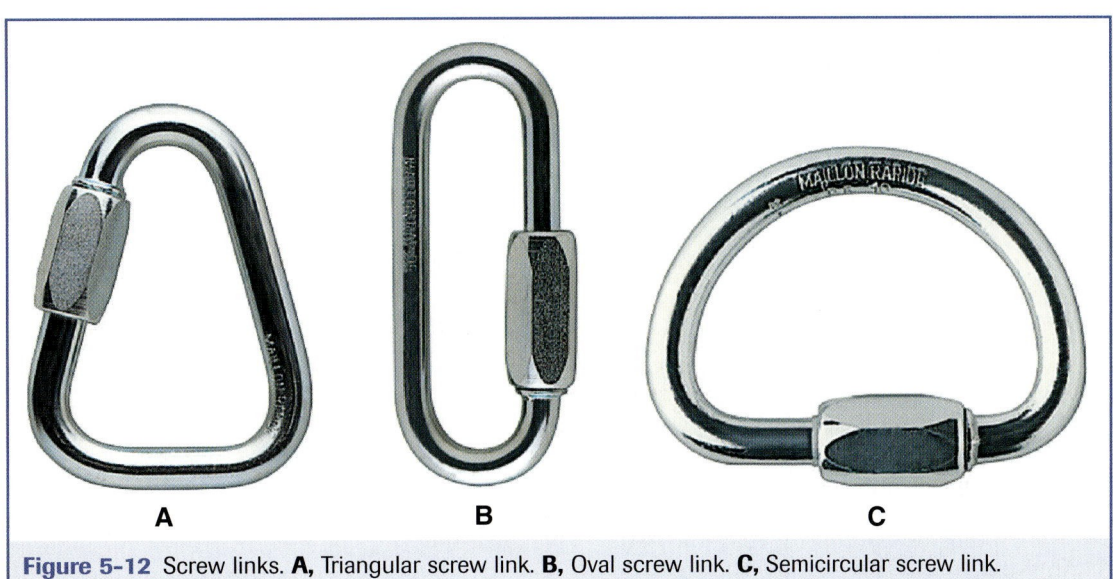

Figure 5-12 Screw links. **A,** Triangular screw link. **B,** Oval screw link. **C,** Semicircular screw link.

If your carabiners have gotten wet, dry them in a warm place. Use a preservative and lubricant such as LPS-1 or WD-40 on critical areas such as hinge pins, springs, latches, and locking knobs to help prevent corrosion. Wipe off excess lubricant before storing the carabiners. Box 5-2 presents solutions to various carabiner problems.

Descenders

A more complete discussion of the use of **descenders** can be found in Chapter 9. The following section is a brief review of the equipment used in rappelling and lowering.

Descenders, also generally called *rappel devices,* are braking devices. The user places one on the rope and attaches it to the seat harness to descend the rope at a controlled speed. Some of the same equipment can be used as braking devices to lower people or equipment under control; such lowering operations may be required during rescue activities. Although many different descenders are available (Box 5-3), they all work on the same principle: the descender creates friction with the rope running through it to produce a controlled descent. In most cases the user controls the speed of the descent by pulling on the section of rope below the descender.

Box 5-2	Troubleshooting Carabiner Problems

PROBLEM

Sticking gates or gates that close sluggishly.

SOLUTION

This problem may be caused by contamination with dirt or by corrosion. Pressurized air can be used to clean the mechanism. *Do not use oil or grease-based lubricants because they attract more dirt and grit.* Lubricate the gate mechanism with LPS-1 or WD-40.

PROBLEM

Carabiner gate has a broken spring.

SOLUTION

The carabiner should be discarded.

PROBLEM

The latch mechanism is broken.

SOLUTION

The carabiner should be discarded.

PROBLEM

The carabiner is bent (this usually is the result of overloading or of loading the carabiner without closing the gate completely).

SOLUTION

The carabiner should be discarded.

Box 5-3	Guidelines for Purchasing a Descender

1. Make sure the descender is sized properly for the diameter of rope you will be using.
2. The descender should create enough friction to give you absolute control over the descent without using brute strength. You should be able to go as slowly as you like and be able to stop at any time.
3. Keep in mind that in a real situation, hardware and equipment make you significantly heavier than your "street weight." You may also be wearing gloves.
4. Check to see that the descender has a lock-off function so that you can secure yourself and remain stopped on the rope with hands off the device.
5. Be sure the descender is strong enough to have an adequate safety factor (see p. 27 for information on how to calculate a safety factor).
6. The descender must be adequate for the length of descent needed.
7. The descender must be able to double as a lowering device if necessary.

Types of Descenders

Figure 8 Descender

A **figure 8 descender** (also simply called a *figure 8*) is a one-person rappel device roughly shaped like the numeral 8 but having rings of unequal size. The smaller ring (or lower one when in use) is clipped into a seat harness with a carabiner or screw link. The larger ring (or upper one when in use) is the one through which the rope passes to create friction (Figure 5-13). All figure 8s are made of metal. Most are made of machined or forged-aluminum alloy that is anodized for greater resistance to wear from the rope.

Some figure 8s are constructed of steel. Their primary advantage is resistance to wear. Steel figure 8s will outlast several aluminum versions, therefore they are particularly appropriate for heavy duty uses such as that seen in training departments. The disadvantages of steel models include weight (steel is heavier than aluminum), higher cost, and generation of less friction than aluminum figure 8s.

Figure 8s are made by a number of different manufacturers and come in a variety of shapes and sizes. They also are a commonly used rappel device and are relatively inexpensive compared with some more complicated pieces of equipment.

Disadvantages

- With most models, once on the rope, the rappeller cannot create a wide range of friction in the device.
- With all models, long rappels (more than approximately 150 feet) are more difficult to control.

Conventional Figure 8 Descender

Conventional figure 8 descenders are mostly found in small sizes and typically have a rounded or slightly squared large ring. They are used primarily in recreational activities such as climbing.

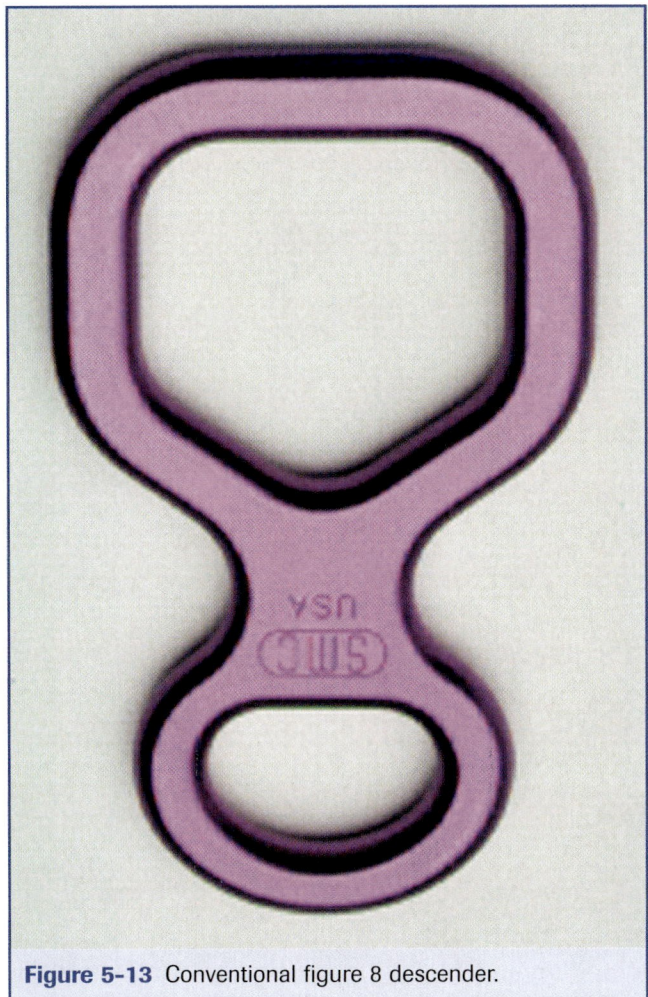

Figure 5-13 Conventional figure 8 descender.

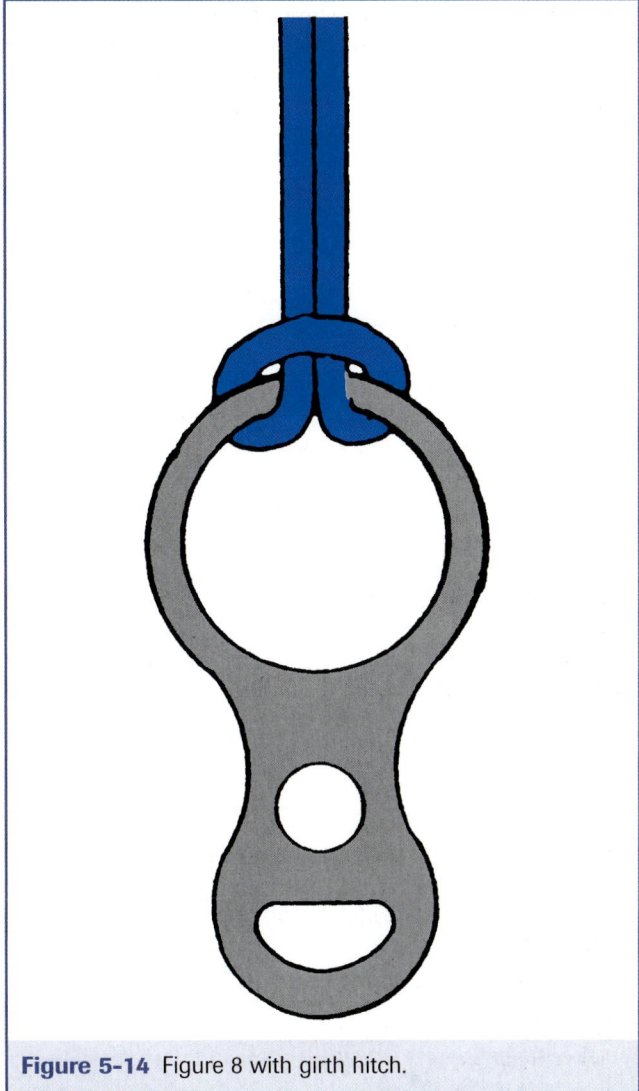

Figure 5-14 Figure 8 with girth hitch.

Advantage
- These descenders are fairly compact and lightweight; they generally are favored by climbers and others for whom size and weight are primary considerations.

Disadvantages
- Smaller models do not dissipate heat easily.
- Smaller models do not take larger diameter ropes.
- All models twist the rope.
- In conventional models, the rope can slip around the large ring to form a girth hitch (Figure 5-14); if this happens during a rappel, the user may be trapped on the rope. This can be a difficult situation from which to extricate oneself alone (see Chapter 9 for ways to prevent this problem and Chapter 10 for possible ways to extricate oneself).

Figure 8 Descender with Ears

The "ears" in a figure 8 descender with ears are projections fabricated into the large ring (Figure 5-15). These devices are sometimes called *rescue 8s*. They are specifically designed so that the rope contours better around the large ring and does not slip over it to form a girth hitch. This type of figure 8 is found in larger sizes.

Advantages
- The rope is less likely to slip around the large ring to form a girth hitch.
- Most models are available in larger sizes, which dissipate heat better.
- These descenders accept large ropes.
- They are easier to lock off.

Disadvantages
- Figure 8s with ears are bulkier and slightly heavier than the smaller conventional figure 8s.
- As with all figure 8s, the figure 8 with ears twists the rope.
- As with all figure 8s, the rappeller, once on rope, cannot create a wide range of friction.
- As with all figure 8s, the figure 8 with ears is more difficult to control on longer rappels.

Brake Bar Racks

A *brake bar rack* (also called a *Cole rack* or a *rappel rack*) is a descending device that offers a great amount of control and the

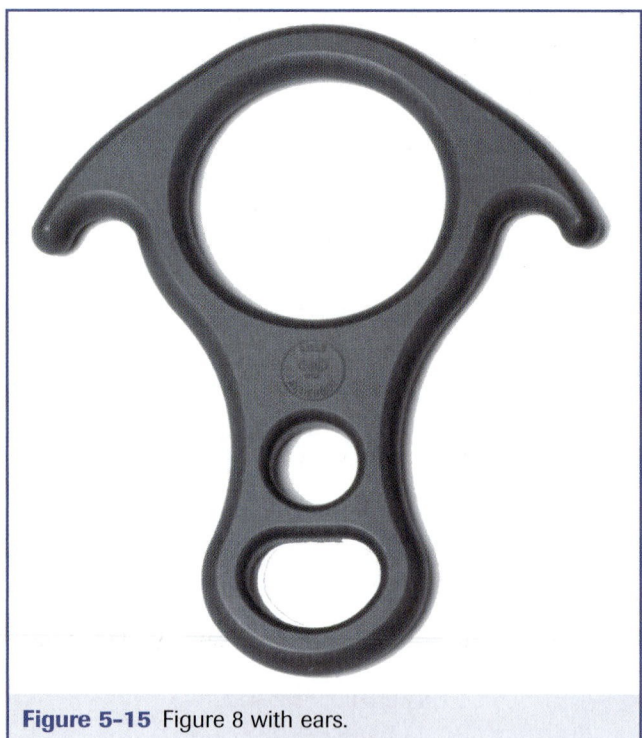

Figure 5-15 Figure 8 with ears.

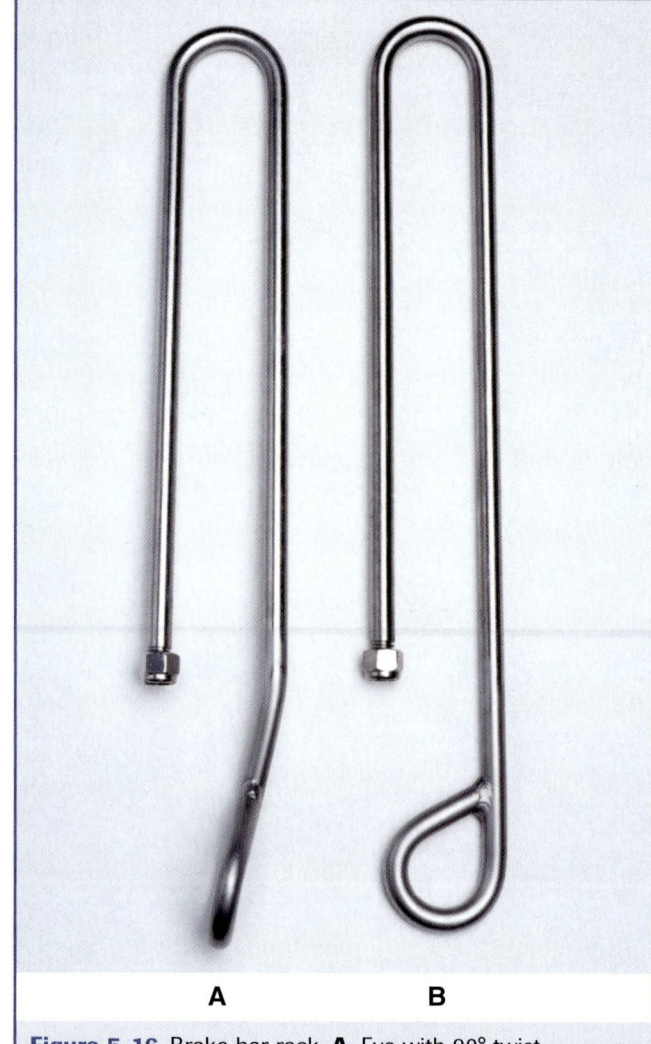

Figure 5-16 Brake bar rack. **A,** Eye with 90° twist. **B,** Straight eye.

ability to vary greatly the amount of friction (Figures 5-16 and 5-17). It also can be used for very long rappels.

The brake bar rack consists of two primary elements:

1. An inverted U–shaped frame, one leg of which is longer than the other. Most frames are made of stainless steel, but there are also titanium versions. The titanium models are very lightweight but more expensive. The end of the longer leg has an eye through which a carabiner can be clipped.

2. A series of bars with a hole drilled in one end so that the bars slide freely on the long side of the frame. On the opposite end the bars are notched so that the end of the bar can clip into the short side of the frame. The rope is woven through the bars. Under tension, the rope keeps the bars in place on the frame.

Friction for rappelling may be controlled by the control hand on the rope below the rack, by varying the bar spacing with the other hand, and by varying the number of bars engaged on the rope. (For more detailed information about use of the rack for rappelling, see Chapter 9.) Most brake bar racks are made of hollow steel bars, although aluminum bars are used in some older designs.

When a brake bar rack is used correctly, the bars are the only elements that wear out. They must be replaced from time to time. Depending on the bars' requirements for friction, they can be purchased in a variety of sizes. Larger bars tend to create greater friction than small-diameter bars.

In the most common configuration, the rack is arranged with a 1 inch (25.4 mm) in diameter grooved top bar to keep the rope in the middle of the bars as it runs through the device. The remainder of the rack usually is filled out with five aluminum bars, each 7/8 inch (22 mm) in diameter.

A device that is increasing in popularity is the *hyper-bar*. A hyper-bar is a top *tie-off bar* that is larger diameter and extends out to one side (or both sides in some designs) to make it easy to add friction or to tie off the rope (Figure 5-17).

Several short versions of the rack, with four or five bars, are available. These are designed to be compact for individuals who have limited pack space or who need to save weight. They are not recommended for rescue work because they provide less friction and have less versatility than the six-bar rack.

For rappelling, the brake bar rack works most efficiently with the open side of the rack toward the ground. Some seat harnesses have a horizontal D ring as a clip-in point; this positions the open side of the rack facing the rappeller's side. To compensate for this, some versions of the rack have a quarter turn in the eye so that the rack remains with the open side toward the ground (see Figure 5-16).

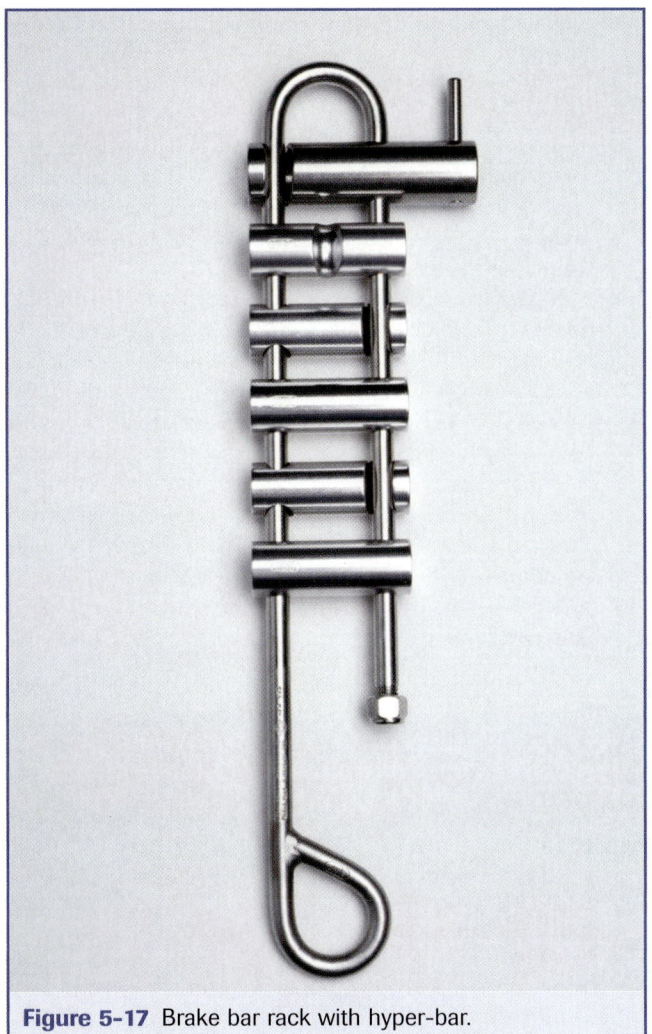

Figure 5-17 Brake bar rack with hyper-bar.

Box 5-4 | **Characteristics of the Standard Rack**

ADVANTAGES

- ❏ Allows friction to be varied greatly even after the rappel has begun
- ❏ Welded eye version is very strong
- ❏ Can be used as a lowering device
- ❏ Does not twist rope
- ❏ Can be easily attached to rope without detaching the rack from the seat harness
- ❏ Takes large-size ropes
- ❏ Can use two ropes at the same time

DISADVANTAGES

- ❏ Bulkier and heavier than some other rappel devices
- ❏ May take slightly longer to lace onto rope

Personal Versus Rescue Versions of the Rack

Rack frames are designed in different configurations to meet the specific needs of the user. In some personal versions of the rack, the eye at the end of the long side is formed by twisting the steel bar around itself. Because large loads could cause this type of eye to untwist, this style of rack should not be used for loads of more than one person. For larger loads, such as those encountered in rescue operations, a rack with a welded eye is used.

Other Types of Brake Bar Racks

In another version of the rack, the legs of the U are equal in length. When this type of rack is in use, the ends of the U point up and are secured with nuts, and the attachment to the seat harness is in the curve of the U. The most common version of this type of rack has three fixed and three slotted bars. The primary reason for this design is that the rack remains straight when loaded. The major disadvantage is that when loaded, the degree of friction cannot be varied by disengaging or engaging bars (Box 5-4).

Other Descenders

Hundreds of other types of descenders are available. Among them are the following:

- Stop (Petzl, France)
- I'D (Petzl)
- Friction Plate (Blitz)

As with all gear you use in the high angle environment, it is your responsibility to obtain specific information about the characteristics of each device and how to train in its use.

Emergency Descent

Some emergencies in the high angle environment may require an immediate descent, even when a person has no hardware specifically designed for rappelling. One improvisation that has commonly been used in the past is the *carabiner wrap,* which involves wrapping the rope several turns around the carabiner to create friction and then attaching the carabiner to the seat harness.

The carabiner wrap is not recommended as a rappelling technique. Many injuries and some deaths have occurred in rappelling attempts using the carabiner wrap. These failures usually resulted because the rope wraps slipped out of the carabiner gate.

Other methods of emergency descent are preferable to the carabiner wrap. Chapter 9 presents a review of emergency rappel techniques.

Rope Grabs

Rope grabs, which are devices that grip the rope, have a variety of uses in the high angle environment. In this book, the term **rope grab** refers to a device used for personal safety, for ascending the rope (**ascenders**), and for hauling systems. (In industry and construction, some types of rope grabs are also used for personal protection against falls.)

Many rope grabs are mechanical devices made of metal that use a camming action to grip the rope; these are sometimes called *hard cams.* Rope grabs can also be made of rope or webbing formed into a hitch that grips the rope; these are sometimes called *soft cams*. The most commonly used soft cam is the **Prusik,** but several other hitches can be used as rope grabs.

Light-Use Ascenders

Light-use ascenders (also called *personal ascent devices*) are rope grab devices used to travel up (ascend) a fixed rope. They all work on the same principle: if the ascender is correctly attached to the rope, its gripping action allows the climber to slide it freely in one direction (up). The ascender then locks in place when the climber correctly applies a downward force (e.g., body weight) to it.

For this system to work, at least two ascenders usually must be used. You attach the ascenders to yourself with rope or webbing sling. You then ascend the rope by raising one ascender while supported by the other ascender as it locks on the rope. By alternating this action, you are able to proceed up the rope.

This is the basic principle of ascending, although the technique has dozens of variations, many using three ascenders for added security (see Chapter 10 for specific details on ascending techniques).

Light-use ascenders are designed for ascending with only one person's body weight, not for hauling systems in which forces are multiplied. They work partly through a cam action, which pivots inside the ascender frame and also grips the rope with a toothed cam (Figure 5-18). Many light-use ascenders have a handle equipped with a safety catch, which releases the cam so that the ascender can be placed on a rope with only one hand.

Many light-use ascenders are used in pairs, usually with right- and left-handed models. For additional security, many people include a third ascender in the system. Most light-use ascenders cannot be used on rope larger than ½ inch (12.5 mm) in diameter.

The following are some of the current manufacturers and models of light-use ascenders:

- Clog (Wales): The frame is made from rolled aluminum.
- CMI (Franklin, West Virginia): Three models are available: (1) the Large Ultrascender; (2) the Small Ultrascender (a smaller, lighter version); and (3) the Expedition (which has an extra large handgrip).

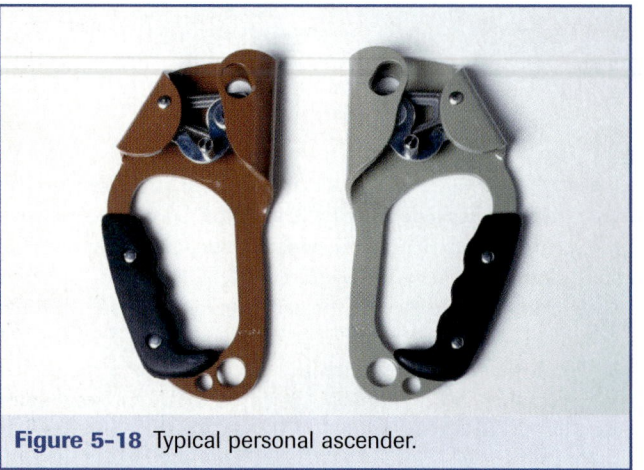

Figure 5-18 Typical personal ascender.

- Jumar (Switzerland): The frame is fabricated from cast aluminum.
- Petzl (France): All Petzl devices are fabricated from rolled aluminum, and three models are available: (1) the Ascension; (2) the Basic (a compact, handleless design that has a toothed cam and is available only in a right-handed model); and (3) the Croll (a toothed cam version that is designed to lie flat against the chest, attached between a seat harness and a chest harness).
- PMI (LaFayette, Georgia): Three models are available: (1) the CAT (a model with a handle); (2) the Chest CAT (a compact, handleless design that has a toothed cam and is available only in a right-handed model); and (3) the Short CAT (a toothed cam version that is designed to lie flat against the chest, attached between a seat harness and a chest harness).
- SRT (Australia): The frame is machined from extruded aluminum, and several models are available for different-size ropes (i.e., 8 to 11 mm and 8 to 16 mm).

Box 5-5 presents a list of questions you should ask when purchasing personal ascenders.

Box 5-5	**Questions to Ask When Purchasing Light-Use Ascenders**

- ❑ What size rope are they designed for?
- ❑ What is their strength rating and how is it determined?
- ❑ Can they be operated easily (placed on and taken off the rope) with one hand?
- ❑ Do they have a secure safety catch to prevent them from accidentally coming off the rope?
- ❑ Can they be used easily while wearing gloves?
- ❑ Are they comfortable in the hand when used as a rope grab device?

▨ *Warning*

Light-use ascenders may damage or cut through rope sheath with loads as low as 1,200 pounds (544 kg). Consequently, personal ascenders should never be loaded with more than the weight of one person and should never be shock loaded.

General-Use Ascenders

General-use ascenders (Figure 5-19) are rope grab devices designed for use with heavier loads than those used with light-use ascenders. General-use ascenders can be used as personal ascenders and also can serve in hauling systems as progress capture devices and rope grabs. Most general-use ascenders do not have handles. Initially you may find general-use ascenders a little more difficult to operate than other types of ascenders

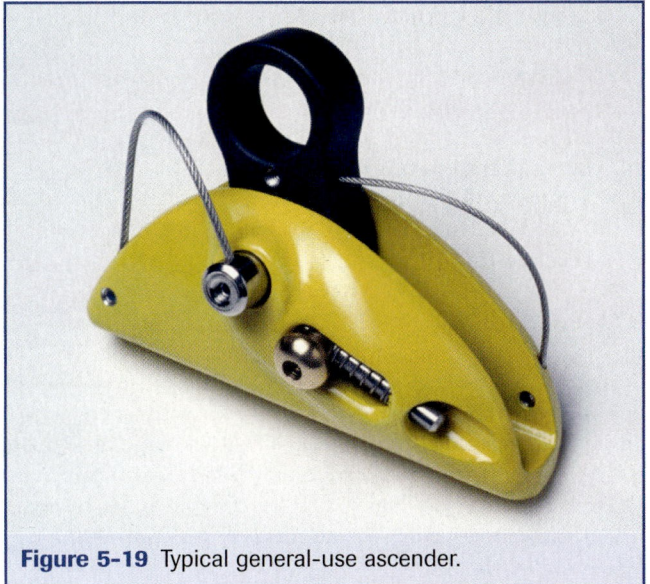

Figure 5-19 Typical general-use ascender.

because they must be taken apart to be placed on the rope. However, once they have been assembled on the rope, they tend to stay there.

On wet, muddy, or icy ropes, general-use ascenders tend to hold better than other types of ascenders. The teeth on the cams are designed to hold well on the rope while causing a minimum of damage to the rope sheath. However, under high loads or severe shock loading, any general-use ascender may damage the rope.

The three major manufacturers of general use ascenders are Gibbs (which has models available in aluminum and stainless steel in sizes to accept $\frac{1}{2}$-inch [12.5 mm] and $\frac{5}{8}$-inch [16 mm] rope); Petzl (Rescucender); and PMI (Progressor, which is available in two models; one has a removable cam for rescue work, and the other has a fixed cam for those who need an adjustable safety that can't come off the rope).

Characteristics of General-Use Ascenders

Advantages
- Hold better than other ascenders on wet, icy, or muddy ropes.
- Have great strength.
- Cam action does not tear rope sheaths as easily as some other types of ascenders.

Disadvantages
- Must be taken apart to be put on and taken off rope.
- Require two hands to put on and take off rope.

Rope Grab Devices for Belaying and Hauling

Light-use ascenders should not be used in hauling systems and other rescue rigging involving loads greater than one person's body weight. Most general-use ascenders should not be used as belay devices because they tend to damage the rope under high weight loading and shock loading. (See Chapters 12 and 16 for discussions of rope grab devices used for rescue.)

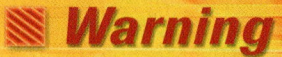

Warning

Any cam-type ascender can cut the rope or slip at much less than the rated strength of either the rope or the cam.

Hardware for Anchoring
Rock Anchors (Artificial Anchors)

Artificial anchors constitute a family of hardware used to create anchors where no natural anchors (e.g., trees or rocks) are available around which rope or webbing can be placed.

Artificial anchors go directly into the rock (and in some cases into ice or snow). Most often, they are placed in cracks or gaps in the rock. However, in some cases they are physically driven into the rock to act as permanent emplacements.

The ability to place reliable artificial anchors is an art involving a number of subtleties, such as the character of the rock itself, the nature of the cracks or gaps in the rock, and the direction of loading on the anchor. This kind of knowledge depends very much on hands-on instruction and experience. These finer points of the placement of artificial anchors are beyond the scope of this book. Individuals who want to develop these skills should consult qualified instruction manuals and literature (some of which are listed in Appendix A).

Pitons

Pitons have been used in mountaineering for many years as a means of anchoring. A ***piton*** is a thin, metal spike with an eye to which a carabiner or webbing can be attached. Pitons are driven into a rock crack with a hammer. Because pitons tend to damage some types of rock and because the use of passive and active cams and chocks has grown, pitons are not used as often as in the past.

Caution

It is very difficult to drive pitons without permanently defacing the rock. Consequently, in some areas, such as state and federally managed parks, the use of pitons is prohibited. Also, many in the rock-climbing community consider the use of pitons to be bad etiquette.

Bolts

Bolts are a means of establishing a permanent anchor in a wall, usually when no other anchors are feasible. Although different designs of bolts are available, most work on the same principle (Figure 5-20):

1. A hole is made in the rock with either a separate drill or, in some designs (called *self-driving*), with a drill that uses part of the bolt itself as the bit.

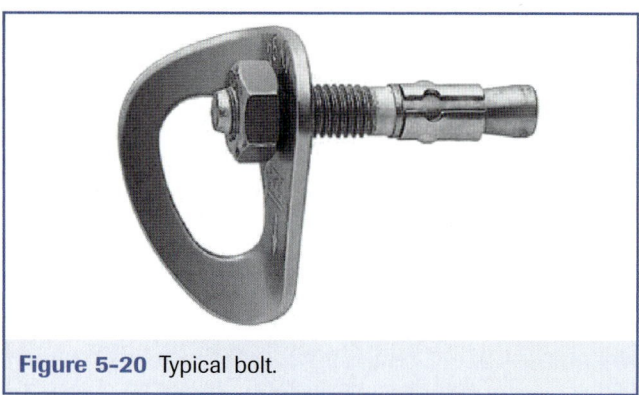

Figure 5-20 Typical bolt.

2. The bolt is set in the hole by causing an element in it to expand, either through a screwlike action or by hammering on the bolt. Some bolting systems use glue for greater security.

3. A *hanger* is attached to the bolt, through which a carabiner can be attached.

For strength and long life, all bolts and components should be made of stainless steel. (The CE standard on bolts requires that they be made of stainless steel.)

▧ Warning

Setting a bolt causes a permanent change in the rock. Either the bolt remains fixed in place or is broken out (chopped), which defaces the rock. In many managed areas, such as state and federal parks, setting of bolts is forbidden. Also, many in the rock-climbing community consider the improper use of bolts to be bad etiquette.

Bolts set previously by unknown individuals at an unknown time are, consequently, an unknown factor. Because of the varying techniques that can be used for setting bolts and because the rock may weather around them, bolts of unknown quality should not be trusted for anchors.

"Clean" Hardware

Other types of anchoring hardware have been developed, partly because pitons and bolts deface the rock. These other types initially were known collectively as "clean" hardware. Although clean hardware generally does not deface rock, it may not be as secure as pitons and bolts.

In rescue operations, environmental concerns take a secondary role to the needs and safety of the rescuers. Consequently, little choice may be available on the location or types of anchoring used. The most solid anchor in the safest location may be what you have to choose in rescue.

Clean hardware is manufactured by a number of different companies. Some of these devices may have very specialized uses, and some with similar designs may go by different names.

Among the basic types of clean hardware for anchoring are the following:

- Nuts, chocks, or stoppers, which work by being wedged in a rock crack that bottlenecks (Figure 5-21)
- Hexcentrics, which can work by both a wedging and a cam action (Figure 5-22)
- Spring-loaded camming devices (Friends, Camalots), which work by a spring-loaded, opposed cam action (Figure 5-23)

Belaying

Belaying is protecting a person from falling by managing an unloaded rope (the belay rope) in a way that secures the person on the rope in case the individual's main line rope or support fails. The belay rope is attached to the person being belayed and is controlled by the belayer. The difference in belaying techniques relates mainly to the manner in which the rope is held, or belayed.

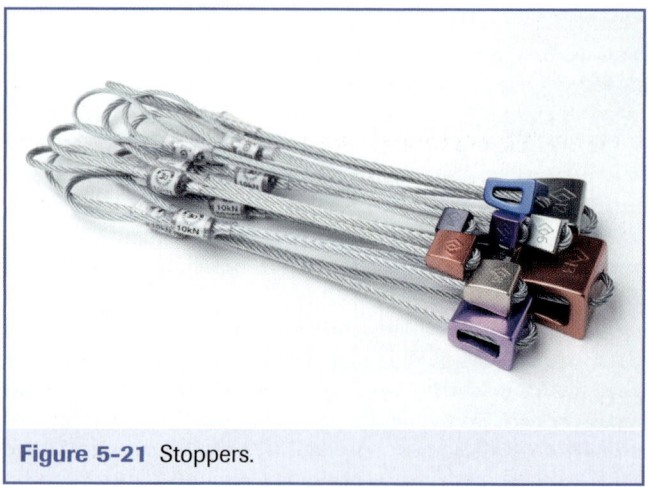

Figure 5-21 Stoppers.

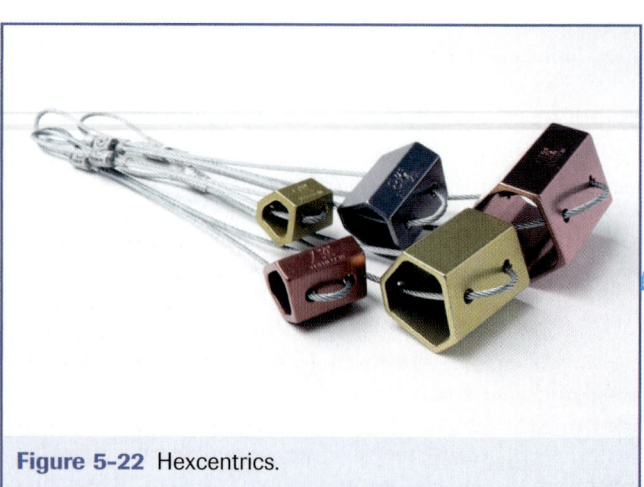

Figure 5-22 Hexcentrics.

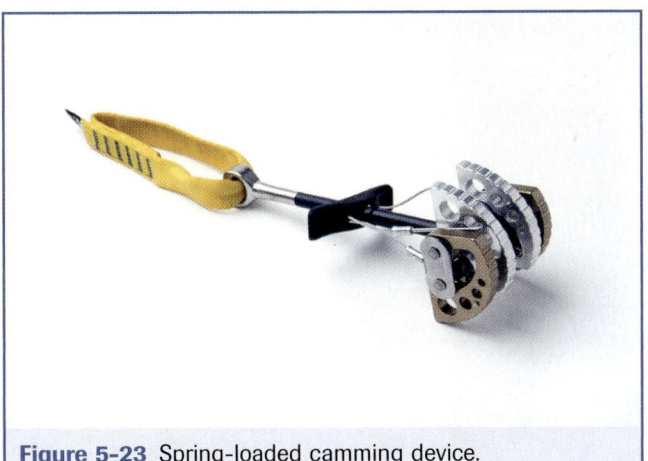

Figure 5-23 Spring-loaded camming device.

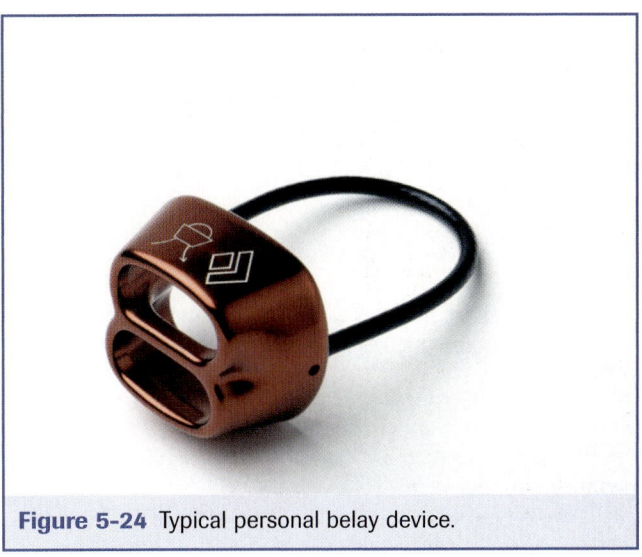

Figure 5-24 Typical personal belay device.

The oldest belay technique is the *body belay,* which involves running the belay rope around the body of the belayer (usually around the waist). In this way, the rope can be brought tight if the person on the end of the rope (the climber, rappeller, worker, or rescuer) falls. The rope is held by friction around the belayer's body. Body belaying has significant disadvantages:

- The force of the fall may cause the belayer to lose control of the rope and drop the climber.
- The force of the fall can easily injure the belayer.
- The belayer can become entangled in the rope. If the belayer does catch the climber, he or she must hold the individual until the climber can become secure.

Because of these problems, alternatives to body belaying have been developed and are preferable.

Belay Devices

Belay devices are equipment used to belay a person exposed to falling. In most belay devices, a bight of rope is fed through the unit. One end of the rope goes to the climber or the person who might fall. The other end of the rope is controlled by the belayer.

Some belay devices work through friction generated when the device presses the rope against a carabiner. An example of this type is the belay plate. The plate consists of a small metal plate with one or two holes. A bight of rope is fed through the plate and secured with a carabiner on the opposite side. The carabiner is clipped into an anchor. When the two strands of rope are pulled apart, a high degree of friction is created on the rope. This stops the fall of the climber.

One example of a belay, or brake, plate is a Sticht (Salewa, Austria). The oldest belay plate design is a *Sticht plate,* which has almost become a generic term. It comes in several different configurations, depending on the specific needs of the user.

Another example of a belay device that works through friction is an Air Traffic Controller (ATC) by Black Diamond (Salt Lake City, Utah). The ATC can be used with ropes ranging from 8.5 to 11 mm in diameter.

Some personal belay devices work through a camming action on the rope (Figure 5-24). An example of this type is the GriGri (Petzl).

The TRE belay device works with a combination of friction (like a Sticht plate) and a spring-loaded rod to increase the force supplied by the belayer's hand.

A more recent belay innovation is the 540° Rescue Belay (Traverse Rescue, Wilmington, Ohio). This mechanical belay device simplifies rescue belaying for heavy loads. Its symmetric design allows either end of the rope exiting the device to be used as the load line, and it has an integrated load release lever. The device is simple to operate, but it can be sensitive to rope size (a problem when ropes are not marked with the true size) and conditions, such as ropes that are too stiff, dirty, or worn.

The 540° Rescue Belay comes in two sizes: small, which is engineered to work with rope sizes of 10.6 to 11.6 mm (nominal $^7/_{16}$ inch), and large, for ropes 11.5 mm to 13 mm (nominal $^1/_2$ inch) (see Chapter 12 for information on how to use the 540° Rescue Belay).

Other Belay Alternatives

Another system for belaying requires only a large locking carabiner, something to anchor it to, and a rope. This is called the *Münter hitch* (or *Italian hitch*). When properly tied and operated, Münter hitches can work as personal belay systems for falls with a low fall factor but not with large loads or high fall factors.

The ability to catch a load with a Münter hitch varies, depending on the rigging situation. For example, it may be easier to catch a load with a Münter hitch if the rope runs across an edge or face or through directional pulleys. These elements in a high angle system add friction and thus help absorb the force of a falling load.

If more than one person is on the load, the potential load can be mitigated by rigging separate belays so that only one person ends up on each Münter hitch belay.

No belay device or technique is perfect for all rescue loads and in every rescue environment. Great caution must be exercised in choosing any belay device for rescue loads. Before you put the device to use, test it under realistic conditions that you will encounter in your own rescues. (See Chapter 8 for more information about the Münter hitch.)

A belay system often used in rescue belaying is the *tandem Prusik belay* (see Chapter 12).

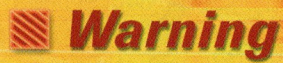

Warning

A personal belay device may not be the most appropriate device for catching loads of more than one person's body weight.

Before using any device or system to belay a rescue load, you should test it under conditions similar to those you will encounter in an actual rescue situation. This ensures that you will be able to catch the load when it falls. (See p. 100 for an example of the belay practice system; also see Chapter 12 for further information on rescue belaying.)

Pulleys

Although a **pulley** is designed primarily to reduce rope friction, this capability makes it useful in a number of functions in the high angle environment. Pulleys also can be used to:

- Change the direction of a running rope
- Position a rope more conveniently, such as to an area where people using the rope will be less exposed to falling, where there is less rock fall, or where rescuers might have more room
- Reduce abrasion on a rope (e.g., a pulley could be used to hold a rope up from a rock or to bring it away from other rope or webbing)
- Develop a mechanical advantage in hauling systems (see Chapter 18)

In certain situations, such as "big wall" climbing, lightweight pulleys often are used for such activities as hauling gear bags. Because weight is a primary consideration and the pulley is used for low-stress activities, these lightweight pulleys often are made of plastic or nylon.

However, in certain high angle systems, and particularly in rescue hauling, the rope is under such stress that heat friction can cause a pulley to melt and fail. Therefore when life support activities are involved, only all-metal pulleys should be used.

Other Characteristics of Pulleys for High Angle Activities

The following are other important characteristics of pulleys used in high angle work:

- Ideally, the *sheave* (wheel) should have a diameter at least four times the diameter of the rope (Figure 5-25). (See Chapter 3 for a discussion of the 4:1 rule.)
- *Side plates* should be movable so that the pulley can be placed on the rope anywhere along its length without the end of the rope having to be fed through the pulley.
- If rope abrasion is a concern, pulleys with side plates that extend beyond the edge of the sheave far enough to protect

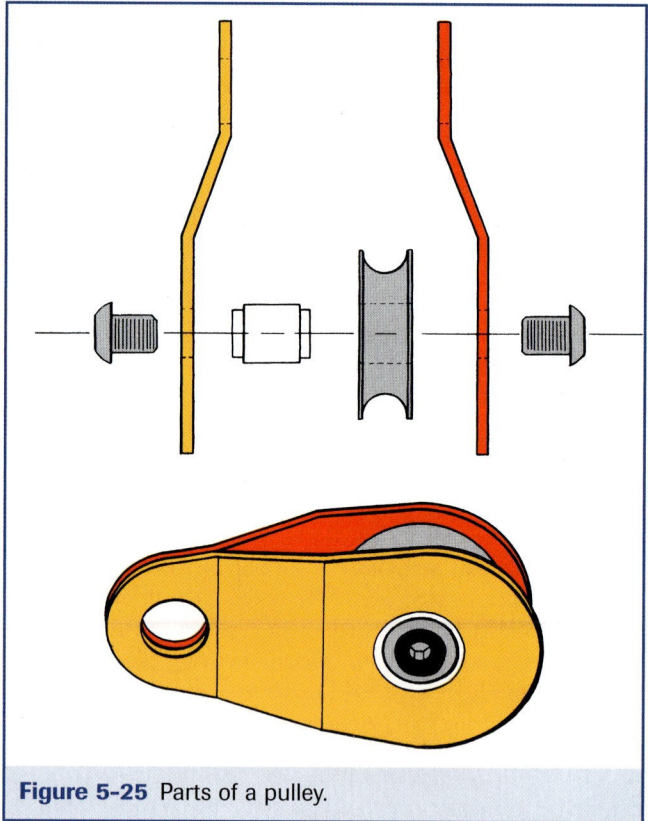

Figure 5-25 Parts of a pulley.

the rope should be used. The side plates generally are the weakest part of a pulley. Therefore pulleys for higher tensile strength rope (larger than 1/2 inch) should have stronger side plates. Pound for pound, steel side plates are stronger than those made of aluminum.

- *Axles* should have rounded bolt heads that will not snag rope, other gear, or rock.

Bearings

Most pulleys for high angle work have one of two types of bearings, bronze bushing or a ball bearing.

Bronze bushing

Advantages
- Less expensive than a ball bearing
- Can be taken apart to be cleaned
- Very strong

Disadvantage
- Can be contaminated by dirt and grit

Ball bearing

Advantages
- Turns slightly more freely than the bronze bushing.
- Some are sealed to prevent contamination by dirt and grit.

Disadvantages
- Slightly more expensive.

- Does not take stress, such as sudden blows, as well as the bronze bushing; also, it is damaged when the hardened steel balls dent the bearing races (technically called brinelling).

Specialized Pulleys

A number of pulleys for the high angle environment have been designed for specific tasks. One of these is the *knot-passing pulley* (Figure 5-26). The large sheave on this type of pulley is designed so that knots connecting lengths of rope can pass over it easily. Other specialized pulleys are the Kootney Carriage, tandem pulleys, and the Prusik minding pulley.

Edge Rollers

Edge rollers are important devices for reducing the friction generated by rope going over an edge. This not only helps with the work being done, as in hauling systems, but also helps prevent abrasion damage to the rope. (See Chapter 4 for descriptions of edge rollers and other rope protection equipment.)

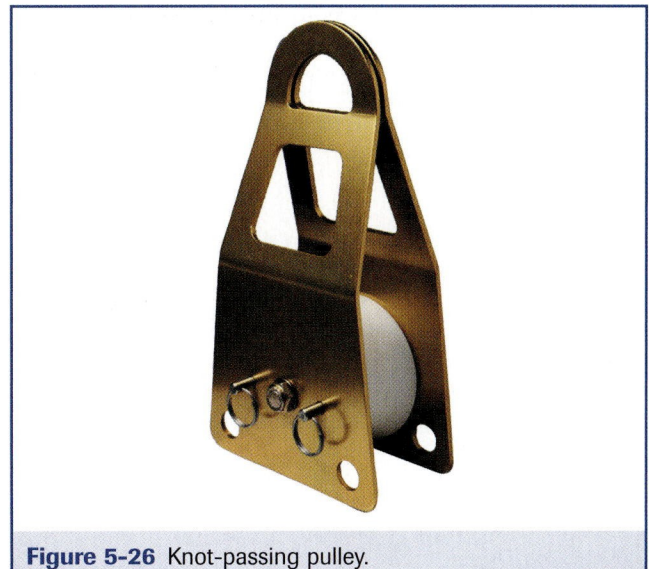

Figure 5-26 Knot-passing pulley.

Evaluation Exercises

Cognitive and Affective Exercises

1. All of the following would be situations in which the rope would come out of a nonlocking carabiner except:

   A. The carabiner presses against a rock.
   B. A rope or piece of webbing pulls across the gate.
   C. The carabiner is reversed and opposed with another.
   D. The carabiner presses against the edge of a wall or cliff.

2. To reduce the risk of a rope coming out of a gate in a nonlocking carabiner, you should use which technique:

   A. Opposition and alignment
   B. Reversed and opposed
   C. Reversed and aligned
   D. Münter hitch

3. All the following are stronger along the spine than along the gate except:

   A. Locking oval carabiner
   B. Nonlocking D carabiner
   C. Locking modified D carabiner
   D. Locking D carabiner

4. A locking carabiner can come unlocked under which of the following circumstances:

   A. Rubbing against a cliff face
   B. Vibration

C. Rope running across the gate
D. All of the above

5. A carabiner's *manner of function* refers to its design to load along the long axis of the carabiner:

   A. False
   B. True

6. Solutions to three-way loading of a carabiner on a seat harness include:

   A. Using a pear-shaped locking carabiner and placing the harness points in the large end and the device or rope in the small end
   B. Using a triangular screw link
   C. If using a sport harness, tying into the rope directly
   D. All of the above

7. A carabiner loaded with the gate open is a problem because of all of the following except:

   A. The locking mechanism may jam.
   B. The rope may slip out.
   C. A device (rappel or ascent) may slip out.
   D. The carabiner may fail completely.

8. Advantages to using a figure 8 descender include:

   A. It does not dissipate heat rapidly.
   B. Smaller models do not take larger diameter ropes.
   C. It is fairly compact and lightweight.
   D. The rope can slip around the ring and into a girth hitch.

9. Disadvantages of the brake bar rack include:

   A. Friction can be varied even after use has begun.
   B. The rack will not twist rope.
   C. It is bulkier and heavier than a figure 8.
   D. It can be used as a lowering device.

10. A personal ascender should not be used for which of the following purposes:

    A. Personal ascent of a rope
    B. As a cam in a mechanical advantage system
    C. As a personal grab device on a fixed line
    D. Hauling a 75-lb (34 kg) pack up a face

11. Examples of artificial anchors include all of the following except:

    A. Rock horn
    B. Stoppers
    C. Bolts
    D. Pitons

12. Disadvantages of using bolts include:

    A. They result in a permanent change in the rock.
    B. Bolts set by unknown individuals may not be secure.
    C. Bolts may have to be "chopped" to remove them.
    D. All of the above.

13. Some anchoring devices are known as "clean"; these include all the following except:

    A. Pitons
    B. Passive cams
    C. Active cams
    D. Nuts

14. Disadvantages of body belaying include all of the following except:

    A. The force of the fall may result in loss of control.
    B. The belay is quicker than other methods.
    C. The belayer may become entangled in the rope.
    D. The force of the fall may injure the belayer.

15. Of the following, which might be an alternative to body belaying:

    A. Use of a bowline knot
    B. Use of a figure 8 device in reverse
    C. Use of a Münter (Italian) hitch
    D. Use of a carabiner brake bar system

16. Pulleys may serve all the following functions except:

    A. Changing direction
    B. Working in mechanical advantage systems
    C. Reducing abrasion on a rope
    D. Acting as a belay device

Psychomotor Exercises

17. Using a locking carabiner, attach it between two ropes and load it along its long axis.

18. With a locking carabiner in front of you, identify the following:

    A. Spine
    B. Latch
    C. Gate
    D. Hinge

19. Using a conventional figure 8, attach it to the rope appropriately.

20. Using a six-bar brake rack, attach it to the rope appropriately.

6

Knots

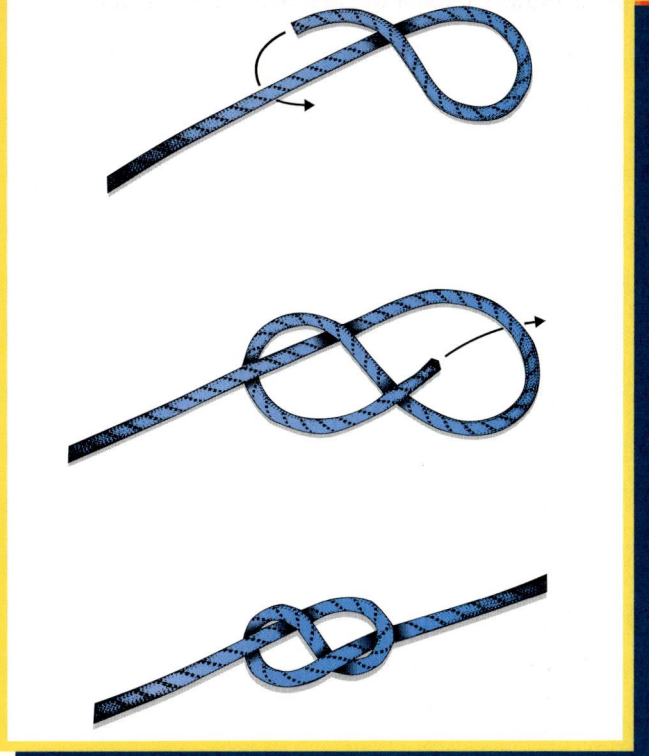

Objectives

On completion of this chapter, you should be able to:

1. Explain why it is necessary to have proficient knot skills before entering the high angle environment.
2. Discuss why it is necessary to practice knot tying continually.
3. Describe the qualities of a good knot.
4. List the ways in which knots affect rope strength.
5. Describe the functions of the following knots:
   - Simple overhand
   - Simple figure 8
   - Figure 8 on a bight
   - Figure 8 follow-through
   - Figure 8 bend
   - Ring bend (water knot)
   - Double overhand backup
   - Grapevine (double fisherman's knot)
   - Bowline on a coil
   - Interlocking long tail bowline
6. Demonstrate that you can tie the following knots correctly:
   - Simple overhand
   - Simple figure 8
   - Figure 8 on a bight
   - Figure 8 follow-through
   - Figure 8 bend

- Ring bend (water knot)
- Double overhand backup
- Grapevine (double fisherman's knot)
- Bowline on a coil
- Interlocking long tail bowline

The material in this chapter conforms to guidelines published by the National Fire Protection Association (NFPA), specifically standard 1983-01, *Standard for Fire Service Life Safety Rope and System Components* (2001), standard *1670, Standard on Operations and Training for Technical Rescue Incidents 2004 edition,* and standard 1006, *Professional Qualifications for Rescue Technicians* (2002). NFPA standards are revised regularly, and readers are advised to review the latest version of these standards.

Key Terms

Back-Up (Safety) Knot A second knot used to secure the tail of a primary knot; also known as a *safety* or *keeper* knot.

Bend A class of knot that joins two ropes or webbing pieces.

Bight The open loop in a rope formed when the rope is doubled back on itself.

Foundation Knot A simple knot that is tied as the first step in tying a more complex knot; examples are the overhand knot and the simple figure 8 knot.

Hitch A knot that attaches to or wraps around an object or rope in such a way that when the object or rope is removed, the knot falls apart.

Knot A fastening made by tying rope or webbing together in a prescribed way. Knots include bights, bends, and hitches.

Safety Knot See Back-Up Knot.

Stopper Knot A knot tied in a rope to help provide bulk. For example, a simple figure 8 knot may be tied in the bottom end of a rope to prevent a person from rappelling off the end, or it may be tied in the top of the rope to prevent the rope from accidentally slipping through equipment.

Knots in the High Angle Environment

The high angle technician must be able to tie knots correctly, confidently, and without hesitation and must know the ways these knots are used. If you go into the high angle environment without these knot skills, you may be a danger to yourself, to a rescue subject, and to your fellow rescuers.

Knots are the links that join many elements in the high angle system. Among other functions, knots are used in the high angle environment for:

- Anchoring
- Tying ropes together
- Tying webbing together
- Tying loops in rope and webbing
- Tying people directly into ropes
- Creating certain belay systems
- Dealing with emergency situations (e.g., devising an emergency seat harness)
- Backing up other knots
- Keeping rope ends from pulling out of equipment
- Ensuring personal safety (e.g., preventing a rappeller from rappelling off the end of a rope)
- Creating emergency ascenders
- Tying safety lines
- Improvising when other elements of a system fail
- Extricating yourself from unexpected difficulties

You must practice your knot-tying skills continually so that you remain proficient and can tie a specific knot instantly when necessary. To maintain good high angle skills, you should own at least two lengths of rope, each several feet (or a couple of meters) long, so that you can continually practice knot tying.

Group training sessions for high angle rescue work typically should begin with a review of knots. Individuals who do not maintain their knot-tying skills should be denied group certification and should not be allowed in the high angle environment. Failure to learn simple but essential skills, such as knot tying, may indicate lack of motivation.

Because many activities take place under severe environmental conditions, every high angle rope technician should be able to tie knots under stress, in the dark, when cold, using only one hand, and with diminished physical ability.

There are thousands of knots, but in this chapter the number explored is reduced to those necessary for major situations encountered in the high angle environment. Note that certain specialized knots are not reviewed in this chapter, but rather are discussed in sections associated with the special skills requiring use of the knot. For example, the Münter **hitch** (also known as the Italian hitch) is reviewed in Chapter 8, and the Prusik is covered in Chapters 10 and 13.

The Qualities of a Good Knot

Although knots vary in their specific use, all good knots have certain characteristics in common, including the following:

- They are relatively easy to tie.
- It is easy to determine if they have been tied correctly.
- Once tied correctly, they remain tied.
- They have a minimal effect on rope strength.
- They are relatively easy to untie after loading.

How Knots Affect Ropes

Every knot diminishes the strength of rope somewhat. The reason for this is that in any sharp bend of a rope less than four times the diameter of the rope, the rope fibers on the outside of the bend carry most of the load on the rope. The fibers on the inside of the bend carry very little of the load or none at all (Figure 6-1). (See the discussion of the 4:1 rule, p. 40).

Some knots, such as bowlines, have sharper bends, resulting in greater strength loss in a rope than occurs with knots such as figure 8s that have more open bends (Box 6-1). Ultimately, the strength of knots, along with other elements of a high angle system, must be taken into consideration when deciding on a

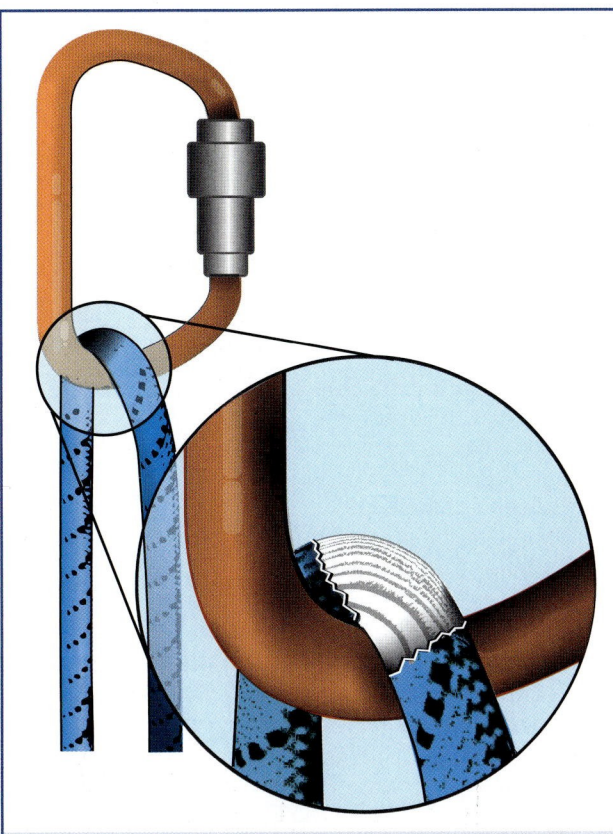

Figure 6-1 Effect of bending rope.

Box 6-1	**Examples of Strength Loss in Rope Tied with Typical Knots***

7/16-inch (11 mm) Static Rope

Average Percentage of Original Strength

Bowline knot: 74%
Figure 8 knot: 78%

1/2-inch (12.5 mm) Static Rope

Average Percentage of Original Strength

Bowline knot: 73%
Figure 8 knot: 80%

*These results are the average of four tests done with new PMI ropes 7/16 inch and 1/2 inch in diameter that were made in July 1990. Other test results may vary, depending on a number of factors such as the design of the rope, the manufacturer, and the test conditions.

rope load ratio or a system safety factor for a rope. (See Chapter 3 for additional discussion of safety factors.)

Knots should be removed from a rope before the rope is put away and stored, for the following reasons:

- Leaving a knot loaded and tied in a rope over a long period may cause permanent strength loss in the rope.

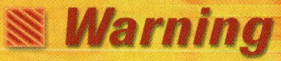

An improperly tied knot, or incorrect application of a knot, could result in serious injury or death.

- Knots left in a rope over a long period tend to set and become more difficult to untie.

Backing Up Knots

It is good practice to back up knots with a **back-up (safety) knot**. Although an overhand knot often is used for this purpose, a more secure backup is the double overhand knot (see Figure 6-12; also see p. 74 for instructions on tying a double overhand back-up knot). A back-up knot is a particular concern when the rope is stiffer, such as static kernmantle ropes, or if the knot is going to be flexed a great deal. The backup should be tied as close as possible to the main knot it is for which it is serving a safety purpose.

NOTE: For clarity, many knots in this manual are not shown with backup knots. However, it should be assumed that in each case the knot has a backup.

Dressing Knots

After a knot has been tied, it should be *dressed* (the strands aligned and uncrossed) and *compacted* (all ends pulled down so that the knot is compact). This ensures that the knot has its greatest holding power, yet maintains as much rope strength as possible.

Also, dressing knots makes it easier to identify them and confirm that they have been tied correctly.

Specific Knots for the High Angle Environment

Overhand Knot (for Rope and Webbing)

Uses

- As a **foundation knot** for beginning other knots, such as the ring bend (water knot).
- As a backup to secure other knots.
  Figure 6-2 shows how to tie a simple overhand knot.

The Figure 8 Family

The figure 8 family of knots meets most knot-tying needs in the high angle environment. Many high angle rope technicians prefer figure 8 knots for the following reasons:

- When tied correctly, they tend to be secure and less likely to come apart under loading and flexing.
- It is easy to tell if they have been tied correctly.
- They diminish rope strength less than some other knots.
- It is easy to remember how to tie them.

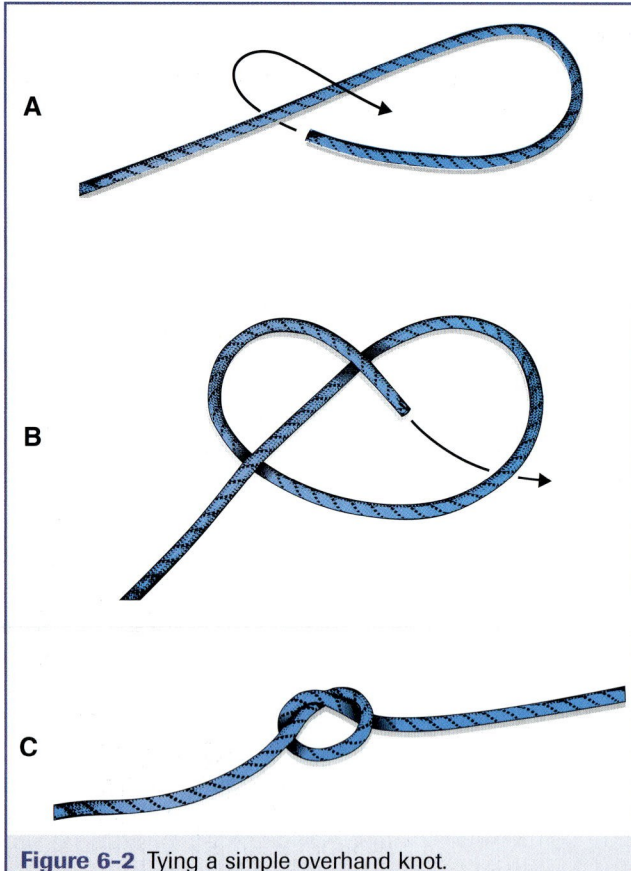

Figure 6-2 Tying a simple overhand knot.

Warning

Figure 8 knots, as with all knots, should be dressed (the strands aligned and uncrossed) and compacted (all ends pulled down so the knot is compact). This ensures that the knot has its greatest holding power, while maintaining as much rope strength as possible.

Simple Figure 8 (for Rope)

Uses

The simple figure 8 knot is used as a **stopper knot** for certain types of security; for example:

- Tied in the bottom end of a rope to prevent a person from rappelling off the end.
- Tied in the top of a rope to prevent it from accidentally slipping through equipment.
- As a foundation knot for beginning the figure 8 follow-through or the figure 8 bend.

Figure 6-4 shows how to tie a simple figure 8 knot.

Caution

❏ Do not mistake the overhand knot for a half hitch (for comparison, a half hitch is shown in Figure 6-3).
❏ When used as a back-up knot, the overhand knot must be pulled down tightly and close to the knot it is backing up (see Figure 6-7).

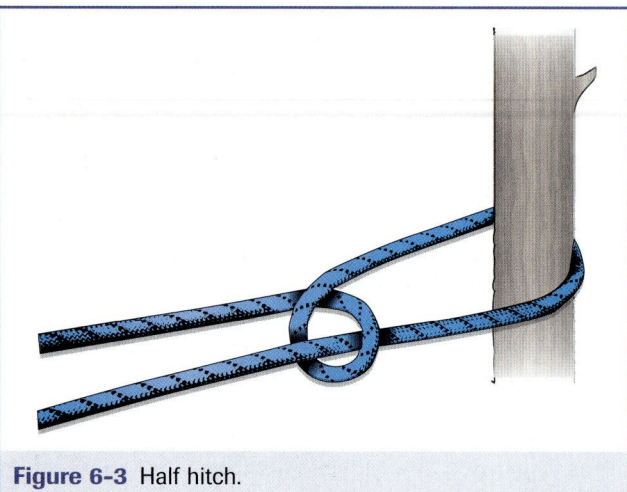

Figure 6-3 Half hitch.

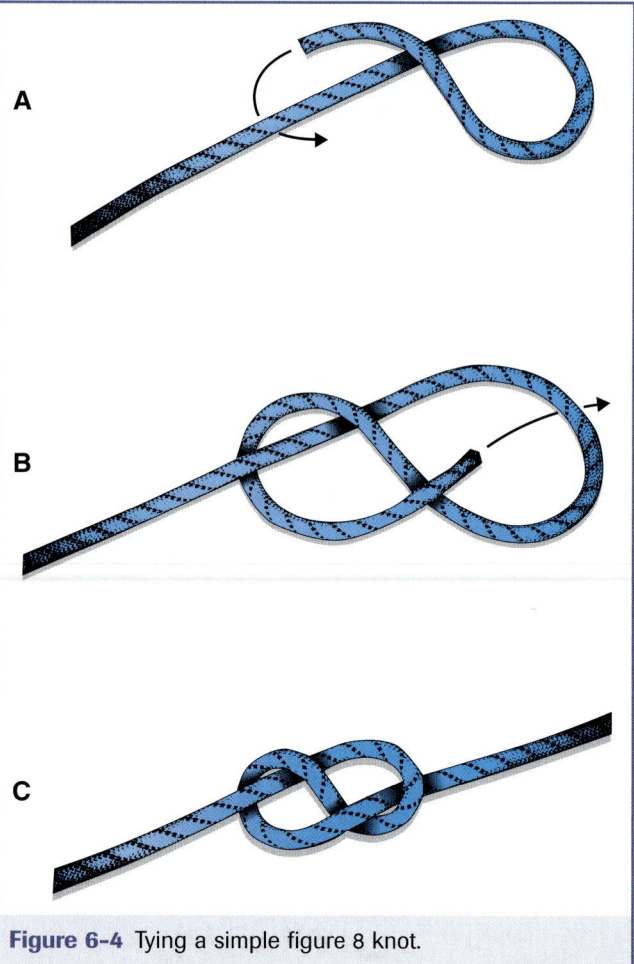

Figure 6-4 Tying a simple figure 8 knot.

Caution

Do not confuse the simple figure 8 knot with the simple overhand knot. Compare the simple figure 8 knot with the overhand knot shown in Figure 6-2; note the extra step in tying the simple figure 8. When you hold this knot up by either end of the rope, it should have the rough appearance of the numeral 8.

Figure 8 on a Bight (for Rope)

Note that a **bight** is simply the loop formed when the rope is doubled back on itself. Creating a bight is the first step in tying this knot. You can do this in the middle of the rope, or a bight can be created at an end, as shown in Figure 6-5, *A*.

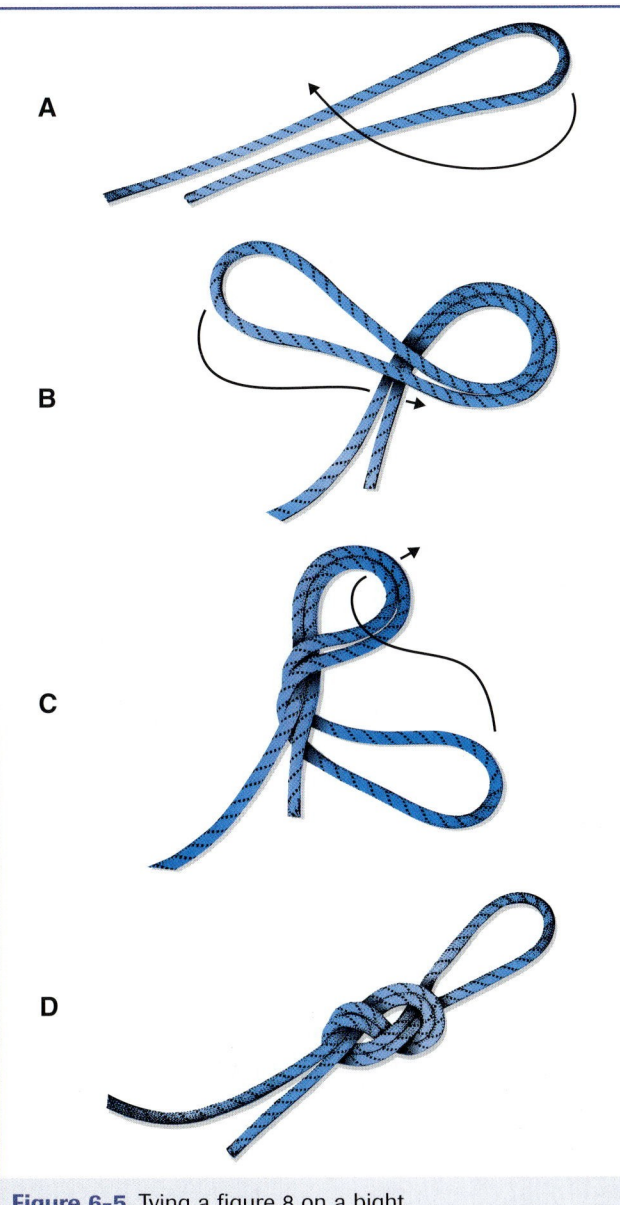

Figure 6-5 Tying a figure 8 on a bight.

Uses

A figure 8 on a bight is used as a secure loop in a rope for clipping into, for such needs as:

- Safety lines
- Persons being lowered
- Litter and other rescue equipment
- Anchor lines

Caution

Be careful that you tie a figure 8 on a bight and not an overhand on a bight (the latter knot is shown in Figure 6-6).

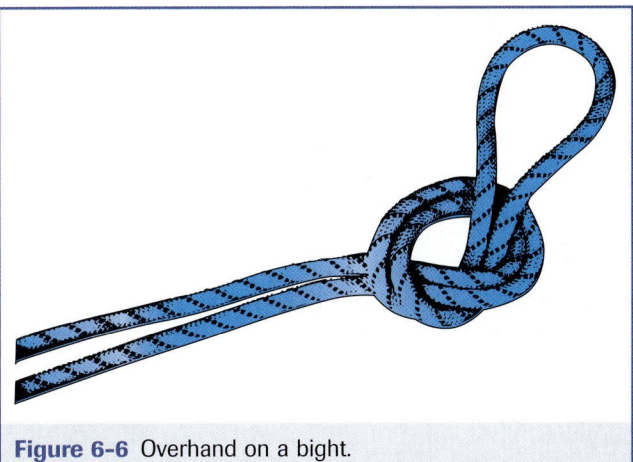

Figure 6-6 Overhand on a bight.

Optional Approach: Bowline Knot

Many authorities experienced in the high angle environment feel that the figure 8 family of knots is preferable to the bowline family; these ropeworkers maintain that a figure 8 knot has the following advantages:

- More likely to be tied correctly.
- More likely to be remembered.
- Easier to tell quickly if it is tied correctly.
- Remains stable if loading on it comes from a direction different from that intended.
- More likely to remain tied after repeated loading and unloading.
- Less likely to invert and become untied when pulled across an obstruction or when the tail of the knot is pulled.
- Weakens the rope less than a bowline.

However, because of the long tradition of using the bowline, some individuals have a passionate attachment to its use. Figure 6-7 shows a correctly tied simple bowline and an overhand back-up knot.

If local policy dictates the use of a bowline instead of a figure 8 knot for tying a loop in a rope, you should obtain instruction in the tying of a bowline from qualified personnel.

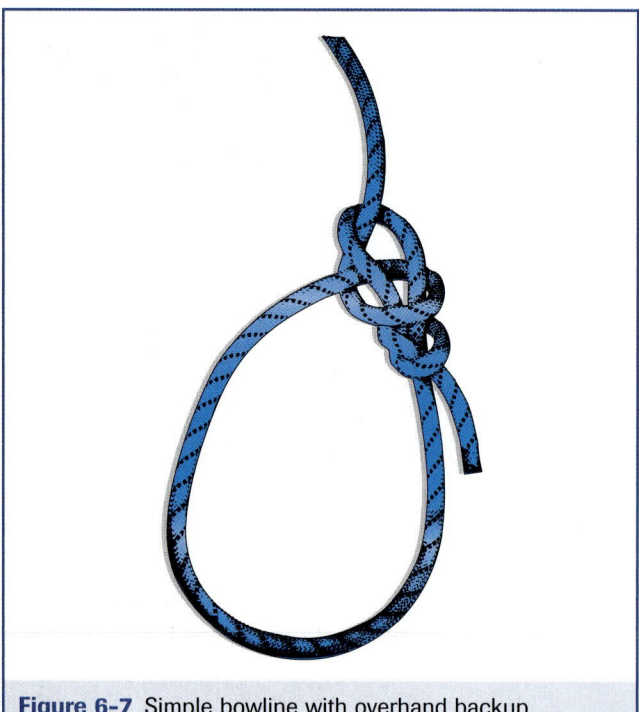

Figure 6-7 Simple bowline with overhand backup.

Warning

If you decide to use a bowline, make certain that it is tied correctly and do the following:

- Make sure the tail of the knot ("bitter end") is backed up with an overhand or other keeper knot.
- Do not use a bowline on a moving rope. If the bowline snags, the knot may invert, changing the direction of the load on it, and fail. Do not load the tail of a bowline, because that also can cause it to fail.

Figure 8 Follow-Through

A figure 8 follow-through (Figure 6-8) is used to create a loop at the end of a rope when a figure 8 on a bight cannot be tied. For example, you may need to anchor to an object closed at both ends (e.g., a structural beam) or to a tall object (e.g., a tree), situations in which you cannot get a simple loop *over an end* of the object. You therefore tie a figure 8 follow-through *around* the object (Box 6-2).

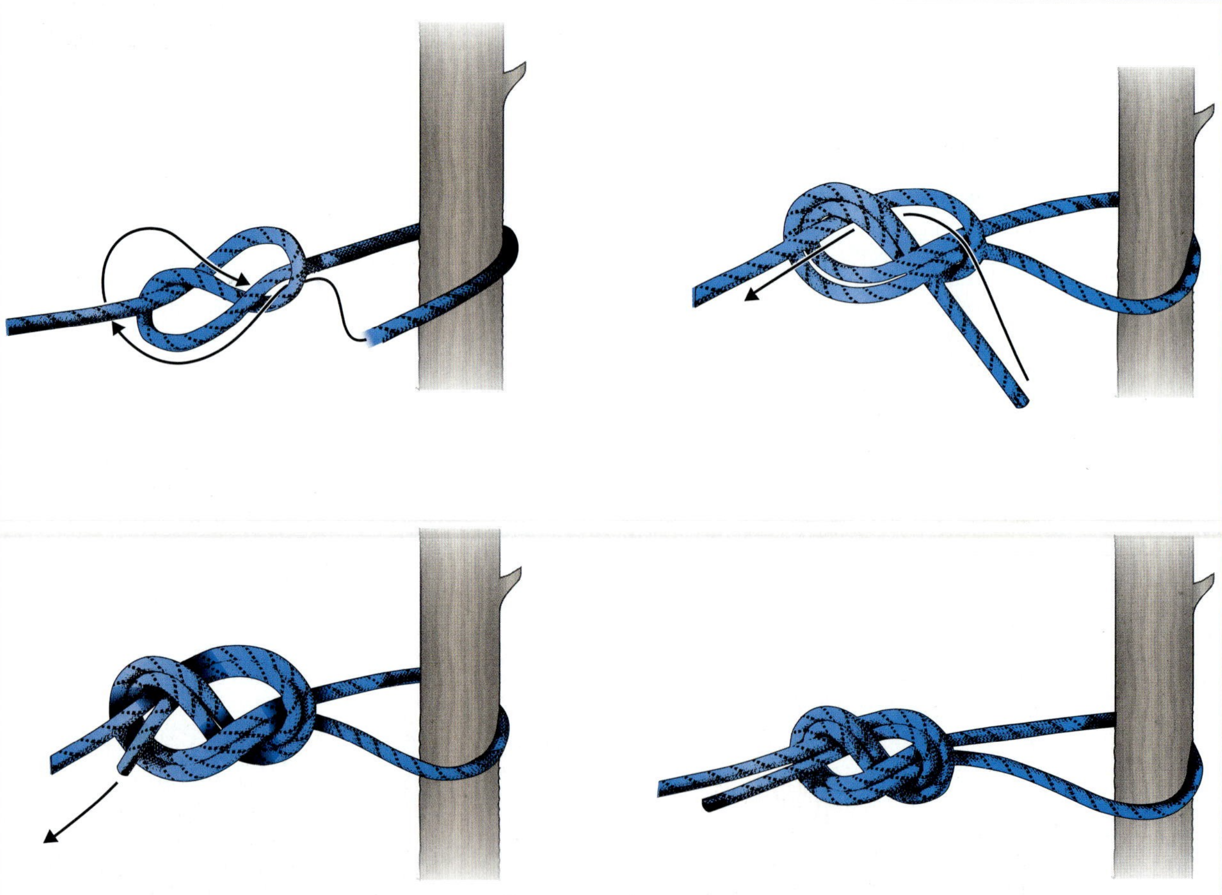

Figure 6-8 Tying a figure 8 follow-through knot.

Box 6-2	**Suggestions for Tying a Figure 8 Follow-Through Knot**

1. Note that the figure 8 follow-through always begins with the tying of a simple figure 8 knot as a foundation well back from the end of the rope.
2. After the simple figure 8 has been tied, pass the end of the rope around the anchor point, then follow back through parallel to the first knot. Follow every contour of the first knot with both rope ends going in the same direction.
3. Do not confuse this knot with the figure 8 bend (Figure 6-9).

Figure 8 Bend (for Rope)

The term *bend*, as applied to knots, refers to the joining of two ropes (Box 6-3).

Uses

A figure 8 bend is used to join two ropes or the two ends of one rope for the purposes of:

- Connecting two pieces of rope.
- Creating a loop of rope by joining the two ends of one rope.

Figure 6-9 shows how to tie a figure 8 bend knot.

Box 6-3	**Suggestion for Tying a Figure 8 Bend Knot**

First try tying this knot using two ropes of different colors. This will make it easier to distinguish the different strands of rope.

Note that the figure 8 bend always begins with the tying of a simple figure 8 knot as a foundation.

The next step is to follow the contour of the first knot exactly, with the rope ends approaching from opposite directions.

⚠ *Caution*

1. Note that the figure 8 bend always begins with the tying of a simple figure 8 knot as a foundation.
2. The next step is to follow the contour of the first knot exactly, with the rope ends approaching from *opposite* directions.

Optional Approach: Grapevine Knot

Another knot that can be used to join two rope ends securely to form a longer rope or to form a loop is the grapevine knot (also known as the *double fisherman's knot*) (Figure 6-10). This knot is very secure, but it may be more difficult to learn and to tell whether it is tied correctly. The grapevine knot can be difficult to untie after it is loaded, particularly in softer hand ropes.

The grapevine knot should be used to join only ropes of a similar diameter. It should not be used for webbing, for ropes of greatly unequal diameters, or for materials that may tend to untie or creep back through the bends of the knot (Box 6-4).

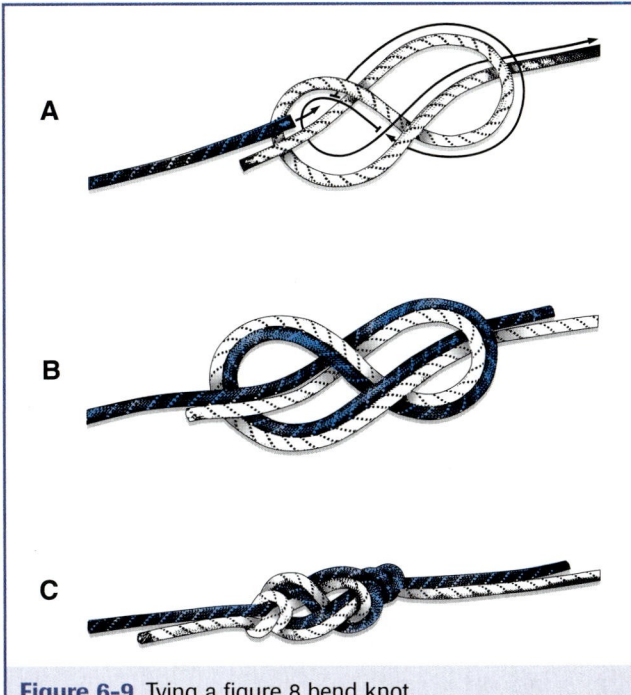

Figure 6-9 Tying a figure 8 bend knot.

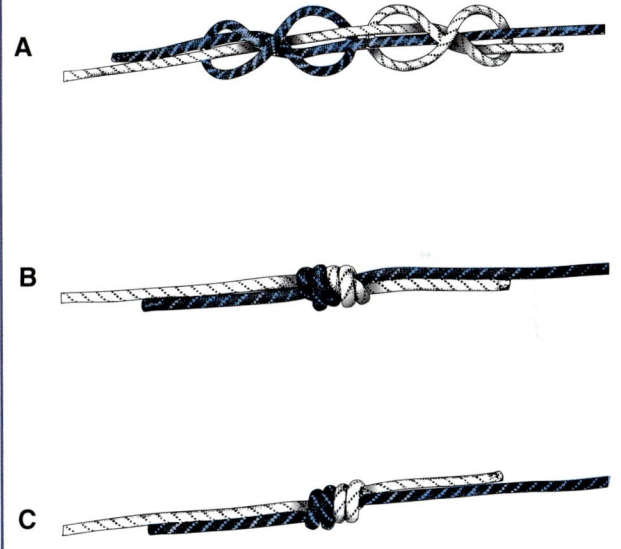

Figure 6-10 Tying a grapevine knot (also known as a double fisherman's knot).

Box 6-4	**Suggestions for Tying a Grapevine Knot**

The tail of each rope, when tied correctly, should end up on the side of the knot opposite the side it entered. The two turns from each half of the knot should lie flat against one another on one face of the knot and appear as a double X on the other face (see Figure 6-10, *B, C*).

Ring Bend (Water Knot)

The ring bend (water) knot, also known as the *overhand bend*, is used only for webbing.

Uses

The ring bend knot is used to join two pieces of webbing or the two ends of one piece of webbing for the purposes of:
- Forming a longer piece (joining two pieces of webbing).
- Forming a loop (tying together the two ends of one piece of webbing) (Box 6-5).

Figure 6-11 shows how to tie a ring bend (water knot) in webbing.

Box 6-5	Suggestion for Tying a Ring Bend Knot

First try tying this knot using two pieces of webbing of different colors. This will make it easier to distinguish the different pieces of webbing as you tie the knot.

⚠ *Warning*

The ring bend is to be used only for webbing. Do not use it for rope. Because of the flat nature of webbing, it tends to contour over itself. Rope does not have this quality, and a water knot in rope may easily come out.

⚠ *Warning*

1. Always have at least 2 inches (50 mm) of webbing in the ends of ring bends *after they are tied and pulled tight.* Although webbing contours well in a ring bend, it tends to be slippery. For additional insurance, back up both sides of the knot with an overhand knot (see Figure 6-11, *E*) or sew loose ends down sufficiently to keep them from working through the knot.
2. A ring bend in webbing should be inspected frequently because over time it tends to work loose.
3. Make sure the webbing follows flat through the knot. A twist in the webbing inside the knot will allow the knot to slip at relatively low loads.

Double Overhand Knot (for Rope)

Use

The double overhand knot is used to back up other knots (this knot is essentially one half of a double fisherman's knot). Figure 6-12 shows how to tie a double overhand knot.

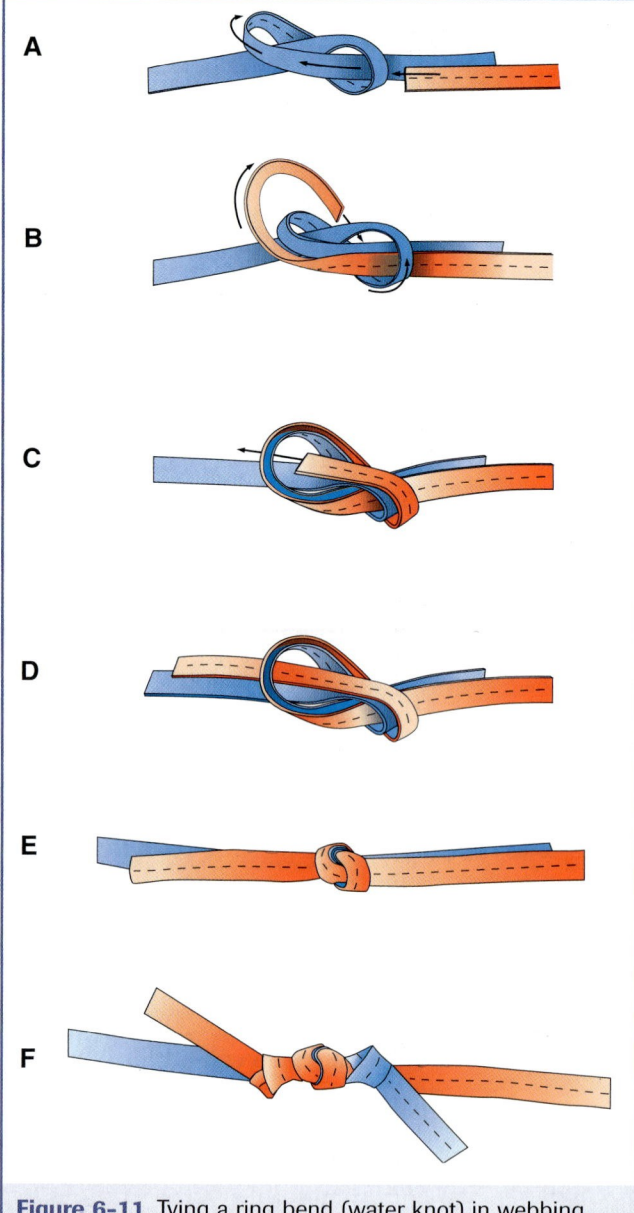

Figure 6-11 Tying a ring bend (water knot) in webbing.

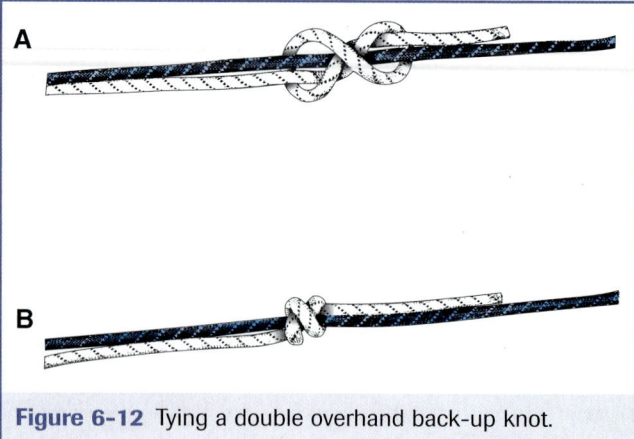

Figure 6-12 Tying a double overhand back-up knot.

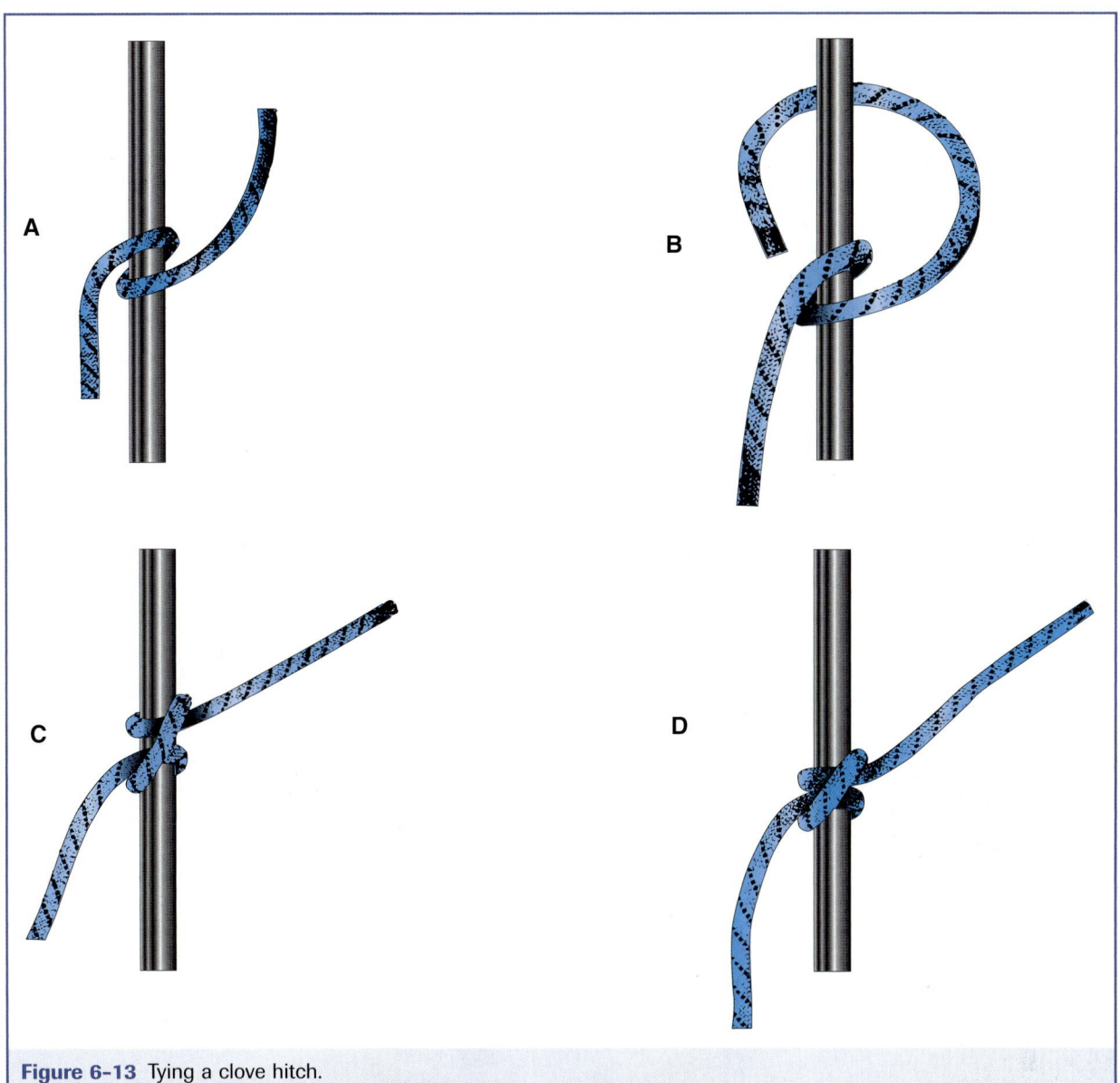

Figure 6-13 Tying a clove hitch.

Clove Hitch (for Rope or Webbing)

Use

A clove hitch is used for anchoring to rounded anchor points, such as litter rails. Figure 6-13 shows how to tie a clove hitch. This method uses the working end of the rope; the clove hitch can be wrapped around an object that is closed on both ends, such as a litter rail.

Bowline on a Coil (for Rope)

Uses

The bowline on a coil is used to create an improvised litter spider (see Chapter 17), using four loops as the spider legs. Figure 6-14 shows how to tie a bowline on a coil.

Interlocking Long-Tail Bowline (for Rope)

Uses

An interlocking long-tail bowline is used for lowering litters and for raising operations (it is used to bring the main line and the belay line to a single point, such as the main attachment point on a litter bridle, at the same time providing tails to back up the litter and the litter attendant). Figure 6-15 shows how to tie an interlocking long-tail bowline.

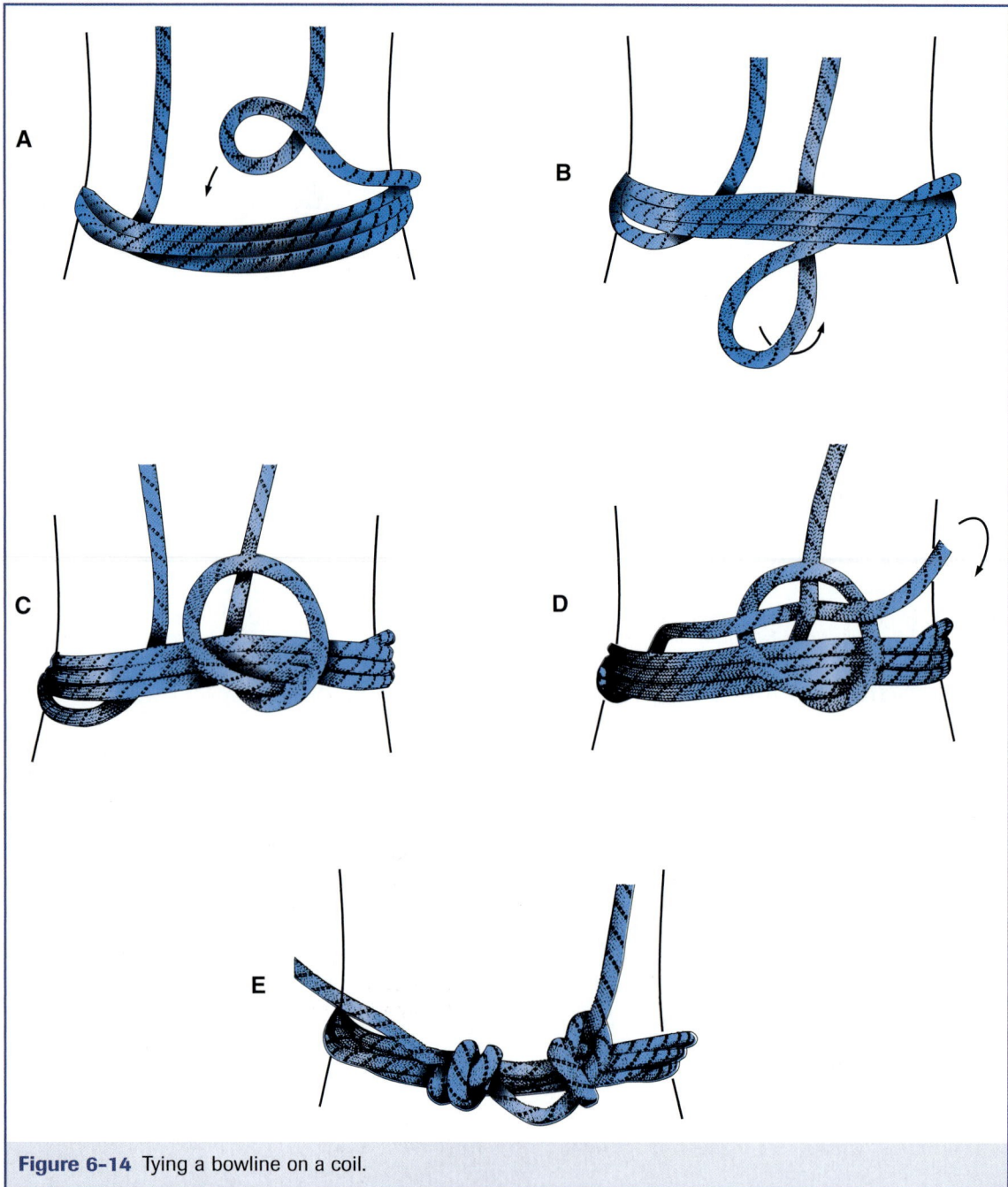

Figure 6-14 Tying a bowline on a coil.

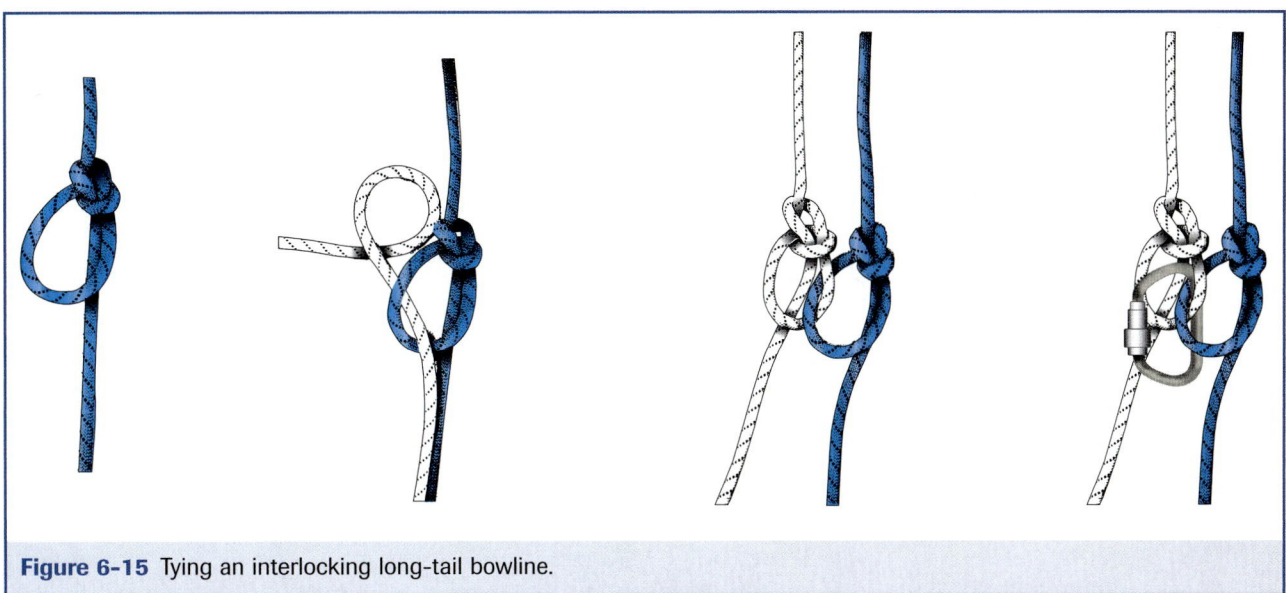

Figure 6-15 Tying an interlocking long-tail bowline.

Evaluation Exercises

Cognitive and Affective Exercises

1. Which of the following are uses for knots in the high angle environment:

   A. Anchoring
   B. Tying ropes and webbing together
   C. Tying a person's seat harness directly to the rope
   D. All of the above

2. Qualities of a good knot include all the following except:

   A. It's easy to tie.
   B. It's easy to determine if the knot is tied correctly.
   C. It's hard to untie after loading.
   D. It has minimal effect on rope strength.

3. Describe a use for each of the following:

   A. Overhand knot
   B. Simple figure 8
   C. Figure 8 on a bight
   D. Figure 8 follow-through
   E. Figure 8 bend
   F. Ring bend (water knot)
   G. Double overhand back-up knot
   H. Grapevine (double fisherman's knot)
   I. Bowline on a coil
   J. Interlocking long-tail bowline

Psychomotor Exercises

4. Tie the following knots in a well-lighted room:

   A. Overhand knot
   B. Simple figure 8
   C. Figure 8 on a bight
   D. Figure 8 follow-through
   E. Figure 8 bend
   F. Ring bend (water knot)
   G. Double overhand back-up knot
   H. Bowline on a coil
   I. Interlocking long-tail bowline

5. Tie the following knots while blind-folded or with your hands under a table:

   A. Overhand knot
   B. Simple figure 8
   C. Figure 8 on a bight
   D. Figure 8 follow-through
   E. Figure 8 bend
   F. Ring bend (water knot)
   G. Double overhand back-up knot

6. Put on your storm clothing, step into a cold shower with the lights off, and tie the following knots:

   A. Overhand knot
   B. Simple figure 8
   C. Figure 8 on a bight
   D. Figure 8 follow-through
   E. Figure 8 bend
   F. Ring bend (water knot)
   G. Double overhand back-up knot

7

Anchoring

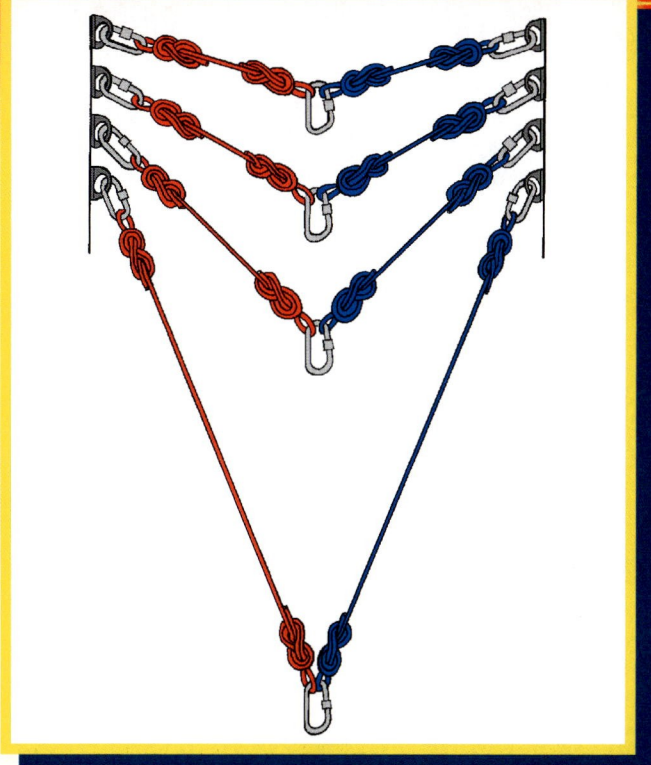

Objectives

On completion of this chapter, you should be able to:

1. Describe the purpose of anchoring in rope rescue.
2. Explain the forces created on anchors, demonstrate ways to reduce or magnify those forces and, given an example of an anchor system, estimate the forces on that system.
3. Explain how to avoid overloading an anchor system.
4. Given an example of a rope rescue site, select anchor placement.
5. Explain the purpose of directionals and demonstrate how to set up a directional.
6. Select the most appropriate knots for use in anchor systems.
7. Give examples of the use of the tensionless hitch in anchor systems.
8. Use the following knots in an anchor system:
   - Tensionless hitch
   - Figure 8 on a bight
   - Figure 8 follow-through
   - Ring bend (water knot)
9. Give examples of the ways rope and webbing are used in anchoring systems.
10. Identify the areas on a building that would be either suitable or unsuitable anchor points and demonstrate secure anchor construction in a building.
11. Discuss the parts of a vehicle that are either suitable or unsuitable anchor points and demonstrate secure anchor construction in vehicles.
12. Give examples of situations requiring multiple anchor points.
13. Explain the angles on a multipoint anchoring system that can create unacceptable forces.
14. Explain the concept of load-sharing anchors.
15. Correctly tie a load-sharing anchor using two anchor points.
16. Correctly tie a load-distributing anchor using a webbing loop on two anchor points.
17. Correctly construct a load-distributing anchor system using three or more anchor points.
18. Explain the concept of a picket system and demonstrate the construction of such a system.

The material in this chapter conforms to guidelines published by the National Fire Protection Association (NFPA), specifically standard 1006, *Professional Qualifications for Rescue Technicians* (2002). NFPA standards are revised regularly, and readers are advised to review the latest version of this standard.

Anchor (n) A secure tie-in point for attaching a line; (v) the act of attaching a line to an anchor.

Anchor Point A single secure connection for an anchor; an anchor point is used either alone or in combination with other anchor points to create an anchor system capable of sustaining the actual or potential load on a rope rescue system.

Anchor System One or more anchor points rigged to provide a structurally sound connection for elements of a rope rescue system.

Artificial Anchors The use of specially designed hardware to create anchors where good natural anchors do not exist.

Backing Up The creation of a secondary or redundant system designed to provide added security, and the creation of one or more additional independent anchors to sustain the high angle system should the initial anchors fail. Backing up may be done at the same anchor point if it is very solid or at other anchor points.

Back Tie A connector from a primary anchor to a second, back-up anchor.

Bombproof Jargon for an anchor or anchor system believed to be very secure.

Directional A technique for repositioning a rope at a more favorable angle than would exist by running the rope directly to the anchor.

Load-Distributing Anchor System (LDA) An anchor system established from two or more anchor points that (1) maintains near-equal loading on the anchor points despite direction changes on the main line rope and (2) reestablishes near-equal loading on remaining anchor points should one or more of them fail. This system is sometimes referred to as a self-equalizing anchor.

Load-Sharing Anchors An anchor system established from two or more anchor points that distributes the load among the anchor points but does not adjust to direction changes on the main line.

Master Attachment Point The point where rigging comes together for maximum strength.

Multipoint Anchor Anchors involving two or more anchor points.

Pendulum (v) To swing on a rope.

Anchors and the High Angle System

Anchors are the means of securing the ropes and other elements of the high angle system to something solid. The place where the anchors are connected is the **anchor point**. Anchor points take a number of forms. They can be manmade (e.g., structural beams) or natural (trees or rocks). Or they might be **artificial anchors** (e.g., nuts, chocks, hexcentrics, and cams) that people have placed in rock walls. On buildings, the most secure anchor points are structural parts such as integral beams and columns. In some situations, the only available anchor points may be on vehicles.

Anchoring is to the high angle system what a foundation is to a building. Without suitable, secure anchors, the remainder of the high angle system (ropes, hardware, and other gear) is in danger of failing, no matter how well established they are. Just as a solid foundation is the primary concern before construction of a building, you must have a suitable, secure **anchor system** before you rig the rest of the high angle system.

Anchor Points

The anchor point is the single secure connection for an anchor. The specific kind of anchor point that you use depends on the high angle environment in which you are working.

Natural Anchors

The most commonly used natural anchors are trees and rocks, around which webbing or rope can be wrapped. However, both have the potential for failure. Before using a tree as an anchor,

you should examine it for weakness, such as possible rot. Even a tree with sound wood may not be a good anchor if the root system is shallow or thin or if the tree is in wet soil. Boulders weighing tons can be pulled over by the stresses of anchor systems.

Anchors on Structures

In industrial and urban settings, anchors often must be established on structures. You must do this carefully to make sure the anchor is structurally sound. On some modern buildings, it often is difficult to find any anchor points at all.

Some examples of deteriorated structures are:
- Corroded metals
- Weathered stonework
- Deteriorated mortar in brickwork

Some examples of inherently weak structural features include:
- Vents constructed of sheet metal
- Flashing
- Gutters and downspouts
- Brickwork without bulk (e.g., small chimneys)
- Fire hydrants

When you rig anchors on buildings, choose anchor points that are inherently part of the building's structure or specifically constructed to support high loads. Some examples of such anchor points would be:
- Structural columns
- Projections of structural beams
- Supports for large machinery
- Stairwell support beams
- Brickwork with large bulk (e.g., corner walls)
- Anchors for window-cleaning equipment

> ## ⚠ *Warning*
>
> - Do not confuse window washer eyebolts with guy wire hooks. Window cleaner eyebolts are substantial (usually ¾-inch [19 mm]), closed eyebolts in structural concrete. Guy wire hooks are used to stabilize items such as signs and antenna; they are not designed for life support.
> - Many window washer eyebolts are designed to be pulled vertically with cantilevered rigging; these may fail if pulled sideways. Always back up window washer eyebolts with other anchors.

Less Obvious Anchors

Some buildings, particularly new ones, at first may appear to have no anchor points. However, after some practice in working this type of problem, riggers may find some unexpected but good anchors.

Elevator and Machine Housings

Elevator and machine housings often are larger than what is expected for an anchor point. However, by taking a length of rope, running it around the housing several times, and tying the ends together with a figure 8 bend, you may be able to create a secure anchor point for several lines.

Scuppers (Roof Drain Holes)

Many buildings have low parapets with drain holes set in them at roof level. You can create an anchor point by running rope or webbing through the drain hole and back over the top of the parapet.

If possible, you should use the scupper on the side of the building opposite the one over which you will run the main line. This allows space on top of the building for rappellers to rig into the rope and to set other rigging, such as lowering and raising systems.

The more substantial parapets are those constructed of reinforced concrete. If the parapet is constructed of brick or block, riggers should make sure that several brick or block courses are involved and that the mortar is in good condition. Even under the best of conditions for a brick or block parapet, it would be wise to rig with at least two anchor points. Be sure to pad all sharp edges.

Wall Sections between Windows and/or Doors

If windows and/or doors are close enough together, you can use them to create a substantial anchor point. Pass the anchor rope or webbing through an open window or door, around the intervening wall, and back through an adjacent window or door to tie off the rope or webbing. The anchor wall should be on the side opposite where the main line will run out of the building. This provides more safe space for rappellers to rig into the rope or to set rigging, such as lowering and raising systems.

Stairwell Beams

If you anchor to stairwell beams, make sure they are the structural members; these are the open steel beams to which the stair risers are anchored.

Artificial Anchors

Artificial anchors are special types of hardware specifically designed for creating anchor points or "protection" in places where no natural anchors are available. Many artificial anchors are inserted into rocks or spaces in rock. These types of hardware include nuts, chocks, hexcentrics, and cams. If such devices are to serve as safe, effective anchors, they must be placed by a person with a great deal of skill and practice in their use.

Bolts are a type of artificial anchor commonly used in rescue operations. However, placing bolts takes time, and a great deal of practice and training are required to learn to set them correctly. They also do permanent damage to the rock, which is frowned on in managed areas such as parkland. (See Chapter 5 for more details on artificial anchors.)

Placement of Anchors

Regardless of the type of anchor, placement of secure anchors depends very much on good judgment, which is developed through experience and practice. Although their specifics may vary from place to place, all anchors share certain characteristics.

Strength of Anchors

Anchors must be able to sustain the greatest anticipated force on the high angle system as calculated through the safety factor (see Chapter 3, p. 27, for the method for calculating a system safety factor). Anchors so strong they are able to withstand any force the high angle system can deliver to them are said to be *bombproof*.

If the potential anchor point cannot sustain the anticipated forces, it must be abandoned for another, more substantial one or joined with one or more other anchor points (multiple anchors are described later in this chapter).

An anchor's ability to withstand the necessary forces of a system depends on a number of factors, including the following:

- *The condition of the anchor.* A live tree, for example, usually can withstand greater forces than a dead one.
- *The structural nature of the anchor point.* A load-bearing structural column in a building generally can withstand greater forces than a handrail.
- *The location of force on the anchor point.* A tree with the force pulling on it near the ground generally can withstand greater force than a tree on which the stress is located higher up.

Direction of Pull on an Anchor Point

Always consider the direction of pull on the anchor point. Try to set anchors that are in line with the direction of pull. Also consider the effects if the direction of pull changes. Some anchors are rigged so that they are strong only when the pull comes from one direction. If the direction of pull changes, the anchor could weaken or fail.

Positioning of Anchors

The position of an anchor affects the high angle activity. This is particularly true in rescue activity. Ideally, the anchor should be close to and directly above the subject to be rescued. However, in some circumstances it might be preferable to have the anchor off to the side, such as when:

- Rocks or other dangerous objects might fall on the rescue subject or rescuers.
- Conditions exist between the anchor point and the rescue subject that could endanger rescuers or damage equipment such as rope.
- A flashover and fire erupt from a window.
- A hostile or deranged person is in the area.
- No suitable anchors are available directly above.

In any high angle activity, it often is desirable that segments of the high angle system, such as the belay rope, be off to the side to avoid rope cross or tangles. However, if the *primary anchor* (the one bearing the greatest load) is off at an extreme angle, problems could arise for those attempting to manage the rope work. For example, they might have to make a wide swing on the rope, or **pendulum**, to reach their objective. However, some anchoring techniques may solve such a problem.

Directionals

A **directional** is a technique for bringing a rope into a more favorable position or angle. Directionals can be created in many ways, and each method must be judged on its advantages and disadvantages specific to a given situation. Figure 7-1 shows two trees, wide apart, that could serve as strong anchors at the top of

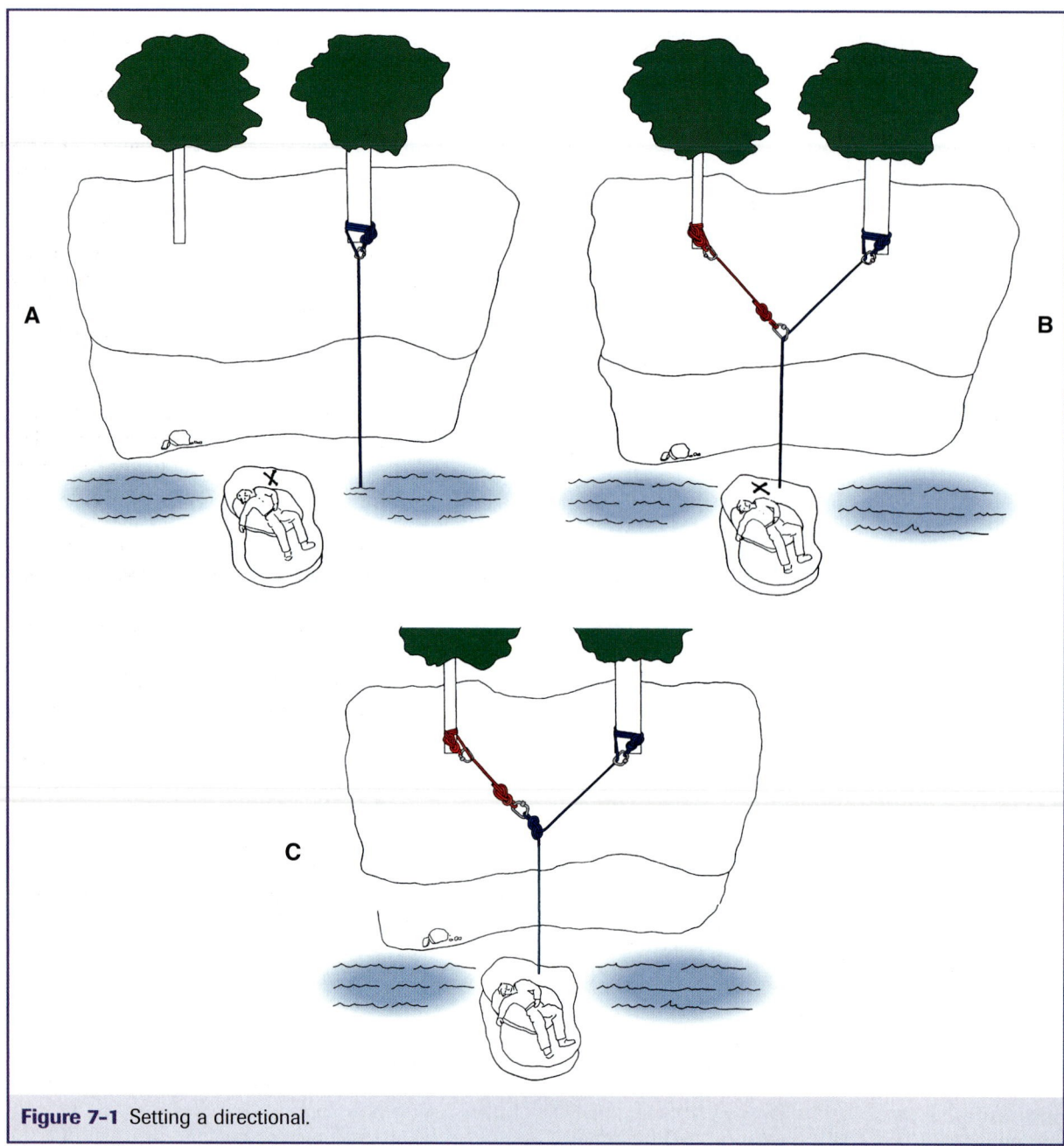

Figure 7-1 Setting a directional.

a cliff. However, say, for example, that you want to use the rope to reach spot X on the ground that is between the trees:

1. If you anchor the rope to either of the two trees (as has been done to the tree on the right in Figure 7-1, *A*), it would be difficult for you to reach spot X without a significant pendulum.
2. Now, say you add a secondary anchor, a directional, to the smaller tree on the left (Figure 7-1, *B*). In the end of this second rope, you tie a figure 8 on a bight knot and clip a locking carabiner into the figure 8 knot. Finally, you clip this locking carabiner across the main anchor rope. Thus the main rope is now at a better angle for you to reach X. One additional advantage with this approach is that the main rope runs freely through the carabiner so that as the exact position of the activity moves back and forth, the angle can change slightly.
3. A less desirable alternative would be to tie a figure 8 overhand knot in the main line and clip it directly into the carabiner on the directional (Figure 7-1, *C*). This would prevent the main line from sliding freely through the carabiner. It would also create a ***multipoint anchor***, but without the advantages of the example in no. 2 above (see Figure 7-1, *B*). When the rope moved to one side or the other, it would impose a great deal of loading on one anchor but very little on the other.

Location of Directionals

When you establish anchors and directionals, you must keep in mind how safe and accessible they are for the high angle personnel who work with them. In Figure 7-1, for example, you could possibly make some improvements by changing the location of the anchors and the directional. If anchor points, such as the trees, were available far enough back from the edge of the drop, you could rig the anchor system and the directional on the top. As a result:

1. Those rigging the anchors and the directional would be in less danger of falling.
2. The rigging would be more accessible and therefore more under the control of the rescuers.

⚠ Warning

1. Depending on the angle the primary anchor rope makes with the directional rope, greater forces could be exerted on the anchor system than if only a single anchor were used (see Figure 7-1, *B*). A directional, in effect, creates a multiple anchor system. (See the discussion later in this chapter on how multiple anchors create forces on the system, depending on the angles the ropes create.)
2. Depending on the specific situation, if the directional fails, a significant pendulum could result. This could cause the main line to drop along with the load, resulting in shock loading to the anchor, rope, and other system components. In addition, the rope could be severely damaged or cut.

---

3. With the rope running over the edge, not all the weight would be directly on the anchor. Part of it would be taken by the edge of the drop. (The drawback would be possible abrasion on the rope.)

Backing Up Anchors

Anchor systems present a number of opportunities for failure, including the following:

- *Uncertain strength of anchor points.* Anchor point failure is the most common cause of anchor system failure. It rarely can be determined for certain what kind of stress an anchor point will take.
- *Failures in human judgment and experience.* Knots may be tied incorrectly, or carabiner gates may be left unlocked.
- *Equipment failures.* Abrasion and cutting of rope and webbing and stressing of both hardware and software can occur.

Because of the potential for anchor system failure and because the rest of the high angle system depends on anchors, it is good practice to back up anchors. ***Backing up*** is the creation of redundant anchors for safety. There are two primary methods of backing up an anchor:

1. Backing up to the same anchor point (Figure 7-2, *A*). Do this only if you are absolutely certain the one anchor point can sustain any forces to which it might be subjected by the high angle system (i.e., it is bombproof). This type of backup is used when the possibility of failure exists in other portions of the anchor system (e.g., carabiners, knots, and slings).
2. Backing up to a separate anchor point (Figure 7-2, *B*). This requires a multiple anchor system. If the direction of loading will be shifting from side to side, you should make the multiple anchor system load sharing (load-sharing systems are explained later in this chapter).

The specific method of backing up the anchor system and the number of anchor points you need depend on a number of variables, including:

1. *The condition of the anchor points.* If the potential exists for failure of one of them or of the equipment attached to it, more than one anchor point is needed.
2. *The nature of the high angle operation.* If both a main line and a belay line are used, for example, you should use separate anchor systems. If the main line and the belay line originate from the same anchor point, the danger exists of line tangles or damage to the rope from rope cross (see Chapter 3 for information on avoiding damage from rope cross). The belay system would also have to be substantial enough to catch a fall, which means you would need a substantial second anchor.
3. *The loads and stresses involved in the system.* These vary in intensity depending on the ways in which the anchors are used, such as for:
   - Supporting only equipment
   - Supporting the weight of only one person
   - Creating directionals that create forces greater than the load *(load amplifiers)*
   - Rescue lowering operations

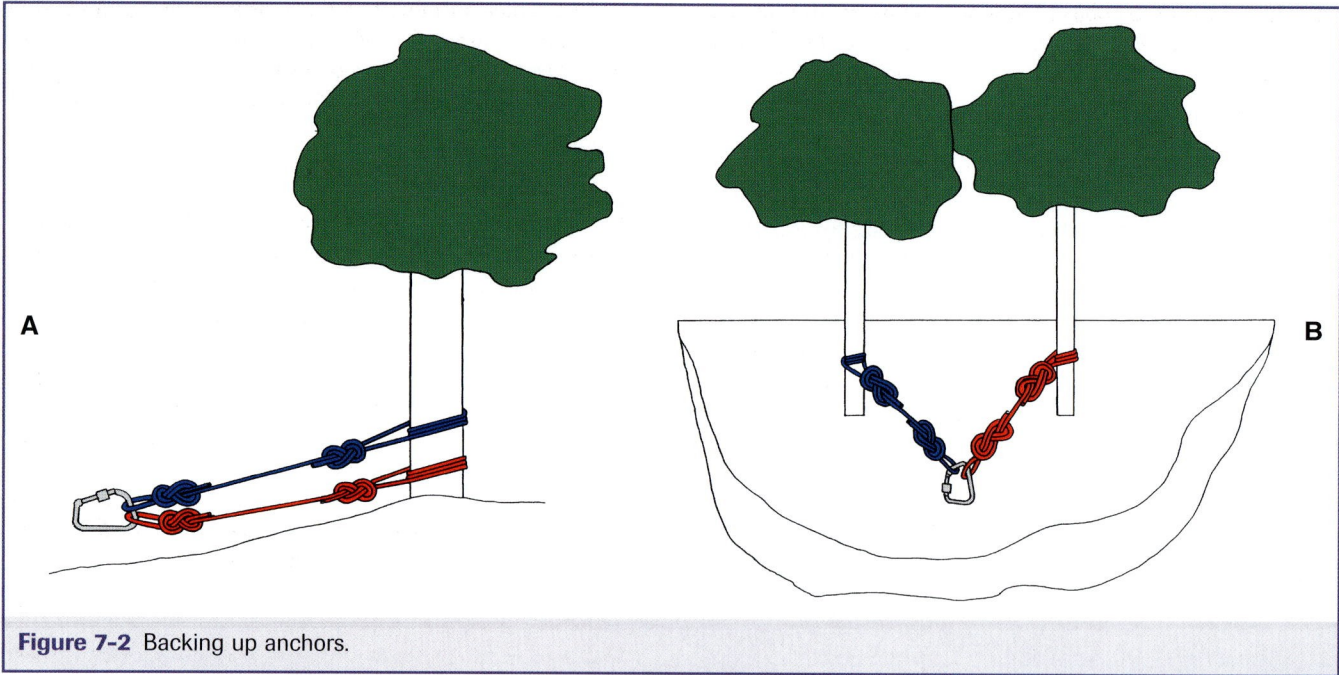

Figure 7-2 Backing up anchors.

- Hauling systems
- Highlines (a system of using a rope suspended between two points to move people or equipment)

Materials for Anchors
Using Rope for Anchors

One of the simplest procedures for establishing an anchor is to connect the main line rope directly to the anchor point. In urgent situations, in which time is critical, this may be the best solution. It also means a simpler anchor system, which reduces the number of components that might fail in a more complicated system.

However, rigging the main line rope directly to the anchor point limits the ability to modify the anchor system, and modifications could become necessary because of the changing conditions that can occur in rescue situations.

A possible solution is to use a separate piece of rope for the anchor system that is as strong or stronger than the main line and attach the main line to it as follows:

1. Attach the anchor rope to the anchor point.
2. Tie a figure 8 on a bight knot in the ends of both ropes where they will meet.
3. Clip the figure 8 knots together with carabiners.

Tie-Offs for Anchor Ropes

Tensionless Hitch One of the most attractive attachments for anchor ropes is the tensionless hitch (Box 7-1), also known as the *high-strength tie-off*. It has advantages as an anchor knot for three reasons:

- It is simple.
- It reduces stress on rope and equipment.
- It can be adapted to changing conditions.

The tensionless hitch is wrapped around an object so that the friction of the wrap takes the load. With enough friction, all the

---

Box 7-1	Procedure for Tying the Tensionless Hitch (High-Strength Tie-Off)

1. Take at least two wraps with the rope around the object to be used as the anchor point (Figure 7-3). The total number of wraps depends on the diameter of the anchor point and the coefficient of friction of the anchor point surface. A smaller diameter and slicker anchor point surface require more wraps, but at least two wraps should be taken on any anchor point. The objective is to have enough rope turns around the object so that no tension exists on the running end of the rope. Rather, the friction absorbs the tension on the turns of rope.

2. Make sure there is no rope cross in the turns. If the anchor is above the load, the rope should spiral upward with the running end at the top. This should be done in case the load has to be lowered slightly, and in effect could be done by using the tree or vertical object as a lowering device.

3. Tie a figure 8 on a bight in the running end of the rope and clip a locking carabiner into the figure 8 knot.

4. Clip the carabiner across the standing end of the rope at the bottom of the spiral. The spiral should be adjusted (this is easier to do with two people) to ensure that there is (1) no slack in the spiral and (2) no sharp angle where the carabiner is clipped across the standing end of the rope.

Alternative Approach

If you do not have a carabiner, you can use a hitch or knot to replace the figure 8 knot and carabiner. Tie off the end in a way that prevents the rope from unwinding around the object and without placing any bends in the loaded section of the rope. The recommended method of figure 8 on a bight and a carabiner is more secure.

force is applied to the object the rope is wrapped around. The end of the rope is tied off without any of the force of the load on the hitch itself; hence the term *tensionless hitch*. When the rope is tied correctly, it is not weakened by a knot and therefore retains its full strength. This assumes that the size of the object is more than four times the diameter of the rope (Box 7-2).

Box 7-2	**Uses of the Tensionless Hitch**

The tensionless hitch can be used on an anchor point around which you can wrap rope; the anchor point must be able to withstand the stress of the forces in the system and must not be damaging to the rope. Examples of such points are trees, columns, and structural beams.

⚠ *Warning*

1. The tensionless hitch works only if adequate surface contact is present between the rope and the object. If the shape of the object does not allow adequate contact, choose another method of anchoring to it. For example, an H-shaped beam has rope contact only in four places; a tensionless hitch will not work in this case.
2. If the anchor point has sharp edges, as are sometimes found on structural beams, the rope should be padded appropriately (see Chapter 4).

Anchoring with the Figure 8 Follow-Through The figure 8 follow-through knot also can be used in rope for anchoring. It has less flexibility for making changes than the tensionless hitch and may result in greater stress on the knot. However, when lighter loads will be placed on the anchor system, the figure 8 follow-through may be preferable because it may be quicker to tie. As with the tensionless hitch, it is used when a loop of rope cannot be placed over the top or around the ends of an anchor point but must be tied around it, such as with a tree or structural column. (See Chapter 6, p. 72, for instructions on how to tie a figure 8 follow-through knot.)

If the vertical member to be used as an anchor point is short enough for you to easily get a loop of rope over it, you can tie a figure 8 on a bight in the end of the rope and place the loop over the anchor. (See Chapter 6, p. 71, for instructions on how to tie a figure 8 on a bight.)

Alternative Approach: Use of a Bowline

If local policy mandates the use of a bowline for tying a loop in a rope, such as for a simple anchor, you must use a bowline in the place of a figure 8 follow-through or a figure 8 on a bight. However, you should take the following precautions:

- Because the bowline is easy to tie incorrectly, carefully inspect the knot to ensure that it is tied correctly. (Figure 6-7, p. 72, shows a simple bowline correctly tied.)
- Back up the bowline with a keeper knot such as the double overhand knot *(barrel knot)*.
- Before loading the bowline, pretension it to tighten it.
- Make sure the bowline is not subjected to loading from a direction other than the intended one.

Use of Webbing for Anchors

Webbing is a convenient material for anchoring. It also is convenient for making continuous loops known as *runners* or *slings*.

Advantages

- Less expensive than rope
- Fewer knots to learn

Disadvantages

- Cannot be tied into as many different knots as rope.
- Does not absorb shock loading as well as most ropes.

Presewn Slings

Properly sewn runners often are used as a quick, convenient means of setting anchors. Two advantages of presewn slings are that they are quicker to use and there is less chance of tying the wrong knot when making a continuous loop. Several brands of presewn slings are available that can be used for anchoring.

Presewn slings are available in a variety of webbing widths and lengths (Figure 7-4). Many of the slings are sewn with loops in both ends. When buying presewn slings, make sure they have adequate tensile strength for the safety factors you are likely to

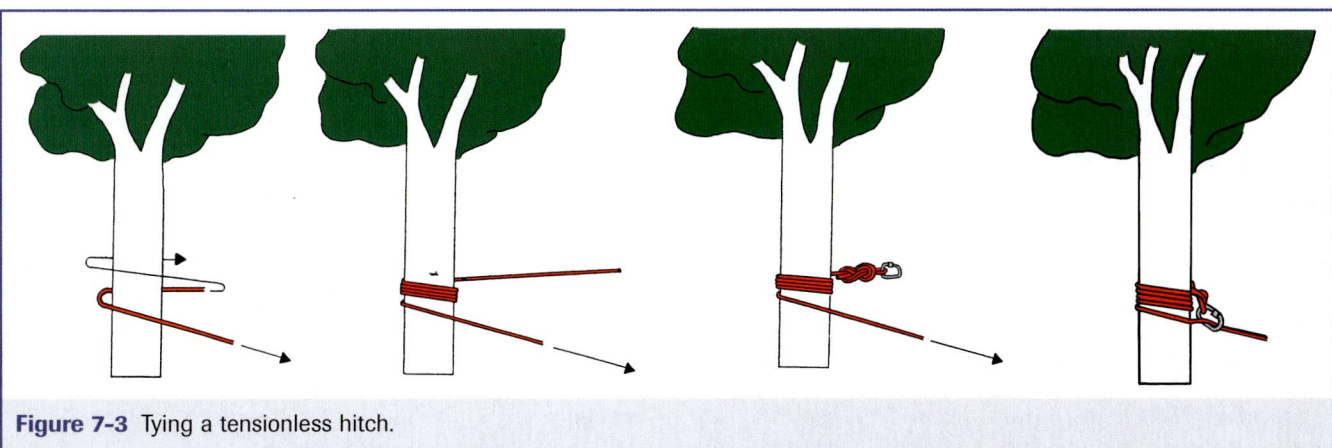

Figure 7-3 Tying a tensionless hitch.

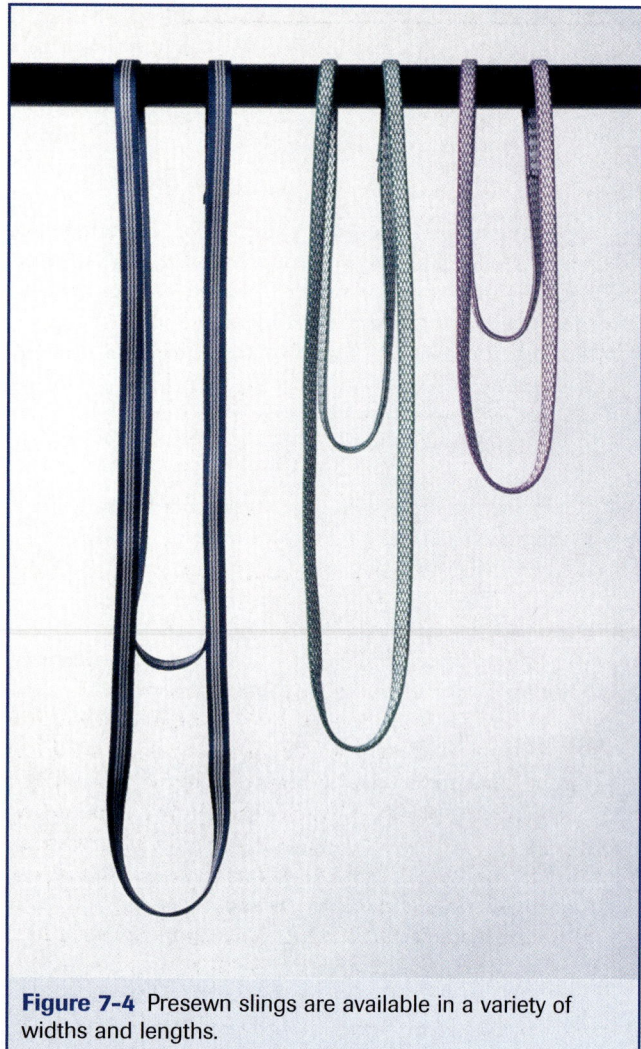

Figure 7-4 Presewn slings are available in a variety of widths and lengths.

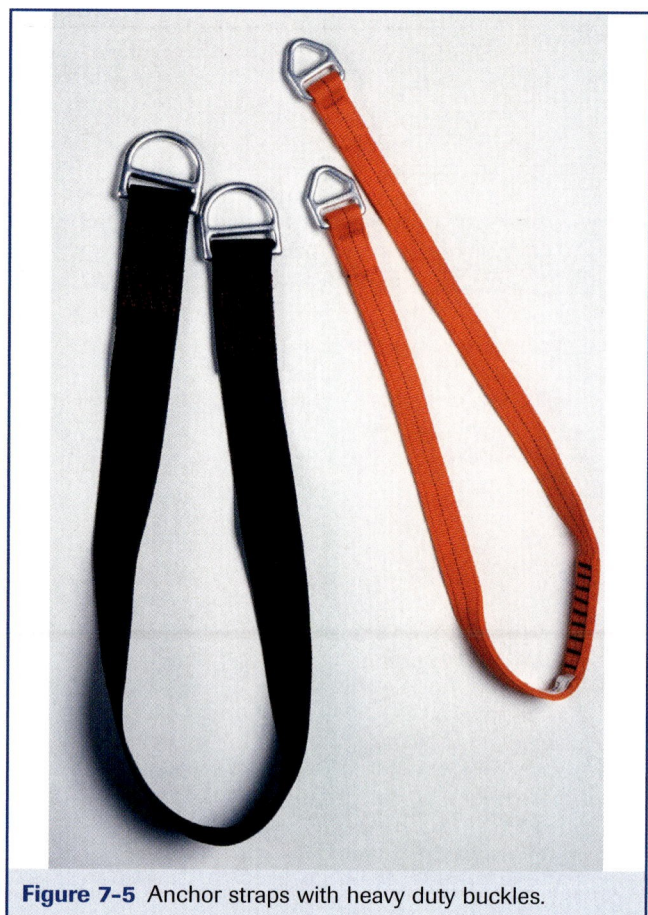

Figure 7-5 Anchor straps with heavy duty buckles.

need. Also, make sure you know how the manufacturer of the presewn slings tests them for strength. Anchor slings can have strength ratings based on being pulled end to end, pulled when rigged using a basket technique, (wrapped around the anchor), or pulled when girth hitched around an object. Before and after you use presewn webbing, always inspect it for wear on the stitching and the web material.

Anchor Straps

Anchor straps are webbing lengths with D rings sewn into each end where a carabiner can be clipped. These straps can be a quick way of setting reliable anchors. Anchor straps come in two basic types. The heavy duty ones (with the NFPA *G* designation) typically have an end-to-end breaking strength of about 8,000 pounds (35.6 kN). The lighter weight versions (NFPA rated *L*) typically have an end-to-end breaking strength of about 4,945 pounds (22 kN). Strap breaking strengths may be higher when the straps are rigged to form a basket.

Some anchor straps have a heavy duty buckle so that the strap can be adjusted to various lengths (Figure 7-5). However, the buckle may slip with a force less than the strap's overall breaking strength. In addition to anchoring, some of these straps can be used for such purposes as litter bridles or as a quick anchor for an edge attendant. As with other presewn slings, make sure the anchor straps you use have adequate tensile strength for your system safety factor. In addition, make sure the manufacturer can provide you with specifications on how much loading causes the adjustable buckle to slip.

Creating Slings from Webbing Lengths

If you do not use sewn runners, you can create a sling from a piece of webbing by tying it into a loop using a ring bend knot (also known as a *water knot, overhand bend, or tape knot*). (See Chapter 6, p. 74, for instructions on how to tie a ring bend knot.)

Placement of Webbing Around Anchor Points

A secure method of placing webbing around an anchor point is to tie it in a loop around the point using a ring bend knot (Figure 7-6). However, if the object used as the anchor point is very large, this procedure can be awkward and time-consuming for one person.

An alternative method is to tie the runner first, wrap it around the anchor point, and then clip the two ends together with a carabiner (Figure 7-7). Such tied runners, however, require double the length of an untied length of webbing.

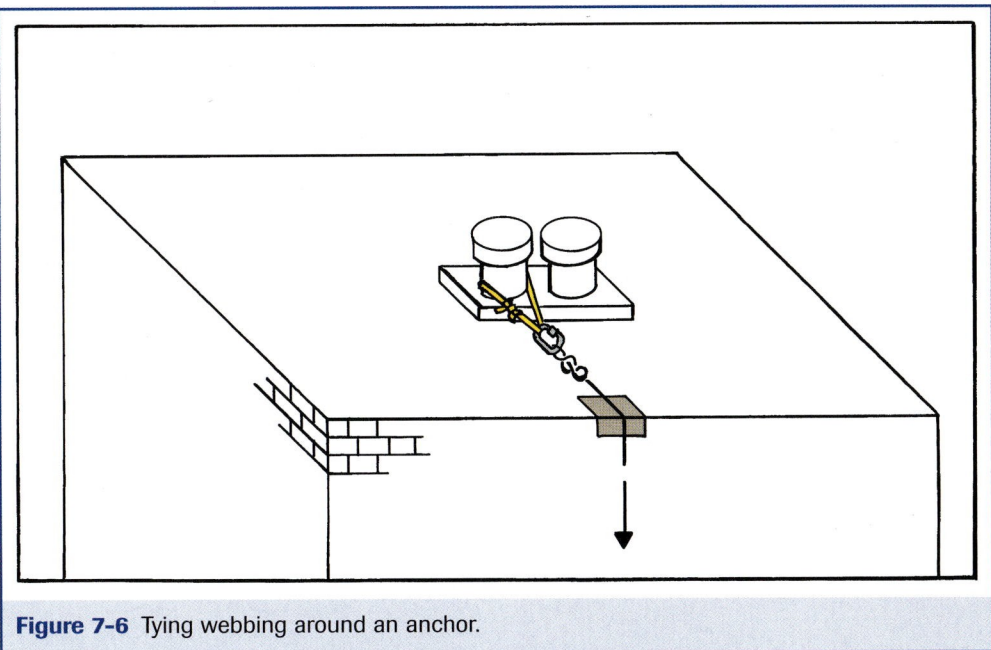

Figure 7-6 Tying webbing around an anchor.

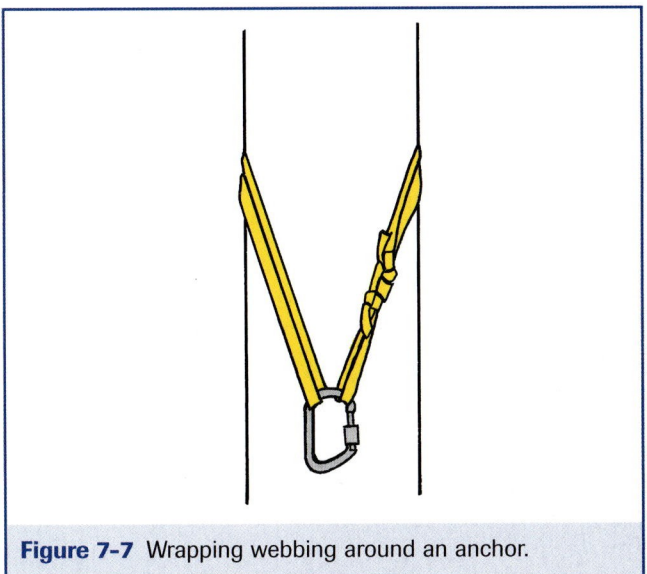

Figure 7-7 Wrapping webbing around an anchor.

Keeping Anchors in Place

It generally is good practice to tie an anchor on a vertical member as low as possible to reduce the stress on it.

However, with a strong enough anchor point, there may be certain conditions in which it would be advantageous to tie the anchor webbing higher up because:

- This usually creates a better angle for a rappeller to get over the difficult edge of a drop.
- Rope abrasion on an edge may be reduced.
- In a rescue operation, a higher angle might improve conditions for lowering a stretcher over an edge.
- Severe friction that is stressing a hauling system may be reduced.

The problem is that a simple loop of webbing around a vertical anchor tends to slip down on the anchor. A conventional method for holding the webbing in place is to tie it around the anchor point in a girth hitch (Figure 7-8, *A*). The drawback to this technique is the temptation to cinch the webbing back on itself (Figure 7-8, *B*). *This should not be done, because it puts potentially dangerous stress on the webbing.*

A stronger alternative to the girth hitch is the *wrap 3, pull 2 system* (Figure 7-8, *C*). In this system, there are three wraps around the anchor with two loops pulled out. Note that for maximum strength, the webbing knot is on the interior loop, where it will incur the least stress.

Anchor Plates

Anchor plates (Figure 7-9) help organize the anchor rigging and prevent it from jamming. They can make the various components easier to see and can make rigging of anchor systems more accurate. Anchor plates commonly are used where multiple lines

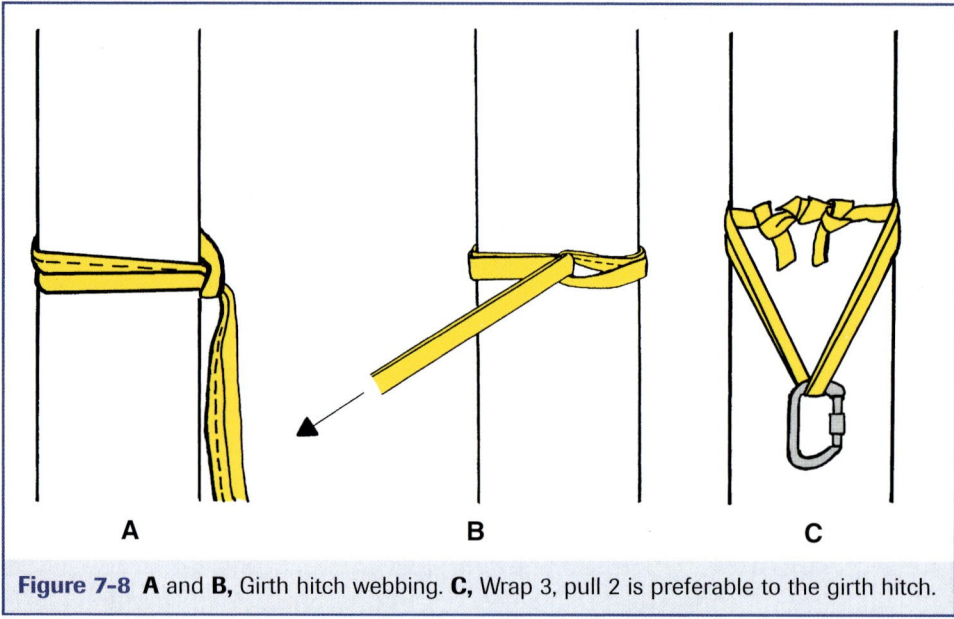

Figure 7-8 A and **B,** Girth hitch webbing. **C,** Wrap 3, pull 2 is preferable to the girth hitch.

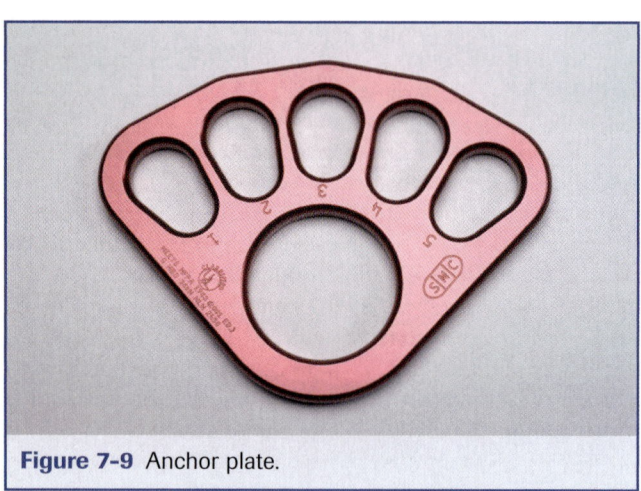

Figure 7-9 Anchor plate.

come together at a common point, for example, where multiple lines need to be clipped into a master attachment point or where multiple anchor lines are collected at one point.

Look for anchor plates that are strong (NFPA rated *G*) and that have contoured edges that are less likely to damage rope and carabiners. The holes should be large enough to accept large locking carabiners easily.

Anchor plates also can be used for other purposes, such as rigging for litters (see Chapter 15).

What to Do When No Anchors Appear to Be Available

Extending Anchors

Although anchors sometimes may not be found nearby, you may be able to establish them by running lengths of rope, sometimes for a few hundred feet, to suitable objects. *This should be done*

only with static rope. Attempting to extend anchors in such a manner with dynamic rope could create a dangerous situation because of the large amount of stretch. Even with static rope, undesirable stretch may occur if only one line is used. Depending on the load, the lines can be doubled, tripled, or quadrupled to reduce the stretch.

An example of a situation in which extended anchors might work would be the roof of a building where (absolutely, positively) no anchor points exist. Often, static rope can be run through a stairwell or the top-floor windows to lower floors where anchors exist.

Using Vehicles for Anchors

A sort of "portable anchor" that usually is available is an emergency vehicle. However, you must observe the following safety guidelines when using a vehicle for an anchor:

1. Park the vehicle on a solid surface. High load forces can drag a vehicle across loose material, such as gravel.
2. Set the parking brakes.
3. If the vehicle has an automatic transmission, set it in "park." If it has a manual transmission, set it in a gear in opposition to the pull (e.g., "reverse" if the pull is from the front).
4. Chock the wheels. Forces created in a high angle system can move a vehicle with its brakes set. If no chocks are available, use spare tires.
5. "Idiot-proof" your portable anchor by removing the ignition key. Further disable the starting system by pulling the coil wire.

Potential anchor points in a vehicle include structural parts, such as axles and cross members. However, be sure to protect rope and webbing from oil and grease. Furthermore, as noted in Chapter 4, rope and webbing also must be protected from destructive substances such as battery acids, which often are found around vehicles.

Some parts of a vehicle are structurally weak and should not be used. These are:

- Bumpers
- Tow hooks (often these have been subjected to intense and unrecorded stress and therefore have the potential to fail)

Portable Anchors

Portable anchors are prefabricated anchors that can be moved from place to place. They usually serve as directionals in places where no anchors are available for attaching a directional, such as in confined spaces or over a space such as a manhole. A common example of a portable anchor is the tripod (see Figure 18-8, p. 286). Another example of a portable anchor is the beam clamp (Figure 7-10). Beam clamps can be quickly attached to overhead structures such as steel beams. Some meet the anchorage requirements for one-person loads set by the American National Standards Institute (ANSI), the Canadian Standards Association (CSA), and the U.S. Occupational Safety and Health Administration (OSHA); 5400 lbf (24 kN). For high loads, two or more beam clamps should be used together as multipoint anchors.

Pickets

A picket system is an alternative in a natural area where no anchors are available. Although a picket system can work very well when correctly rigged, establishing it properly usually takes a great deal of time. In addition, not all soil types can hold pickets securely. Loose, sandy, or muddy soil, or snow, may not hold well regardless of the number of pickets used.

Most picket anchor systems consist of several rows of pickets. Figure 7-11 and Box 7-3 explain the construction of one row.

Multipoint Anchors

Multipoint anchors involve two or more anchor points. Multipoint anchors are used when one anchor point is insufficient to withstand the anticipated forces or when one anchor point is inconveniently placed.

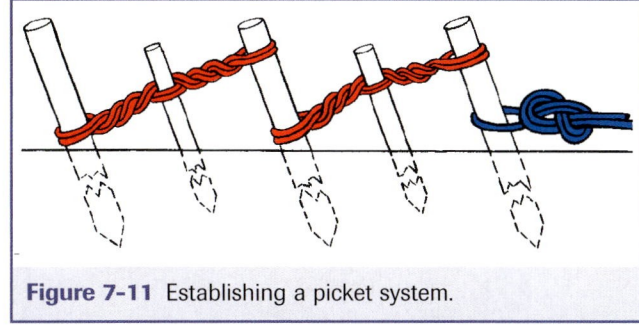

Figure 7-11 Establishing a picket system.

Box 7-3	**Establishing a Picket System**

1. The pickets should have a minimum length of 5 feet (1.5 m) so that a minimum of 3 feet (1 m) is in the ground and a maximum of 2 feet (0.5 m) is above ground.
2. Drive the pickets at an angle of 15 degrees away from the force to be anchored.
3. Connect the pickets in each row by lashing from the top of the first picket (the one closest to the load) to the bottom of the next picket close to the ground. Continue in this manner until all the pickets in the row have been lashed together.
4. Tension the lashings by twisting them with a stick four to six turns. Drive this stick into the ground to secure it.
5. Construct the next rows of pickets as described above.
6. Connect the main line by clipping it to the front picket in each row with a load-sharing anchor system.

Multiple Slings on a Single Anchor Point

By adding attachments to an appropriate anchor point, you can help prevent the collapse of an anchor system caused by the failure of a single item, such as webbing, a carabiner, or improperly tied knots. Figure 7-12 shows the use of two slings of equal length on a single anchor point. This kind of system is used only when the single anchor point is absolutely secure (bombproof). *There is no insurance at all in the additional webbing and carabiners if the anchor point fails.*

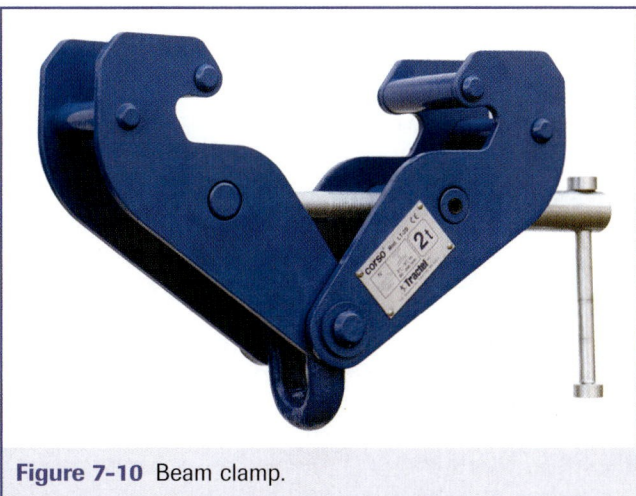

Figure 7-10 Beam clamp.

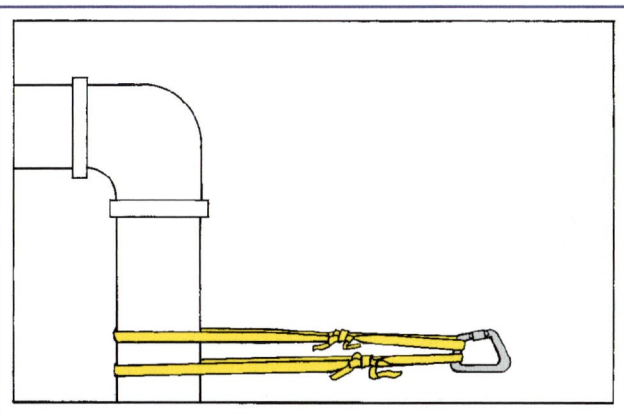

Figure 7-12 Two slings back up one another on a single anchor.

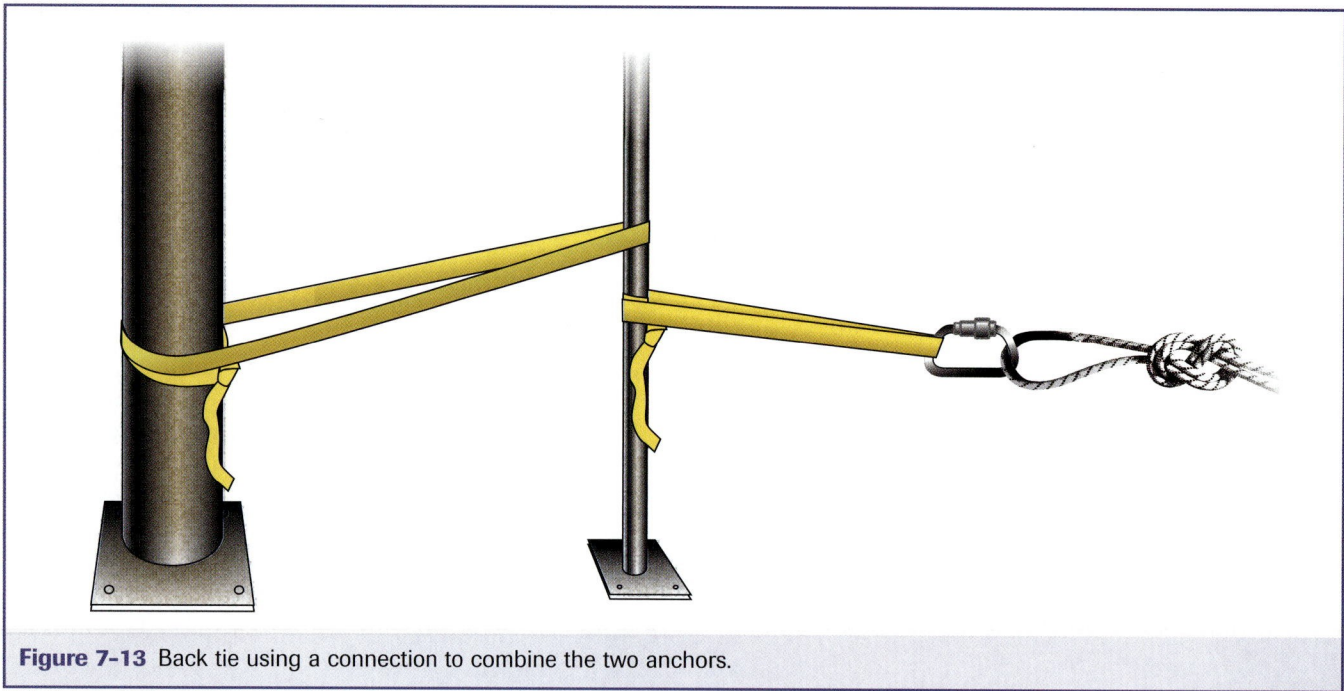

Figure 7-13 Back tie using a connection to combine the two anchors.

Backing Up Anchors

It is good practice to back up single anchors with a second anchor. Backing up is essential when you have an anchor that is in the right position but not strong enough alone for a rescue load. In Figure 7-13 the anchor point on the right is near the edge and in a good position, but it does not have the strength to take the load. You might consider this a *primary anchor.*

Behind the primary anchor and directly in line with it is a second anchor. The strength of this *secondary anchor,* combined with that of the primary anchor, will be enough to sustain the rescue load.

To combine the two anchors, a rope or sling is run between them; this connector is known as a **back tie**.

Two things must be kept in mind when using a secondary anchor:

1. The secondary anchor must be *as strong as or stronger* than the primary anchor.
2. The back tie must have no slack that would allow shock loading, which could cause both anchors to fail.

Pretensioned Back Ties

Anchor systems often have inherent slack caused by rope or webbing stretch and by flexing of anchor points. If such anchor systems receive shock loading, the elements could fail. One way to lessen the chance of shock loading is with a pretensioned back tie. A pretensioned back tie is a method of removing slack in a back-tied anchor system before it is loaded (Figure 7-14).

One technique for creating a pretensioned back tie is to connect with rope two anchor points tensioned with a simple mechanical advantage system. The following steps are used to construct the system shown in Figure 7-14:

1. Place wrap 3, pull 2 webbing attachments on each anchor facing one another.

2. Pace a large locking carabiner in each of the web attachments.
3. Use a length of rope to create a simple 3:1 mechanical advantage system using the carabiners.
4. Start by attaching the rope to the carabiner at the rear anchor.
5. Run the rope through the forward carabiner and back through the rear carabiner, and pull it forward until it almost reaches the front carabiner.
6. Tension the simple hauling system using two people. After the initial tensioning, vector the system by pulling it back and forth sideways to remove additional slack.
7. While maintaining the tension, tie off the system near the front carabiner using half hitches.

NOTE: The pretensioned back ties should be close to in line with the direction of pull of the lowering or hauling system or highline. They should never be more than 15 degrees off to either side.

Load-Sharing Anchors

If anchor points are at all questionable or are inconveniently placed, **load-sharing anchors** may be a solution. The simplest way to create a multiple anchor system for load sharing is to use two anchor ropes or slings of equal length. Run them from different anchor points and clip them together into a single point using one or two large locking carabiners (Figure 7-15). The point where you clip the two lines together with the carabiners is known as a **master attachment point**. In load-sharing anchors, a master attachment point is the point where the multiple lines come together.

Load-Distributing Anchors

A major problem with a fixed, load-sharing anchor system such as that shown in Figure 7-17, *A*, is that the stress on the anchor

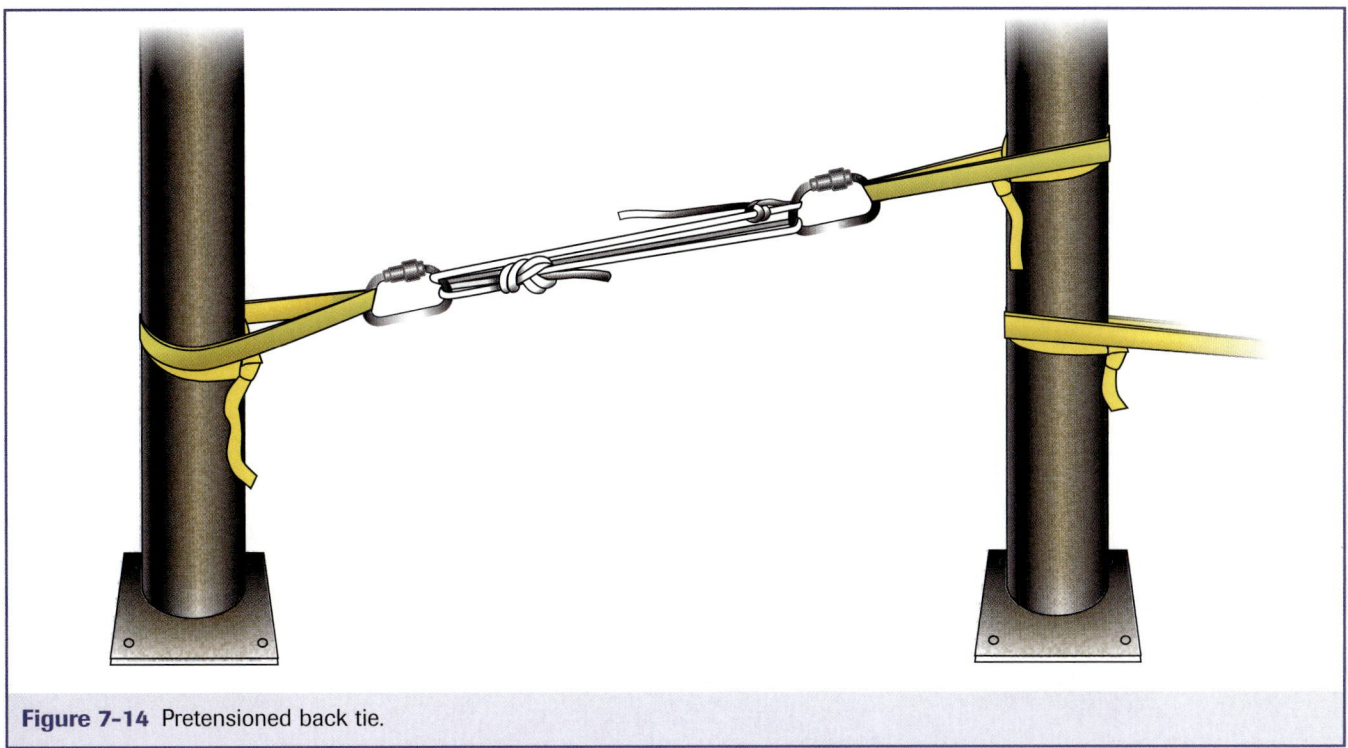

Figure 7-14 Pretensioned back tie.

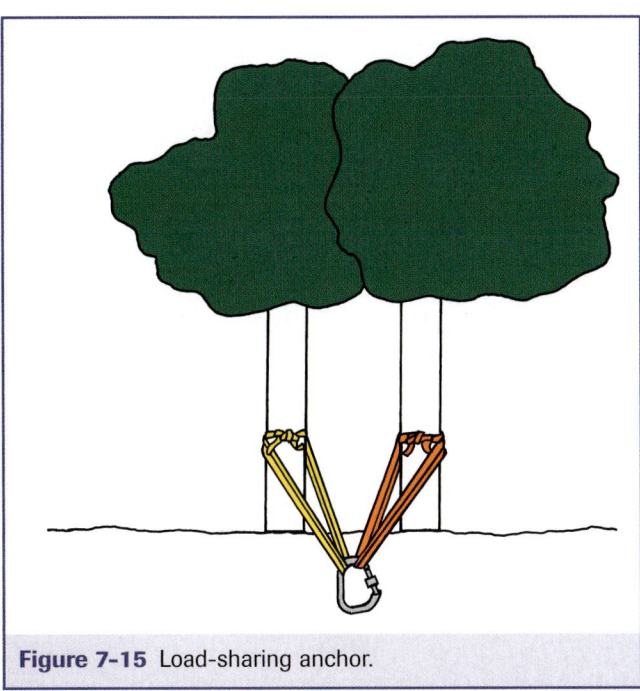

Figure 7-15 Load-sharing anchor.

points is equal only when the force from the main line pulls directly in the center of the angle. This often is not the case in high angle operations. Most of the time, the force pulls to one side or the other (Figure 7-17, *B*). It also may move back and forth from side to side. Obviously, if the possibility exists that either of the anchor points cannot sustain these side-to-side forces, the entire anchor system may fail.

A possible solution to this problem is to create a **load-distributing anchor system (LDA)**. This type of system, when correctly constructed and when conditions are right, can have some important advantages:

1. The forces on anchor points should remain distributed and shared by all anchor points, whatever the direction of pull.
2. If any anchor point fails, the system should readjust to help redistribute loading on the remaining anchor point or points.

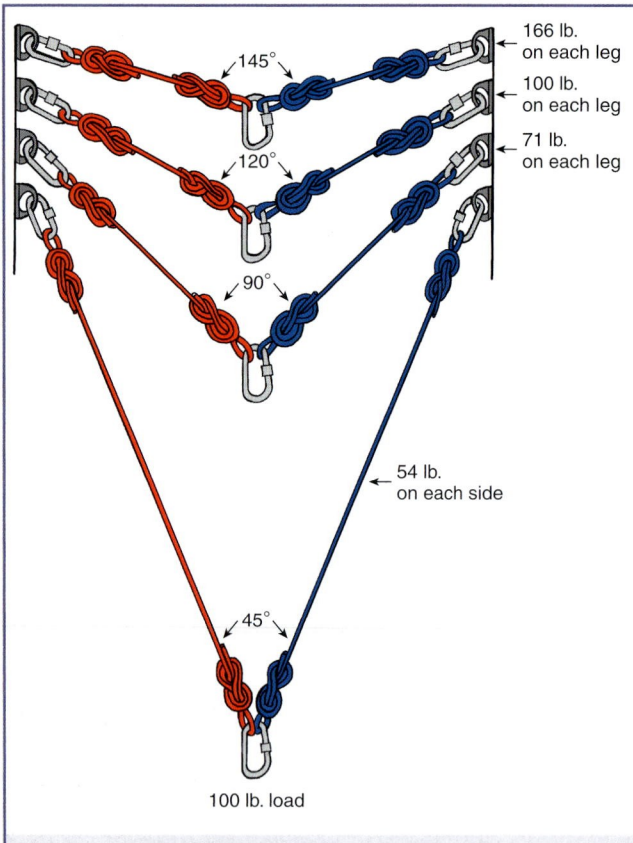

Figure 7-16 Relationship between anchor sling tension and a 100-pound (45 kg) load at different angles.

LDAs are sometimes called *self-equalizing anchors*. However, it is important to note that no anchor system can be made completely "self-equalizing" because:

- With the angles involved in rigging any LDA, the elements of the system are subject to varying forces, and the system therefore can never be completely equalized.
- In a shock loading situation, redistribution of forces does not occur instantaneously. During this transition to redistribution, some elements of the LDA system receive greater loads than others.

It is critical that all rescuers realize that LDAs are not for casual use in rescue. Because of their complexity and potential for failure, these systems should be used only when there are no other options, such as load-sharing or extending anchors.

Load-distributing anchors may be the only option, particularly in natural environments where rescuers are using artificial anchors. They also can be used in low-load situations when it is known in advance that the angle of the pull will be changing, such as in a low angle litter evacuation (see Chapter 16) in which the litter must be walked around an obstacle.

The following guidelines can help ensure the best distribution of forces and adaptation to shock loading with failure of an anchor point:

- Keep the angles small, both to reduce magnification of forces on anchors and to help the system readjust to the new loading.

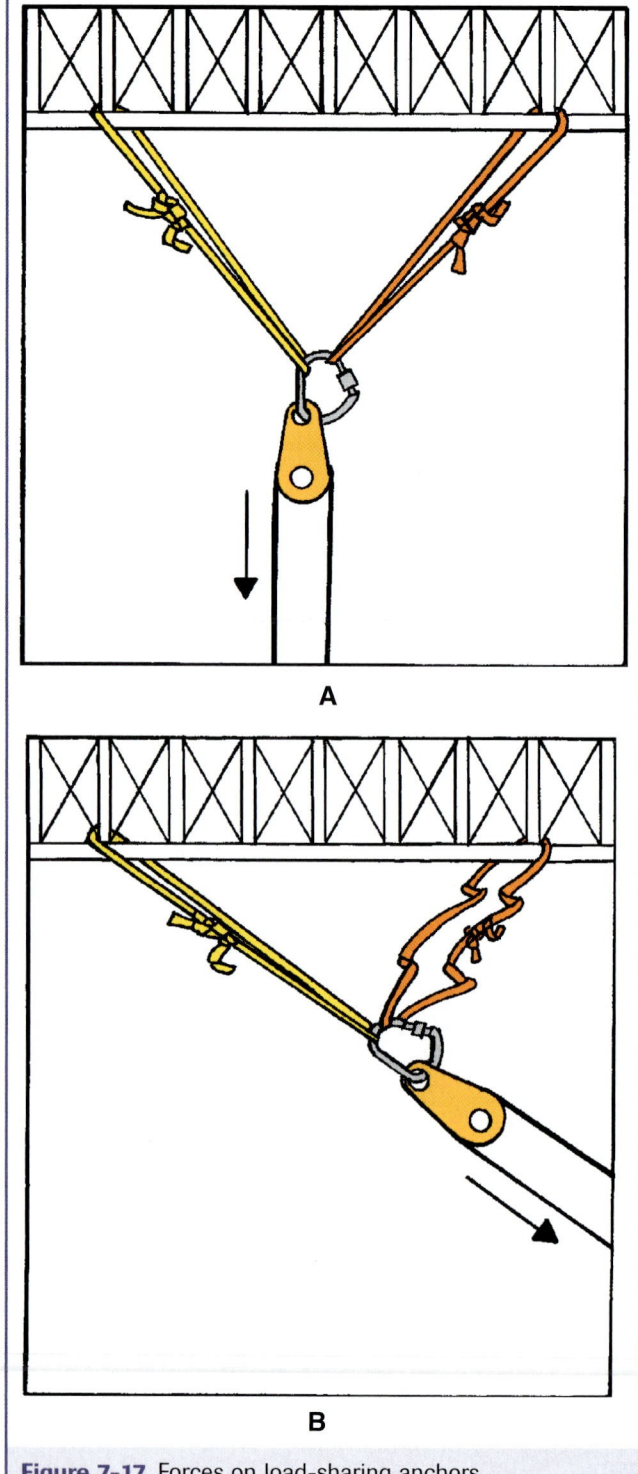

Figure 7-17 Forces on load-sharing anchors.

- Design the systems so that as little drop as possible would occur should any anchor fail. One way to do this is to keep the anchor legs as small as possible.
- Do not use bulky rope or webbing and adjust the system so that knots are less likely to run through carabiners when the system readjusts.

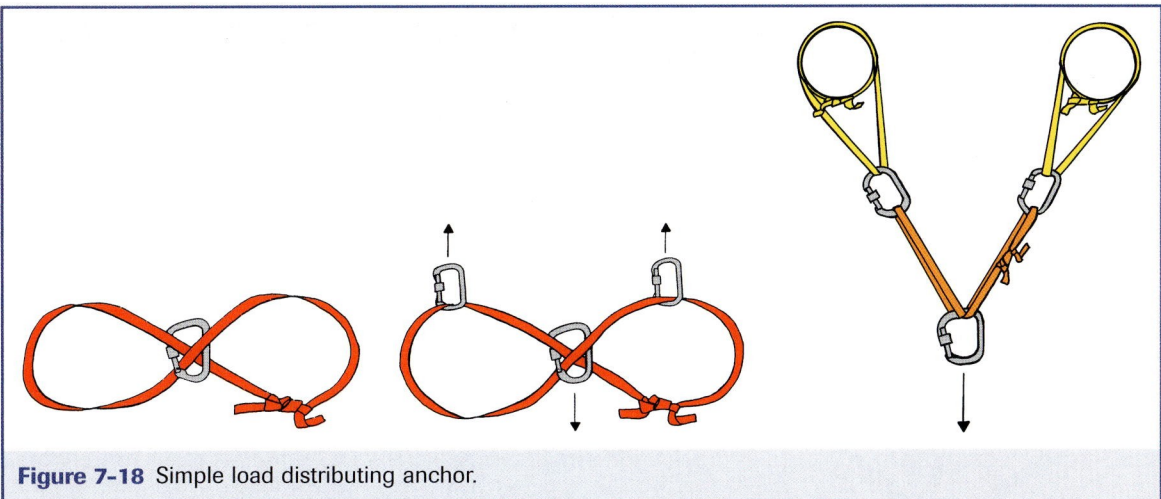

Figure 7-18 Simple load distributing anchor.

- Use Kevlar or Spectra in an anchor system only if you include shock-absorbing materials somewhere in the system; rope and webbing made of materials such as Kevlar and Spectra do not have the shock-absorbing qualities of materials such as nylon.
- Make all the anchor points in a load-distributing system as bombproof as possible.

Simple Two-Point, Load-Distributing Anchor System One of the simplest self-equalizing anchors involves two anchor points and uses a sling and a carabiner.

Creating a Simple Two-Point, Load-Distributing Anchor (Figure 7-18)

1. Configure a loop of webbing or rope in the shape of an **8**.
2. Clip a large locking carabiner across the inside loop.
3. Take each end of an outside loop and clip it into an anchor point.
4. Clip the carabiner on the inside loop into the main line. This will be the focal point for the anchor system.
5. Make sure the angles made by the sling do not exceed the critical ones described in the Warning box on p. 91.
6. Before loading the system, test it by hand. One at a time, simulate failure of each one of the anchors to make sure the system catches the load.

Whatever the direction of the pull, the central carabiner should slip along the sling to equalize the forces. Should one anchor point fail, the webbing should set itself to pull on the other anchor point.

Tying a Load-Distributing Anchor System Using a Two-Loop Figure 8 (Figure 7-19)

1. Create a large loop by using a length of rope and tying the two ends together using a figure **8** bend (or double fisherman's knot).

2. For ease of operation, set the circle of rope on the ground or the floor.
3. Place the knot at about 3 o'clock or 9 o'clock on the circle so that it remains out of the way.
4. Take a large bight of rope and flip it back inside the circle about two thirds of the way up.
5. The lower section of the circle is now doubled, so that there are four strands of rope.
6. Gather these four strands of rope together and tie a figure **8** knot with them.
7. At the top of the circle, there is now a large loop with a smaller loop inside. To reduce shock loading, keep the size of the large loop to a minimum, with a circumference of no more than 8 feet. At the bottom of the circle is a much smaller loop created by tying the figure **8** from the four strands.
8. Take the larger loop at the top of the circle and clip it into all the anchor points using a locking carabiner at each point.
9. Take the smaller loop at the bottom of the large loop. Using locking carabiners, clip this to the larger loop between each anchor point.
10. Take the small loop below the knot created from the four strands. Clip this into the main line using one or two large locking carabiners. This is the focal point for the anchor system.
11. If the system is tied correctly, should any one point fail, the load should be redistributed among the remaining anchor points. The system should also distribute the load among all points whatever direction the load is coming from.
12. The riggers should inspect the system to make sure it will indeed perform in this manner before the system is loaded by people. If any problems are noted, such as a knot jamming, the system must be adjusted so that it will work as intended.

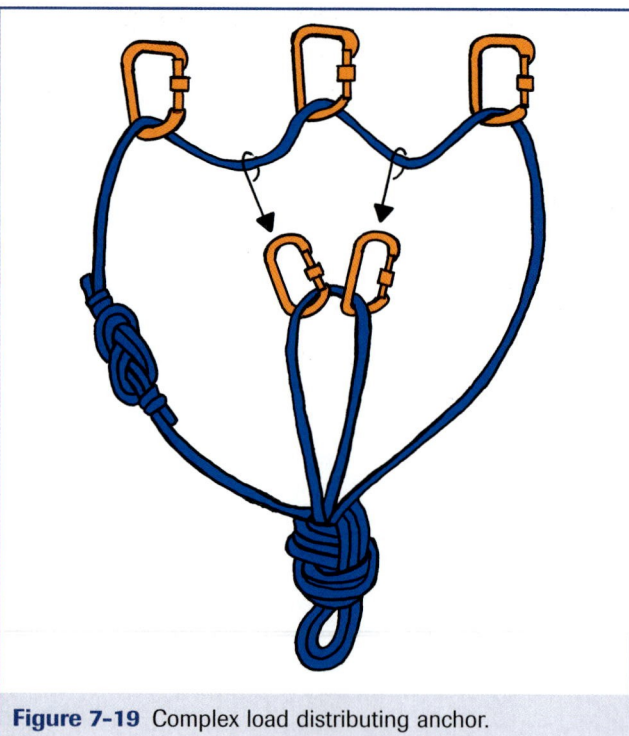

Figure 7-19 Complex load distributing anchor.

Evaluation Exercises

Cognitive and Affective Exercises

1. Name three factors that affect the ability of an anchor point to withstand the forces of high angle activity.

2. Give three situations in which anchors should not be set directly above the high angle activity, but rather off to the side.

3. What is the purpose of a directional in an anchor system?

4. What would be the possible disadvantage of tying the main line directly into an anchor point?

5. What are three advantages of using the tensionless hitch, or high-strength tie-off, in an anchor system?

6. When a tree is examined for use as a potential anchor point, attention should be paid not only to the soundness of the wood but also to the nature of the _____.

7. Why is it imprudent to leave knots tied in webbing (unless each runner is carefully inspected before use)?

8. How should webbing be tied to hold it in place on a vertical anchor point?

9. Name two typical reasons why anchor points on buildings may be inadequate.

10. List three potential anchor points on buildings that are inherent parts of the structure.

11. Name the parts of a vehicle that:

    A. Should not be used as anchor points.
    B. Might be used as anchor points.

12. Give two situations in which complex anchors are used.

13. Ideally, the angle between the legs of an anchor system should not be more than _____ degrees, and they should never be more than _____ degrees.

14. Describe two ways to reduce the potential for shock loading when rigging LDAs.

Psychomotor Exercises

15. Create a directional on an anchor system that initially was set at an inconvenient angle.

16. Set a tensionless hitch (high-strength tie-off) on a tree or column for a downward pull.

17. Perform the following correctly:

    A. Tie a runner from webbing in a simple loop around a vertical anchor point.
    B. Tie a loop from a rope around the same anchor point.

18. Using an internal loop, set a runner tied from webbing around a tree or column so that it will not slip down.

19. Correctly set an anchor on a building using an anchor point that is an integral part of the structure. (NOTE: If a training tower or similar structure is used, the student should not use any anchor points previously prepared, such as ring bolts.)

20. Using webbing or rope on an anchor system with two anchor points, demonstrate the following:

    A. The angle that the two legs of the anchor should not exceed.
    B. The angle that the two legs must not exceed.

21. Correctly tie a load-sharing anchor using two anchor points.

22. Correctly tie a load-distributing anchor using a webbing loop on two anchor points.

23. Correctly set a load-distributing anchor system using three or more anchor points.

8

Belaying of One-Person Loads

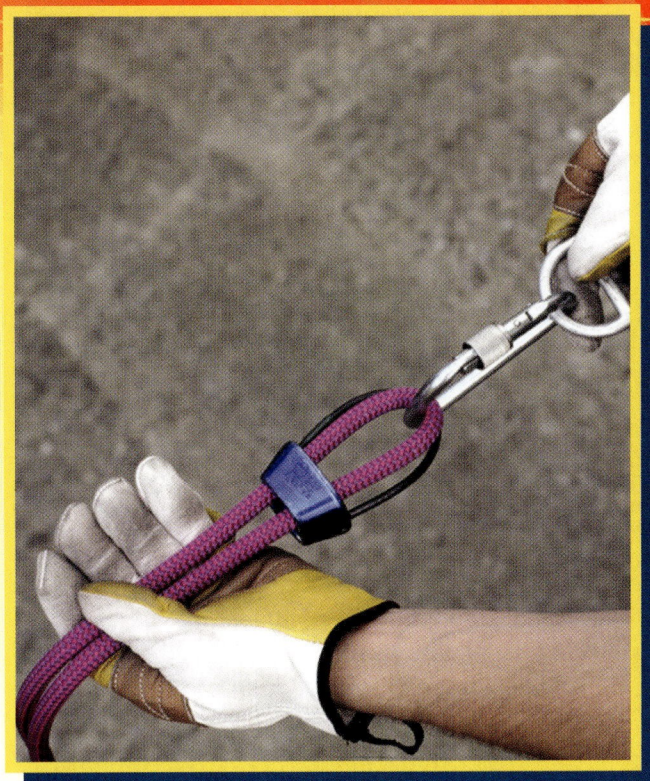

Prerequisites

Before attempting the activities described in this chapter, you must have demonstrated that you can properly:

1. Use and care for rope.
2. Use and care for other equipment needed in the high angle environment.
3. Tie correctly and without hesitation the knots necessary for safe, effective work in the vertical environment (see Chapter 6).
4. Apply the principles of anchoring and rig a secure anchor.

Objectives

On completion of this chapter, you should be able to:

1. Define belaying.
2. Distinguish between belay of one-person and belay of a rescue load.
3. List the elements of a belay system.
4. Describe situations that might require a belay.
5. Repeat from memory and in sequence the belay voice communications.
6. Belay a person using a Münter hitch.
7. Belay a person using a one-person belay device.
8. Discuss why it is necessary to have both complete knowledge of and thorough practice in belaying before attempting to belay a person in an actual high angle situation.

The material in this chapter conforms to guidelines published by the National Fire Protection Association (NFPA), specifically standard 1006, *Professional Qualifications for Rescue Technicians* (2002). NFPA standards are revised regularly, and readers are advised to review the latest version of this standard.

Key Terms

Belay To protect against falling by managing an unloaded rope (the belay rope) in a way that secures one or more individuals in case the main line rope or support fails.

Belay Device A braking mechanism through which a secondary line, also called the belay line, is rigged. The device must allow free run of the belay rope through it when the system is operating correctly; it must exert a slowing or stopping action on the belay line if an uncontrolled descent or fall occurs on the main line.

Belayer Person responsible for operation of the belay.

Belay Line The line attached to one or more individuals that provides protection against a fall or system failure.

Belay Plate A common type of belay device; it is a simple metal plate with one or more slots for rope that is used in conjunction with a carabiner to exert friction on a belay rope.

Lowering The process and system by which a load is lowered while controlled from above. A lowering rope is weighted through its entire operation and moves consistently in a downward direction.

Münter Hitch A type of running knot commonly used in belaying that slips around a carabiner to create friction against itself. It is also known as the Italian hitch or half ring bend.

Belaying
Belaying Is a Serious Commitment

The word **belay** comes from the days of sailing vessels. On those ships, hefty belaying pins were set into the rails of the vessel. When sailors raised heavy objects, such as sails, they would attach a rope to the object and then take a turn of the rope around the belaying pin to prevent the line from slipping away from them.

In the high angle environment, the principle is the same except that the purpose of modern belaying is to keep a person or load from falling. The person is attached to a rope, and the rope is managed in such a way, or *belayed,* as to keep the person from falling far enough to be injured.

The ability to belay is a critical skill for anyone operating in the high angle environment. If you accept the assignment as a belayer, you have made a very serious commitment. It means that the well-being, perhaps even the life, of the person at the end of the rope is in your hands. Saying that you can belay when you cannot or allowing your attention to lapse from the job of belaying could result in severe injury or death for the person at the end of the rope.

One-Person versus Rescue Belay

The techniques and equipment discussed in this chapter are designed for belaying of one person (light duty loads). They should not be attempted with loads of more than one person; these larger loads are commonly known as *heavy duty* or *rescue loads.*

All belay devices and techniques perform somewhat differently in practice. Some are better for belaying light duty loads, such as a one-person load; some create insufficient friction for catching heavier loads of more than one person or even one heavy person (see Chapter 13 for information on belaying heavy duty loads). *Know the limitations of the system or systems you use.*

The Belay System

The following elements constitute a one-person belay system (Figure 8-1):

- An anchor attached to the belay device. The anchor should be able to hold the highest potential shock load that could result from the fall of the person being belayed.
- A person tied to a rope who is at risk of falling (this may be a person rappelling, ascending, or climbing; a climber is used in this example).
- A harness worn by the climber that is attached to the rope. The harness should be able to hold the climber safely, causing minimal injury, when the person is caught by the rope.
- A **belay device**. A belay device is in essence a braking mechanism. A secondary line called, the **belay line**, is run through the belay device. The belay line is controlled so that in the event of an uncontrolled descent or fall by the person or load being belayed on the main line, the belay device, under the control of the belayer, exerts a slowing or stopping action on the line.
- The **belayer**. This individual controls the belay device and the rope. The belayer's main duty is to ensure proper activation of the belay system. Most of the time, the belayer will not be braking the rope. He or she engages the device only if the climber falls. However, the belayer must also manage the rope so that excessive slack does not increase the shock load to the rope if the climber should fall.

Situations Requiring a Belay

A belay may be called for any time exposure to the danger of falling arises. A belay would be required in the following situations:

- A person is rock climbing or mountaineering in hazardous terrain. Should the climber slip, a proper belay can hold the individual.
- A rescue situation involves the danger of falling. For example, a belay line would be attached to a rescuer attempting to aid a person threatening to jump from a bridge.

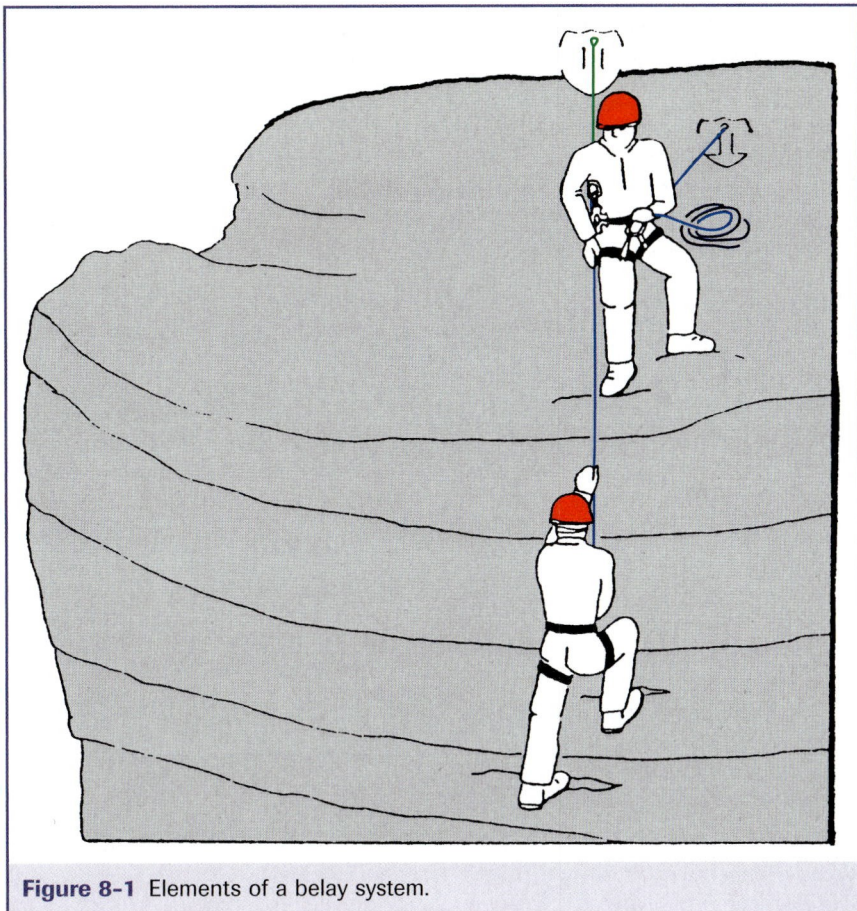

Figure 8-1 Elements of a belay system.

- A person is crossing an area not generally dangerous but which includes a small area of exposure to falling.
- A person is unsure of himself or herself in attempting a new skill, such as rappelling for the first time.
- A person's physical or mental capabilities are diminished; for example, because of injury, vertigo, exhaustion, or hypothermia.
- Environmental factors, such as possible rock falls or areas slick with ice, increase the danger of falling.
- One or more people are being lowered by rope, such as in a rescue.
- One or more people are being raised by rope, such as in a rescue.

Decisions on When to Belay

In some cases the need for a belay is not completely clear-cut, such as in the following situations:

- A person who is very experienced in the high angle environment is rappelling or ascending. He or she may feel that a belay would only be a hindrance.
- A belay might cause a greater problem than not having one. For example, several rope lines may already be involved, and an additional line from a belay could cause entanglement.
- A free drop is involved, in which the load may spin. A belay line could entangle the main line and stop everything from moving.

Judgments about these situations must be made locally by well-trained and experienced individuals. At a minimum, belays should be used any time the combined potential for and consequences of a fall are unacceptable to the situation. As a general rule, if you are not sure, it is probably best to belay (Box 8-1).

Belay Failure: The Human Element

Numerous climbing accidents have occurred because of belayer failure. Such accidents often are caused by one factor or a combination of two factors:

1. The belayer's attention drifts momentarily just as the person on the rope falls.
2. Because of insufficient training, the belayer does not automatically perform the correct actions.

Because of the potential for belay accidents, some organizations adopt a philosophy that a belay should catch when the belayer is "hands free." However, this is not effective in every case, because it does not always provide the most efficient or maneuverable system. It can also be counterproductive, because a human's natural reaction at the moment of truth may not necessarily be to let go.

One basic principle about human nature is this: *In a sudden emergency, humans respond with what is instinctive.* Such emergency situations could relate to driving experience under the threat of a vehicular accident or to weapons training in a law

Box 8-1 | A Belay Is Not the Same As Lowering

Belays and lowerings (see Chapter 16) involve different techniques and different equipment and are used for different purposes, although they may be used together. Do not confuse the two.

BELAY

A belay is a safety to catch people if they should fall. A belay rope can be run either way (up or down) while it is being used for a belay. A belay rope does not have weight on it unless a fall occurs on it or "tension" is called for in special cases. Depending on the activity, the belay rope may be maintained with some slack in it. A belay uses specialized equipment, such as a belay plate, or special knots, such as the **Münter** hitch.

If a fall occurs, a good belay system should have the ability to lower the load a short distance to a point where it can be stabilized.

LOWERING

A **lowering** is the controlled lowering of individuals and equipment using rope through a lowering device and hardware such as the large ring of a figure 8 descender or a brake bar rack (neither of which should be used for a belay). A lowering rope goes one way–down. A lowering rope has weight on it throughout the lowering operation.

enforcement confrontation. *Belaying is a similar activity in that it must be thoroughly learned under realistic conditions, followed by constant practice, until it becomes instinctive.* Otherwise, the belayer may fail to take the correct action when the emergency suddenly occurs. Such failure could result in severe injury or death.

It is not enough to have intellectually learned belaying. That is, it is not enough to have read about belaying, to have watched it, or even to have practiced the hand positions.

You must have combined both the mental and physical experience of the actual belay situation.

Caution

Hand Protection

In belaying, the belayer must wear gloves to protect his or her hands from rope friction. This must be done for two reasons:
- To protect the hands from possibly severe rope burns from a running rope.
- To prevent pain caused by grasping a running rope and to allow the belayer to hold the rope firmly.

Suggestion

Discarded truck tires often work well as the weight for a belay practice system. They are inexpensive and are less likely to damage concrete or asphalt floors when they drop.

Belay Practice System

Figure 8-2 shows an overall view of a belay practice system for one person (see Chapter 13 for information on belaying a rescue load). The practice system consists of the following elements:
- A weight or a dummy weighing at least 200 pounds (91 kg) to simulate the weight of a falling person (see the Suggestion box above).

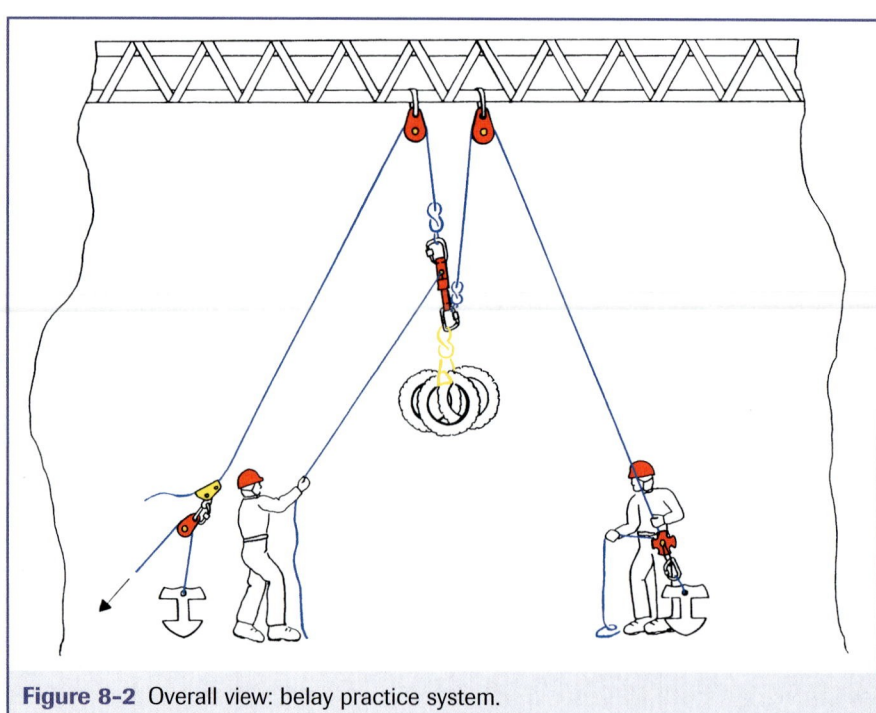

Figure 8-2 Overall view: belay practice system.

- A method of raising the weights. A winch may be the easiest and most convenient way of doing this. However, a mechanical advantage hauling system can be used for raising the practice weights (Figure 8-3).
- A belay station, where a belayer is located.
- An instructor's station.
- A rope, under the control of the instructor, that triggers the weight's fall. The triggering mechanism can be created from a seat belt buckle, a parachute harness release, or a military helicopter harness release (Figure 8-4 and Box 8-2).

Such a belay practice system, which simulates the forces of a falling climber, is essential to the instruction of belaying. This system is very simple and inexpensive to construct. Details on the system for hauling the weight and on the triggering mechanism are shown in Figures 8-3 and 8-4.

Box 8-2	**Belay Practice System Procedure**

The procedure for practicing belaying is as follows:
1. The belayer and the instructor take their stations.
2. An assistant begins to haul the weight up.
3. The student belayer "belays" the raise by keeping slack out of the rope.
4. At some point, without warning, the instructor pulls the line that triggers the fall of the weight.
5. The student belayer attempts to arrest the fall of the weight.

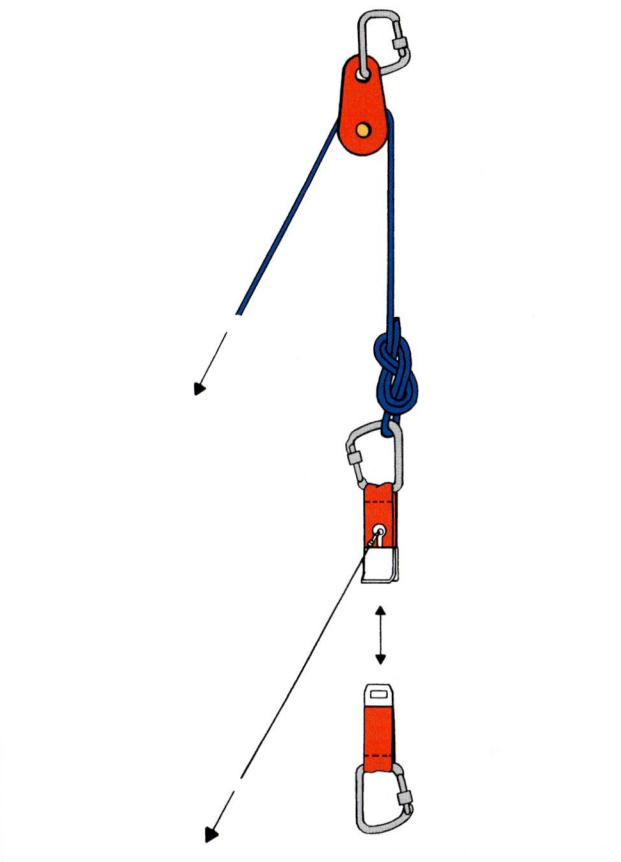

Figure 8-4 Trigger: belay practice system.

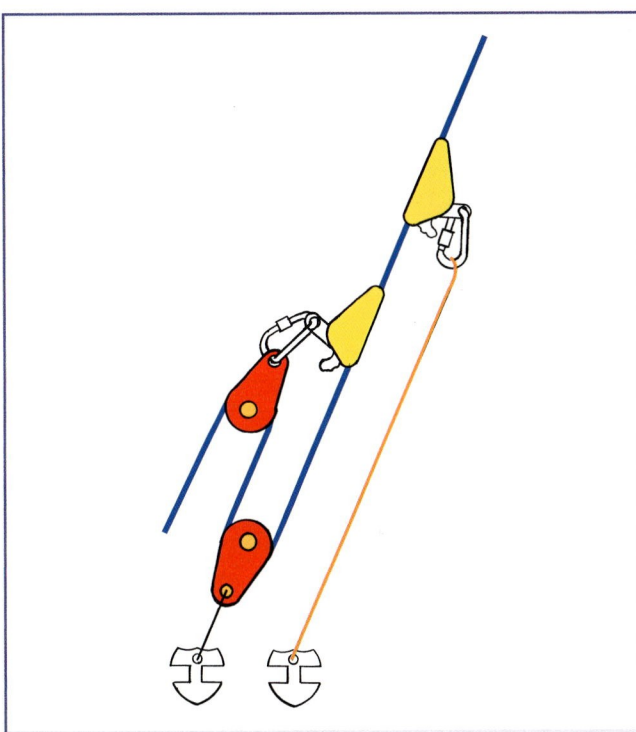

Figure 8-3 Hauling: belay practice system.

⚠ Warning

Beware of directional carabiners or pulleys in belay systems. The directional anchor and the anchor hardware, such as carabiners, pulleys, and slings, endure almost twice the impact force to which the climber or belayer is subjected, because the anchor must hold both the fall and the offsetting force of the arrest by the belayer. These two forces added together, minus system friction, are what the anchor must handle in a belay run through a directional.

Belaying Signals

When you are belaying, it is essential that you use the standard voice signals (also called *commands* or *calls*). Otherwise, even momentary confusion could cause an accident.

In climbing and mountaineering, a group of voice signals has been standard usage in belaying for years. These same calls work well in both the work and rescue environments.

The voice signals are exchanged between a climber (or rappeller) and the belayer to ensure that both are ready.

The standard belay signals, in sequence, are as follows:
1. **Climber:** "On belay?" *(I am about to climb [or rappel]; are you ready to catch me if I fall?)*

Warning

When the weight falls and the belay catches, the belay rope comes taut with great force. To avoid injury, the belayer and others around the belayer must take the following precautions:

1. Be aware of the position the rope and belay device will take when the belay catches and stay out of this path. Otherwise, the impact of the rope and/or belay device can cause serious injury.
2. Keep fingers, hair, and clothing free of the rope near the belay device. Otherwise, these could be swept into the belay device, possibly causing injury and impeding the belay.
3. One-person belay devices are designed for catching one-person loads and may not be the most appropriate device for catching rescue loads.

2. **Belayer:** "Belay on." *(I am ready to catch you if you fall.)*
3. **Climber:** "Climbing (rappelling)." *(I am starting to climb [rappel].)*
4. **Belayer:** "Climb (rappel) on." *(Go ahead.)*

Once a climber is in place and no longer needs the belay, the climber initiates an exchange to end the belay:

5. **Climber:** "Off belay." *(I am in a secure place now. I no longer need the belay.)*
6. **Belayer:** "Belay off." *(I am no longer belaying you.)*

When the climber and belayer are not within sight of each other, they can extend this sequence to include an "off rope" statement by the climber (which is repeated by the belayer). This helps the belayer know when to start pulling on the rope, when to hang onto the rope because it might disappear, or when the rope has been cleared for other needs:

7. **Climber:** "Off rope." (I am finished with the rope.)
8. **Belayer:** "Off rope." (I understand that you are finished with the rope.)

Some additional signals can aid communication between the climber and the belayer during the belay cycle; for example, at times when the belayer is holding the rope too tightly:

Climber: "Slack." *(There is too much tension on the rope; I cannot move as well as I would like.)*

Belayer: (No verbal response is required, only the action of letting an appropriate amount of slack into the rope.)

The converse problem is too much slack in the rope; for example, the climber may be at a particularly tricky point and may need the support of the rope to make a move:

Climber: "Tension."

Belayer: (No verbal response is required, only the action of taking slack out of the rope.)

Consistency of Communications

It is important to emphasize that once these voice communications have been agreed upon, they must not be changed without prior agreement. Otherwise, some confusion in communication could result, and this, even if brief, could be dangerous.

It is also important that all people involved discuss and clarify their understanding of the signals, even if they know one another and have worked together before. Slight variations in interpretation can cause accidents.

NOTE: Well-entrenched traditions of belay signals may differ, depending on the geography and culture. What is important is that the climber and belayer agree on the terminology to be used.

Make Yourself Heard

For the belay voice signals to work, they must be heard by those involved. Do not be timid when you use them. Wind, falling water, machinery, or other conditions can make voice communications difficult to hear. The belay signals require at least shouting, perhaps yelling, to be effective. If the required response to a command is not received, repeat the command louder.

Belaying Techniques

A number of one-person belaying techniques are used in the high angle environment. They all work essentially the same way: they create a braking action on the rope to prevent the person at the end of the rope from falling far enough to be injured.

In this chapter some of these one-person belay techniques are examined in detail. These techniques are among those considered to be simple to learn and easy to use and to pose less danger to the belayer and the person on the rope.

The Münter Hitch

The **Münter hitch** is the subject of some controversy because it may be insufficient to control heavy duty loads. However, because of its versatility, it can be useful for belaying light duty loads. When using the Münter hitch, it is easy to reverse rope direction without unclipping the rope, and no extra equipment is required other than a carabiner. The ideal carabiner for use with a Münter hitch is one specifically designed for this purpose, usually called an HMS (an acronym for the German word *Halbmastwurfsicherung*) or Münter hitch carabiner. The HMS carabiner has a pear-shaped design with gentle curves that allow the Münter hitch to move freely back and forth through the carabiner. A more angulated carabiner, such as a D design, can cause jamming of the Münter hitch (although this type of carabiner can be used, with care, in a pinch). Factors to consider when using a Münter hitch are (1) where the force will ride on the carabiner in the event of a failure and (2) how the rigging can be done so as to reduce the probability of the moving rope opening the carabiner gate.

Warning

As with all belay techniques, the Münter hitch belay must be practiced on level ground and with a weight or dummy drop before it is attempted with a person in the high angle environment. This practice must be done under the guidance of a qualified instructor.

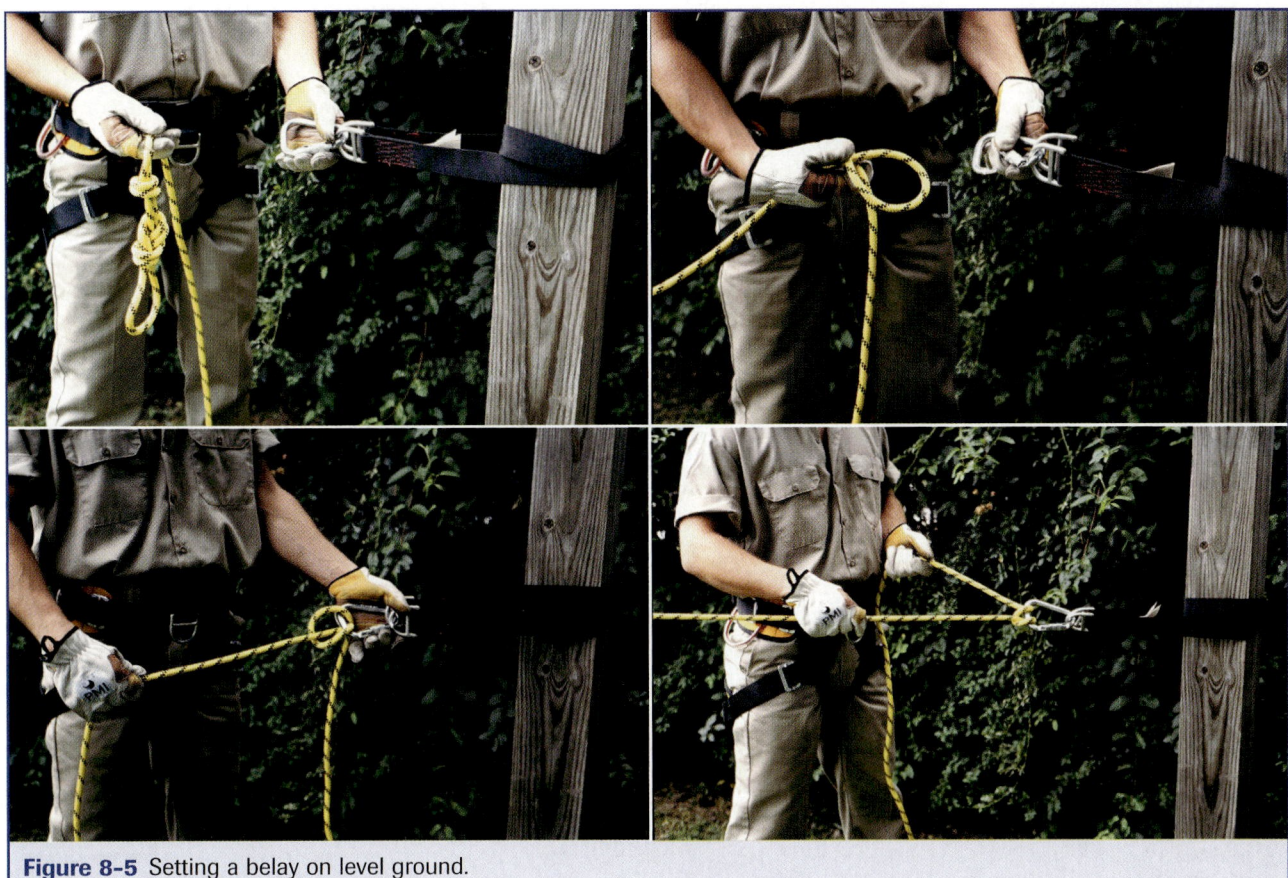

Figure 8-5 Setting a belay on level ground.

Procedure for Belaying a Person with the *Münter* Hitch

Setting the Belay on Level Ground (Figure 8-5)

1. Tie a piece of webbing or rope sling into a secure anchor (see Chapter 7).
2. Clip a large locking carabiner into the anchor sling.
3. Tie a Münter hitch near the end of the rope where the person being belayed will be. Although a Münter hitch can be tied in several ways, Figure 8-6 shows a simple method that is easy to remember.
4. Clip the HMS carabiner across the portion of the Münter hitch that has two sections of rope parallel to one another. Lock the carabiner.
5. Always remember that the Münter hitch runs in both directions. This means that if the person on the rope is moving away from you, the loop in the bight will be on the side of the carabiner toward the climber. If you are pulling up rope (the climber is moving toward you), the loop will be on the side of the carabiner facing you.

Practicing the Münter Hitch Belay on Level Ground (Figure 8-7)

Preparation

1. Face the climber. Take the rope on the side of the carabiner away from the climber in your dominant hand (e.g., the right hand for right-handed individuals). *This is your brake hand.*

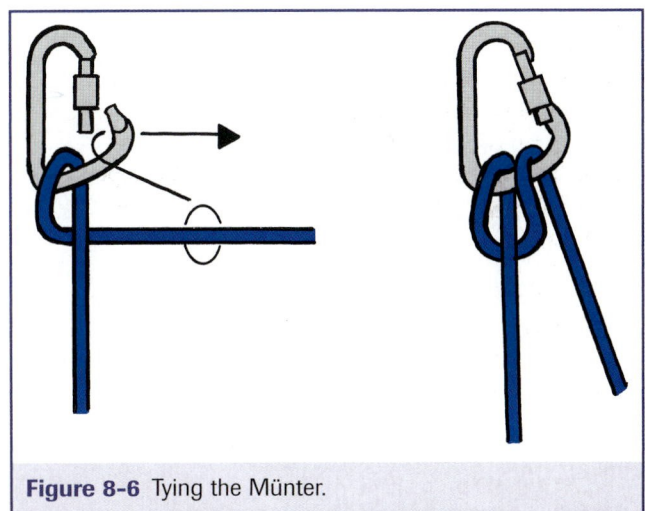

Figure 8-6 Tying the Münter.

You must not take this hand off the rope when the person is "on belay" unless the belay is tied off.

2. Take the rope on the side of the carabiner near the climber in your nondominant hand (the left hand for right-handed individuals). This is your *guide hand,* which is used to help manipulate the rope. The guide hand needs no more force than what the index finger, middle finger, and thumb can provide to manipulate the rope. The guide hand does not provide braking force.

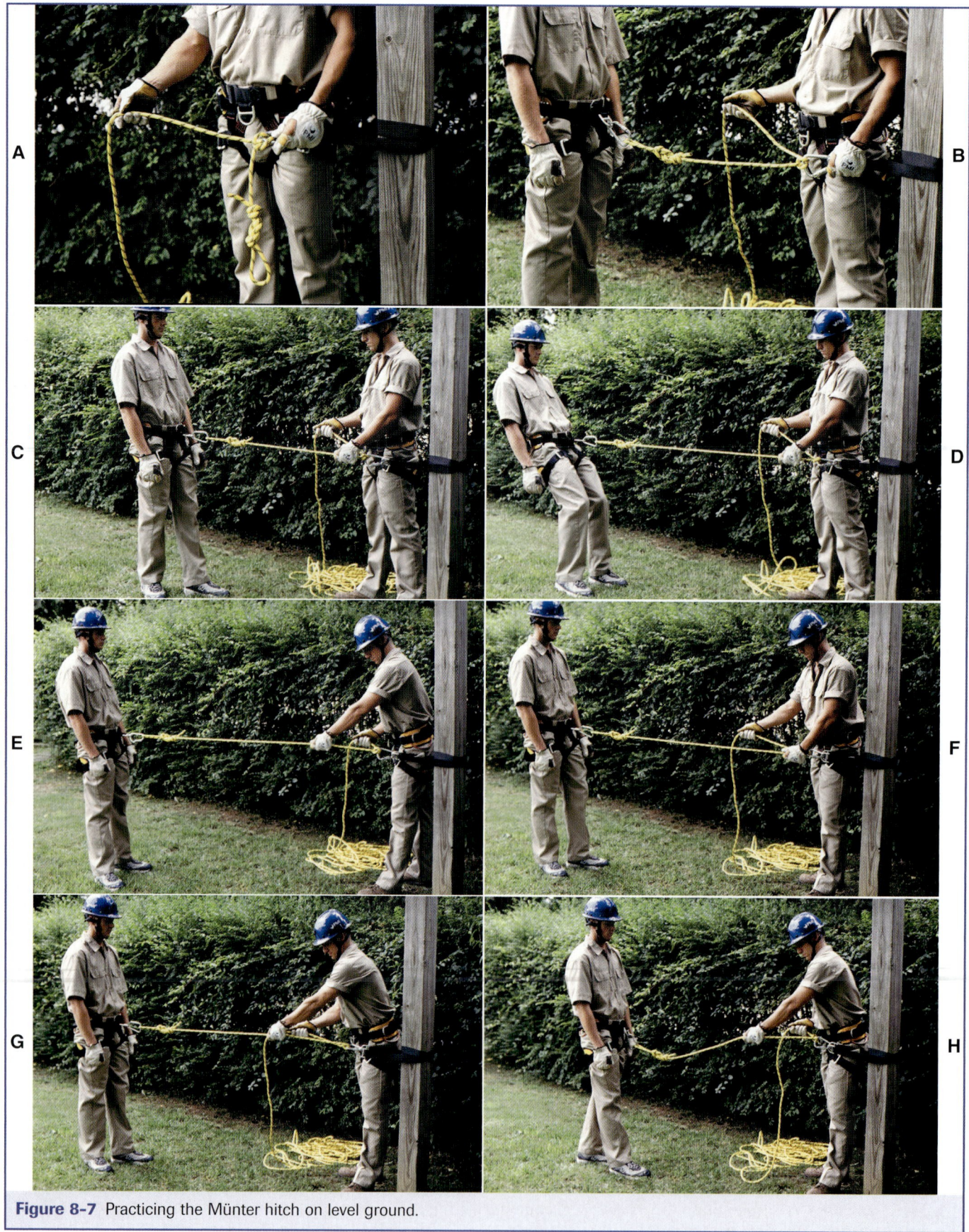

Figure 8-7 Practicing the Münter hitch on level ground.

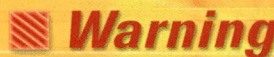

Warning

When anchoring yourself as a belayer, *never* place yourself into the system. That is, do not belay with a device clipped to the front of your harness and the anchor clipped to the back of your harness. Should the climber fall and the system shock load, you could be severely injured, possibly suffering a fractured pelvis. You could be disabled or incur a life-threatening injury.

Attaching the Climber

3. Now, have a partner wearing a seat harness clip into the end of the rope (Figure 8-7, *A*).

4. Remove slack in the rope between the carabiner and the climber by pulling it out with the brake hand. The starting hand positions for letting out rope is with the brake hand about 3 feet (1 m) from the carabiner and the guide hand about 1 foot (.3 m) from the carabiner (Figure 8-7, *C*).

5. Begin the belay voice signals. The person on the rope says, "On belay." If the belayer is ready, he or she responds, "Belay on." The person on rope then says, "Climbing," and the belayer answers, "Climb on."

6. Have the person on the rope begin slowly walking backward. As this evolution proceeds, continue with the appropriate commands (see belaying signals given previously).

7. With the guide hand, pull the rope out from the carabiner and feed it to the climber; allow the climber to set the rate of rope run. As your brake hand approaches within 1 foot (0.3 m) of the carabiner, slide it back *while still holding the rope*. Then slide the guide hand back to its original position. Continue this hand shuffle as the climber moves away from the belayer. *Never take the brake hand off the rope.*

8. Now, to give a feel of the control you have, hold the rope firmly with the brake hand, stopping the person on the rope from going farther.

9. In an area where the climber will not slip, have the person firmly plant his or her feet on the ground and lean back from the rope. Hold the rope firmly with the brake hand (Figure 8-7, *D*).

10. To get a feel of the control, slowly let a few inches of rope out with the climber leaning against the rope (Figure 8-7, *E*).

Reversing Direction

11. Have your partner walk slowly toward you. The problem now is to take in rope while keeping the person safely on belay.

12. Have your brake hand on the rope about 1 foot (.3 m) from the carabiner (Figure 8-7, *F*).

13. Place your guide hand on the rope about 3 feet (1 m) from the carabiner.

14. As slack comes into the rope, pull it out by pulling with the brake hand. Also pull the rope with your guide hand to reduce friction on the Münter hitch and help ease the rope through the carabiner (Figure 8-7, *G*).

Note that reversing the Münter hitch can sometimes take a bit of effort. It can be difficult to get the hitch to pop back through the carabiner and reverse direction. This is most easily done when the Münter hitch is in the middle of the rounded portion of the carabiner.

Just as your guide hand approaches your brake hand, grasp both sides of the rope with your guide hand. *Do not cross hands.*

15. Holding both lines in place with the guide hand, move your brake hand up the rope toward the carabiner *without taking it off the rope*. When the brake hand is back to its original position, about 1 foot (.3 m) from the carabiner, hold the rope again with the brake hand and slide the guide hand back to its original position, about 3 feet (1 m) from the carabiner. Repeat this hand shuffle as the climber walks to you (Figure 8-7, *H*).

16. Continue the procedure until the person on the rope reaches your position.

17. Exchange the voice signals that conclude the belaying cycle *(Person on rope: "Off belay," Belayer: "Belay off.")*.

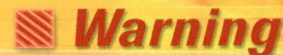

Warning

For maximum friction (maximum control) when using the *Münter* hitch, keep the braking side of the rope close to the rope going to the load. That is, to provide maximum friction, keep the angle of the rope as small as possible.

Practicing the Belay with a One-Person Weight or Dummy

Now practice belaying with a Münter hitch using the belay practice system with a one-person dummy or weight shown in Figure 8-2. First practice this procedure with the weight falling as it is raised. Then practice it with the weight falling as it is lowered.

In an actual belay situation, of course, it is preferable to keep the climber in view. However, this does not always happen in real life. Therefore it is best to practice while facing away from the weight or dummy so that you cannot visually anticipate the fall. This will sharpen your skills at catching an unexpected fall.

As each fall of the dummy or weight comes onto your rope and you catch it, lower it to the ground using the Münter hitch.

Warning

Moving the hand positions on the rope is one of the most critical operations in belaying. Remember: *The person at the end of the rope could fall at any time while you are belaying.* If you do not have your brake hand on the rope at all times, ready to grasp it in an instant, you may drop the person and cause severe injury or death.

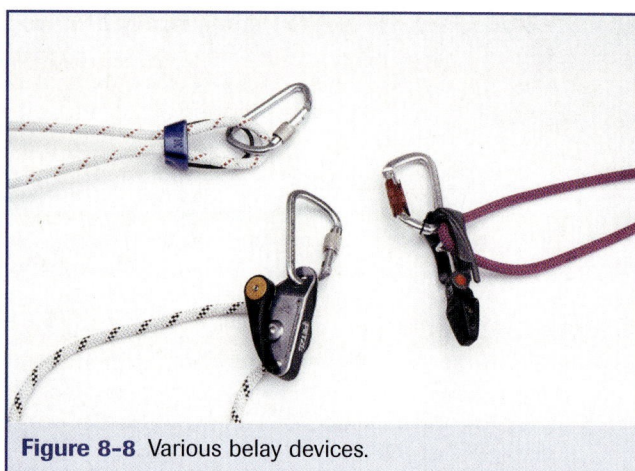

Figure 8-8 Various belay devices.

Using a Free Running Belay Device

Another way to belay a one-person load is to use a slot-type, free running belay (or brake) device. Figure 8-8 shows various designs of one-person belay devices. Many traditional belay devices use a variation of the belay plate design. The **belay plate**, combined with a carabiner, creates rope friction on the device so that the belayer can control the belay line.

Some early plate devices have two slots of the same size. They are designed for belaying with both single- and double-rope systems. Other early plates have two slots of different sizes. They are designed for people who might be using an 10.6 mm rope on one occasion and a 9 mm rope another time. Modern free running belay devices, such as the Air Traffic Controller (ATC) (Black Diamond) are really not plates at all but operate on the basic principle of the early belay plates. These newer devices can also work with a range of rope diameters.

Belay plate–type one-person belay devices are designed only for use with kernmantle ropes (either static or dynamic). *They are not designed for use with laid ropes.*

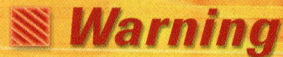

Warning

When the weight falls and the belay catches, the belay rope comes taut with great force. To avoid injury, the belayer and others around the belayer must take the following precautions:
1. Be aware of the position the rope and belay device will take when the belay catches and stay out of this path. Otherwise, the impact of the rope and/or belay device can cause serious injury.
2. Keep fingers, hair, and clothing free of the rope near the belay device. Otherwise, these could be swept into the belay device, possibly causing injury and impeding the belay.
3. One-person belay devices are designed for catching one-person loads and may not be the most appropriate device for catching rescue loads.

For this practice session, use a one-person belay device such as the ATC. A variation of the belay plate design, the ATC uses friction to create control of the rope. The friction occurs when the belayer pulls the rope, forcing the ATC back against the carabiner. This results in greater friction from the rope on the carabiner and the ATC.

Belaying with the ATC
Rigging the One-Person Belay Device (ATC) (Figure 8-9)

1. Tie a webbing or rope sling into a secure anchor (see Chapter 7).
2. Clip a locking carabiner into the end of the loop.
3. Take a bight of rope near the end of the rope where the person to be belayed will be.
4. Push a few inches (or centimeters) of the bight through the hole in the smaller end of the tapered plate of the ATC.
5. Clip the loop of the rope and the ATC's wire cable through the locking carabiner.

Warning

Belaying with a one-person belay device must be practiced on level ground and with a weight or dummy drop before it is attempted with a person in the high angle environment. This practice must be done under the guidance of a qualified instructor.

Practicing the Belay with the ATC on Level Ground (Figure 8-10)
Preparation

1. Take the rope on the side of the belay (or brake) device away from the climber in your dominant hand (e.g., the right hand for a right-handed individual). *This is your brake hand. You must not take this hand off the rope when the person is "on belay" unless the belay is tied off.*
2. Take the rope on the side of the brake device nearest the climber in your nondominant hand (the left hand for right-handed individuals). This is your *guide hand.* You will use it to help manipulate the rope.
3. To stop the rope from running out, pull back on the rope with the brake hand so that the angle of the rope strands is approximately 180 degrees. Keep the guide hand in position to help maintain control of the rope. Note that this forces the ATC device against the carabiner, creating friction on the rope. To maintain the braking action, hold the rope tight with your brake hand.

Attaching the Climber

4. Now, have a partner wearing a seat harness clip into the end of the rope.

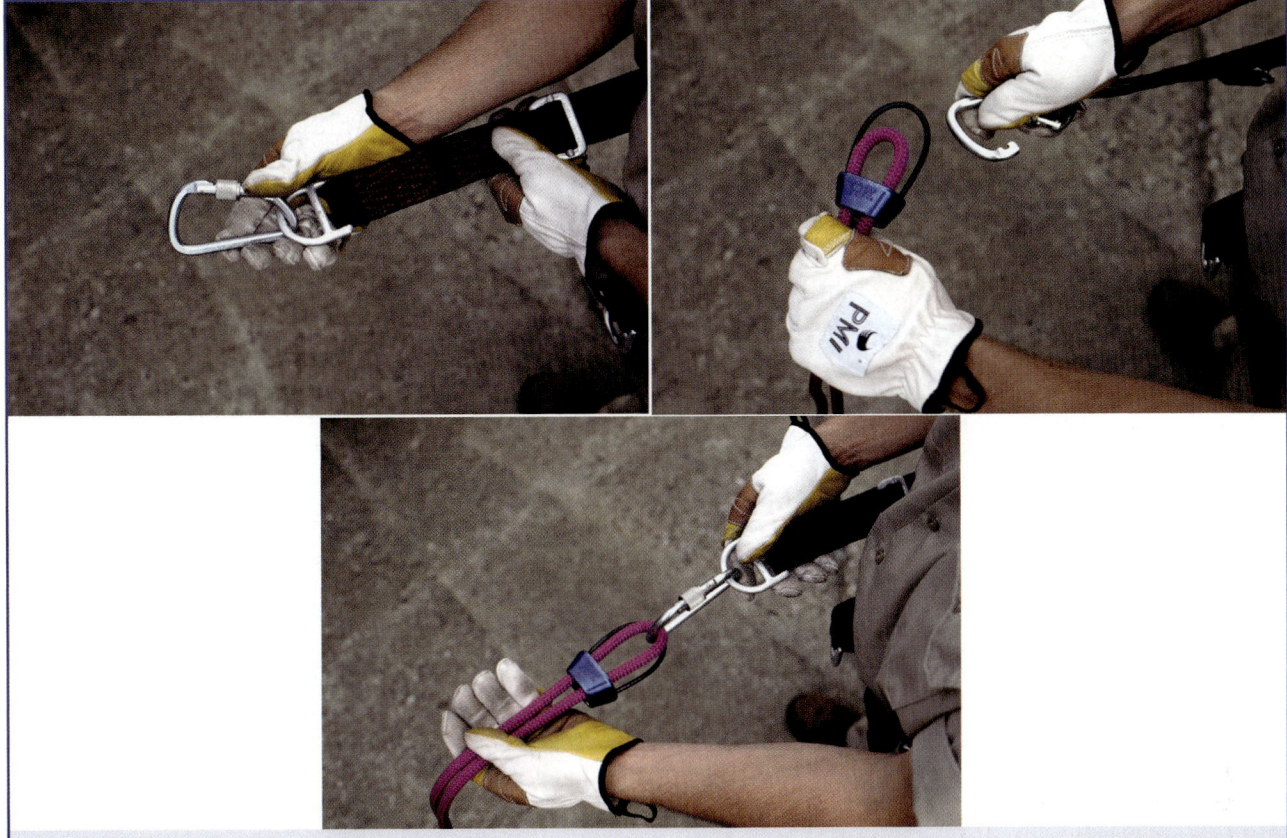

Figure 8-9 Rigging the one-person belay device.

5. Remove slack in the rope between the belay device and the climber by holding the rope strands at a narrow angle and pulling the slack out with the brake hand.
6. Begin the belay voice signals. *(The person on the rope says, "On belay." The belayer, if ready, responds, "Belay on.")*

Practicing with the Climber

7. Have the person attached to the rope begin slowly walking backward (Figure 8-10, *B*).
8. Feed rope into the belay device with the brake hand and pull it with the guide hand. Maintain just enough slack so that it is noticeable and it allows the climber freedom of movement.
9. Now, initiate a braking action. Pull back on the rope with the brake hand so that the angle of the rope strands is approximately 180 degrees. Keep the guide hand in position to help maintain control of the rope (Figure 8-10, *C*).
10. In an area where the climber will not slip, have the person firmly plant his or her feet on the ground and lean back from the rope. Hold the rope firmly with the brake hand.
11. Stop feeding rope through with the brake hand. The device should lock, holding the climber in place.
12. To get a feel of control, slowly let out a few inches (or centimeters) of rope with the climber leaning against the rope. Do this by bringing the two sides of the rope toward each other and by moving your brake hand toward the belay device (Figure 8-10, *D*).

⬛ Warning

Moving the hand positions on the rope is one of the most critical operations in belaying. Remember: *The person at the end of the rope could fall at any time while you are belaying.* If you do not have your brake hand on the rope at all times, ready to grasp it in an instant, you may drop the person and cause severe injury or death.

Reversing Direction

13. Now, have your partner walk slowly toward you. The problem now is to take in rope while keeping the person safely on belay. To practice control of rope tension, do not allow the rope between the climber and the belay device to touch the ground.
14. Keep your brake hand on the rope about 1 foot from the belay device.
15. Place your guide hand about 3 feet (1 m) from the belay device (Figure 8-10, *F*).
16. As slack appears in the rope, pull the slack out by pulling the rope with the brake hand. Your guide hand can help move rope toward the belay device.
17. At some point, your brake hand will have pulled so much rope that you will have to move this hand back toward the

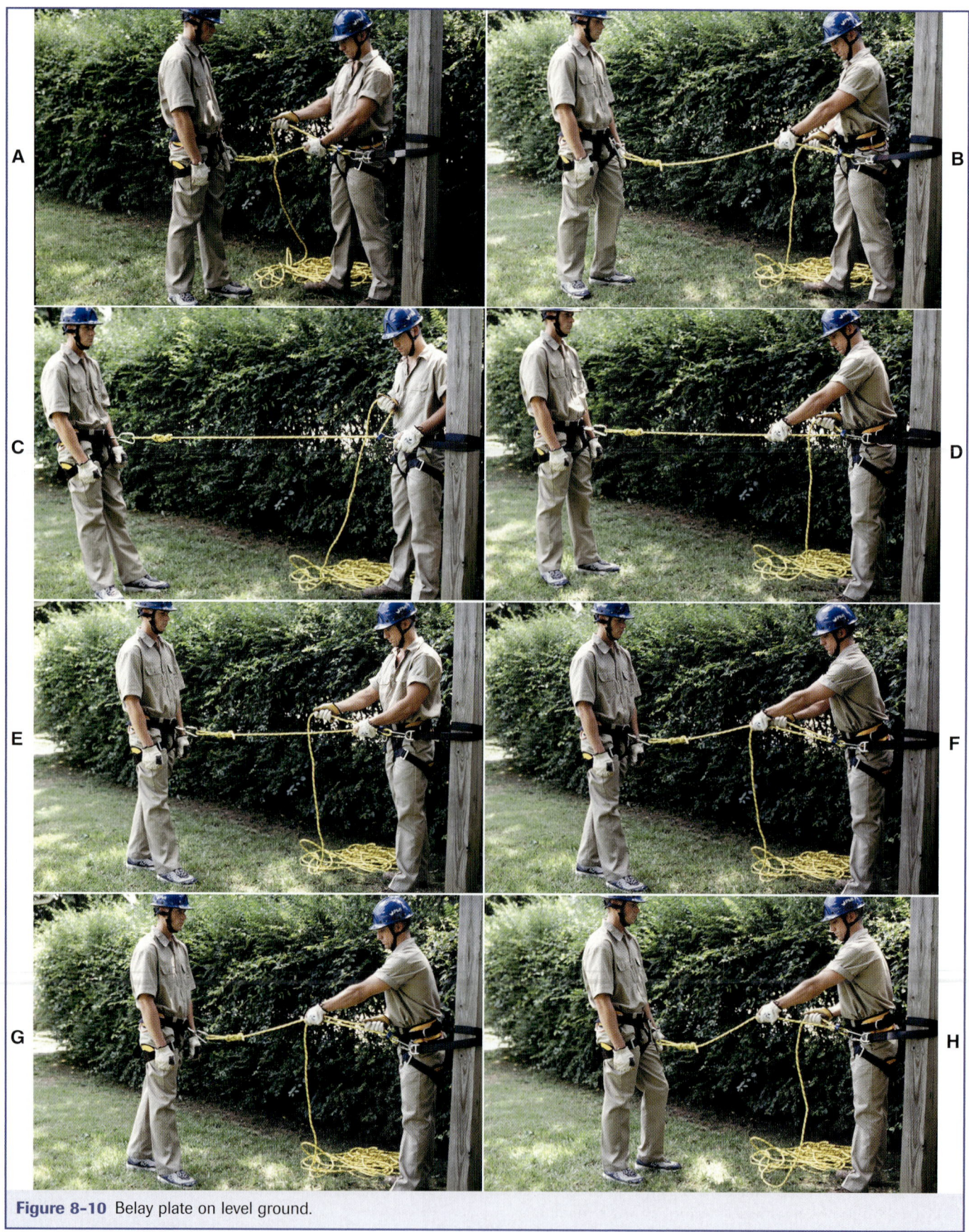

Figure 8-10 Belay plate on level ground.

braking device. While gripping the rope with the brake hand, slide the guide hand back toward the belay device and below the brake hand. Hold the rope on the free (standing) part of the rope in your guide hand extended away from the body. Use two or three fingers of the guide hand to grip the free (standing) part of the rope. Keep the brake hand in the ready to brake position.

18. Using the guide hand, grip the standing end of the rope to provide back tension against the brake hand, and then slide the brake hand back toward the belay device, *all the while keeping the brake hand in the ready to brake position* (Figure 8-10, *G*).

19. Continue the procedure until the person on the rope reaches your position (Figure 8-10, *H*).

20. Exchange the voice signals that conclude the belay cycle. *(Person on rope: "Off belay." Belayer: "Belay off.")*

▩ *Warning*

When the weight falls and the belay catches, the belay rope comes taut with great force. To avoid injury, the belayer and others around the belayer must take the following precautions:

1. Be aware of the position the rope and belay device will take when the belay catches and stay out of this path. Otherwise, the impact of the rope and/or belay device can cause serious injury.
2. Keep fingers, hair, and clothing free of the rope near the belay device. Otherwise, these could be swept into the belay device, possibly causing injury and impeding the belay.
3. One-person belay devices are designed for catching one-person loads and may not be the most appropriate device for catching rescue loads.

Practicing with the ATC Using a Belay Weight or Dummy

Now practice belaying with the ATC using a belay weight or dummy as shown in Figure 8-2. Practice first with the weight or dummy falling as it is raised and then practice with the weight or dummy falling as it is lowered. In each case, as the weight comes onto your belay line, lower it to the ground with the brake plate.

In an actual belay situation, it is preferable to keep the climber in view. However, this is not always possible. Therefore it is best to practice while facing away from the weight or dummy so that you cannot visually anticipate the fall. This will sharpen your skills at catching an unexpected fall.

Belay Plates in Figure 8 Descenders

Some figure 8 descenders are designed with a belay plate either in the small ring or between the two rings. However, you should use figure 8 belay plates with caution for the following reasons:

- The slot in the figure 8 may not be the correct size for the rope you are using.

▩ *Warning*

Do not use the figure 8 descender as a belay device with the rope wrapped in the large ring as for rappelling or lowering. The large ring is not designed with enough friction to stop a rope that is shock loaded from a fall.

- Some figure 8s have slots that are not well designed for use as a belay plate.
- A figure 8 is not as well balanced as some devices and may not be as easy to use.

Assisted Catch Belay Devices

Some personal belay devices are designed to provide an *assisted catch*. That is, in the event of sudden loading, a mechanical action helps brake the rope. Popular devices include the GriGri (Petzl) and the TRE Sirius. Assisted catch devices are designed to stop a falling climber more quickly than free running devices. *They should always be used with dynamic rope.* Always belay with these devices in such a way that you are not relying on the assisted catch. *You should always consider your brake hand to be the primary source of belay activation and arrest.*

Belaying with the TRE

Rigging the Assisted Belay Device (TRE) (Figure 8-11)

1. Read the user instructions supplied with the TRE.
2. Tie a webbing or rope sling into a secure anchor loop (see Chapter 7).
3. Attach the TRE to the locking carabiner using the supplied rubber O ring to secure the TRE in the small end of the carabiner.
4. Clip the locking carabiner with the TRE into the end of the loop, making sure the TRE is not limited in range of motion by other objects near the anchor point.
5. Open the TRE by pressing the locking slide toward the release lever with your finger. Release the crossbolt arm by pulling it forward.
6. Take a bight of rope near the end of the rope where the person to be belayed will be.
7. Push a few inches (or centimeters) of the bight through the rope slot in the TRE, loop the rope over the crossbolt, and close the device by returning the crossbolt to the original position.
8. Note the graphics on the device. The rope exiting the slot on the hand icon end must go to the belayer, and the rope exiting the slot on the climber icon end must go to the load or person being belayed.
9. Check that the device operates properly. The belayer holds the brake end of the rope while the climber firmly pulls on the running end of the rope; if the TRE blocks the rope, the device is in the proper position.

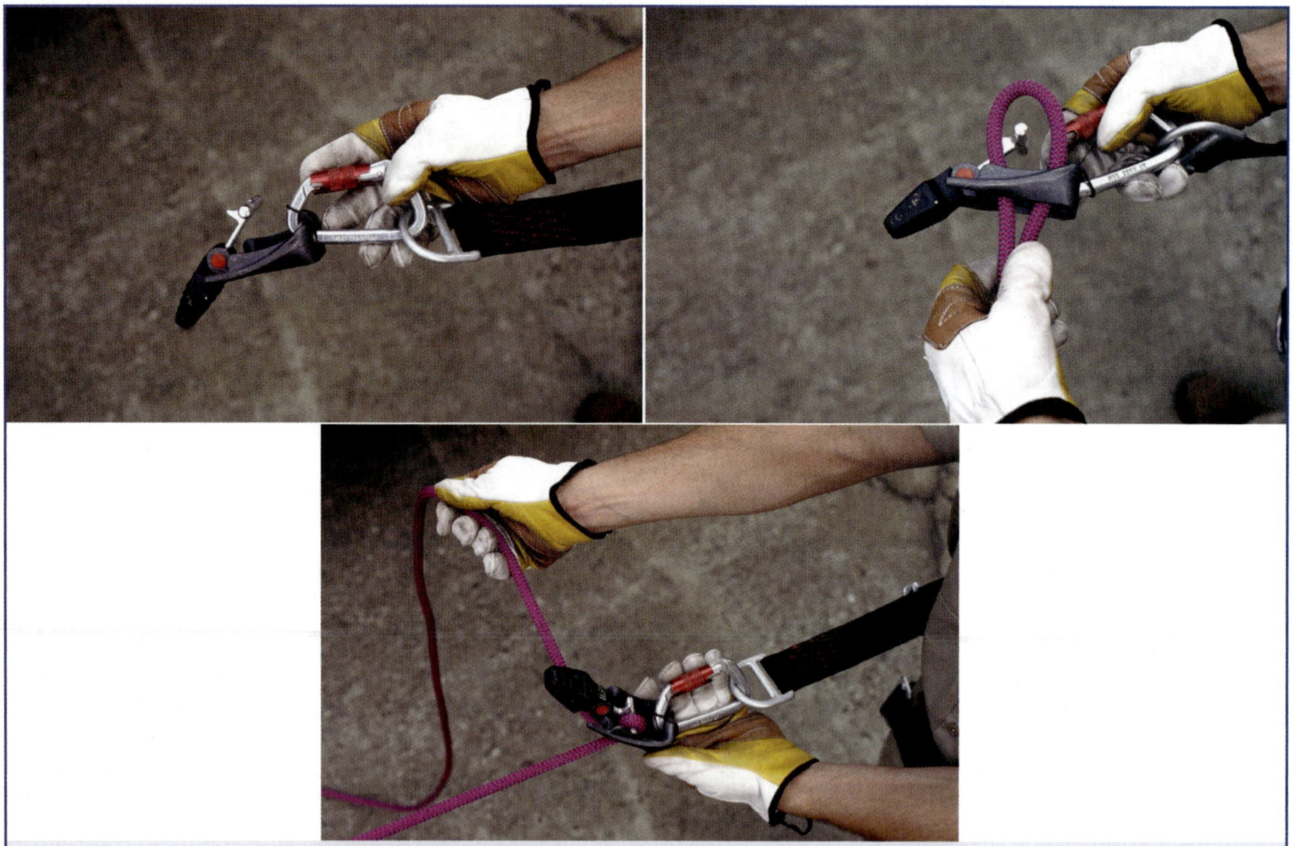

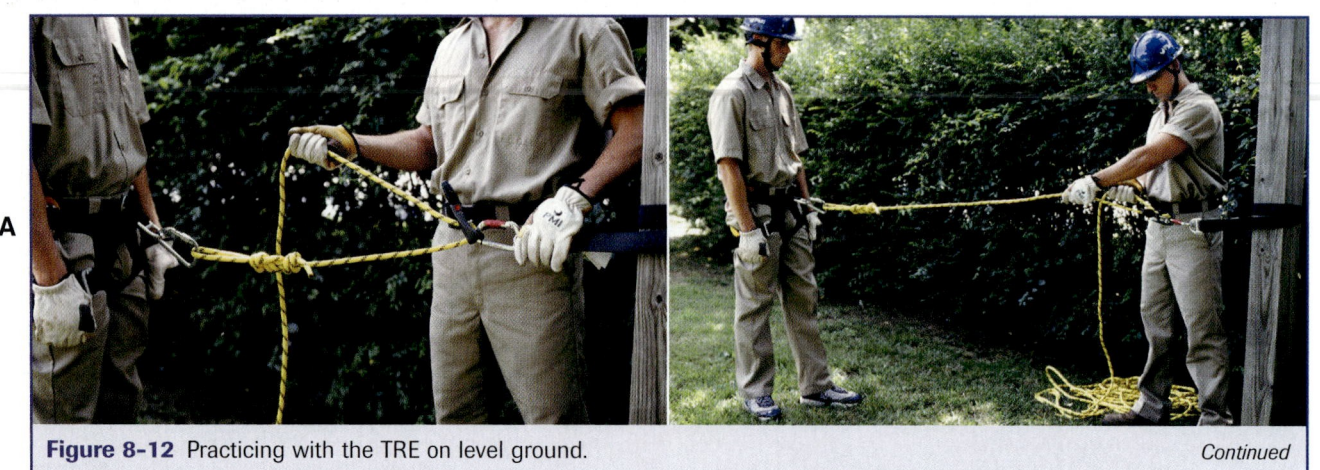

Figure 8-11 Rigging the assisted belay device (TRE).

Practicing the Belay with the TRE on Level Ground (Figure 8-12)

Preparation

1. Face the belay device. Take the rope that comes from the side of the TRE with the hand icon at the slot in your dominant hand (e.g., the right hand for right-handed individuals). *This is your brake hand. You must not take this hand off the rope when the person is "on belay" unless the belay is tied off.*

2. Take the rope on the side of the TRE that runs to the climber in your nondominant hand (the left hand for right-handed individuals). This is your *guide hand*. You will use it to help manipulate the rope.

3. To stop the rope from running out, pull back on the rope with the brake hand. Keep the guide hand in position to help maintain control of the rope. Note that this forces the crossbolt of the TRE to pinch the rope against the slot of the TRE, causing friction on the rope. To maintain the braking action, hold the rope tight with your brake hand.

A

B

Figure 8-12 Practicing with the TRE on level ground.

Continued

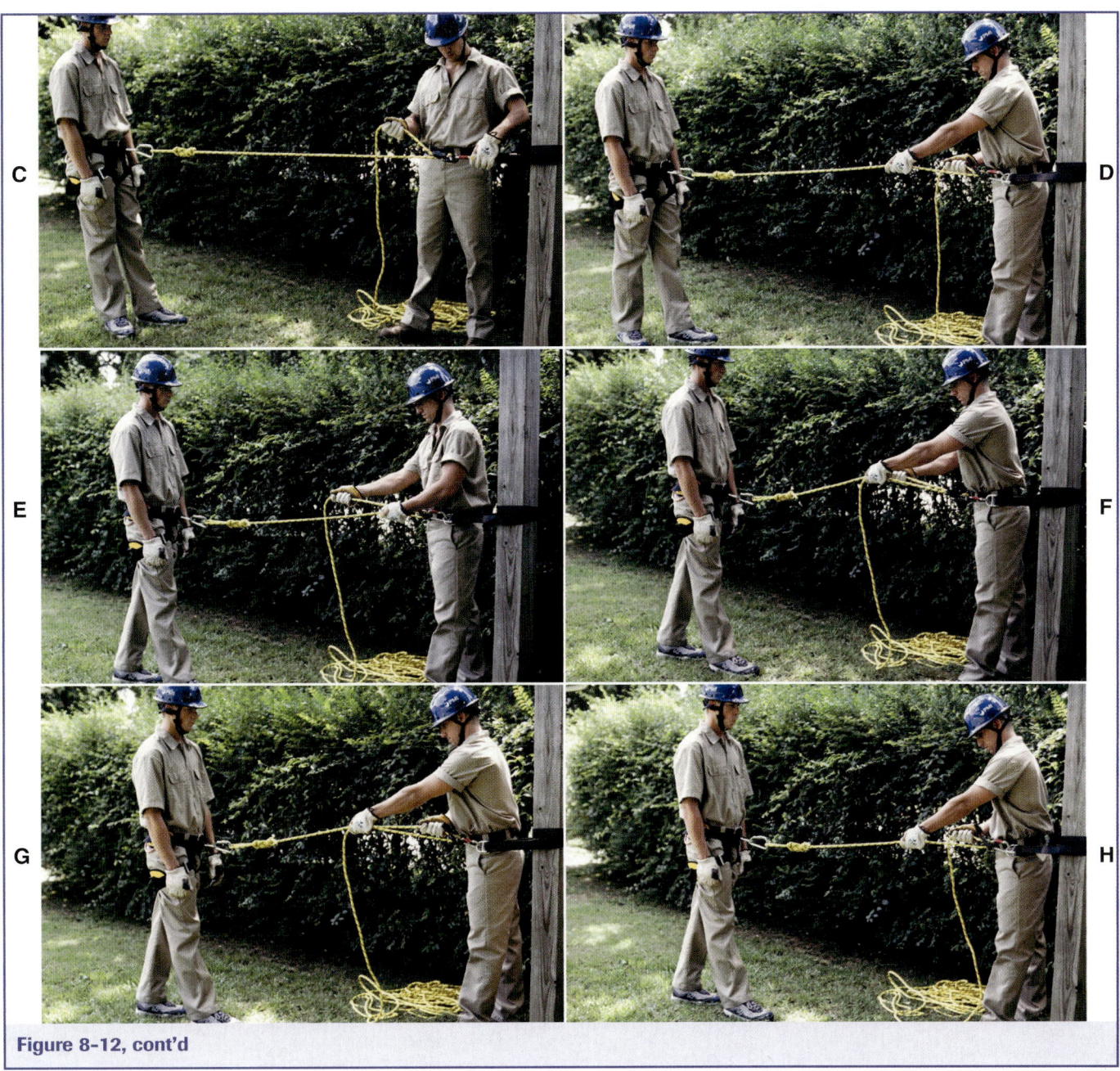

Figure 8-12, cont'd

Attaching the Climber

4. Now, have a partner wearing a seat harness clip into the end of the rope (Figure 8-12, *A*).

5. Remove slack in the rope between the belay device and the climber by holding the rope strands at a narrow angle and pulling the slack out with the brake hand (Figure 8-12, *B*).

6. Begin the belay voice signals. *(The person on the rope says, "On belay." The belayer, if ready, responds, "Belay on.")*

7. Have the person attached to the rope begin slowly walking backward.

8. Feed rope into the belay device with the brake hand and pull it with the guide hand. Maintain just enough slack so that it is noticeable and it allows the climber freedom of movement.

9. Now, initiate a braking action. Pull back on the rope with the brake hand. Keep the guide hand in position to help maintain control of the rope. To maintain the braking action, hold the rope tight with your brake hand. Keep the guide hand in position to help maintain control of the rope.

10. In an area where the climber will not slip, have the person firmly plant his or her feet on the ground and lean back from the rope. Hold the rope firmly with the brake hand (Figure 8-12, *C*).

11. Stop feeding rope through with the brake hand. The device should lock, holding the climber in place.

12. To get a feel of control, slowly let out a few inches (or centimeters) of rope with the climber leaning against the rope. Do this by bringing the two sides of the rope toward each other and by moving your brake hand toward the belay device.

Reversing Direction

13. Now, have your partner walk slowly toward you (Figure 8-12, *D*). The problem now is to take in rope while keeping the person safely on belay. To practice control of rope tension, do not allow the rope between the climber and the belay device to touch the ground.

14. Have your brake hand on the rope about 1 foot (.3 m) from the belay device.

15. Place your guide hand about 3 feet (1 m) from the TRE.

16. As slack appears in the rope, pull the slack out by pulling the rope with the brake hand. Your guide hand can help move rope toward the belay device (Figure 8-12, *E*).

17. At some point, your brake hand will have pulled so much rope that you will have to move this hand back toward the braking device. While gripping the rope with the brake hand, slide the guide back toward the belay device and below the brake hand. Hold the free (standing) part of the rope in your guide hand extended away from the body. Use two or three fingers of the guide hand to grip the free (standing) part of the rope. Keep the brake hand in the ready to brake position (Figure 8-12, *F*).

18. Using the guide hand, grip the standing end of the rope to provide back tension against the brake hand; then slide the brake hand back toward the belay device, all the while keeping the brake hand in the ready to brake position (Figure 8-12, *G*).

19. Continue the procedure until the person on the rope reaches your position (Figure 8-12, *H*).

Warning

When the weight falls and the belay catches, the belay rope comes taut with great force. To avoid injury, the belayer and others around the belayer must take the following precautions:

1. Be aware of the position the rope and belay device will take when the belay catches and stay out of this path. Otherwise, the impact of the rope and/or belay device can cause serious injury.

2. Keep fingers, hair, and clothing free of the rope near the belay device. Otherwise, these could be swept into the belay device, possibly causing injury and impeding the belay.

3. One-person belay devices are designed for catching one-person loads and may not be the most appropriate device for catching rescue loads.

20. Exchange the voice signals that conclude the belay cycle. *(Person on rope: "Off belay." Belayer: "Belay off.")*

Practicing with the TRE Using a Belay Weight or Dummy

Now practice belaying with the TRE using a belay weight or dummy as shown in Figure 8-2. First practice a belay with the weight or dummy falling as it is raised and then practice with the weight or dummy falling as it is lowered. In each case, as the weight comes onto your belay line, lower it to the ground with the brake plate.

In an actual belay situation, it is preferable to keep the climber in view. However, this is not always realistic. Therefore it is best to practice while facing away from the weight or dummy so that you cannot visually anticipate the fall. This will sharpen your skills at catching an unexpected fall.

Warning

Practice with the belay device you will be using. The devices are different and require skill to operate smoothly and correctly. The only way to gain that skill is actual practice with the device you will be using.

Additional Cautions for Belayers
Arranging the Belay Direction

The main elements of the belay system—the anchor, the belay device, and the climber—must be in as direct a line as possible so that the instant the climber falls, the force comes directly onto the belay device and the anchor. If these elements are not in a direct line, any or all of the following could happen:

- The belay device could fail to work properly.
- The belayer could be thrown off position.
- The anchor could fail.
- The system could be shock loaded.

Also, the belay rope must not be around or against the belayer or any other person, because that individual could be injured by the rope's suddenly coming taut.

Maintaining Proper Slack in the Belay Rope

As belayer, it is critical that you maintain a proper amount of slack in the belay rope. If a climber is on the rope, a rope that is too taut can interfere with the climber's movement. If the belay is a safety for a separate lowering system, a too taut rope could interfere with the brakeman's actions. Good judgment on the amount of slack to allow in the belay rope is another skill that develops with practice in belaying. The rope should have at least some *visible* slack, but not so much that intense shock loading of the rope would occur during a fall.

Securing the Belayer

If the belayer is near a place where he or she could fall, the belayer must be secured to an anchor by a safety line.

If you are the belayer, connect your safety line to an anchor separate from the belay if possible. This helps to ensure that you, as the belayer, are not endangered by a climber's fall and that whatever happens, you will remain stable to continue the belay or otherwise assist the climber.

Bottom Belay (for Rappelling Only)

A bottom belay is a pull on the rappel rope from a position below the rappeller (Figure 8-13). In essence, it is a substitute for the rappeller's control hand. A bottom belay can be performed by an individual at the bottom of the belay or by a second rappeller on a separate line who is lower than the belayed rappeller. Pulling on the belayed rappeller's line increases friction on the rappeller's descender. This method is commonly used to assist a rappeller who is in danger of losing control.

A bottom belay is not a substitute for the belays previously described. It should be used only when a top belay is not available and in an emergency.

Bottom belays have significant drawbacks, including the following:

- The rope can easily slip out of the grip of the person at the bottom.

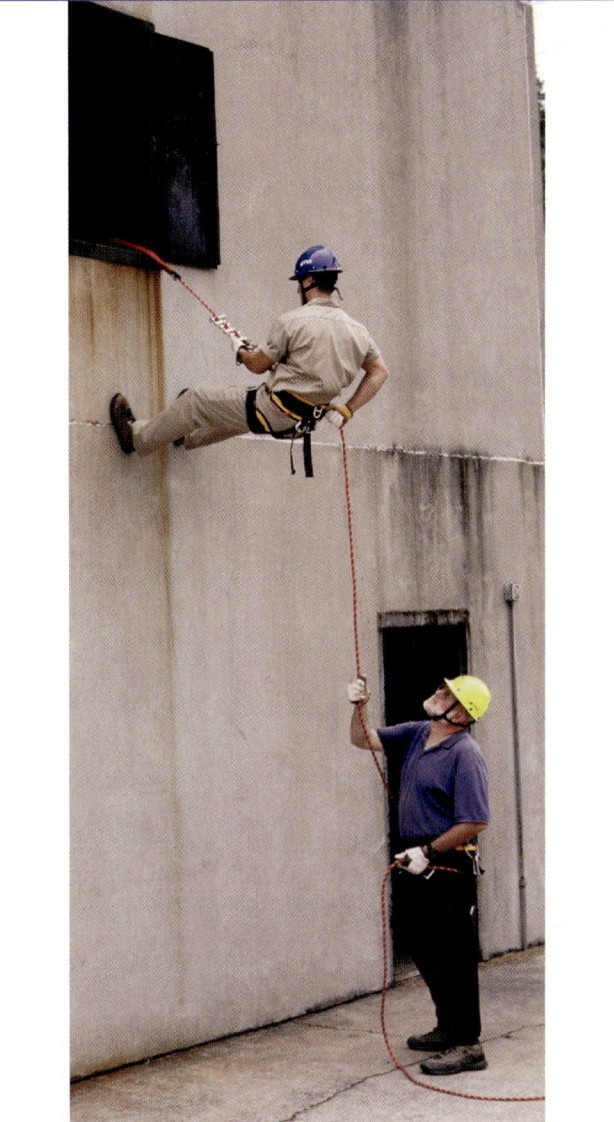

Figure 8-13 Bottom belay.

- The belayer can exert only as much pressure as his or her body weight. This often is sufficient if the belayer is directly below the rappeller and the rappeller has not gained too much momentum out of control. However, it frequently is not effective if applied from an angle or from so far beneath the rappeller that the pull is rendered ineffective by stretch in the rope.
- A bottom belay is not effective with all rappel devices.
- A person doing a bottom belay is in danger of being hit by objects such as rocks dislodged by the person or rope above.
- A bottom belay does not provide backup for failure of the main line rope, anchor, or rappel device, but only for an out of control rappel.

Body Belays

An additional technique for belaying is known as the *body belay*. With this technique, the belayer creates friction by running the rope around his or her body, usually around the waist. Except in emergencies this technique is not recommended, for the following reasons:

- It is not as easy to stop a fall as with a belay device.
- It can injure the belayer.

- The belayer's ability to hold a fall is only as strong as his or her pain threshold.
- If the belayer is at the top of a drop, he or she could be pulled over.
- The belayer can become entangled in the rope.
- If the climber falls, the belayer may be entrapped in a position from which he or she cannot assist the climber.

Evaluation Exercises

Cognitive and Affective Exercises

1. List the six elements of a belay system.

2. Describe six situations in which a belay might be required.

3. Describe how a belay differs from a lowering in the following:

   A. Purpose
   B. Technique
   C. Equipment

4. With you playing the role of a belayer and another person playing the role of a climber, recite from memory the cycle of belay voice communications. Reverse roles.

5. List three reasons why belay plates on figure 8 descenders may pose problems.

6. List the conditions in which a bottom belay can be used.

Psychomotor Exercises

7. On flat ground, rig a Münter hitch belay system. Using a partner tied into the rope, have him or her walk away from you in a belay cycle.

8. Repeat the above with the partner approaching you.

9. Repeat numbers 7 and 8 using a personal belay device.

10. Using a belay dummy and weight fall, rig a Münter hitch belay and simulate a situation in which a climber falls as the rope is being let out.

11. Using a belay dummy and weight fall, rig a Münter hitch belay and simulate a situation in which a climber falls as a rope is being taken in.

12. Using a belay dummy and weight fall, repeat numbers 10 and 11 using a one-person belay device.

9
Rappelling

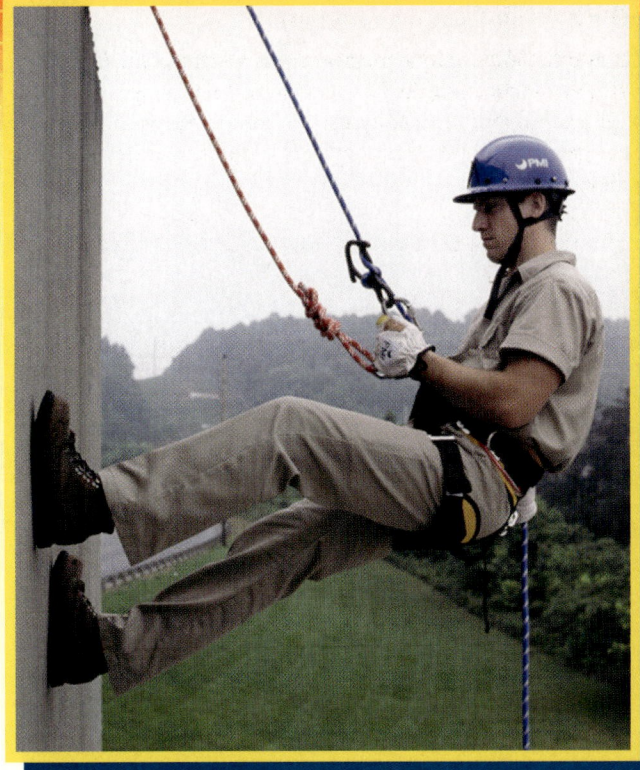

Key Terms

Arm Rappel (Guide's Rappel) A type of rappel in which the rope wraps around both outstretched arms and across the person's back. The technique is sometimes used in sloping terrain. It does not give enough control for vertical situations.

Body Rappel (*Dulfersitz* Rappel) A type of rappel that uses the body as friction by running the rope through the legs, across one hip, over the opposite shoulder, and to a braking hand. Because of the discomfort involved and the potential injury to body parts, this rappel has largely been supplanted by other techniques.

Brake Bar Rack A rappel device that consists of a series of short metal bars fixed to and sliding along a U-shaped metal rack with an eye at one end for attachment.

Brake Hand The hand that grasps the rope to help control the speed of descent during a rappel. The dominant hand (e.g., the right hand in a right-handed individual) usually is the brake hand.

Carabiner Wrap A rappel technique that uses several rope wraps around a seat harness carabiner to create friction and control the descent. It generally is not considered a safe or secure technique for rappelling.

Descender A rappel device that creates friction by means of a rope running through it; it is attached to a rappeller to control descent on a rope. Most descenders can also be used as a fixed brake lowering device. Also called a *descent control device*.

***Dulfersitz* Rappel** See Body Rappel.

Figure 8 Descender A commonly used descender made roughly in the shape of a figure 8.

Guide Hand The hand that cradles the rope to help balance the rappeller. The nondominant hand (e.g., the right hand in a left-handed individual) is usually the guide hand.

Locking Off The technique of jamming a rope into a descender or tying off securely so that the rappeller can stop the descent and operate hands free of the rope.

Münter Hitch Rappel A limited-use rappel technique involving a Münter hitch attached to the seat harness carabiner.

Rappelling Controlled descent of a rope using friction to obtain the control. Normally the friction is created by rope running through a descender.

Rappelling

Rappelling is the controlled descent of a rope using the friction of the rope through a descender as the means of control. It is a necessary skill for operating safely in the vertical environment. Learning safe, controlled rappelling skills is a step toward developing vertical competency.

To the inexperienced, rappelling may appear to be a spectacular act. However, the ability to rappel does not by itself indicate that a person is skilled and knowledgeable in the vertical environment. Rappelling is not the ultimate goal for a high angle technician; it is just one personal skill, which must be used in combination with other skills for activities in the vertical environment. For example, rappelling may be the means of travel in a controlled descent of a vertical face. It also may be combined with other essential vertical skills for performing a rescue.

⬛ Warning

It is essential that from the beginning, anyone learning to rappel maintain absolute control of the descent. Among the ways of ensuring this control are the following:
- Avoid rapid, bouncing rappels that can lead to loss of control, damaged rope, overloaded anchors, and injuries.
- Use a top belay.
- Learn under the guidance of a qualified, experienced instructor.

Importance of Control

An important sign of a person's competence in rappelling is *control*. Evidence of control includes the ability to:
- Control the descent with minimal physical effort
- Rappel in a controlled manner so that the rope is not damaged by heat buildup in the rappel device and anchors are not damaged by shock loading
- Stop the rappel any time
- Tie off securely and operate hands free of the rope and rappel device
- Operate in any body position, including the inverted position

How Rappelling Works

All techniques for rappelling use friction with the rope to slow the rate of descent. Both the ***body rappel (Dulfersitz rappel)*** and the ***arm rappel (guide's rappel)*** use friction of the rope on the body to slow the descent. This friction, and the resulting heat and discomfort, can make these techniques unpleasant to use. Because of this discomfort and the potential dangers, these techniques are no longer widely used.

Most modern techniques use *rappel devices*, or ***descenders*** (also known as ***descent control devices***), which are attached to the rappeller, usually by means of a seat harness carabiner. The rope runs through the device to create friction so that the heat and pressure are directed into the device and not the rappeller's body. A well-designed rappel device also offers more control of the descent than does a body rappel.

With most rappel devices, the rate of descent is controlled by pulling on the part of the rope below the device. This increases friction by increasing rope tension and pressure on metal parts of the device. The rappeller usually exerts this controlling action with the dominant hand (e.g., usually the right hand for a right-handed person). This hand is known as the **brake hand**.

The rappeller's other hand cradles the rope above the device or (with some descenders) the device itself. *This hand does not support body weight by grasping the rope.* With most rappel devices, this hand is known as the **guide hand**, which helps balance the rappeller. In some rappel devices it may also help control the descender.

Rappels Using Body Friction
Arm Rappel

Figure 9-1 shows the arm rappel, which sometimes is used for short distances on low angle slopes. The user sets up the rappel by having his or her upper back to the anchored rope while facing uphill. The rappeller then wraps both extended arms around the rope. The friction and rate of descent are controlled by varying handgrips.

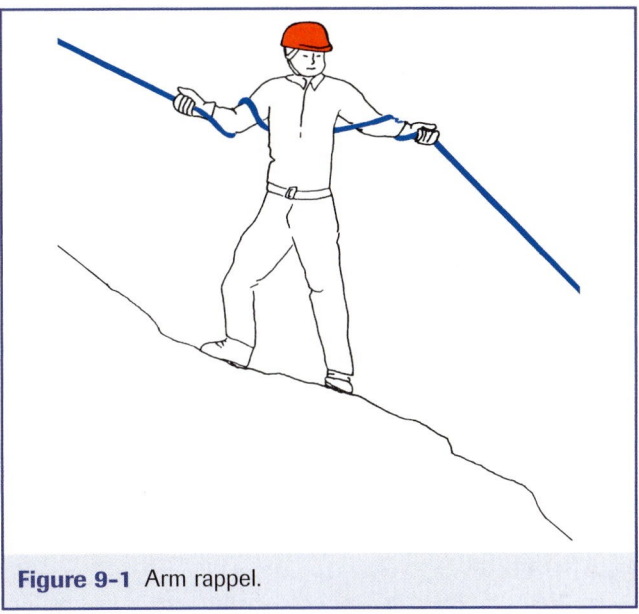

Figure 9-1 Arm rappel.

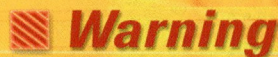

Warning

Use the arm rappel only on short, low-angle slopes; it does not produce enough friction to control full body weight adequately in a completely vertical situation. Because of the potential for rope abrasion injuries on the arms and hands, use this technique only when you are wearing long-sleeved shirts and gloves. Make sure your rope is long enough so that you end up in a safe zone at the end of the rope.

Body Rappel (*Dulfersitz* Rappel)

Figure 9-2 shows a procedure for wrapping the rope for a body rappel:

1. The rappeller straddles an anchored rope, facing the anchor.
2. The part of the rope below the rappeller is brought around one hip (i.e., the side with the dominant arm).
3. The rope then is brought across the chest and over the opposite shoulder.
4. The rope now is brought down across the back to the braking hand (the dominant hand), which is on the same side as the hip where the rope runs.
5. The rappeller controls the descent by (dominant) hand strength and by bringing the rope across the torso with the brake hand.

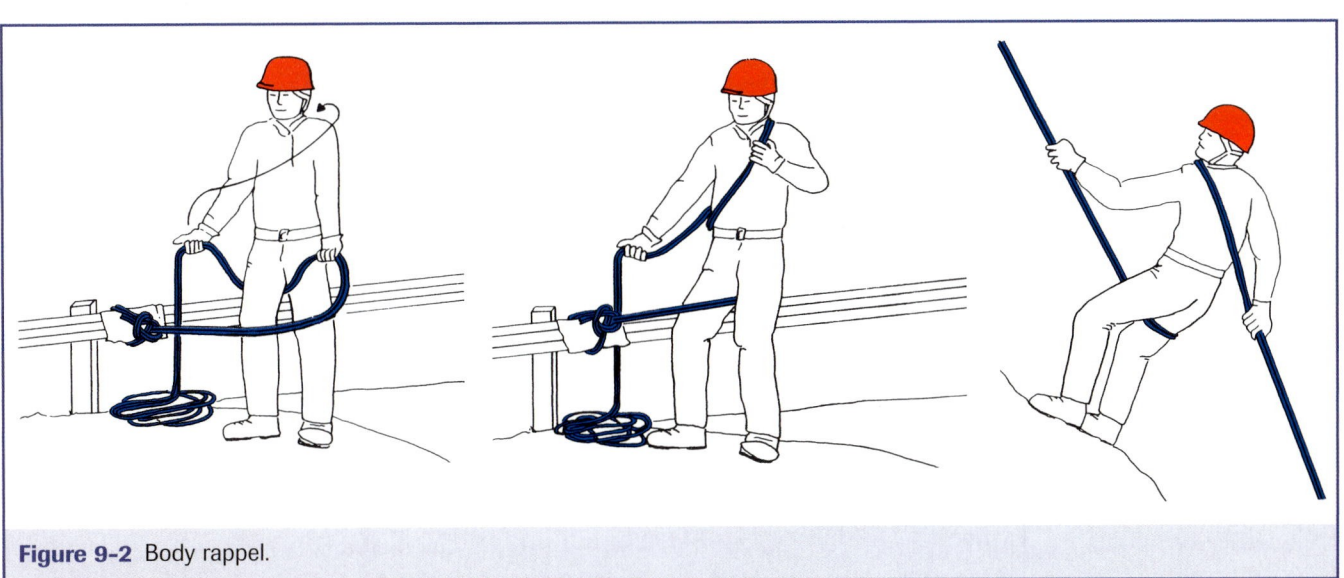

Figure 9-2 Body rappel.

As mentioned in the warning box below, one danger of the body rappel is that on high angle rappels, the rope can become unwrapped from the leg. Therefore the wrapped leg must be kept lower than the unwrapped leg and the upper body.

The body rappel technique can cause considerable pain, possibly severe enough to prompt the rappeller to let go to relieve the pain.

⚠ Warning

The body rappel must be practiced on a low-angle slope before it is attempted on a steep slope. It should not be used as a general practice, but rather only in case of emergency, when no hardware is available for use as a rappel device.

The body rappel technique presents two potential dangers:

1. The rope could come unwrapped from rappeller's leg. Consequently, the rappeller would lose friction with the rope and may fall free to the ground. This is a particular danger on a vertical face.
2. Rope abrasion and pressure can injure body parts, particularly the crotch and shoulder. Thick padding in these areas is recommended.

Mechanical Rappel Devices
Figure 8 Descenders

One design of a conventional *figure 8 descender* is shown in Figure 9-3 (see Chapter 5 for more details on materials and the various designs). The larger ring of the figure 8 may be rounded or squared off, depending on the specific design. The larger ring creates friction on the rope; the smaller ring attaches to a seat harness carabiner.

Most conventional figure 8 descenders are found in smaller sizes. Because they are compact and lightweight, smaller figure 8s are often used by climbers and other individuals involved in recreational activities.

Although the conventional figure 8 is a strong device for rappelling, it has significant drawbacks in some situations (Box 9-1).

Box 9-1	**Drawbacks of Figure 8 Devices**

Figure 8 devices have a number of drawbacks; for example:

❑ You cannot use the smaller version with larger diameter rope.

❑ You may find it difficult to use the smaller figure 8 descender double wrapped (double wrapping of a figure 8 descender is explained on p. 125).

❑ When you are rappelling with the conventional figure 8, the rope wraps can slip up and around the larger ring, forming a girth hitch (Figure 9-4).

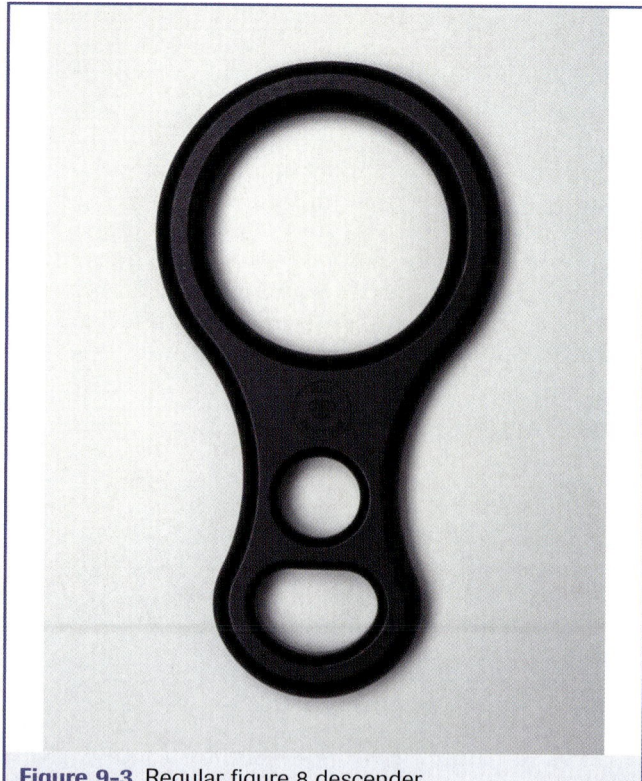

Figure 9-3 Regular figure 8 descender.

The Girth Hitch Problem

Accidental girth hitching of the figure 8 ring tends to occur under two circumstances:

1. When the rappeller attempts to ease over a difficult edge or ledge, and the edge catches a wrap of rope on the bottom of the figure 8. The weight of the rappeller forces the wrap over

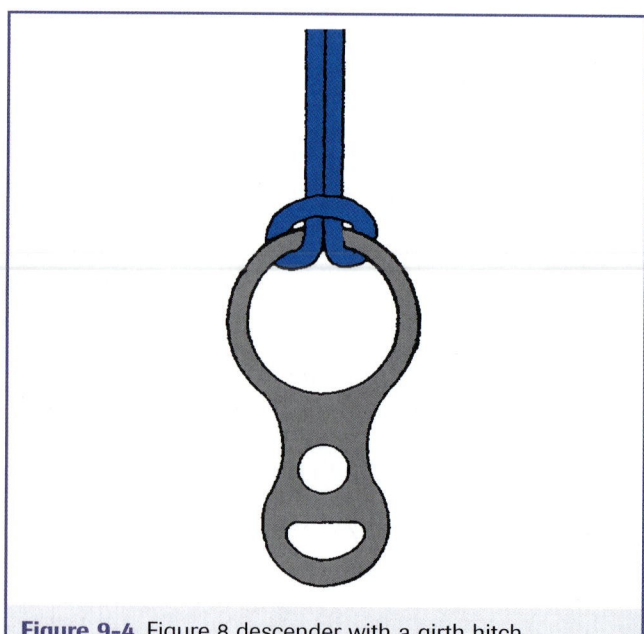

Figure 9-4 Figure 8 descender with a girth hitch.

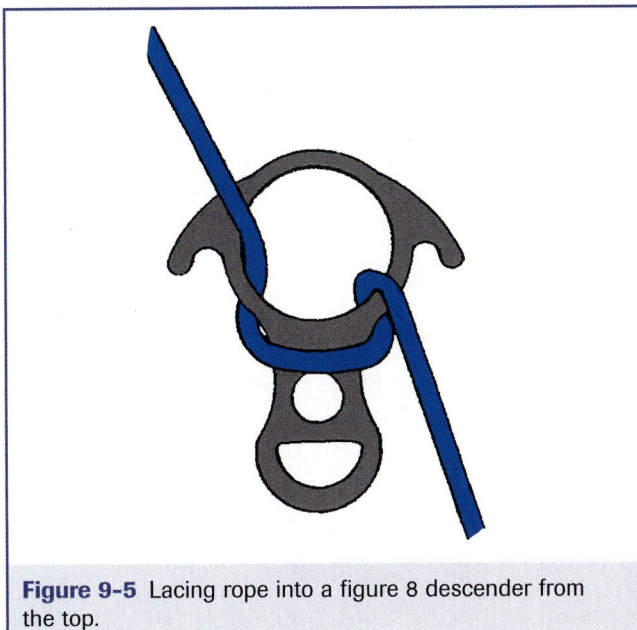

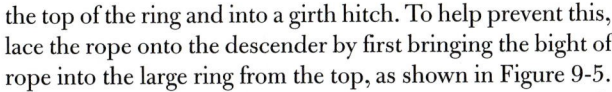

Figure 9-5 Lacing rope into a figure 8 descender from the top.

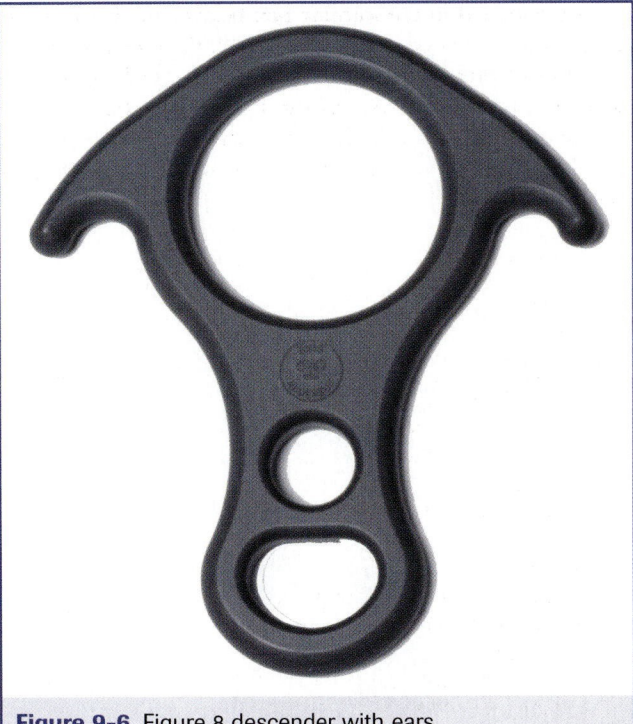

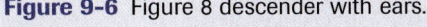

Figure 9-6 Figure 8 descender with ears.

the top of the ring and into a girth hitch. To help prevent this, lace the rope onto the descender by first bringing the bight of rope into the large ring from the top, as shown in Figure 9-5.

2. When a rappeller allows momentary slack in the rope, such as when rappelling over ledges or uneven faces or in bouncing rappels. These situations cause a momentary slack in the rope wrap, allowing it to slip over the large ring.

Girth hitching of the figure 8 immediately stops the rappel and prevents the rappeller from descending farther. Movement can begin again only when the rappeller can remove his or her weight from the girth hitch long enough to slide it back over the large ring. Without the appropriate skills and equipment, this is a difficult and hazardous position from which to escape. Rappellers with good upper-body strength might be able to extricate themselves forcefully by lifting the body weight from the figure 8. However, it is easier and usually safer to set an ascender or Prusik knot on the rope above the figure 8 and step into an attached sling. (See Chapter 10, p. 160, for possible ways of extricating yourself from this kind of situation.)

The best solution to the problem of a girth hitch on a figure 8 descender is prevention. One way to prevent a girth hitch is to use a figure 8 with ears (Figure 9-6). The "ears" (protrusions on the larger ring) primarily serve to prevent the rope from slipping over the larger ring to form a girth hitch. However, the ears also help to contour the rope around the ring and to hold the rope in place when *locking off*. Consequently, unless space and weight are strong considerations, the figure 8 with ears is preferable for most rappellers.

Rappelling with the Figure 8 with Ears

Using the Figure 8 with Ears on Level Ground (Figure 9-7)

PREPARATION

1. Don a sewn, manufactured seat harness with thigh supports and a front tie-in point.

Warning

1. Rappelling techniques must be learned and practiced under the guidance of a qualified instructor.
2. These techniques must be practiced first on level ground and then on short and moderate slopes before they are used on a steep face.
3. Everyone practicing rappel techniques on a steep face or in any other area where a severe fall is possible must use a top belay.

2. Clip a large locking carabiner or screw link into the seat harness tie-in point. If the carabiner or screw link is in a vertical plane after being clipped on, make sure the gate is toward your body (this helps prevent friction against a vertical face from opening the gate).
3. Establish a secure anchor point.
4. Firmly attach a main-line rappel rope to the anchor point.

ATTACHING THE FIGURE 8

5. Take a figure 8 with ears in your guide hand (Figure 9-7, *A*).
6. Face the anchor with the rope running past you on your brake hand side.
7. On the rappel main line near the anchor, take a bight of rope in your brake hand. Push it through the large ring of the figure 8 descender *from the top* (Figure 9-7, *B*).
8. Bring the bight of rope around the end of the small rung of the figure 8 descender and across the waist of the rappel

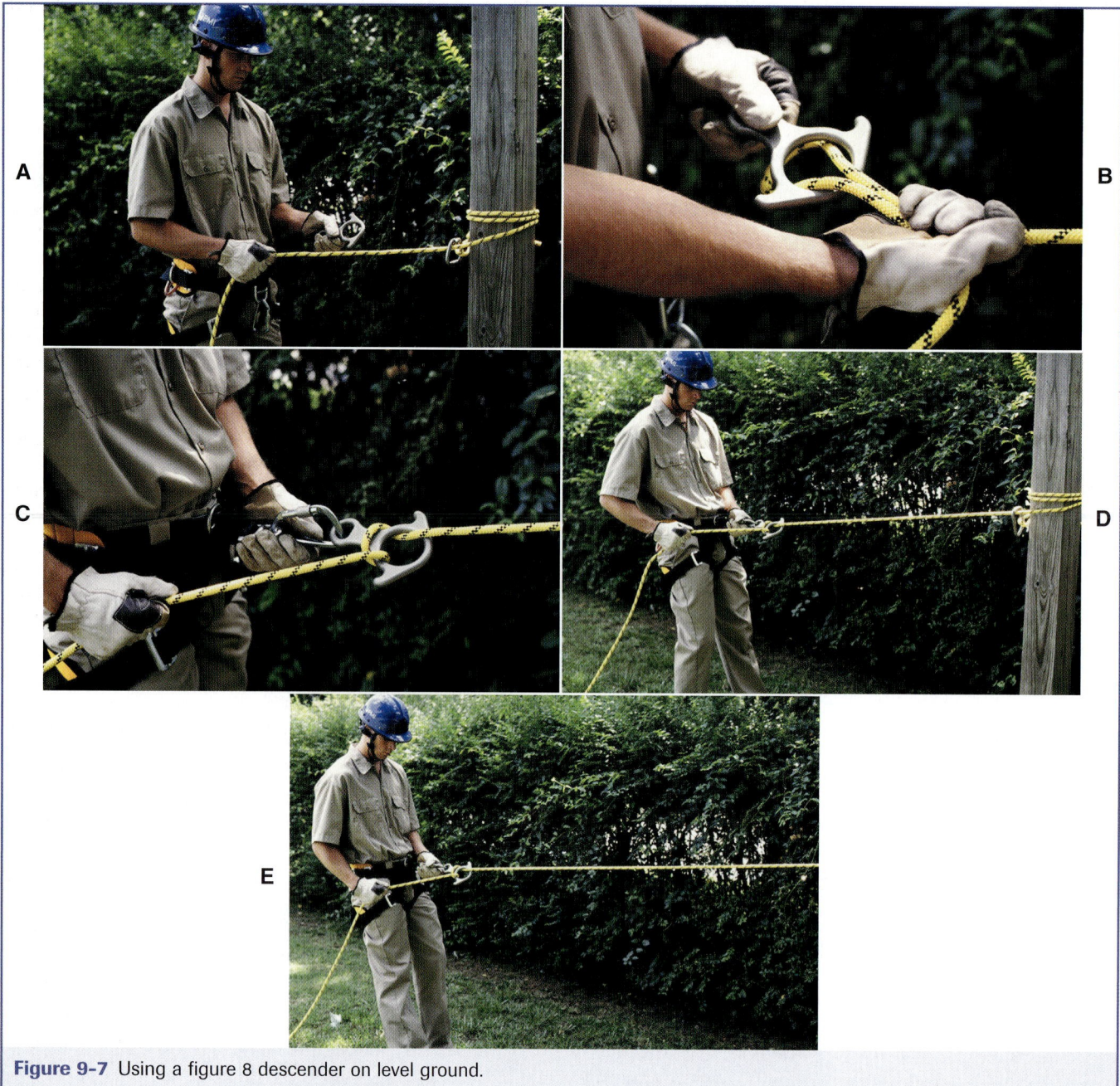

Figure 9-7 Using a figure 8 descender on level ground.

device. Snug the rope around the figure 8 descender by pulling on the piece of rope on the side of the descender away from the anchor (i.e., the running end). If the figure 8 descender will be in a horizontal plane when it is clipped into your seat harness, the rope should run across the top of the waist of the figure 8 descender. If the figure 8 descender will be in a vertical plane once it is clipped into your seat harness, the rope should lie across the side of the descender near your brake hand (Figure 9-7, *C*).

NOTE: When you must slide over a difficult edge to rappel, the figure 8 descender could get caught on the edge. You will be less likely to jam on the edge if the rope is on the side of the descender away from the edge. Also, if you are using a conventional

figure 8 descender and keep the rope on the side away from the edge, the rope is less likely to be pushed up over the larger ring and form a girth hitch.

9. Clip the small ring of the figure 8 descender into your seat harness carabiner. Lock the carabiner (Figure 9-7, *D*).

10. Take the running part of the rope (the part on the lower side of the figure 8 descender) in your dominant hand (e.g., the right hand on right-handed individuals). This is your *brake hand*. For the brake hand, the cardinal rule is: *when rappelling, never take your brake hand off the rope unless the descender has been securely tied off.*

11. With your nondominant hand (e.g., the left hand for right-handed individuals), lightly cradle the rope above the figure

8 descender. This is your guide hand. This hand is not for supporting your weight, but rather to help you balance yourself. For the guide hand, the cardinal rule is: *when rappelling, do not support your weight with the guide hand because you could be thrown off balance.*

12. Now, by pulling down on the rope with your brake hand, pull the slack out of the rope between the figure 8 descender and the anchor. If this is difficult, you can help the process with your guide hand (Figure 9-7, *E*).

13. Grasp the rope below the figure 8 descender with your brake hand and pull it taut against your hip, with your hand about 6 inches (15 cm) below your hip. This is the best position to assume that will provide extra stopping power by using the friction of the rope against your hip. (You should not keep the rope against your hip constantly, however, because it may abrade the webbing of your seat harness.) Keeping the rope taut with your brake hand, swing the rope out about 2 feet (0.7 m) from your hip at an angle that is comfortable for your arm.

NOTE: Now is the time for a safety check. Have your instructor check your rigging, carabiners, descender, gloves, and so on.

STARTING THE RAPPEL

14. Lean back from the anchor so that the rope between the figure 8 descender and the anchor becomes taut. Always remove the rope slack between your descender and the anchor before beginning a rappel.

15. As you lean back against the rope, begin to walk backward, using your brake hand to let the rope slip slowly through the figure 8 descender; keep your guide hand lightly on the rope above the rappel device. As you let the rope slip through your brake hand, keep the same distance on the rope between your hand and the figure 8 descender.

LOCKING OFF (FIGURE 9-8)

16. Gripping the rope with the brake hand, allow the rope to slide through the descender until the brake hand is about 1 foot (0.3 m) from the rappel device (Figure 9-8, *A*).

17. *Using your brake hand, hold the rope taut* and with a continuous, smooth motion, pull the rope in an arc from the rappel position straight out in front of you. Pass the brake side of the rope below the main line and then to a point where the rope and your hand are 180 degrees from the rappel position (Figure 9-8, *B*).

NOTE: This may be a little difficult to do while standing on flat ground. When a rappeller is suspended by the rope on a steep slope or vertical face, the movement is much less awkward to perform. This has to do with the angle of the rope and anchor in relation to the figure 8 and the rappeller.

18. *Maintain a firm grip on the rope with your brake hand.* Then, using the brake hand, take the strand of rope the hand is holding and pull it down farther toward you to trap it between the strand of rope that goes to the anchor and the large ring of the figure 8 descender (Figure 9-8, *C*). *The*

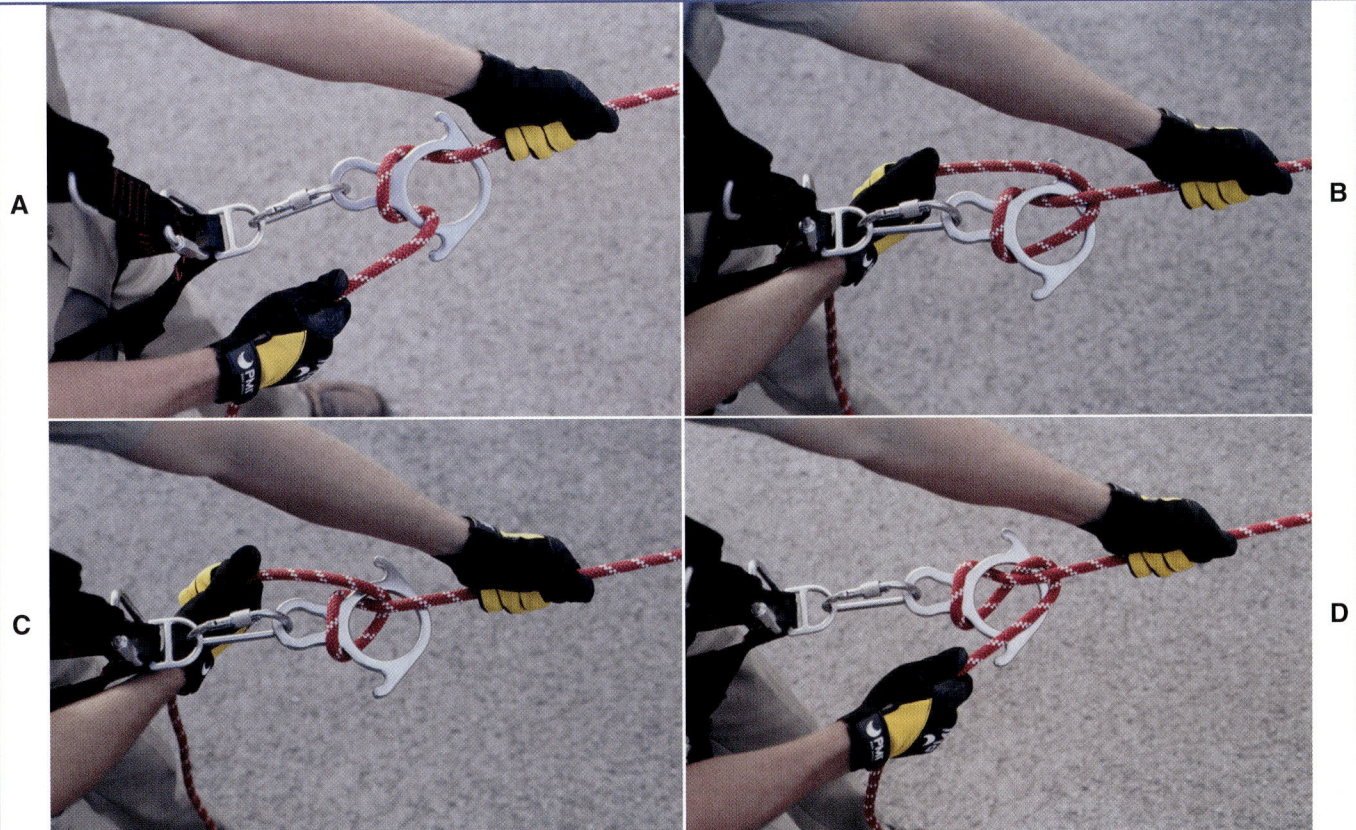

Figure 9-8 Locking off a figure 8 descender.

braking side of the rope must be firmly trapped between the rope that goes out of the descender to the anchor and the large ring of the figure 8. For this to happen, there must be tension on the rope between the figure 8 descender and the anchor.

UNLOCKING

19. *Take the rope firmly in your brake hand.* In a smooth, continuous motion, pull the rope first straight toward the anchor and then in an arc back to the rappel position. You will hear a slight "pop" and feel a slight bump as the rope unlocks from the rappel device (Figure 9-8, *D*). *Keep the rope firmly in your brake hand.* Continue rappelling.

Rappelling with the Figure 8 Descender on a Slope (Figure 9-9)

PREPARATION

1. Establish a secure anchor point at the top of a short slope of about 45 degrees (if a slope is not available, use a stairway). Attach the rappel rope securely to the anchor point.

2. Establish an anchor point for a belay. Attach an anchor sling securely into the anchor point. Clip a large locking carabiner into the end of the anchor sling.

3. Have a belayer take position. If a Münter hitch is being used for belay, have the belayer create the hitch in the belay rope and clip it into the belay carabiner. If the belayer is using a mechanical belay device, attach it to the rope and clip it into the belay anchor carabiner. Make sure the carabiner gate is locked.

NOTE: Keep a proper distance between the belay anchor rope and the main-line rappel rope. As noted elsewhere in this book, it is good practice to keep rope strands (such as the belay line and the main-line rappel rope) apart to prevent tangling and damage to the rope from heat fusion as a result of rope cross. However, the distance between the rappel line and belay anchors should not be too great. If the anchors are separated by too great a distance, and the main-line rappel anchor fails but the belay catches, the possibility of a *pendulum fall* exists (this is a sudden swing on the line that could result in injury to the rappeller or damage to the rope).

4. Clip into the belay rope. Initiate the belay cycle with the belay voice signals *(Rappeller: "On belay." Belayer [if ready]: "Belay on.")* (Figure 9-9, *A*).

5. At a secure point, where you are in no danger of falling, follow steps 5 through 14 under Using the Figure 8 with Ears on Level Ground (pp. 119-121) to lace the figure 8 descender onto the rope (Figure 9-9, *B* and *C*).

NOTE: Do a safety check on all equipment and rigging. In particular, inspect carabiners for sideloaded gates and unlocked gates and anchor slings needing adjustment. Make sure that loose clothing is tucked in, hair is not in danger of being caught, and the helmet chin strap is secure.

BEGINNING THE RAPPEL

6. Begin to back down the slope, controlling your descent with the brake hand and following steps 14 through 18 (p. 121). Keep the following principles in mind (Figure 9-9, *D*):
    - Keep your body generally perpendicular to the slope.
    - Keep your feet apart, about the width of your shoulders.
    - Keep your knees relaxed and slightly flexed.
    - Take slow, deliberate steps backward.
    - Keep your body slightly turned in the direction of the brake hand, looking down slope to select a path of travel.
    - Use your guide hand for balance. *Do not support your weight with the guide hand.*
    - *Never take the brake hand off the rope unless the belay device has been securely locked off.*

7. When part way down the slope, stop the rappel and lock off the figure 8 descender as described in steps 16 through 18 (left column) (Figure 9-9, *E* and *F*).

8. Unlock (step 19, left column) and continue the rappel to the end of the slope.

9. Conclude the belay cycle with the belay voice communications. *(Rappeller: "Off belay." Belayer: "Belay off.")*

> ## ⬛ Warning
>
> 1. Rappelling techniques must be learned and practiced under the guidance of a qualified instructor.
> 2. These techniques must be practiced first on level ground and then on short and moderate slopes before they are used on a steep face.
> 3. Everyone practicing rappel techniques on a steep face or in any other area where a severe fall is possible must use a top belay.

Rappelling Down a Vertical Face with a Figure 8 Descender (Figure 9-10)

PREPARATION

1. Choose a short vertical face (about 20 feet [6 m]) on which the top breaks over gradually into a steep face. On the first try, do not choose a face with a sharp edge.

2. Establish a secure anchor (see Chapter 7) a safe distance from the edge. If possible, have the anchor point high above the edge; this will assist any rappeller going over the edge. Attach the main-line rappel rope securely to the anchor point.

3. Establish a separate anchor for a belay a safe distance from the edge. Attach a sling securely to the anchor point. The anchor point and sling should be established so that the belayer, when taking position, has a good field of view of the top and face but is not in danger of falling over the edge. In the end of the sling, clip a large locking carabiner.

4. Have a belayer take position to belay. If the danger of falling exists, have the belayer secure himself or herself to a safety line. If a Münter hitch is to be used for the belay, have the belayer tie the Münter hitch into the belay rope and clip it into the belay carabiner. If the belayer is using a mechanical belay device, attach it to the rope and clip it into the belay anchor carabiner.

5. Clip into the belay rope with a knot or locking carabiner. Initiate the belay cycle with the belay voice signals *(Rappeller: "On belay." Belayer [if ready]: "Belay on.")* (Figure 9-10, *A*).

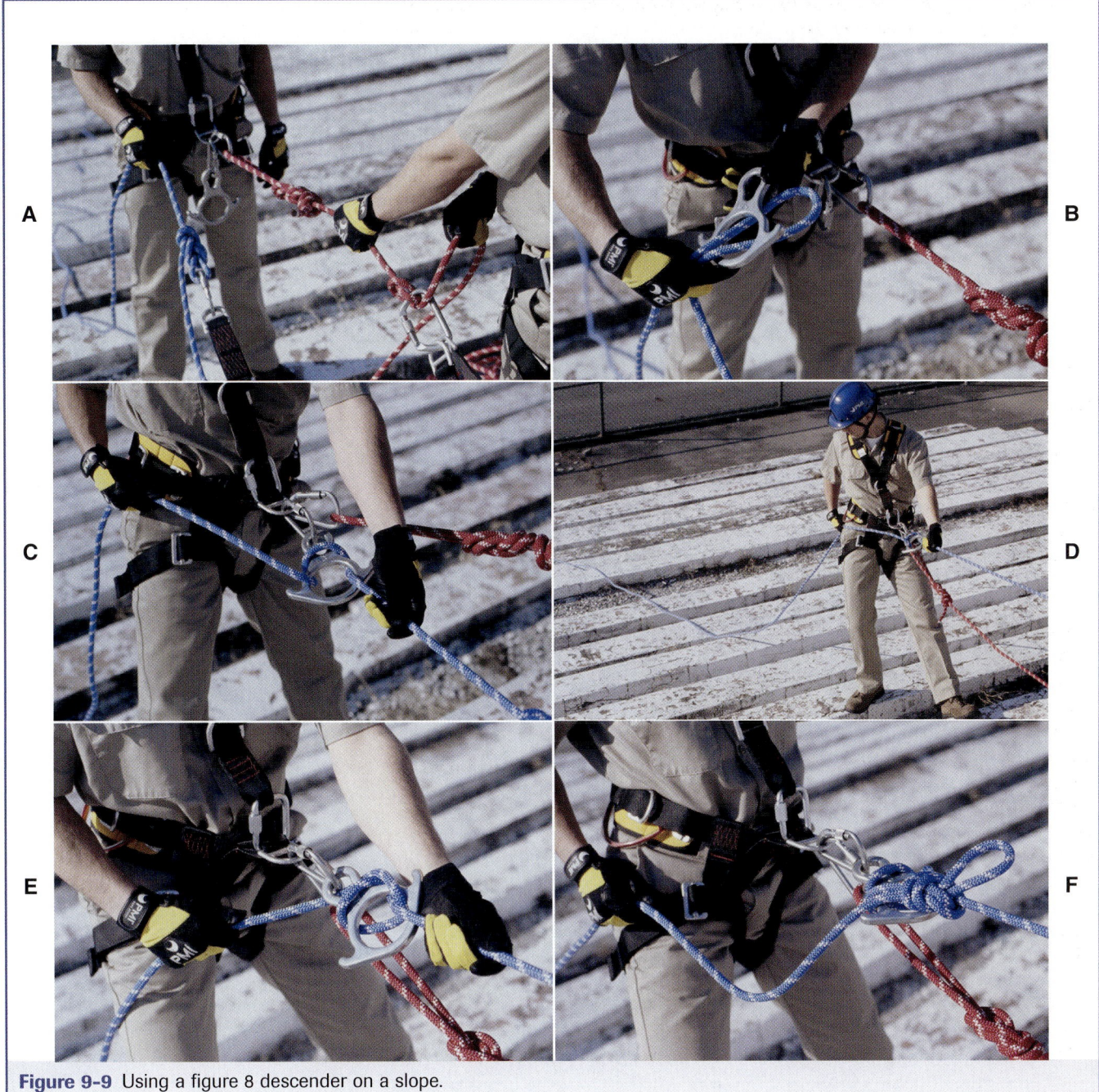

Figure 9-9 Using a figure 8 descender on a slope.

BEGINNING THE RAPPEL

6. At a secure point, where you are in no danger of falling, follow steps 7 through 14 under Using the Figure 8 with Ears on Level Ground (pp. 119-121) for attaching the figure 8 descender to the rope (Figure 9-10, *B*).

7. Make sure the slack is out of the rope between the figure 8 descender and the anchor. Do a safety check on all connectors (e.g., carabiners) and on the seat harness, the anchor, and other rigging. Make sure no loose clothing or hair can be caught in the descender. Make sure your helmet is on securely.

8. Slowly begin backing toward the edge. Keep the following principles in mind:
   - *Keep your body generally perpendicular to the slope.* To do this, you must deliberately lean out as the slope becomes vertical. At first, this may seem an unnatural stance, but this position is necessary to prevent your feet from slipping out from under you (Figure 9-10, *E* and *F*).
   - Keep your feet about shoulder width apart for balance. This helps prevent your being pulled to one side.
   - Keep your knees relaxed and slightly flexed.
   - Take slow, deliberate steps backward.

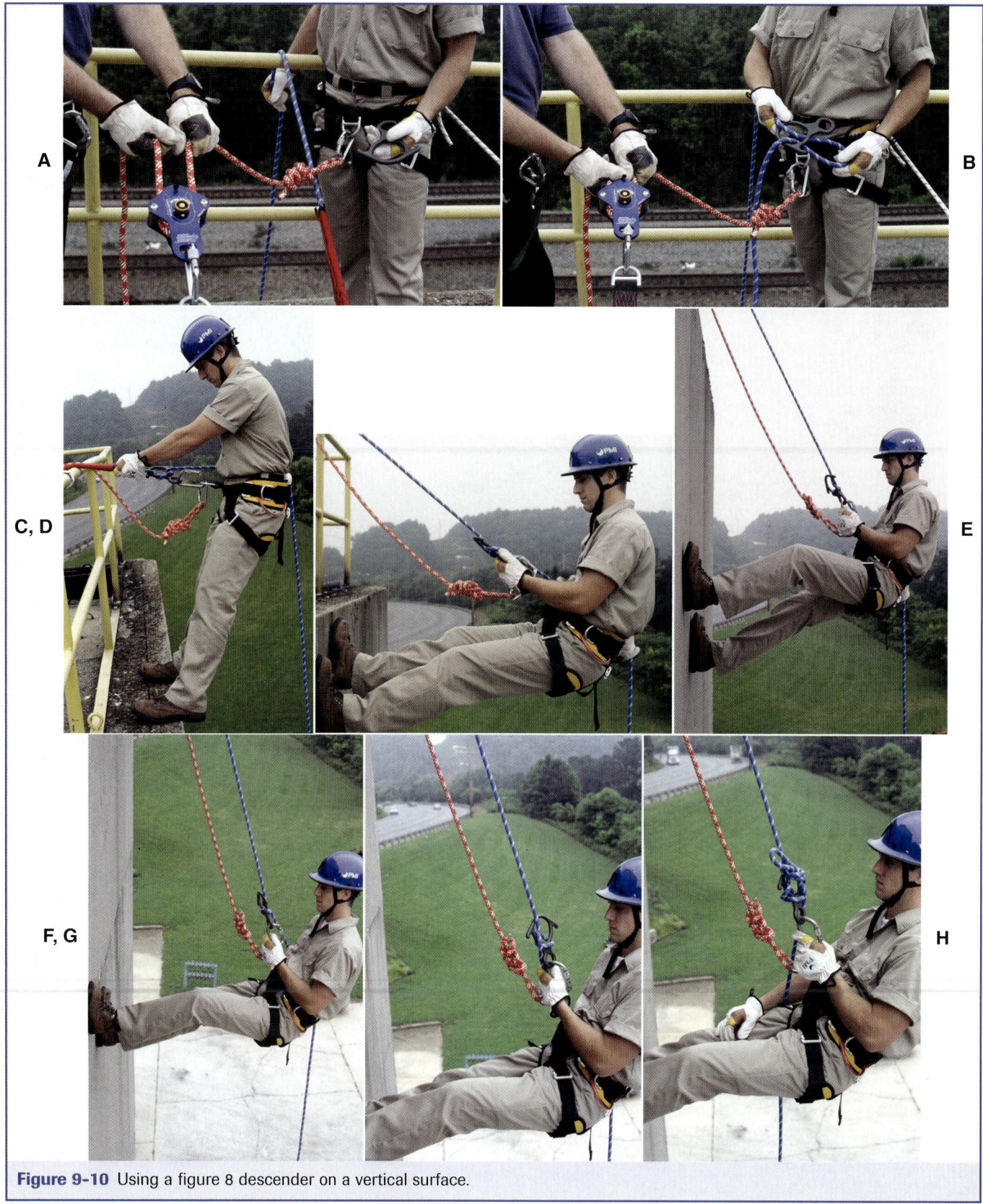

Figure 9-10 Using a figure 8 descender on a vertical surface.

- Keep your body slightly turned in the direction of the brake hand, looking down slope to pick a path for your descent.
- Use your guide hand for balance. *Do not support your weight with your guide hand.*
- *Never take your brake hand off the rope unless you are securely locked off.*

NOTE: The belay, as it is normally used, is for the safety of the rappeller. It is not to be used by the belayer to control the rappeller's rate of descent, nor is it to be used to share the load when the rappeller is in a controlled descent. To learn proper control of a rappel device, students must learn to control their full weight, with no control coming from the belayer. Therefore it is important that the belay line have a small amount of slack as the rappeller descends. Only if the rappeller loses control or requests assistance (e.g., by calling, "Tension") does the belayer control the rappeller's weight and/or rate of descent.

9. As you move over the edge, more of your weight is held by the rope. This means that you need to exert greater effort for control with the brake hand. As the rope is weighted, you may feel pulled to the right or left. Step slightly in that direction until you feel a better balance (Figure 9-10, *E, F*).

10. If you slip, fall over, or even turn upside down, *keep calm. Hold tight with your brake hand until you orient yourself.* Then, slowly, place your feet against the face and rebalance yourself.

LOCKING OFF

11. Midway down the face, stop the rappel and lock off. On a vertical face, with your weight on the rope and descender, you will find it more difficult to trap the rope between the main line and the large ring of the figure 8 descender (Box 9-2). Hold the brake line steady and pull it across and

---

Box 9-2 | **Locking Off a Large Figure 8 Descender**

1. Trap the brake side of the rope between the line going to the anchor and the large ring on the descender.
2. Pull the brake side of the rope firmly down toward the seat harness carabiner, across the surface of the figure 8, and around behind the ears. Do not bring the rope through the large ring of the figure 8; it should be between the line going to the anchor and the large ring and above the line first locked off. Make sure the rope lies firmly around the device and there is no slack.
3. Bring the brake side of the rope down and around the figure 8 again and then behind one ear, but do not place it between the line going to the anchor and the large ring. Instead, form a large bight of rope from the brake side of the rope.
4. Bring the bight up parallel with the rope going to the anchor.
5. Tie an overhand knot with the bight onto the rope going to the anchor.
6. Make sure that the overhand knot is well contoured and that there is no slack in the knot.

---

down with deliberate force until it is securely trapped (Figure 9-10, *G*).

A MORE SECURE LOCK OFF FOR THE FIGURE 8 DESCENDER

In some vertical situations, a more secure lock off for the figure 8 descender may be desirable, such as when the rappeller may need to be locked off for a long period, when he or she must do a great deal of moving about in one position to manipulate equipment or a rescue subject, or under any other circumstances in which the rappeller feels the need for greater security.

Figure 9-11 shows a technique for more securely locking off a large figure 8 descender (the technique is described in Box 9-2).

To unlock this more secure lock off, untie the overhand knot and unwrap the brake side of the rope from around the figure. *Always keep the rope firmly in your brake hand, with no slack in the rope between your brake hand and the figure 8.*

UNLOCKING

12. Untie the overhand knot. You will find it more difficult to pull the brake side if the rope is out of its trap between the large ring and the standing part of the rope, because in a vertical situation your full weight is involved. Grasp the rope tightly and pull it slowly away from you until you feel a slight jolt, which indicates that it has come unlocked. (You may have to use both hands to pull the rope out of its locked position.) Maintain tension on the rope with your brake hand. *Never take your brake hand off the rope.*

13. Rappel to the bottom (Box 9-3) and complete the belay cycle *(Rappeller: "Off belay." Belayer: "Belay off.")*

GAINING EXTRA FRICTION FROM THE FIGURE 8 DESCENDER

One advantage of the figure 8 with ears is the ease with which friction can be increased, which means greater control of the descent. Figure 8s with ears are larger and therefore have a larger surface area for creating friction. Also, the ears help contour the rope and hold it in place.

DOUBLE WRAPPING A FIGURE 8 DESCENDER (FIGURE 9-12)

Double wrapping of a figure 8 descender must be done before the descender is attached to the seat harness carabiner. Once the rappeller is on rope, double wrapping is no longer possible.

1. Face the anchor with the rappel rope running past you on your brake hand side.
2. At the place on the rappel rope where you want to attach yourself for the rappel, take a bight of rope in your brake hand. Push it through the large ring of the figure 8, downward through the top (if the ascender will be in a horizontal plane) or from the side with the brake hand (if the descender will be in a vertical plane) (Figure 9-12, *A*).
3. Bring the bight of rope around the small ring of the figure 8 and over the waist of the device (Figure 9-12, *B*).
4. Push the bight of rope through the large ring again, between the two strands already there. If you need more rope, pull on the bight (Figure 9-12, *C*).
5. Bring the center of the bight back over the waist and pull the rope strands snug (Figure 9-12, *D*).
6. Attach the figure 8 descender to your seat harness carabiner and lock the carabiner.

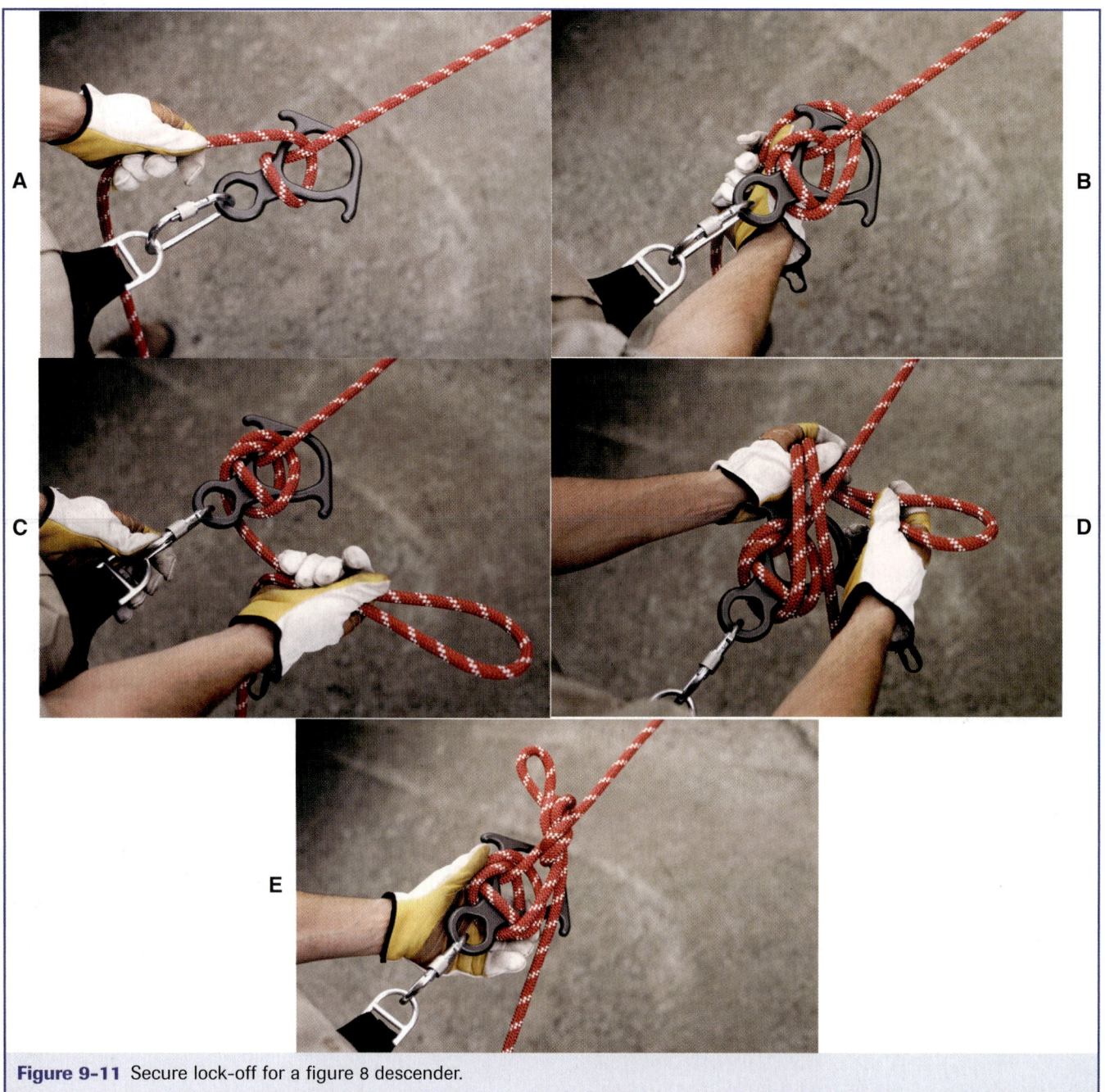

Figure 9-11 Secure lock-off for a figure 8 descender.

Rappelling with a Double-Wrapped Figure 8 Descender

Although a double-wrapped figure 8 descender can give a rappeller added control through greater friction, it requires some increased attention to technique.

The double-wrapped figure 8 descender works more smoothly with the brake hand out to the side (Figure 9-13). This position helps guide the rope into the figure 8 descender. If the hand is closer to the body, the following may occur:

1. The strand of rope running around the figure 8 descender on the brake hand side may begin to cross itself. This poses no danger, but the increased friction will slow the rate of descent, and the descent also may feel a little rougher.

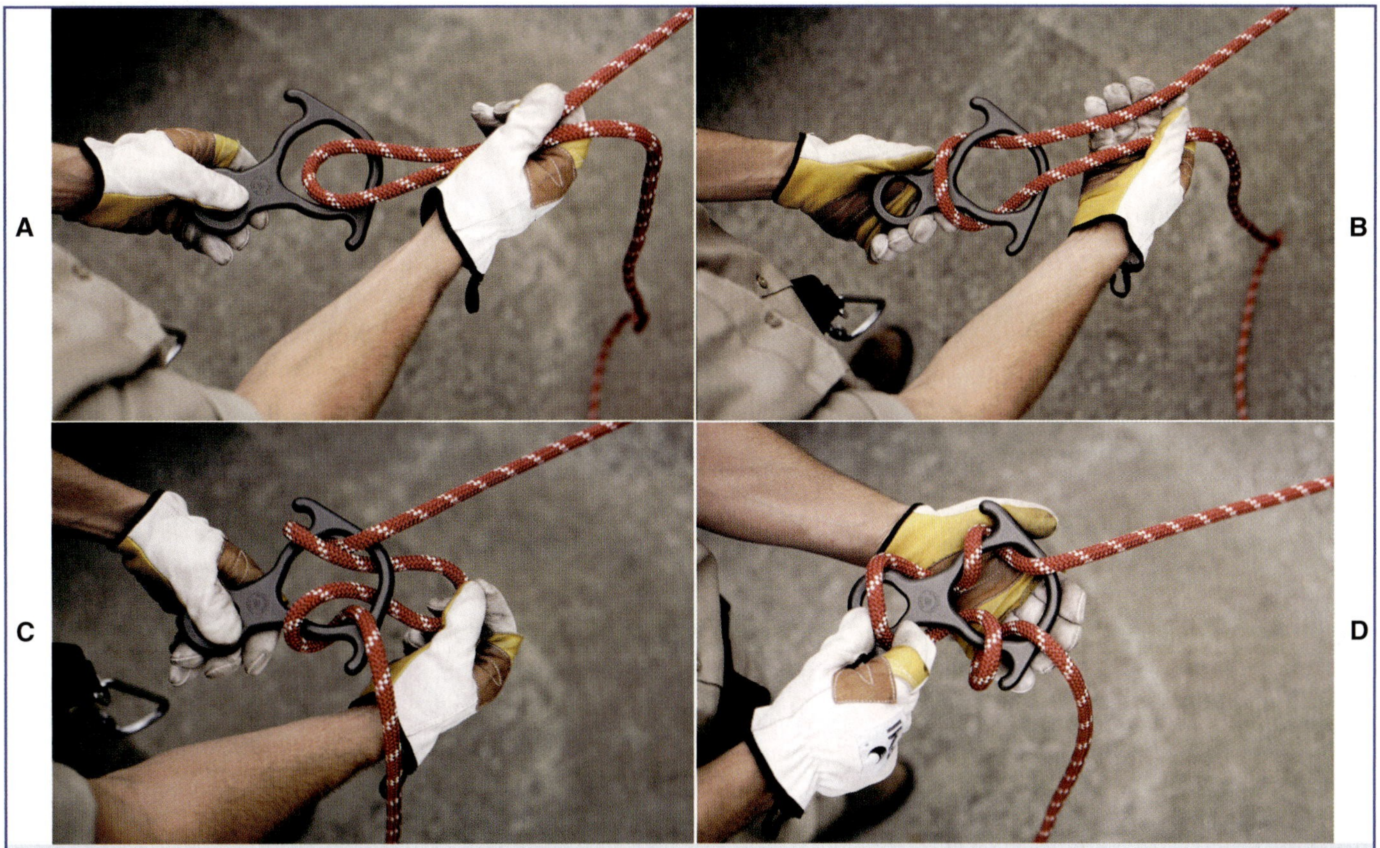

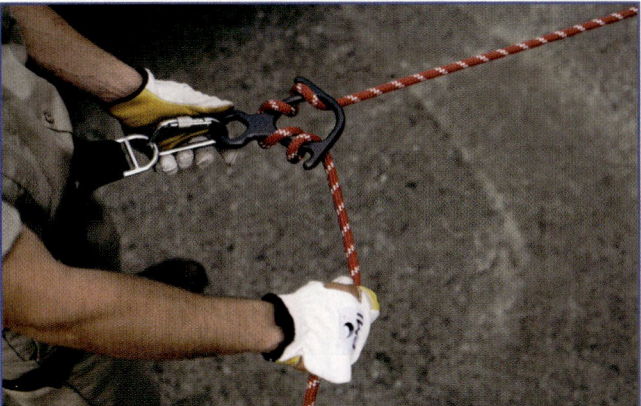

Figure 9-12 Double wrapping the figure 8 descender.

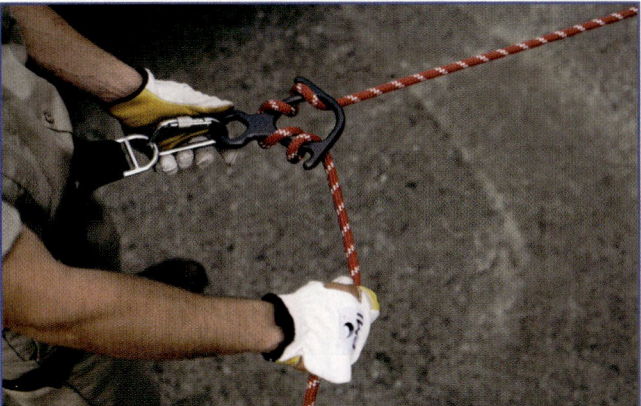

Figure 9-13 Hand position with a double-wrapped figure 8 descender.

2. To uncross the strands, simply bring the brake hand back away from the body. You will feel a slight bump as the rope strands uncross.

GAINING EXTRA FRICTION WHEN ON RAPPEL

A rappel should be done only when the rappeller has friction, and therefore control, to spare. However, if during the rappel not enough friction is generated, some techniques can be used to create additional control.

Increasing Friction with the Body

One technique for increasing friction with the body is to bring the rope sharply against the thigh (Figure 9-14). However, it is not good rappel technique to have to do this continually, for two reasons:

1. The rope may run across the webbing of the seat harness and damage it.
2. This maneuver leaves no extra friction to spare in case it is needed.

Gaining Extra Control with a Spare Carabiner

In some situations you may need more friction than the figure 8 descender may offer, such as when:

- Using a new or wet rope
- Rappelling with extra equipment
- Doing an emergency rescue (pickoff) of another person

The sequence for using a spare carabiner to gain extra friction is as follows (Figure 9-15):

1. Add a second locking carabiner to your seat harness tie-in point. Always place the extra carabiner on the side the rope exits the figure 8 (usually your brake hand side).
2. (If you are locked off) unlock the second carabiner and clip the rope into the carabiner. Lock the carabiner.
3. Firmly grasp the brake side of the rope where it comes out of the second carabiner.
4. Unlock the figure 8.

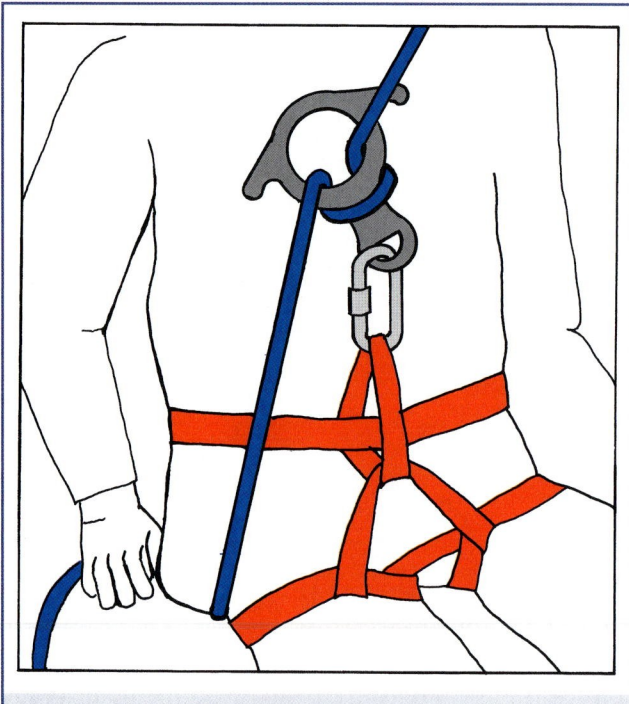

Figure 9-14 Gaining hip friction on a rappel.

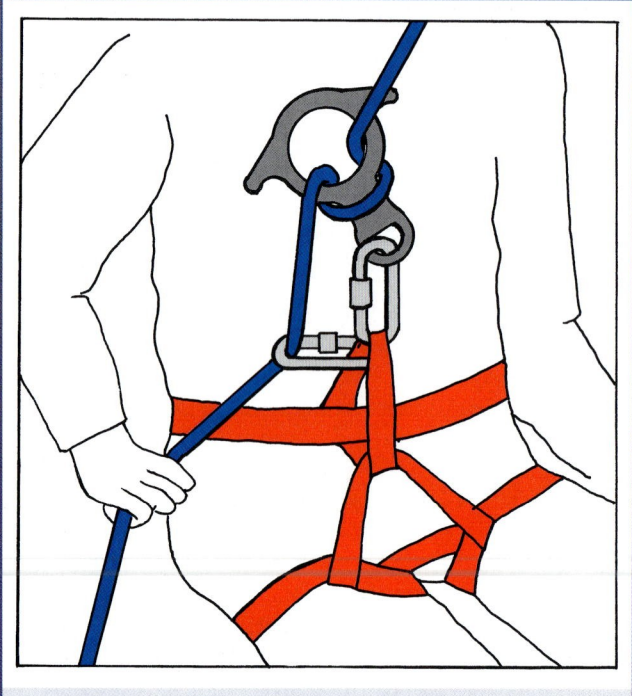

Figure 9-15 Gaining friction with an extra carabiner.

5. Control with the brake hand, using the second carabiner by pulling upward rather than downward as you would if you did not have the spare carabiner.
6. To lock off, raise the rope across toward the guide hand and lock off in the usual way.

Rappel Stance

When most people are learning to rappel, they feel uncomfortable backing over a sharp edge while standing. However in most situations, this is the most effective stance for rappelling. Some rappellers, when intimidated by a difficult edge, may try to "sneaky Pete" their way over the edge by rolling over it on their side or stomach. This type of maneuver should be avoided, if possible, for the following reasons:

- The friction of your body against the edge can unlock the carabiner, causing it to disconnect from your seat harness.
- Your feet or hands can easily become trapped between the rappel rope and the edge.
- Equipment can be damaged; for example, carabiners and seat harnesses can get snagged on the edge.
- On cliffs, this method brushes rocks and other debris over the side and endangers individuals below.

The preferred stance is on both feet (or, as an alternative, on both knees). On particularly difficult edges, some variations can be used.

Getting over the Edge

Usually, the most difficult part of a rappel is getting over the edge. This often has to do with apprehension. However, getting over the edge of a wall or cliff frequently presents a physical challenge as well. Several techniques can help you get started over the edge. *Do not attempt any of the following for the first time without a top belay.*

Variation 1: Butt Thrust (Figure 9-16)

1. Face the anchor. Back up, slowly letting slack through your descender until you are standing with the balls of your feet on the edge.
2. Imagine that something is pushing you at your waist, so that your butt is slowly being thrust back out over the drop and opposite the anchor. *Keep your feet in place.* This should get the weight off your toes and onto the insteps of your feet against the face of the wall (this helps keep your weight pressing against the wall).
3. As this is happening, the rope from the anchor should be coming downward to meet the edge of the drop. When the rope reaches the edge, it will create greater stability for you by completing a three-legged tripod (i.e., the rope on the edge plus your two feet kept shoulder width apart).
4. If you need to help this process of getting the rope down to the edge, you can quickly shuffle your feet down the face of the wall. Taking small steps helps keep your balance.

Variation 2: Knees Over Edge (Figure 9-17)

1. Walk back to the edge with the slack out of the rope.
2. Get down on your knees at the edge of the drop.
3. Lean back, getting your butt back away from the edge.
4. Slide over the edge on your knees. Your toes will hit the wall, and you will stabilize as the rope comes down on the edge. Continue to rappel backward, with your feet shoulder width apart against the wall and your torso parallel to the face.

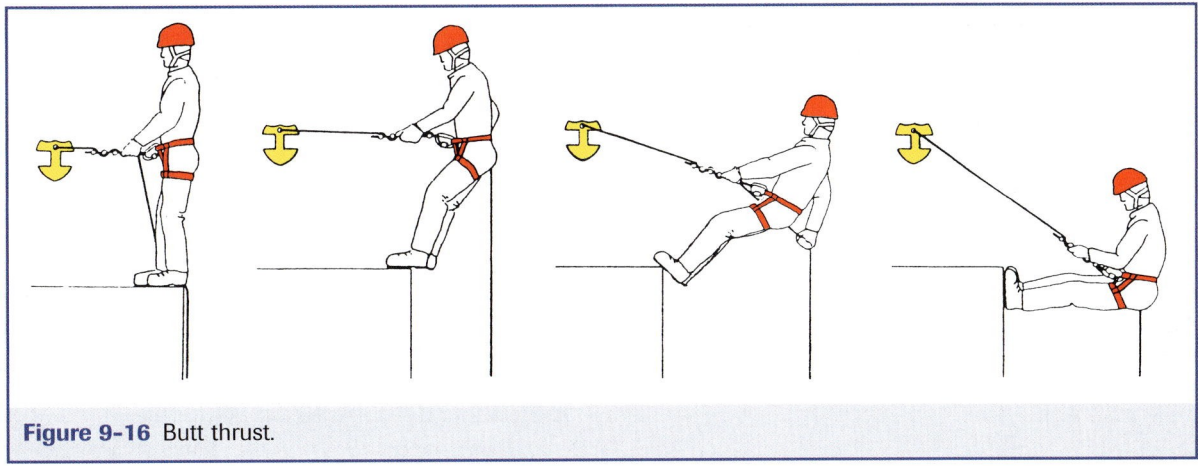

Figure 9-16 Butt thrust.

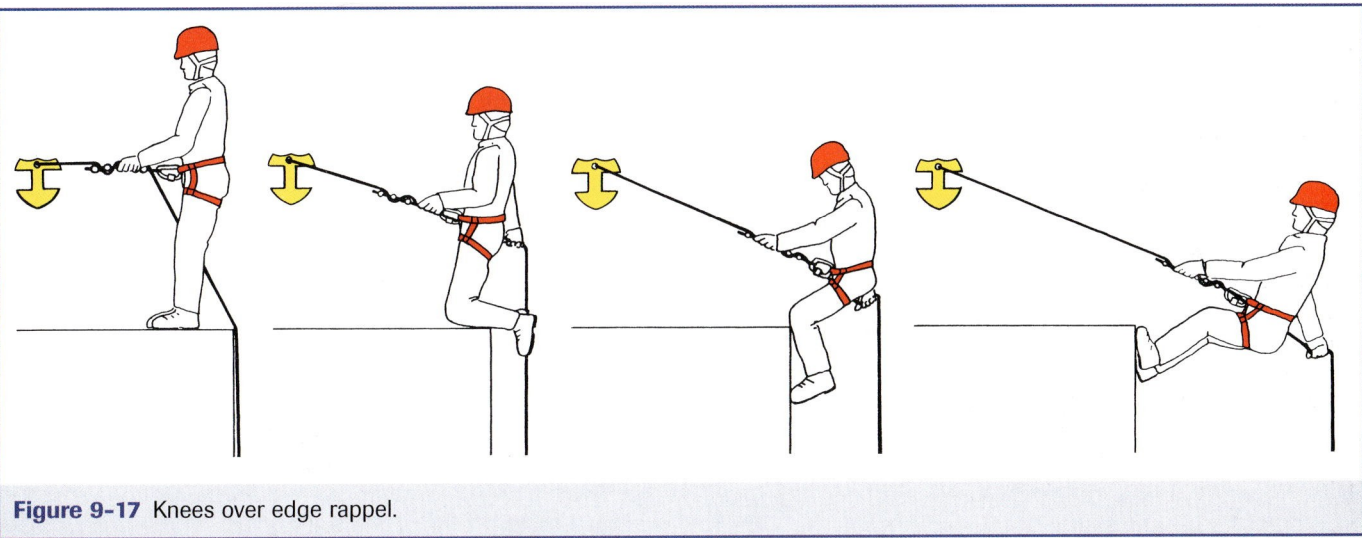

Figure 9-17 Knees over edge rappel.

Clearing the Descender

It is very important that as you clear the edge on a rappel, the descender also clears and does not catch on the edge. Otherwise, the descender may become jammed, and you will be stranded in a precarious position.

When you are backing over the edge in a rappel, therefore, always observe the position of the descender and make sure it is going to clear the edge.

Effect of the Rope Angle on Rappelling

A factor that significantly affects the degree of difficulty involved in rappelling over an edge is the angle the rope forms from the rappeller to the anchor point (Figure 9-18). The effect ranges from greatest difficulty with a horizontal angle (the anchor is level with or lower than the rappeller) to least difficulty with a vertical angle (the anchor is above the rappeller). A vertical angle is rare. Most of the time, a compromise must be found: getting the rope angle as high as possible while maintaining a safe, secure anchor point.

Undercut Edges

An undercut edge is one that is overhung so far back that your legs cannot reach the wall as you start your rappel over the edge. An undercut edge presents the rappeller with a special problem. It requires an advanced technique, which you should attempt only after you have developed full confidence and skill in controlling the descender.

Rappelling from an undercut edge is similar to rappelling from a helicopter skid. It involves keeping your feet on the edge while lowering the rest of your body until your head is well below your feet and the edge of the overhang. Only after you are certain that the rappel device and your torso are far enough below the edge to clear it do you step off the edge. *This often results in a forward pendulum.* Your feet must absorb the shock of the forward motion against the vertical face (if there is one).

The Brake Bar Rack

The ***brake bar rack*** descender has both advantages and disadvantages in rappelling.

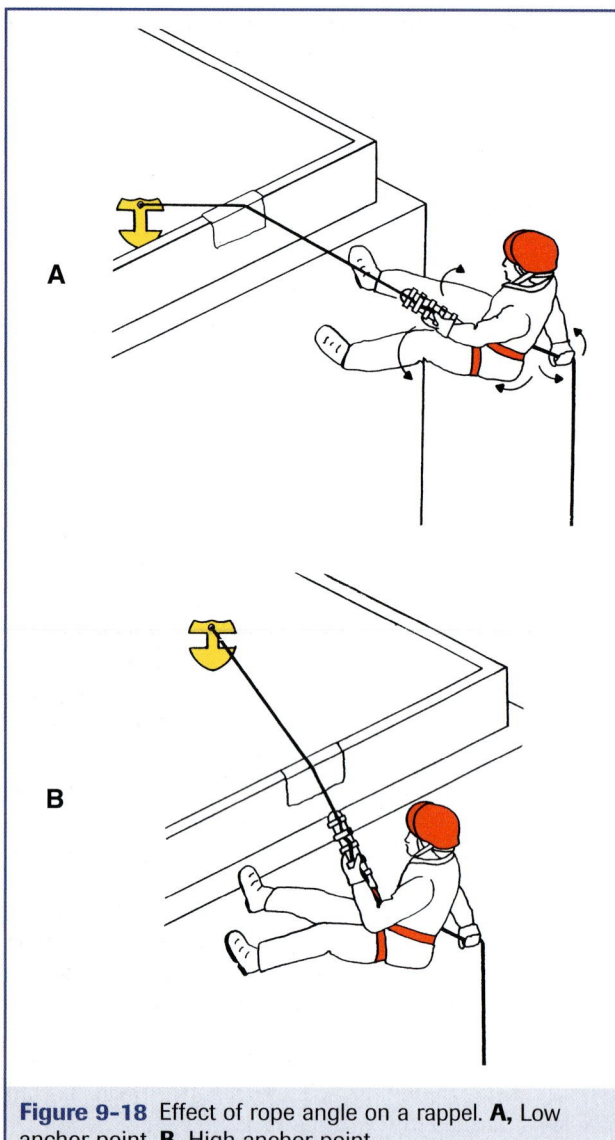

Figure 9-18 Effect of rope angle on a rappel. **A,** Low anchor point. **B,** High anchor point.

Suggestion

A particular technique for getting over the edge can prevent dropping over, pendulum, and potential shock loading of the rappel system: hang an anchored, separate rope loop, sling, or daisy chain over the edge to use as a step.

Before starting over the edge, always rig in your descender and take any rope slack out of it. This will help you weight the rope as quickly and smoothly as possible.

Advantages

- It offers greater friction, and therefore greater control, than most descenders.
- It allows the friction level to be changed after the rappel has begun.

- Because of its variable friction, longer drops can be rappelled more comfortably than with most other descenders.

Disadvantages

- It is somewhat more complex than descenders such as the figure 8, therefore it takes a bit longer to attach to the rope.
- It is somewhat bulkier and heavier than some other descenders.

Rappelling with the Brake Bar Rack

See Chapter 5 for more specific details on the brake bar rack.

Using the Brake Bar Rack on Level Ground

ATTACHING THE BRAKE BAR RACK TO YOUR HARNESS

1. Decide on the number of bars with which you want to begin the rappel. (While learning to use the brake bar rack, always begin a rappel with all six bars engaged; as you become more experienced, you will learn how many bars are needed according to specific situations.) Figure 9-19 shows the brake bar rack in position on a seat harness ready to be put on the rope (the rack is in position for a right-handed individual).
2. If your seat harness carabiner is in a horizontal plane, attach the rack to it with the short leg of the rack down. If you have a seat harness carabiner in a vertical position, attach the rack with the short leg toward the brake hand (e.g., the right hand on a right-handed person).

ATTACHING THE BRAKE BAR RACK TO THE ROPE (FIGURE 9-20)

3. Establish a secure anchor point.
4. Attach the rappel rope securely to the anchor point.
5. Clip the rack into your seat harness carabiner and lock the carabiner (with the gate toward your body).
6. Stand facing the anchor with the rappel rope on your brake hand side.
7. Hold the rack out in front of you in your guide hand.
8. Disengage all bars except the top one on the rack. Do this by sliding them one at a time toward the bottom of the rack (toward the eye). Squeeze the two legs of the rack together with one hand and, with the other hand, flip back each bar.

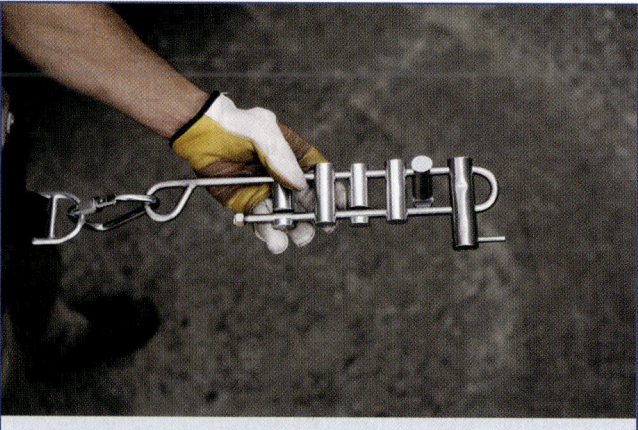

Figure 9-19 Brake bar rack on a harness.

9. Pick up the rope with your brake hand. Guide the rope between the two legs of the rack and across the top bar. *Do not pass the rope between the top bar and the bend of the rack (Figure 9-21). This results in pinching of the rope, making the descent harder to control and causing excessive wear on the rack.*

10. Reach down below the rack, grab the rope, and pull it across the top bar away from you (toward the anchor), pulling the slack out of it (see Figure 9-20, *A*).

11. With the other hand, clip in the second bar at the bottom of the rack and slide it up to trap the rope between it and the top bar (see Figure 9-20, *B*).

12. Bring the free end of the rope back across the second bar, pulling it toward the anchor so that the second bar is snugged in by the force of the rope pulling against it. Note that the rope must be on the side of the bar opposite the notch to hold the bar in place on the rack frame (see Figure 9-20, *C*).

13. Repeat the process with the remainder of the bars until all six have been clipped in (see Figure 9-20, *D-F*).

Operating the Rack for a Rappel

14. In an area with good footing (so that you will not slide down), lean back against the rope. The preferred position for your brake hand is below the rack and off to the side. This position for the brake hand is similar to that for other rappel devices (Figure 9-20, *G*).

15. Your guide hand takes a position different from that used with other rappel devices. Instead of being on the rope above the device, as with other descenders, your guide hand should be resting on the bars of the rack, holding the bar ends between the thumb and fingertips.

16. With your brake hand, pull the rope away from you (using the anchor). The bars, if laced correctly, should all be pulled together toward the top of the rack. This is known as the *quick-stop position*. With a hyper bar you can get even more friction by running the rope over and around the hyper bar extension and pulling it back toward you (Figure 9-20, *H-I*).

17. Bring the rope back to the normal rappel position.

18. With your guide hand, grasp the bottom bar on either side of the rack and push it (along with the other bars) toward the top of the rack. This is the *stop* position for the guide hand. By jamming the bars together in this manner, toward the top of the rack, you increase the friction on the rope and add another element of control.

19. Using the guide hand, pull the bars, one by one, back toward you. As you are doing this, ease your grip on the rope with the brake hand. This increases the "go" mode of the rack by reducing the friction between the bars and the rope. As you lean back against the rope, you may feel it begin to move a bit through the rack and through your brake hand.

20. If you have not moved, disengage the bottom bar. Do this by first swinging the rope with the brake hand in an arc to the opposite side of the rack to uncover the bottom bar (Figure 9-20, *F*). Then squeeze the two legs of the rack together at the open end of the rack that is near you. Unclip the bottom bar. Let it slide down the rack toward the eye and out of the way. Now spread the remaining bars apart along the length of the rack; this reduces the friction even more.

21. If you still have not moved, remove the fifth bar (which is now on the bottom) in the same way that you disengaged the sixth bar. Spread the remaining bars along the length of the rack.

22. Now, reverse the process by clipping bars back in to gain friction. To do this, use your guide hand to squeeze the legs of the rack together and clip the bars in, one at a time, at the bottom, lacing the rope back between them. This is the same process used when you initially laced up the rack on the rope.

Tying Off the Rack (Figure 9-22)

23. Lean back against the rack so that the rope between the rack and the anchor is taut. Start the tie-off process by taking the rope with your brake hand and pulling it away from you, to the top of the rack and toward the anchor (Figure 9-22, *A*).

24. With your brake hand, pull the rope over to the side of the rack and across the top hyper bar (if so equipped) between the rack frame and the pin at the end of the hyper bar so that the rope runs across the top bar (Figure 9-22, *B*).

25. Bring the rope back toward you, pulling it taut so that it locks all the bars together. Bring the rope through the two legs of the rack and across the bottom bar.

26. Pull the rope away from you, toward the anchor, in the same path you did before. Pull it firmly so that all the rope sections are taut and the bars locked together (Figure 9-22, *C*).

27. The rack should now be locked in a "stop" position. With your brake hand extended parallel to the strand that runs to the anchor, hold the rope away from you. At the point the trailing end of the rope crosses your brake hand, form a large bight in the rope using the assistance of your guide hand (Figure 9-22, *D*).

28. Treating this bight as one rope, use it to tie an overhand knot in the line going to the anchor. Cinch the overhand knot firmly against the top bar of the rack. *There must be no slack in the rope running over the bar, nor space between the bars.* The rack is now locked off (Figure 9-22, *E, F*).

Unlocking the Rack

29. When unlocking the rack, *always keep a firm grip on the rope and allow no slack in the brake end of the rope.* To unlock, reverse the locking process. Untie the overhand knot, while maintaining tension on the rope with your brake hand. Slowly lower the rope to return to the "stop" position (see Figure 9-22, *C*).

30. With your brake hand firmly on the rope, pull the brake end of the rope in a 180-degree arc until it is straight out in front of you.

31. Still grasping the rope firmly with your brake hand, use your guide hand to pull the rope straight out to the side, then through a 180-degree arc and back to the normal rappel position.

32. Resume your guide hand's normal position of cradling the bars. If you have not begun to move again, pull the bars apart with your guide hand until the decrease in friction allows you to rappel again.

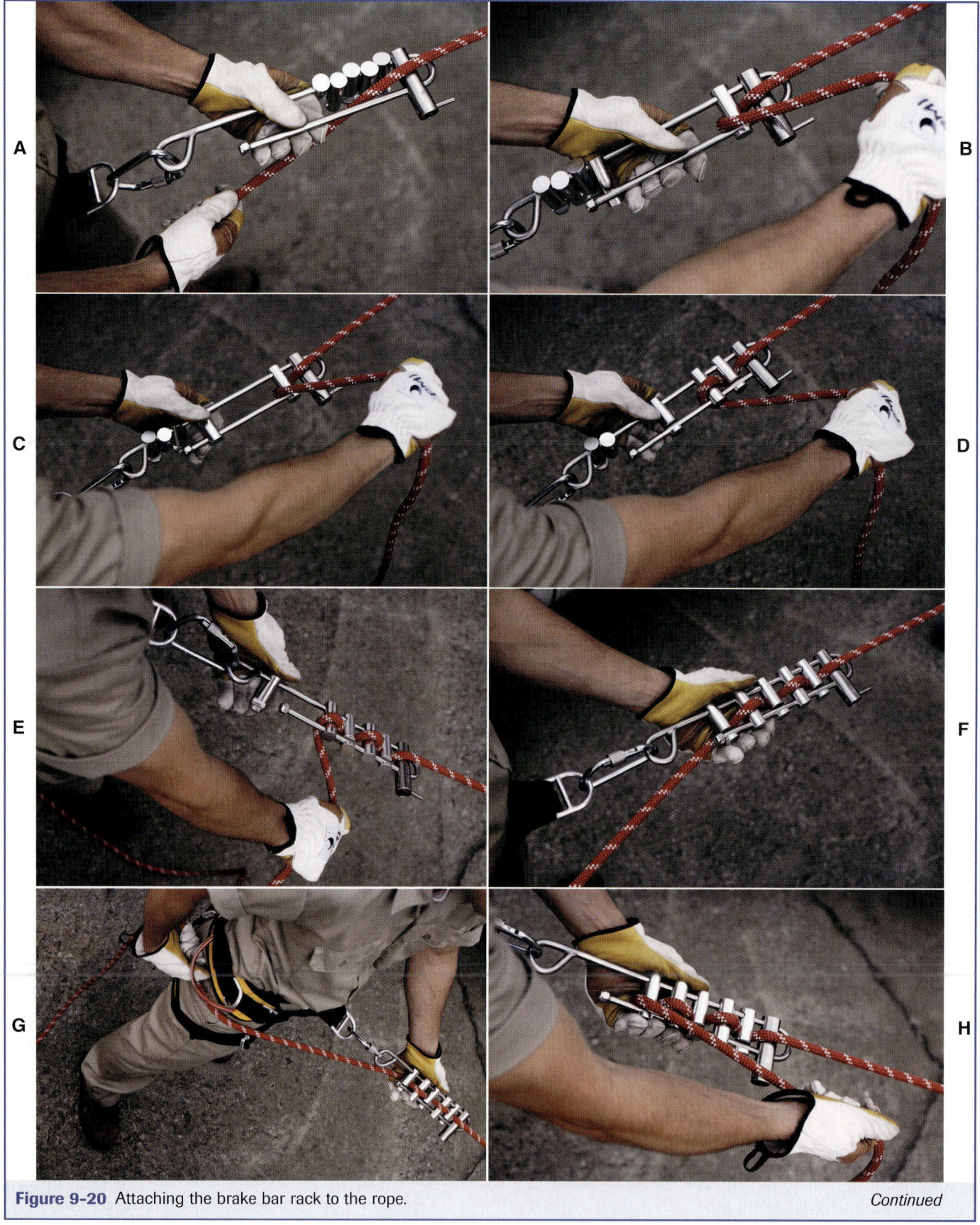

Figure 9-20 Attaching the brake bar rack to the rope.

Continued

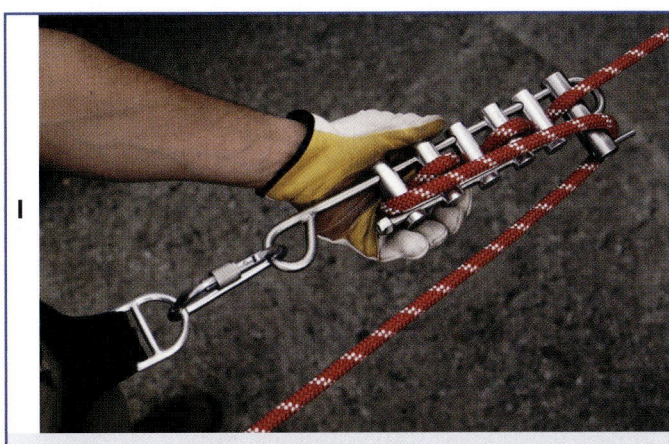

Figure 9-20, cont'd

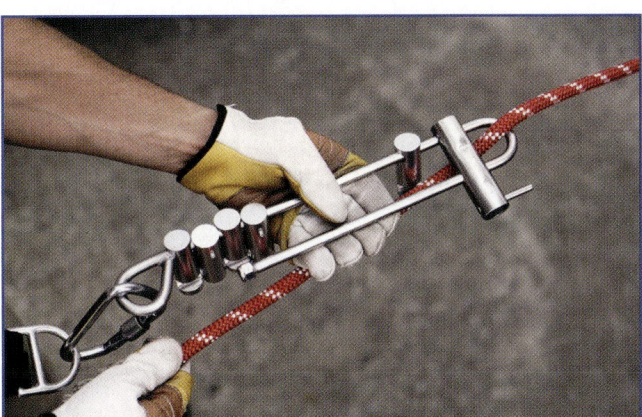

Figure 9-21 Incorrect lacing of the brake bar rack.

GETTING OFF ROPE

33. Getting the rack off the rope reverses the process of putting it on the rope. You may leave the rack attached to your seat harness carabiner while doing this. With your brake hand, pull the rope back in the direction of the anchor so that it uncovers the bottom bar completely.

34. Using your guide hand, squeeze the legs of the rack together and unclip the bottom bar. Let the bar slide to the bottom of the rack.

35. With your brake hand, move the rope back through the leg of the rack, uncovering the next bar up and pulling the rope back toward the anchor. Unclip the next bar up with your guide hand. Continue this procedure until all the bars have been disengaged.

Rappelling with the Brake Bar Rack on a Slope (Figure 9-23)

PREPARATION

1. Establish a secure anchor point at the top of a short slope of about 45 degrees. (If a slope is not available, use a stairway.) Securely attach the main-line rappel rope to the anchor point.

2. Establish an anchor point for a belay. Attach a sling securely to the belay anchor point. Clip a large, locking carabiner into the end of the anchor sling.

3. Have the belayer take position. If a Münter hitch is to be used for the belay, have the belayer tie it in the belay rope and clip the Münter hitch into the belay carabiner. If the belayer is using a mechanical belay device, attach it to the rope and clip it into the belay anchor carabiner.

4. Clip the rappeller into the belay rope. Initiate the belay cycle with the belay voice signals *(Rappeller: "On belay." Belayer [if ready]: "Belay on.")*.

5. In a secure position, where you are in no danger of falling, follow steps 5 through 13 under Using the Brake Bar Rack on Level Ground (p. 131) to lace the rope onto the rack. Make sure there is no slack between the rack and the anchor (Figure 9-23, *A*).

NOTE: Have the instructor do a safety check. Along with checking the other critical elements in the belay system, make sure the bars are secured correctly. Check all connectors, such as carabiners, to make sure they are locked and in position of function. Make sure the seat harness is buckled correctly, and the anchors are secure. Make sure that no loose clothing or hair can be drawn into the rappel device. Make sure your helmet is on securely.

DOING THE PRACTICE RAPPEL

6. Begin backing down the slope, controlling your descent with your brake hand and, if necessary, with the guide hand on the bars. If you are unable to move, use the guide hand to pull the bars down toward you, as described in step 19 (p. 131) (Figure 9-23, *B*).

7. If, after spreading the bars along the length of the rack, you still have not moved, disengage the bars as described in steps 20 (p. 131). *Never have less than four bars on the rack.*

8. Rappel until you are about midway down the slope. With your brake hand, do a quick stop, as described in step 16 (p. 131).

9. Rappel a short distance farther. Now, using your guide hand on the bars, attempt to stop yourself as described in step 18 (p. 131).

10. Relax your guide hand and tie off the rack as described in steps 23 through 28 (p. 131) (Figure 9-23, *D*).

Rappelling with the Brake Bar Rack Down a Vertical Face (Figure 9-24)

PREPARATION

1. Choose a short vertical face (about 20 feet [6 m]) where the top breaks over gradually into a steep face. On the first rappel, do not choose a face with a sharp edge.

2. Establish a secure anchor point safely back from the edge. If possible, have the anchor point high up; this will help the rappeller in going over the edge. Attach the main-line rappel rope securely to the anchor point.

3. Establish a separate anchor point for a belay. Securely attach a sling to the belay anchor point. The anchor point and sling should be established so that the belayer, when in position of operation, has a good field of view of the top and face but

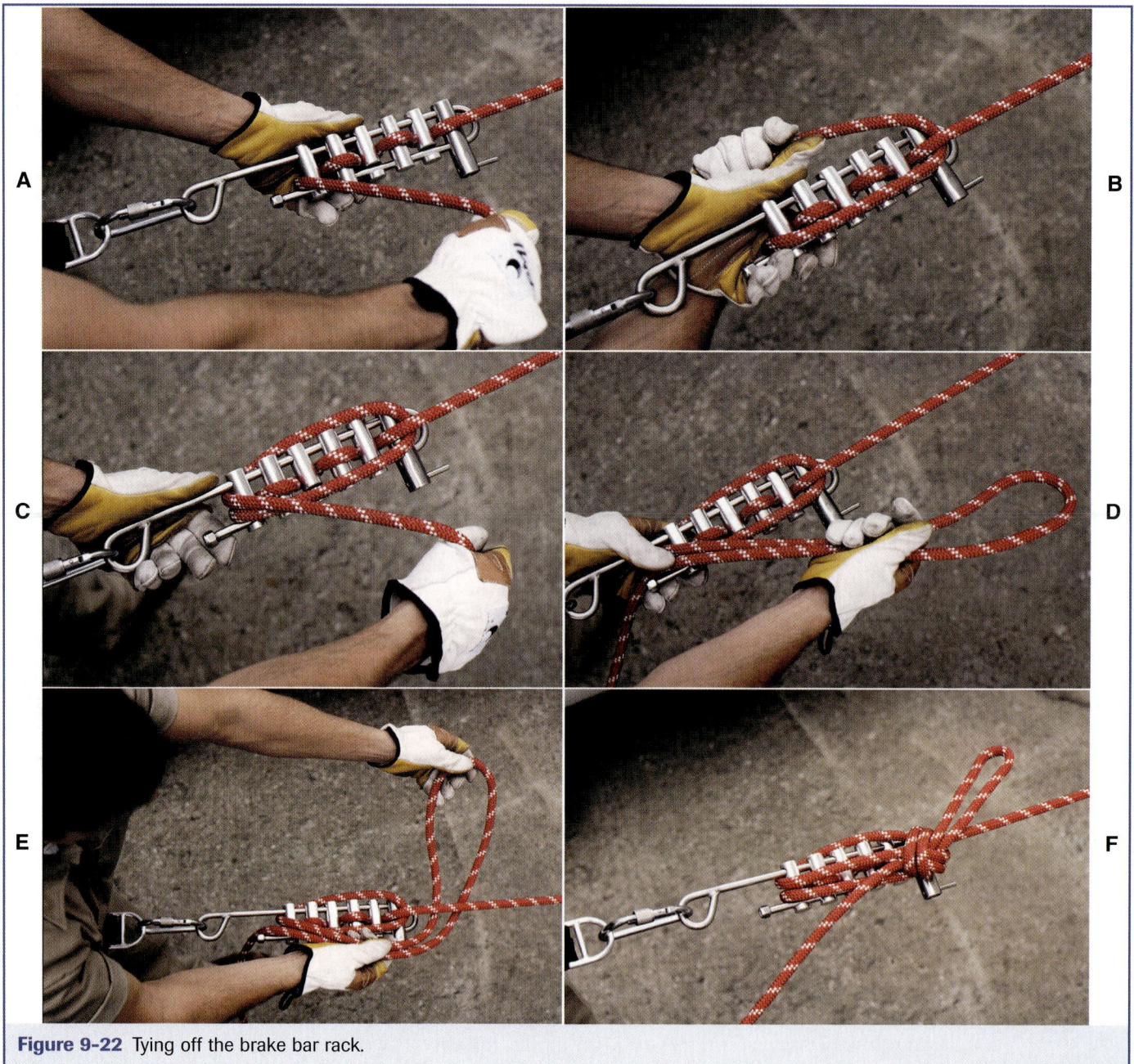

Figure 9-22 Tying off the brake bar rack.

is not in danger of falling over the edge. Clip a large locking carabiner into the end of the belay anchor sling.

4. Have the belayer tie into a safety line and take position. If a Münter hitch is to be used for the belay, have the belayer tie the Münter hitch in the belay carabiner. If the belayer is using a mechanical belay device, attach it to the rope and clip the rope into the belay carabiner.

5. Clip into the belay rope with an appropriate knot or locking carabiner. Initiate the belay cycle with the belay voice signals *(Rappeller: "On belay." Belayer [if ready]: "Belay on")* (Figure 9-24, *A*).

6. In a secure position, where you are in no danger of falling, follow steps 5 through 13 (p. 131 to lace the rope onto the

rack. Make sure there is no slack between the rack and the anchor (Figure 9-24, *B*).

DOING THE PRACTICE RAPPEL

7. Begin backing toward the edge. Because you are on top, there is a great deal of friction in the rack but little weight to pull the rope through. Consequently, you may have to feed the rope through the rack by letting slack with your brake hand. Also, you may have to reduce friction with your guide hand by spreading the bars apart or perhaps by disengaging one or two bars. *Remember: As soon as you start over the edge, your full weight will come onto the rack, and you may need the friction. Be prepared to reengage the bars with your*

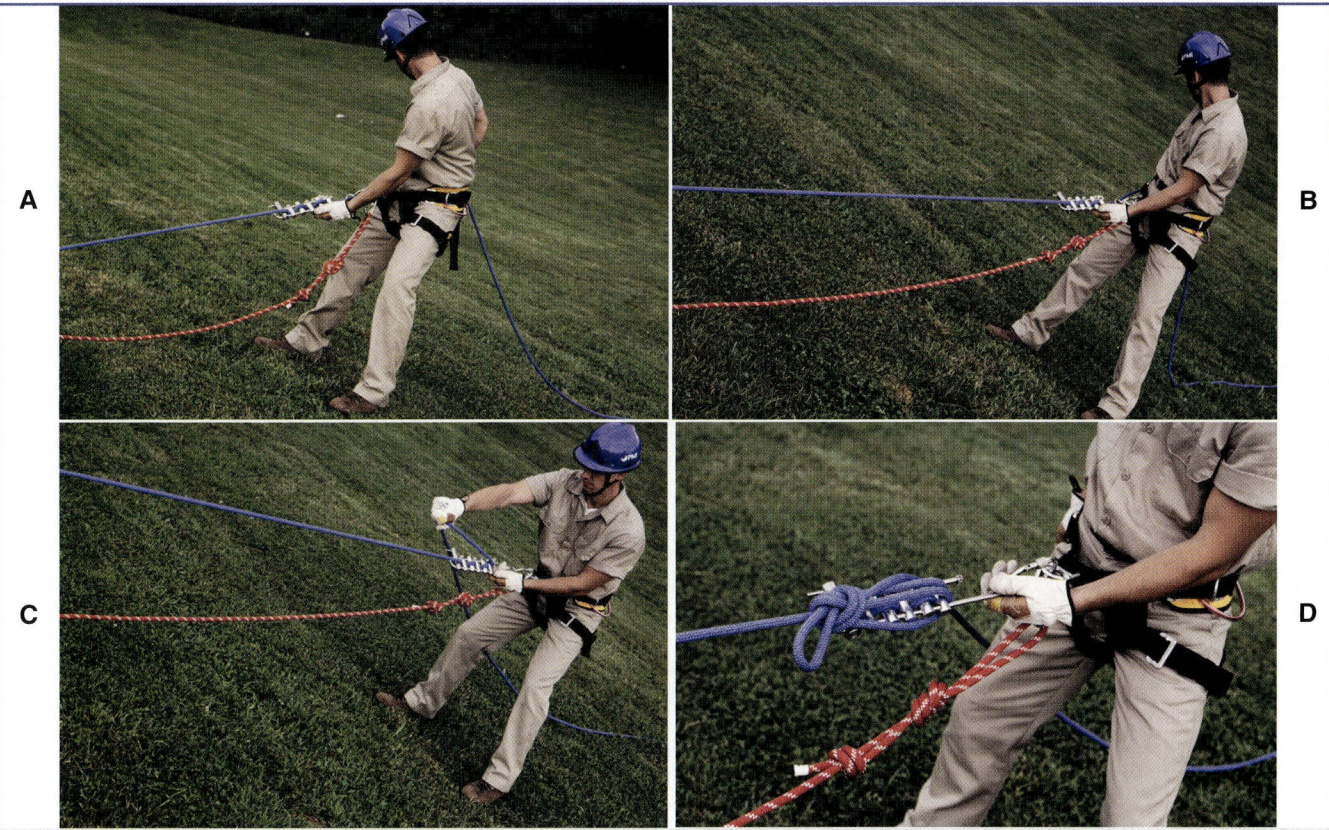

Figure 9-23 Using a brake bar rack on a slope.

guide hand and to establish control with your brake hand (Figure 9-24, *C*).

8. As you go over the edge, keep the following principles in mind:

   - *Keep your body generally perpendicular to the wall.* This means you must deliberately lean out as the wall becomes vertical. At first this may seem unnatural, but it is necessary to keep your feet from slipping out from under you.
   - Keep your feet shoulder width apart for balance. This helps prevent you from being pulled to one side.
   - Keep your knees relaxed and slightly flexed.
   - Keep your body slightly turned in the direction of your brake hand, looking down slope to pick a path for your descent (Figure 9-24, *D*).
   - Use your guide hand for balance and to control the bars. *Do not support your weight with your guide hand.*
   - *Never take your brake hand off the rope unless you are securely locked off.*

9. After you are over the edge, rappel a few feet, then bring the brake side of the rope up through the quick stop position and over the end of the hyper bar and back to the side (Figure 9-24, *F*).

10. Tie off the rack so that you can be hands free of the rope (Figure 9-24, *G, H*).

11. Unlock and rappel a few feet farther.

12. Attempt to stop your descent with your guide hand by jamming the bars up together.

13. Pull the bars apart and rappel to the bottom.

14. Complete the belay cycle with the appropriate voice signals *(Rappeller: "Off belay." Belayer: "Belay off.")*

▨ Warning

A major concern in going over the edge with a rack is the possibility of catching the device on the edge. This can happen with any rappel device. However, because of the rack's length, you need to be particularly careful not to catch it on the edge. If you do catch the rack on the edge, any of the following might happen:

1. The rack could get jammed on the edge, preventing the rope from running through the device and stranding you in that position.
2. The pressure of your body weight could break the carabiner or bend the rack, causing it to malfunction in the future.

The solution to these problems is to avoid edge catch. As you go over the edge, make sure you lean out enough and push back with your feet before you step down so that the rappel device clears the edge before the rope lies across the edge (Figure 9-25).

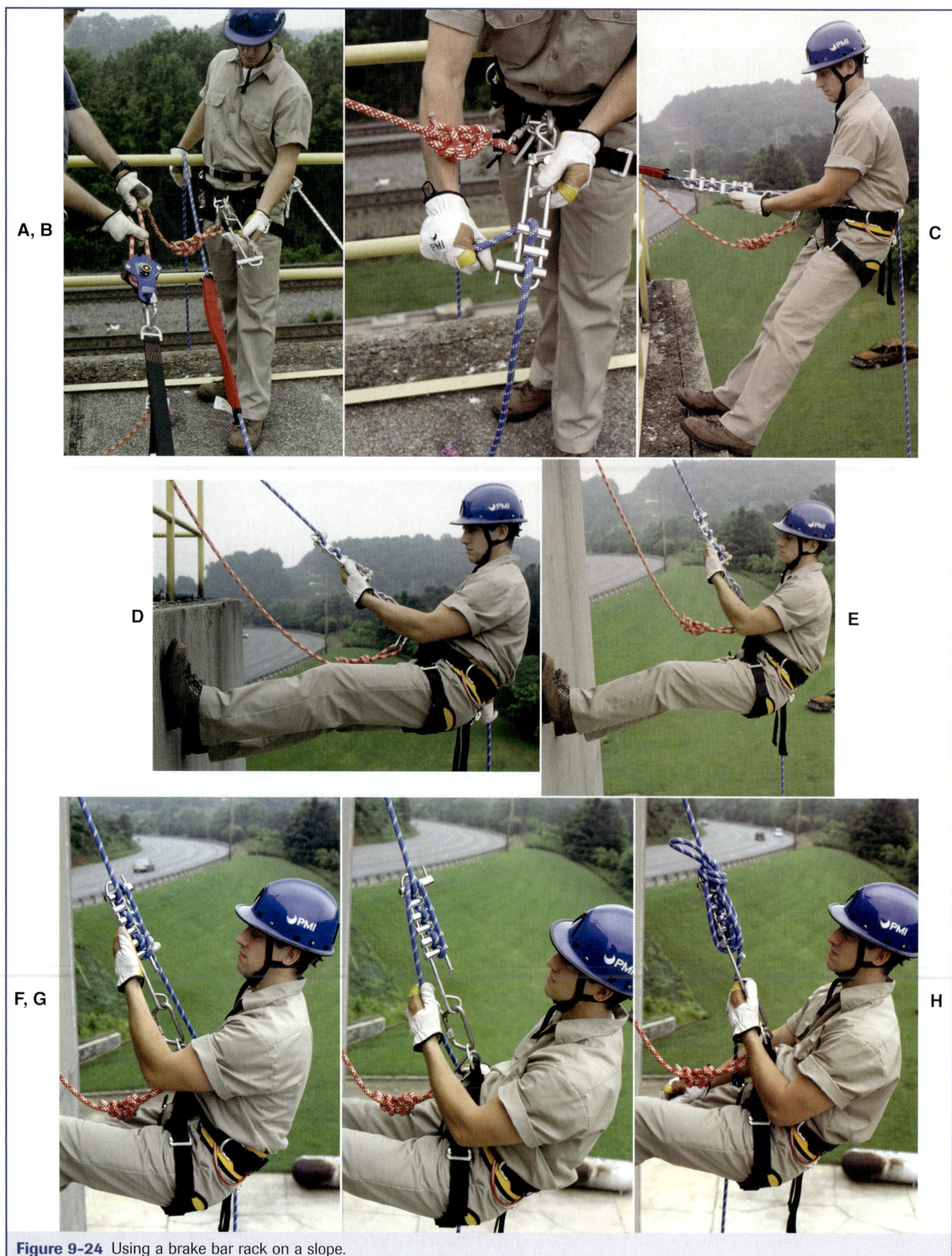

Figure 9-24 Using a brake bar rack on a slope.

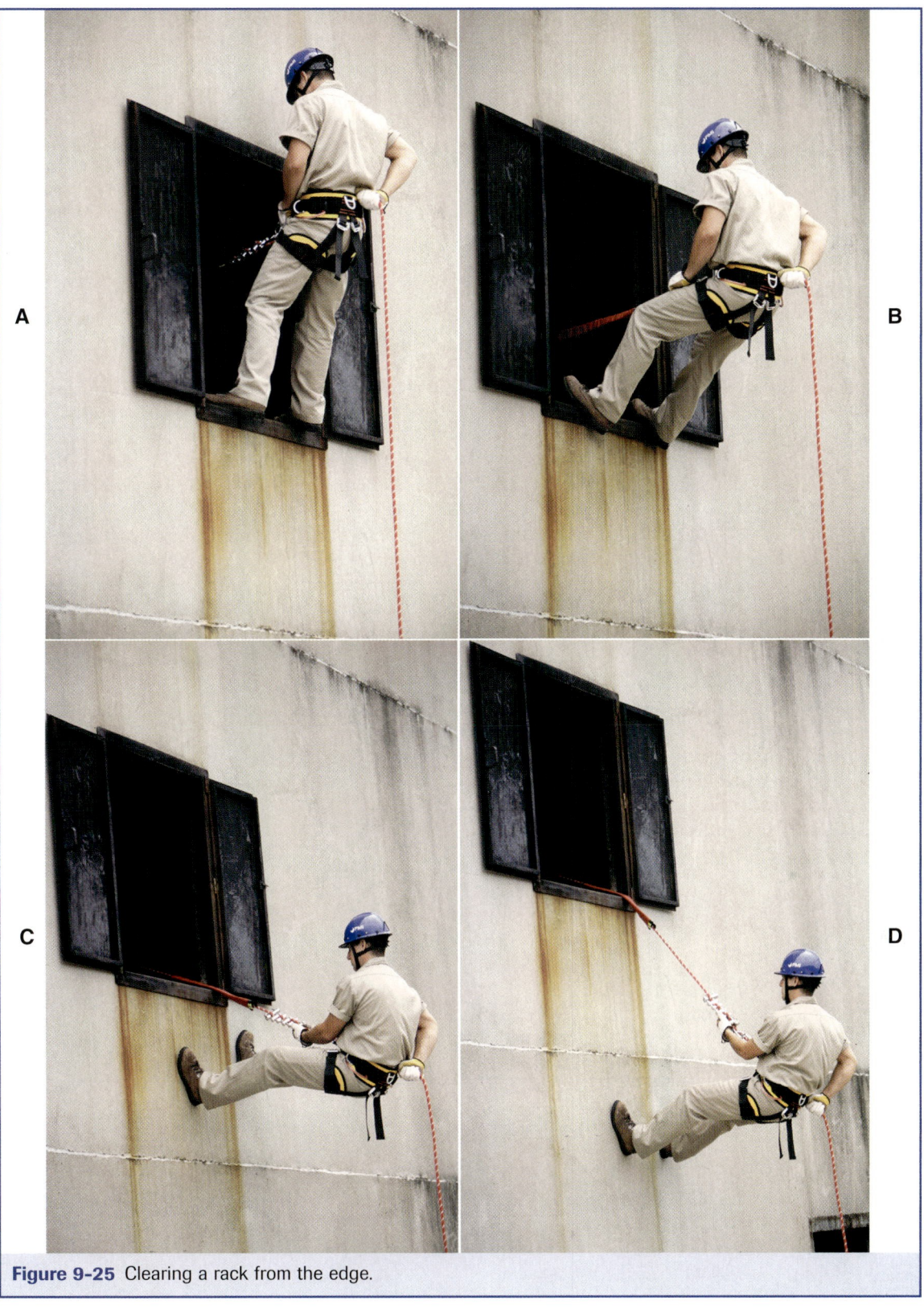

Figure 9-25 Clearing a rack from the edge.

15. Remove the rack from the rope.
16. Immediately move away from the drop zone to lessen your chances of being hit by falling objects and to clear the rope for others.

Emergency Descent Systems

Emergency situations may arise in which a rappel is necessary but the person has no descender. There are possible solutions to this problem.

One solution might be the body rappel, described earlier in this chapter. However, as noted, this technique has some distinct disadvantages and dangers.

A system used in the past is the **carabiner wrap**, which involves wrapping a seat harness carabiner with several turns of the rappel rope to create friction. However, *the carabiner wrap rappel is not considered a satisfactory and safe technique for rappelling,* for the following reasons:

- If the rope wraps are not put onto the carabiner correctly, they can spiral out of the carabiner gate, resulting in a free fall.
- The rope wraps can bear on the carabiner gate and break it.

An alternative to the carabiner wrap might be the **Münter hitch rappel** (Figure 9-26) (also see Chapter 6 and Figure 8-6, p. 103).

Self-Belay Techniques

When belaying of a rappeller by another person is not possible or practical, self-belay techniques may be possible. Most self-belay techniques are based on the use of some type of rope grab device on the main rappel line above the descenders. Usually the rappeller is attached to the device by means of a short sling attached to a chest harness. The self-belay mechanism is triggered by a definitive action by the rappeller, such as leaning over backward.

> ### ▨ *Warning*
>
> The **Münter** hitch rappel, like all other rappel techniques, must be practiced on level ground, on a moderate slope with a rappel, and on a short drop with a rappel. Because the **Münter** hitch rappel wears on the rope and twists it, and also wears on the carabiner, it is a limited-use technique.

The regulations of the U.S. Occupational Safety and Health Administration (OSHA) require that in a work place environment such as high angle window cleaning, a *secondary safety system* be used. This could be, for example, a self-trailing rope grab on a belay or safety line.

Using a Prusik Safety in Rappelling

A traditional means of rappelling self-belay has been to use a *Prusik safety,* which uses a Prusik hitch on the rope; the end of the Prusik loop is connected to the rappeller's harness (see

> ### ▨ *Warning*
>
> Self-belay techniques are not completely automatic safeties; rather, they require some positive action by the rappeller. Remember: In an emergency, a person reacts with an instinctive action. Whether the response is the correct action in a self-belay emergency may depend on how well trained and disciplined the rappeller is.

Chapter 10 for further information on the Prusik knot). The theory is that should the rappeller's descent run out of control, the Prusik knot can be tightened on the main rope to stop the fall. However, the rappeller must avoid certain pitfalls, or the "safety" may not work at all.

For example, in a panic, the falling rappeller may grab for the Prusik knot itself; this does not close the knot, but rather opens it up. The result is a free fall, until the rappeller hits bottom. This usually occurs when the rappeller pulls down on the top of the Prusik knot instead of letting go.

Some precautions can help the rappeller use the Prusik safety as intended:

- Practice using the Prusik safety at a safe height so that your emergency actions become automatic.
- Make sure the Prusik is tight enough and properly dressed so that it will catch when needed.

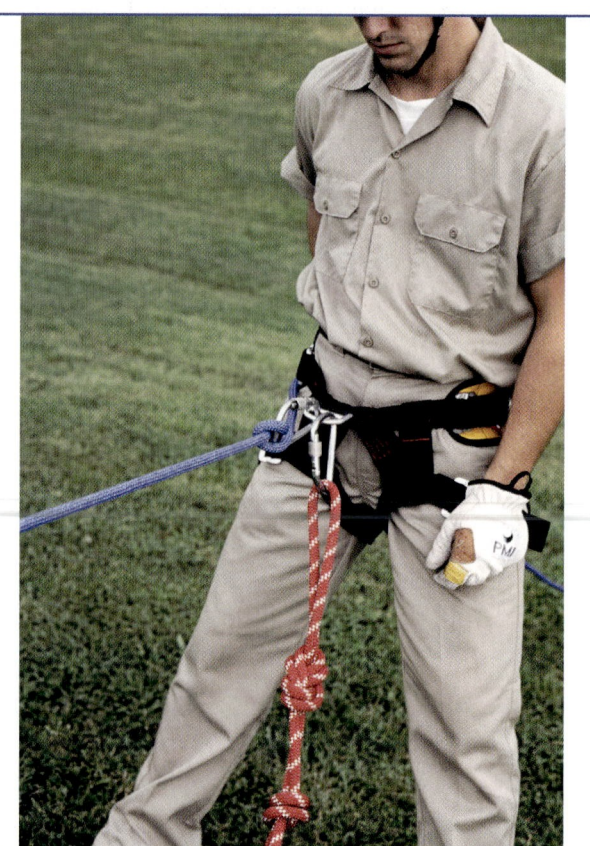

Figure 9-26 Münter hitch rappel.

Place the Prusik safety *under* the rappel device. This means you must make the sling short enough so that it does not jam into the rappel device. An example configuration would have the rappel device connected to the sternal attachment point of a full body harness, with the Prusik sling attached at the waist attachment point. Or the rappel device could be extended upward with an attachment sling to a seat harness. *In all cases, the Prusik hitch must remain in reach at all times but low enough that it doesn't jam in the rappel device.*

There are numerous types of self-belay device systems. Some of them may add complications that can create hazards to the process of rappelling. All of them must be practiced thoroughly before use in the high angle environment.

Protecting the Rappel Rope Below You

In most cases, the rappel rope is simply dropped down the vertical face where the rappeller is about to travel. However, under some circumstances this might not be desirable, such as:

- In tactical operations in which a hostile person below the rappeller could grab the rope (and thereby control the rappeller).
- When a very frightened and unpredictable person is below the rappeller.
- When unstable rocks could be knocked loose by the rope and fall on people below.
- When the rappeller wants to prevent the rope below him or her from being damaged or cut by falling debris and rock.
- When the rope could become tangled or jammed, and the rappeller could not retrieve it.

In such cases it might be desirable for the rappeller to keep the rope with him or her. One way to do this is to attach the rope bag to the rappeller (Figure 9-27). The bag can be attached in a number of ways:

- If it is very light, the bag can be attached to a seat harness equipment sling.

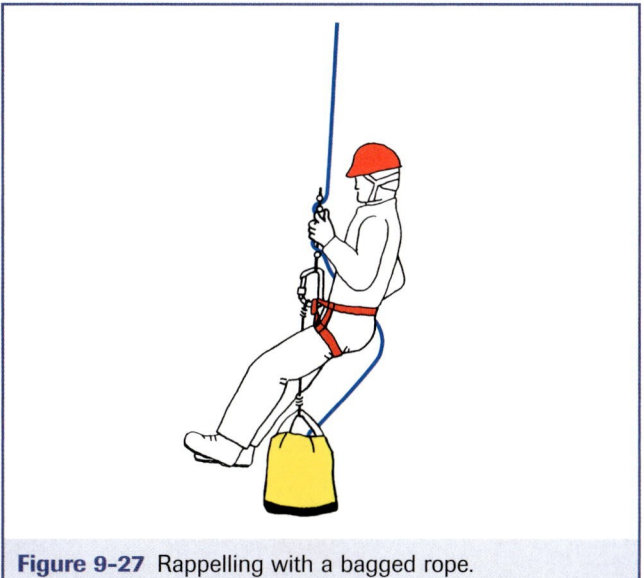

Figure 9-27 Rappelling with a bagged rope.

Warning

1. It is difficult to estimate the length of a bagged rope accurately. When rappelling from a bagged rope, therefore, the danger exists that you could rappel off the end of the rope. Always either tie a stopper knot in the bottom end of a bagged rope or tie the rope end to the bag to avoid rappelling off the end of the line. (See Preventing a Rappel Off the End of a Rope, next page.)
2. Rappelling with a bag attached to your body requires special care to prevent rope tangles that could jam in your descender. You also must be very careful that the bag does not jam in your descender. These are particular problems when rappelling from helicopters, a situation in which a jammed rappel device could leave you stranded on the rope hanging from the helicopter, possibly leading to severe injury or death.

- If the bag is heavy, it can be attached with a carabiner directly into the bottom of the descender.
- Specially designed rope bags have straps that attach to the rappeller's lower leg.

Extricating Jammed Rappel Devices

Rappel devices are notorious for snagging loose material and becoming jammed, perhaps stranding the rappeller in a difficult and painful position that might require a rescue. Possible problems include:

- T-shirts and other loose clothing
- Hair
- Body parts (e.g., loose flesh on an underarm)

The best solution to this problem, of course, is prevention:

- Tuck in shirttails and other loose clothing.
- Keep hair trimmed or tied back and tucked into the helmet.
- Keep flabby body sections (e.g., underarms, stomachs) away from rappel devices.

Extrication Techniques

Avoid using a knife to extricate yourself from a jammed rappel device. It is very difficult to use a knife in such situations without damaging the rope or cutting it completely. If you are trying to cut jammed material from a descender, you probably are under pressure, physically unbalanced and, possibly, also in pain, therefore it is extremely difficult for you to cut away the offending material without also touching the rope with the knife.

Another problem in using a knife involves hair jammed in a descender. Remember that hair is usually attached to scalp. An attempt to cut hair out of a descender could also inflict a significant scalp wound.

One way out of such a situation is to take your weight off the descender by using an ascender or Prusik knot above the descender (see Chapter 10 for a description of this technique).

Preventing a Rappel Off the End of a Rope

In some situations you may face the danger of rappelling off the end of a rope. This usually occurs when you cannot see the bottom of the drop before you begin the rappel. As you near the bottom end of the rope, you may not be paying attention or you may lose control. One form of insurance against rappelling off the end of a rope is to use a *stopper knot*. A figure 8 knot can be tied in the bottom end of the rappel line (or in both strands if you are rappelling on a doubled rope).

An even better knot is a figure 8 on a bight, which forms a loop. This gives you something to stand in while you figure out what to do next.

Evaluation Exercises

Cognitive and Affective Exercises

1. List five characteristics of controlled rappelling.

2. Why are the body rappel and arm rappel uncomfortable to use?

3. The rate of descent in rappelling is controlled by the _____ hand.

4. The _____ hand helps balance the rappeller but does not support weight.

5. The arm rappel should be used only for what situations?

6. What two dangers arise with use of the body rappel?

7. What are the two main drawbacks to using the conventional figure 8 descender?

8. Explain one way to get out of a girth hitch with the conventional figure 8 descender.

9. Give one way to prevent the development of a girth hitch.

10. Describe one way to lace up a figure 8 descender that will help prevent it from jamming if it is caught on an edge.

11. Why should you keep a proper distance between a rappel line anchor and a belay anchor?

12. What is the danger in having too great a distance between a rappel line anchor and a belay anchor?

13. List seven principles to keep in mind when rappelling down a vertical face.

14. Explain one technique for gaining extra friction from a figure 8 descender.

15. What can occur when rappelling on a figure 8 with the brake hand too close to the body?

16. Describe the preferred stance for rappelling.

17. Describe the effect of the angle of the rope from the rappeller to the anchor point.

18. Why is it important that a rappeller not catch the rappel device on the edge of a drop?

19. Name three advantages and three disadvantages of the brake bar rack.

20. In lacing the rope onto the brake bar rack, the rope (should) (should not) be passed between the top bar and the bend of the rack.

21. What is different about the position of the guide hand when using a brake bar rack in contrast to other rappel devices?

22. What is the minimum number of bars that should be used on a brake bar rack?

23. Give two reasons the carabiner wrap rappel is not considered a satisfactory and safe technique.

24. When a self-belay device is used, why should care be taken not to get the connecting sling too long?

25. What should you do to the bottom of your rope to prevent rappelling off the end?

Appendix

Personal Escape Devices and Kits

In recent years, personal escape ropes and kits have become popular with rescuers and others who work at height. Generally, such kits are a prudent idea for those who might be caught with no other means of escape. Recently, organizations such as the National Fire Protection Association (NFPA) have provided standards (e.g., NFPA standard 1983-01) for personal escape equipment to help ensure the safety of such equipment.

Before the widespread acceptance of personal escape kits, many firefighters, ski patrollers, and rescuers carried home-built kits. These often consisted of a standard figure 8 descender and whatever lightweight rope could be found. In many cases this was "commodity rope," such as that found at hardware stores, which is not acceptable for life safety applications. Currently, the pendulum seems to have swung full spectrum in the other direction, with manufacturers now offering extremely high-end equipment.

Personal Escape Rope

As the foundation of most systems, ropes are a critical element in personal escape gear. Fiber choices include polyester, nylon, aramid, and ultra-high molecular weight polyethylene (UHMWPE). Each of these fibers has advantages and disadvantages, but the general characteristics are as follows:

- Polyester has good strength properties, low elongation, and a relatively "slick" finish.
- Nylon has strength properties similar to those of polyester, but it has greater elongation.
- Both polyester and nylon have melting points in the range of 460° F (238° C) to 500° F (260° C).
- Aramid fibers have a high strength-to-weight ratio and high temperature resistance, but the fibers are self-destructive under repeated bending abuse, and aramids disintegrate at a temperature of about 900° F (482° C).
- UHMWPE also has a high strength-to-weight ratio, but the fiber is slippery and difficult to work with, and its melting point is very low (300° F [149° C]).

More important than the melting or disintegration temperature in the selection of an escape rope is the rope's maximum working temperature. Nylon and polyester ropes have a maximum working temperature of 250° F (121° C) to 275° F (135° C). The maximum working temperature for aramid ropes is closer to 350° F (177° C), and UHMWPE ropes have a maximum working temperature of only 150° F (66° C).

When selecting your foundation rope, consider that most of the life of an escape rope is spent in the pocket of your turnouts or in a storage bag—"out of sight, out of mind." Therefore the rope must be durable and dependable, even when folded, squashed, and tossed around in its container. It should also be sufficiently lightweight to carry reasonably easily, so that it is where it is needed when it is needed.

In use, an escape rope must be reasonably strong; that is, strong enough for a user who may weigh nearly 300 pounds (136 kg) with gear and protective clothing, plus an acceptable safety factor. Perhaps more important, the escape rope must have enough elongation to absorb the impact of the user as he or she leaps to safety, possibly with a certain amount of free fall before the person gains control of the descent. The diameter of the rope should be large enough to provide adequate friction with the descent device used and sufficient to go over an edge without fear of parting. Heat resistance is important, but being flame proof may not be as high a priority as some of the other factors mentioned. There doesn't seem to be a common problem of firefighters plunging to the ground because their ropes aren't flame resistant.

The rope should be prerigged with a means of anchoring, either by tying or clipping around an object.

Personal Escape Descenders

Most important, a descender should be made to function effectively with the rope on which it is being used. Some descenders are rope specific, and it is important to know this information to avoid accidental injury or death. Other descenders may not be specific to an individual rope but still must be used on a rope of a certain diameter, construction, or material to operate effectively.

Another important priority with descenders is whether they can be easily attached to or removed from a rope. A descender that is easily attached, such as the SMC Escape 8, works well for training because it can be rigged and rerigged for several descents by several users. Some users prefer a more securely prerigged escape descender, such as the PMI PED, to help overcome potential inadvertent detachment during the urgency of an actual incident.

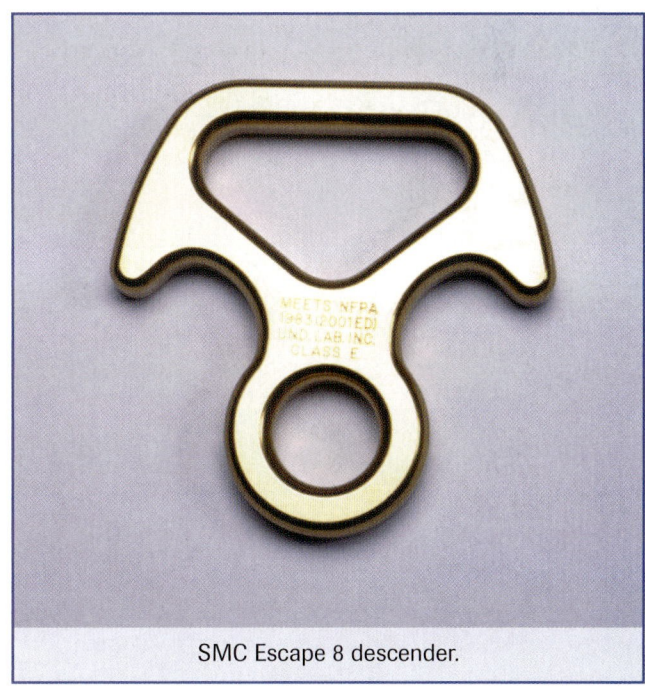

SMC Escape 8 descender.

Escape Belt

The final critical piece of the escape kit is the means of connecting the user to the descender. Some users already will be wearing a work or rescue harness. Some firefighting protective wear now comes with a harness prerigged in the clothing or built into the self-contained breathing apparatus, which helps resolve this step. Without this type of equipment, however, a quick-donning means of attachment is required.

At one time, emergency belts that simply encircled the torso were believed to be better than nothing. More data and several incidents have shown that this is not necessarily the case. A belt, especially a thin, webbing type belt, can be extremely painful and even disabling in use. Wider belts, such as the fire rescue escape device, and harnesses with leg loops are the preferred type of escape wear.

By far, the best course of action is to consult a single manufacturer to obtain your entire escape system. This helps ensure that all components work together effectively.

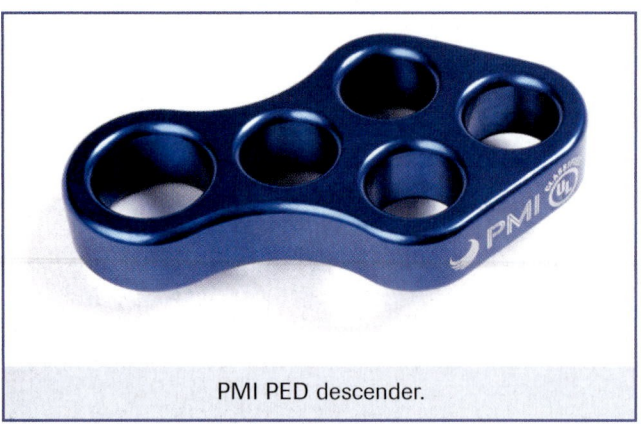

PMI PED descender.

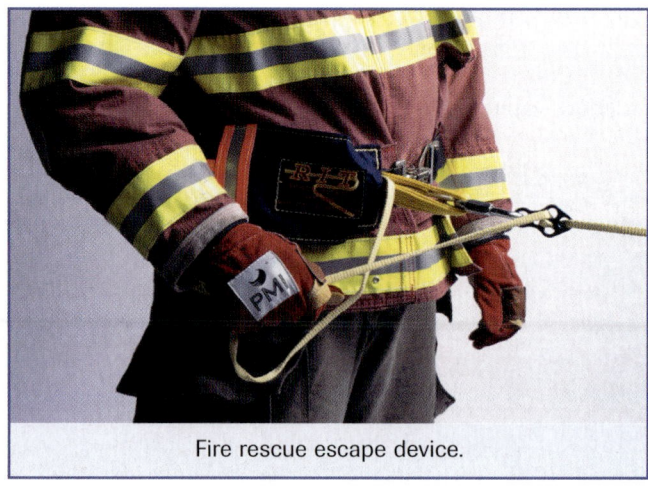

Fire rescue escape device.

10

Basic Ascending Techniques

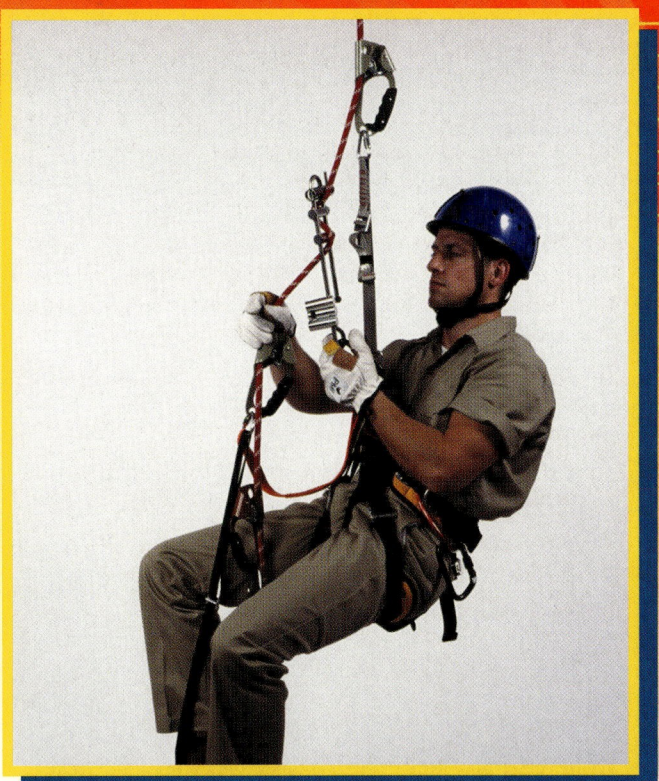

Prerequisites

Before attempting the activities described in this chapter, you must have demonstrated that you can properly:

1. Use and care for rope.
2. Use and care for other equipment needed in the high angle environment.
3. Tie correctly and without hesitation the knots described in Chapter 6.
4. Apply the principles of anchoring and rig a safe, secure anchor.
5. Apply the principles of belaying: safely and confidently belay another person using either a Münter hitch or a one-person belay device.
6. Apply the principles of rappelling: rappel safely, confidently, and under control; tie off the rappel device to operate hands free of the rope; and return to a safe, controlled rappel.

The material in this chapter conforms to guidelines published by the National Fire Protection Association (NFPA), specifically standard 1006, *Professional Qualifications for Rescue Technicians* (2002), and standard 1670, *Operations and Training for Technical Rescue Incidents (2004)*. NFPA standards are revised regularly, and readers are advised to review the latest version of this standard.

Objectives

On completion of this chapter, you should be able to:

1. Describe the principles and purposes of ascending and identify the equipment required for an ascending system.
2. Tie and use a Prusik hitch.
3. Use light-use ascenders.
4. Ascend a fixed rope using an ascending system created from three ascenders.
5. Explain what is meant by an ascending "system" and list the criteria that must be met to create safe, efficient ascending systems.
6. Explain what is meant by "changing over" from ascending to rappelling or from rappelling to ascending and describe the techniques involved in these procedures.
7. Safely change over from ascending to rappelling and from rappelling to ascending.
8. Explain the need for and use of the procedure known as "tying off short" and be able to tie off short while ascending.
9. Describe how you can use ascenders to extricate yourself from a jammed rappel device or other similar emergency.

Key Terms

Ascenders *Rope grab devices* used to ascend a fixed rope or, with specific types of ascenders, to create a hauling system. The two categories of ascenders are (1) light-use ascenders (also called *personal ascenders or personal ascent devices*), which normally are used for no more than one person's body weight, and (2) *general-use ascenders,* which are used both as personal ascenders and in hauling systems for progress capture devices and as rope grabs.

Ascending A means of moving up a fixed rope using either mechanical devices or friction hitches attached with slings to the climber's body.

Ascender Slings Attachments, usually webbing or rope, that connect a climber to the ascenders.

Changeover To transfer from an ascending mode to a rappelling mode or from a rappelling mode to an ascending mode while on rope.

Chicken Loop A safety loop that fits around the ankle to secure the ascender sling and to prevent the foot from slipping out of the sling should an upper connection fail and the climber fall backward.

General-Use Ascenders A mechanical rope grab device that operates primarily by the force of a cam action wedging

the rope against the inside of the device's shell. General-use ascenders are designed to slide in one direction on a rope. They are used for personal ascenders and in hauling systems for progress capture devices and rope grabs.

Hitch A knot that attaches to or wraps around an object or rope in such a way that when the object or rope is removed, the knot falls apart.

Light-Use Ascenders Also called a *personal ascender* or *personal ascent device*, a light-use ascender is a rope grab device used to travel up (ascend) a fixed rope. Light-use ascenders normally are used for no more than one person's body weight.

Prusik Hitch A type of friction hitch used in ascending and belaying. The term *Prusik* also is used by some individuals as a verb, meaning to ascend, even when mechanical devices are used (e.g., to Prusik a slope).

Prusik Loop A continuous loop of rope in which a Prusik hitch is tied.

Tying Off Short A safety technique that creates an extra point of attachment during ascending by tying the person directly into the main-line rope.

The Purpose of Ascending

Ascending a rope is, in essence, the opposite of rappelling. It involves the use of mechanical devices or friction hitches to safely and efficiently climb a fixed rope. *Ascending* is a further development of competency in the vertical environment. If you are only able to rappel, you can travel only one way on the rope: down. Having the capabilities to competently rappel *and* ascend means that you have developed the freedom to travel both down and up the rope.

To further develop competency and enhance your skills in rappelling and ascending, you also must be able to change safely from rappelling to ascending, and vice versa, while on rope. This procedure is known as a *changeover*. To be able both to ascend and to perform a changeover safely and efficiently requires a mix of equipment and the simultaneous use of skills, which means that you must have a thorough knowledge of the equipment and an instinctive use of the skills. These come only through practice of the required techniques.

Along with the development of ascending and changeover skills and a thorough knowledge of the equipment involved comes the ability to extricate yourself from certain difficult situations; for example, you may need to extract yourself from a jammed rappel device without the risk of using a knife.

How Ascending Is Accomplished

Ascending is accomplished through the use of rope grab devices, called *ascenders*. When used properly and secured to the rope, ascenders can be made to slide in only one direction: up.

Types of Ascenders
Friction Hitches

There are several kinds of friction hitches, but the most commonly used type is the Prusik hitch.

Mechanical Ascenders

Mechanical ascenders work by an offset camming action that presses the cam against the rope, preventing the device from sliding down the line. The two types of mechanical ascenders are general-use ascenders and light-use ascenders.

General-Use Ascenders

A *general-use ascender* grips the rope primarily by squeezing it against the inside of the device's shell. Two examples of general-use ascenders are the Rescucender and the Progressor.

Light-Use Ascenders

A *light-use ascender*, which is also called a personal ascender or personal ascent device, works primarily by gripping the rope with a toothed cam and also by pressing the rope against the inside of the shell of the device. Several brands of light-use ascenders are available, including those made by CMI, Petzl, Jumar, SRT, and PMI.

In most cases ascenders are attached to the climber's body by *slings,* which are connectors made of webbing or rope. The slings may be connected by various means to the seat harness, the chest harness, and the climber's feet.

The actual ascending process involves alternating actions on the part of the climber. First, the climber rests his or her weight on the first ascender as it grips the rope, keeping the body weight off the second ascender; the climber then moves the second ascender up the rope. Body weight is shifted to the second ascender and taken off the first ascender, which is then moved up the rope. The climber ascends the rope by repeating this cycle.

For most ascending activities, at least two ascenders are required. The use of three ascenders increases the margin of safety.

The Basics: A Prusik Hitch

Friction hitches were the first type of rope grab devices used in ascending. For the most part, they have been replaced in ascending by mechanical devices. However, it is still important that you know how to tie and use a friction hitch, because you can improvise a friction hitch with rope or cord if you do not have mechanical ascenders. On numerous occasions, the ability to improvise a friction hitch has saved lives by helping people extricate themselves from difficult situations. Friction hitches also have helped people perform a self-rescue after failure of a mechanical ascender. In addition, friction hitches are used in rigging for some rope rescue systems.

Although there are a number of different friction hitches, the one most commonly used is the ***Prusik hitch***.

Selecting Rope for a Prusik Hitch

Diameter

The Prusik hitch works more efficiently if the rope of which it is made is smaller in diameter than the main-line rope to which it is attached. As a general rule, the diameter of the Prusik cord should be two thirds to three fourths the diameter of the main-line rope. This usually works out to an 8-mm Prusik cord to be used on an 11-mm (⁷/₁₆ inch) rope, or a 9-mm Prusik cord for a 12.5-mm (¹/₂ inch) rope.

Avoid extremes. The Prusik cord must be strong enough to support the intended load with a proper safety margin, but it should not be so large that it is hard to get the hitch to "set."

Stretch

The Prusik cord should not be stretchy, otherwise it will be difficult to loosen once it is "set" on the rope.

Construction

Construction of Prusik cord is a compromise between two features:

- A softer braid cord grips better but is more difficult to loosen and move up the rope; also, it wears out faster.
- Harder braid cords are easier to loosen and move up the rope but do not grip as well.

Creating a Prusik Loop

To create a Prusik loop for a seat harness, make a continuous loop from an approximately 6-foot (2 m) length of the type of Prusik cord you have chosen. This can be done by tying the two ends of the cord together in a grapevine knot (double fisherman's knot).

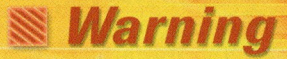

Warning

Materials used for Prusik hitches wear quickly and should be inspected before each use.

Attaching a Prusik Loop to a Rope (Figure 10-1)

The following sequence explains how to tie a two-wrap Prusik onto a rope. This exercise uses a rope anchored vertically so that you can test the tied Prusik to see if it supports your weight; however, a Prusik can be tied onto a rope at any angle.

1. Securely anchor a static kernmantle rope vertically so that it supports your weight.
2. Stretch out the Prusik loop between your two hands with the connecting knot about midpoint.
3. At about eye level, begin to place the loop on the rope by forming a Prusik hitch. Hold the loop against the rope on the side of the rope facing you. Have a smaller portion of the loop (about 6 inches [15 cm]) off to the right of the rope (Figure 10-1, *A*).
4. Bring the larger side of the loop around the main-line rope toward you and pull it through the smaller side of the loop. Make sure the figure **8** bend (or grapevine knot) passes well through and that the coils formed around the main rope are even (Figure 10-1, *B* and *C*).
5. Bring the larger side of the loop through the same path as before. Make sure the coils of the Prusik hitch around the main rope are even and parallel (Figure 10-1, *D*).
6. Tighten the Prusik hitch around the main rope: (1) with one hand, pull the end of the Prusik loop away from the main rope; (2) at the same time, with the other hand, grasp the knot by placing the fingers on the coils of the hitch on the side away from you, with the thumb on the bar portion of the hitch on the side next to you; grasp the hitch with the thumb and pull the bar tight against the rope (Figure 10-1, *E-G*).

Weighting the Prusik Hitch

Now, test the Prusik hitch to make sure it holds.

7. Grasp the end of the Prusik loop and pull down, placing your weight on it. If you are wearing a seat harness, you can clip the Prusik loop into the harness with a carabiner and sit down, with the Prusik loop taking your weight (Figure 10-1, *H, I*).
8. If the hitch begins to slide, set it further by holding it in your hand and pressing it closed, using the thumb as in step 6 above.

The Prusik hitch can be used for a variety of purposes. For example, it can be used to tie onto a rope to hold rope pads in place.

You should practice tying the Prusik under a variety of conditions, and you should be able to tie it with one hand.

Other Uses for the Prusik Loop

As mentioned in Chapter 1, it is a good idea to carry with you a couple of Prusik loops that can be used quickly for unforeseen

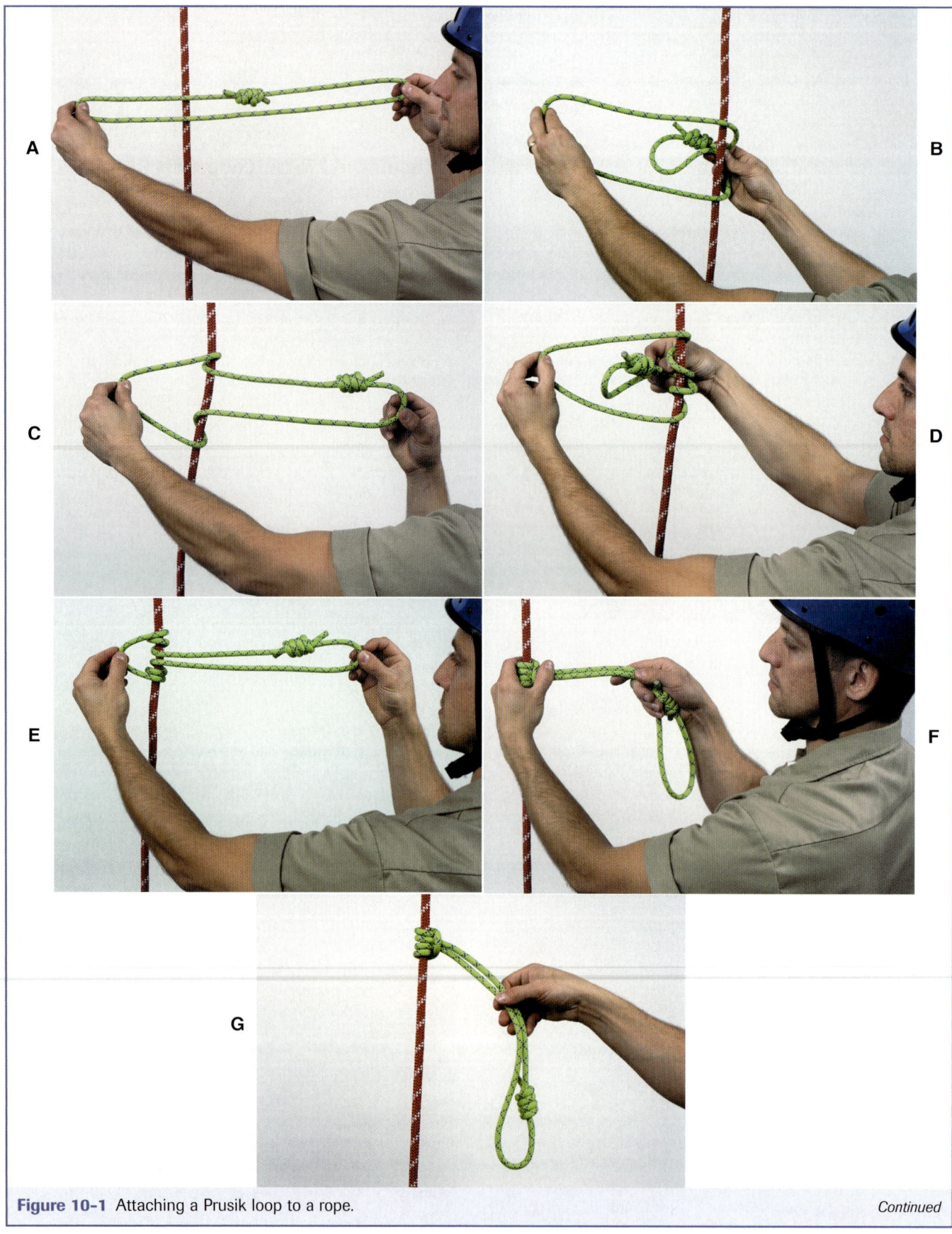

Figure 10-1 Attaching a Prusik loop to a rope.

Continued

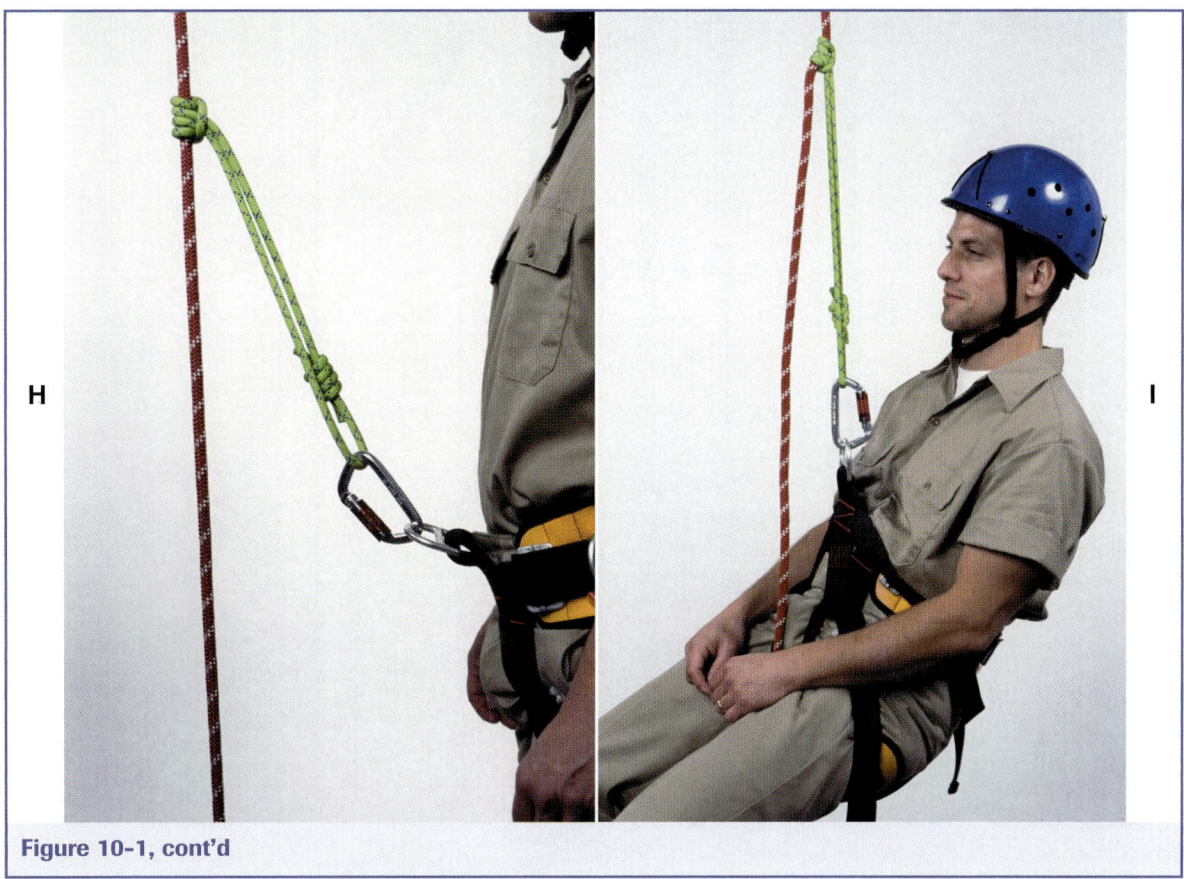

H   I

Figure 10-1, cont'd

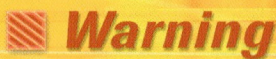

⚠ *Warning*

Never press down on the top of a Prusik or other friction hitch unless you want it to slide down. In a life support situation, downward pressure could release the hitch, causing a fall, which could result in severe injury or death.

needs. For example, if your descent device jams while you are rappelling, you can use a Prusik on the line above the device to get your weight off the rappel device and unjam it (see p. 160 for specific details on using an ascender to unjam a rappel device). A Prusik might also be used as a self-belay on safety lines at the edge of a drop.

Greater Holding Power: The Three-Wrap Prusik

The two-wrap Prusik hitch, described earlier, is adequate for most personal-use vertical applications. However, for greater holding power, such as when the rope is slippery from mud or ice or when greater weight is involved, the three-wrap Prusik may be better (Figure 10-2). The three-wrap Prusik is created by

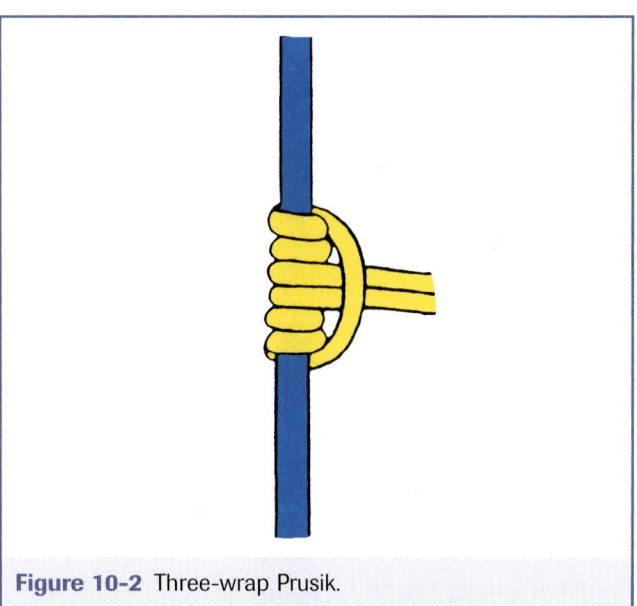

Figure 10-2 Three-wrap Prusik.

running the Prusik sling one more time through the loop. This is known as adding another wrap.

Although the three-wrap Prusik hitch offers the potential for greater holding power, it may be more difficult to manipulate than the two-wrap version. (See Chapter 12 for information on using the three-wrap Prusik for rescue belays.)

Mechanical Ascenders for Personal Use

Most people now use mechanical ascenders for personal ascending. These devices tend to be easier, more efficient, and more convenient than hitches. For personal use, the light-use ascender is the most commonly used mechanical ascender. Figure 10-3 shows a typical light-use ascender with a handle. Although the parts of some models may not look exactly like the ones shown here, these devices all work in essentially the same way.

Parts of the Light-Use Ascender

Frame

The frame (see Figure 10-3, *A*) is the structure to which the parts are attached; it is the part of the ascender that mostly determines the device's strength. The frame may be made of extruded, stamped, or plate aluminum or in some cases from cast aluminum.

Handle

The handle (see Figure 10-3, *B*) may be an integral part of the frame, or it may be attached to the frame with rivets or bolts. In some designs the handle is molded to fit the contour of the hand and can be comfortably used with gloves or mittens. Not all light-use ascenders have handles. Those without handles usually are designed for direct attachment to the climber's body and are operated without using the hands.

Safety Lever

A safety lever (see Figure 10-3, *C*) in the locked position prevents full downward movement of the device's cam. This helps prevent the ascender from coming off the rope accidentally.

Nose

The nose (see Figure 10-3, *D*) forms the inside channel into which the cam pushes the rope so that the ascender stays on the rope.

Tie-In Points

Tie-in points (see Figure 10-3, *E*) are usually an integral part of the frame and are used to fasten a sling that is attached to the climber. Most ascenders have tie-in points at the bottom so that the ascender can support a person hanging below the device. Some ascenders have additional tie-in points at the top. These are used in certain ascending systems in which the ascender is pulled along as the climber advances up the rope.

Right-Handed and Left-Handed Ascenders

Most ascenders with handles are manufactured in right-handed or left-handed models. Some manufacturers color code their ascenders for ease of differentiation. However, the following quick test can help you determine whether the device is a right-handed or left-handed model:

1. Turn the ascender so that the opening for the rope between the nose and the cam is facing you.
2. On a left-handed model, the handle will be to your left; on a right-handed model, the handle will be to your right.

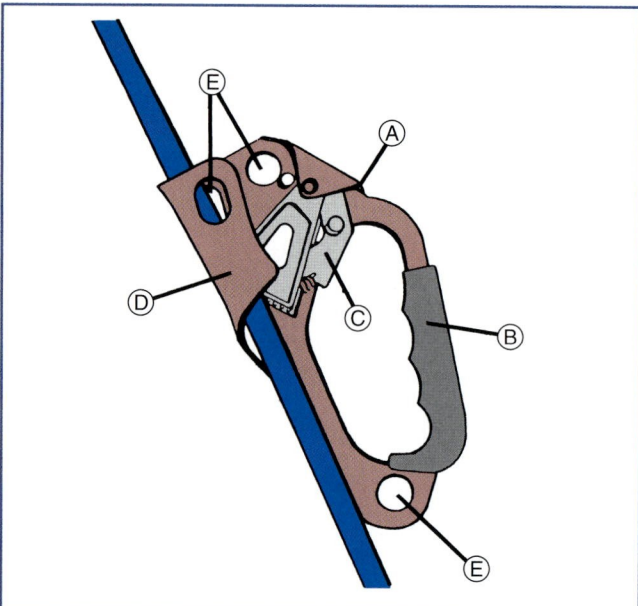

Figure 10-3 Typical light-use ascender (right hand). *A,* Frame. *B,* Handle. *C,* Safety lever. *D,* Nose. *E,* Tie-in points.

Ascender Slings

To be used safely and efficiently, ascenders must be attached to the climber's body with connectors known as ***ascender slings.*** These slings may be made of either webbing or rope. Many prefer rope for the following reasons:

- An appropriately designed rope may abrade less easily than webbing.
- Rope works better than webbing if the sling must go through a roller device (these are used in certain ascending systems).

If you decide to construct your ascender slings from rope, you may be able to use line of a smaller diameter than that normally used for the main-line rope. A sling made of rope $\frac{5}{16}$ to $\frac{3}{8}$ inch (8 to 10 mm) in diameter might be appropriate as long as it has an adequate safety factor.

Most of those experienced in the use of ascenders prefer slings constructed of static rope. Static rope tends to stretch less than dynamic rope and therefore transfers the energy involved in ascending directly to the ascenders rather than absorbing it.

The length of the slings depends on factors such as your body proportions and the type of ascending system you use. These factors are explored later in the chapter.

Attaching the Slings to the Ascender

Because the designs of ascender tie-in points differ, the methods of connecting the slings to the ascender vary, depending on the brand and design used. Consult the manufacturer's instructions for specific information.

When connecting the sling to an ascender, remember that a sharp bend in a rope diminishes the rope's strength (see Chapter 4, p. 40, for an explanation of the 4:1 rule). If the ascender's tie-

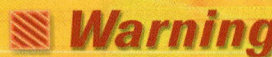

Warning

Light-use ascenders can and do fail when misused. The following conditions are the most common means by which these ascenders fail.

Frame Breakage

Ascender frames constructed of cast aluminum can crack or break when subjected to the high stress of being dropped. Cast aluminum frames can crack under their paint, leaving no outward sign of damage. Previously owned ascenders of any type may have been subjected to stresses that could result in failure. For this reason, do not use a previously owned ascender unless you know its complete history.

Rope Damage

Rope damage occurs when the ascender pulls on the rope with such force that the teeth of the cam tear the rope sheath. Sheath tearing has been known to occur with as little force as 800 pounds (363 kg) on the ascender and rope. For this reason, ascenders with sharp-toothed cams should never be used in situations involving more than one person's body weight. For example, toothed cams, such as are found on light ascenders, should not be used in rescue hauling systems.

Rope Slipping Out of the Ascender

Light-use ascenders are designed to operate most efficiently and safely on vertical ropes and when moved in a direct line with the rope. Light-use ascenders have been known to slip off the rope when pulled away from the rope or torqued on the rope. This can happen when light-use ascenders are used on a rope that is not completely vertical but at an angle, such as when ascending a sloping highline or traversing a rope along a ledge. If the chance exists that the ascender might be used in this way, for which it was not designed, a safety carabiner should be clipped across the ascender and the rope (Figure 10-4). This may not prevent the ascender from slipping from the rope, but the sling will remain connected to the rope via the carabiner.

Warning

Some warn against clipping a carabiner or snap link directly into an ascender with a cast aluminum frame. It is thought that under a severe impact, the carabiner or snap link might cause the cast aluminum frame to crack.

---

in point is wide enough, the sling can be tied directly into it using a figure 8 follow-through knot. If the tie-in point is narrow, such that it would create too sharp a bend in the rope, the rope should be clipped into a carabiner or screw link, which then is clipped directly into the carabiner tie-in point.

A figure 8 on a bight knot is tied in the end of a rope sling that is to be attached to the person. If the sling is to be attached to a seat harness, the knot is connected to the carabiner, which is clipped into the front tie-in point of the seat harness. If the sling is to be attached to the climber's foot, a large loop is needed in the figure 8 knot. This loop should be large enough to slip through a chicken loop (see p. 154) and onto a boot (see Creating an Ascending System later in the chapter).

Using a Light-Use Ascender (Figure 10-5)

The following steps detail the use of a light-use ascender.

1. For this initial exercise, you will need only one light-use ascender with a handle. It may be either a right-handed or left-handed model, depending on which feels more comfortable.
2. Using rope, create an ascender sling. For this exercise, the total length after tying should be only about 2 feet (0.7 m). Attach the sling to a lower tie-in hole of the ascender, either directly or with a carabiner, following the guidelines given previously. Tie a figure 8 on a bight loop in the end of the rope sling that will be attached to you.
3. Don a seat harness and clip a locking carabiner into the seat harness tie-in point.
4. Clip the seat harness into the loop of the ascender. Lock the carabiner.

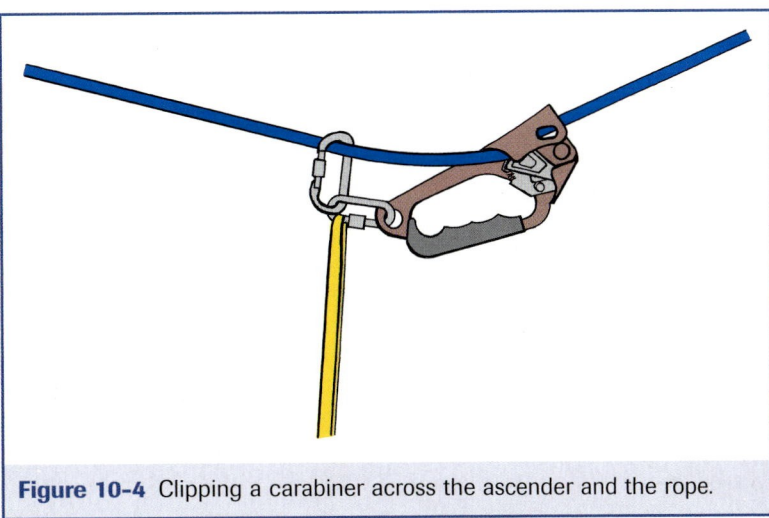

Figure 10-4 Clipping a carabiner across the ascender and the rope.

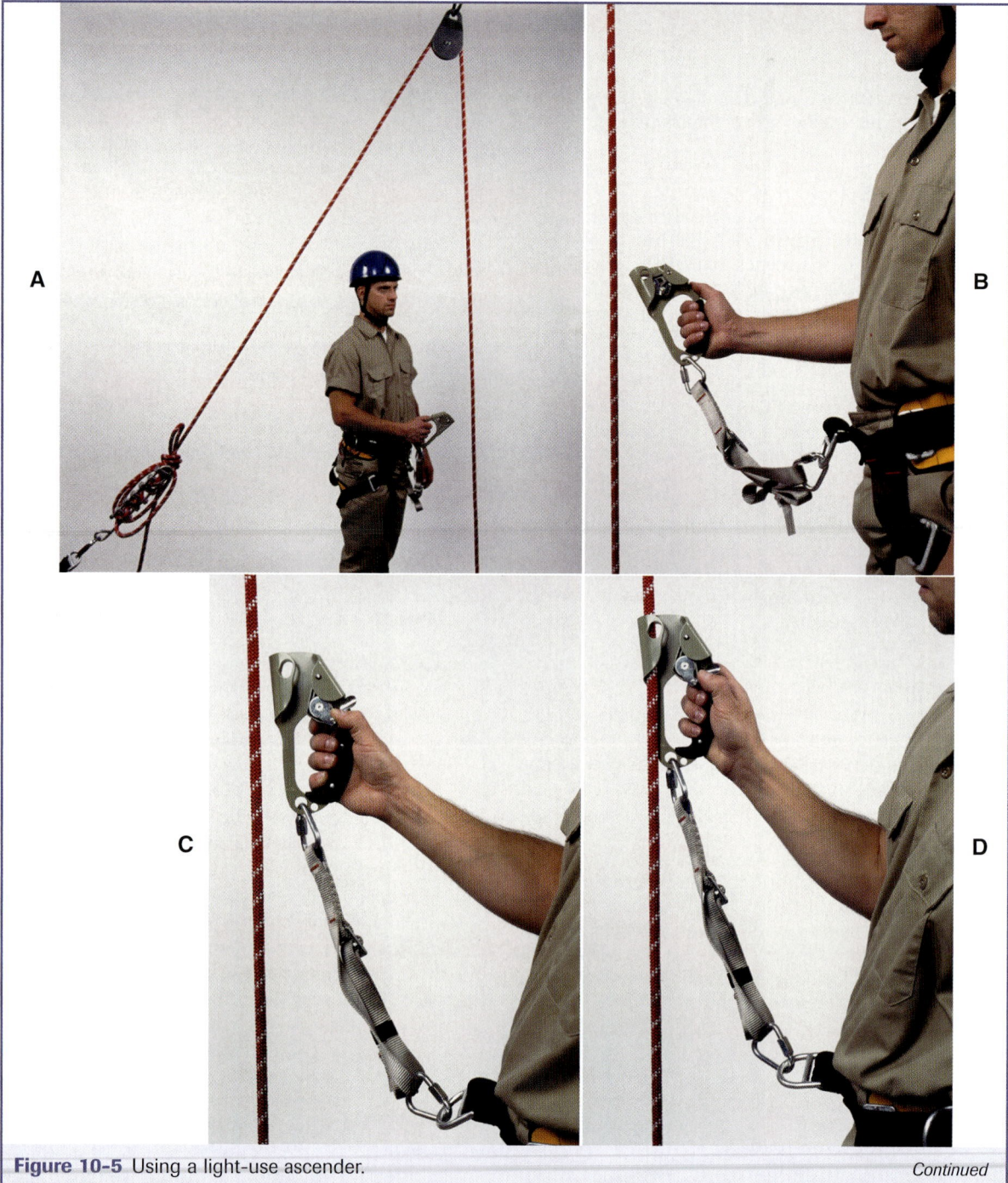

Figure 10-5 Using a light-use ascender.

Continued

Attaching the Ascender to the Rope

5. Securely anchor a main-line static kernmantle rope vertically so that it will support your weight with an adequate safety factor. When you are on the rope, you must have a way to get back down once you have pushed the ascender up as far as it will go (Figure 10-5, *A*).

6. Take the ascender in one hand and press the safety lever so that the cam swings down and open. The literature provided by the manufacturer should give specific instructions for triggering the safety lever, although this usually is done

with the thumb of the hand holding the ascender. On some ascenders, the safety lever can be triggered just by grasping the device's handle. On other ascenders, the hand must grasp the entire ascender, with the handle against the palm and the index and middle fingers around the nose (Figure 10-5, *B* and *C*).

7. Attach the ascender to the rope at about eye level with the nose up. To do this: (1) Hold the cam down with the trigger; (2) position the ascender so that the main-line rope runs in the channel of the nose; (3) release the cam so that it presses

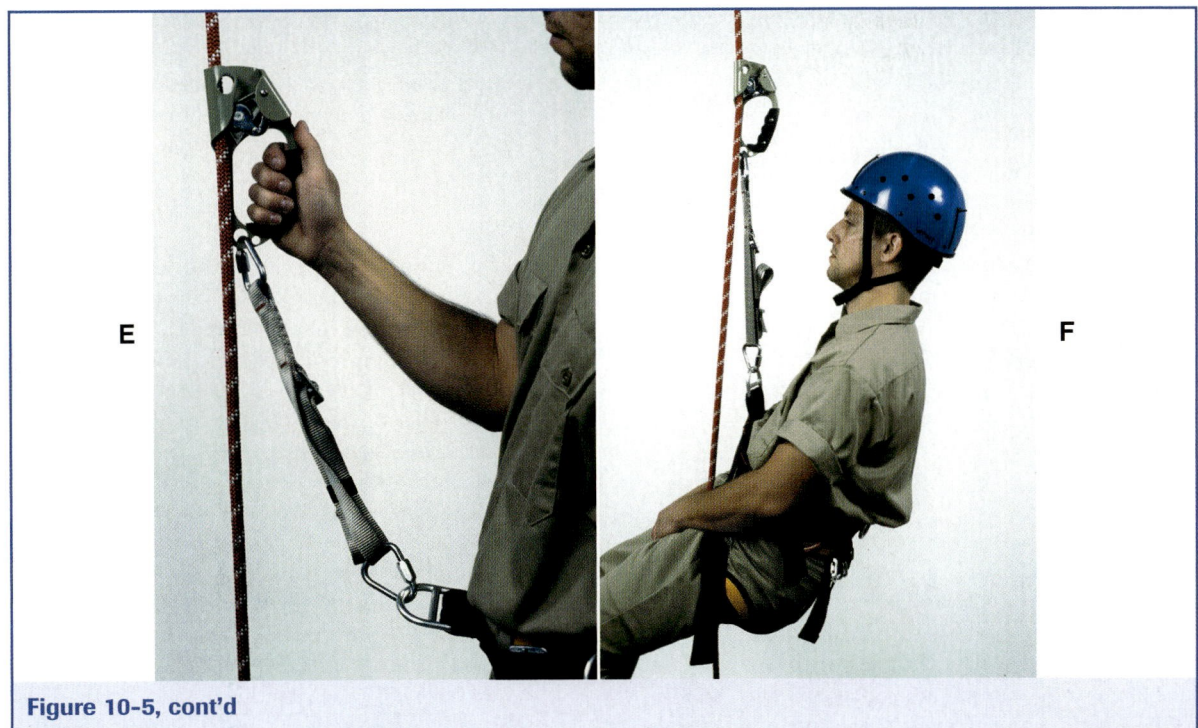

Figure 10-5, cont'd

the rope into the channel of the nose and the ascender remains on the rope; (3) release the safety lever, making sure it now locks the cam on the rope. *When ascending, never touch the safety lever unless you intend the ascender to come off the rope* (Figure 10-5, *D, E*).

8. Sit down so that the sling comes taut and the ascender supports your weight on the rope. If the rope stretches to the extent that you end up on the ground, reset the ascender up the rope so that you are supported (Figure 10-5, *F*).

9. Stand up so that your weight is off the sling and push the ascender up a foot. Then sit down again.

Backing the Ascender Down the Rope

10. Stand up so that your weight is completely off the ascender. Grasp the upper part of the ascender around the nose and use your thumb to move the cam down while slightly lifting the ascender. *Do not touch the safety lever.* Move the ascender down a foot and release the cam so that it reengages the rope. Sit down again on the ascender until it supports your weight.

These 10 steps constitute the basics of using a light-use ascender. Because you used only one ascender, your movement was limited. When using ascenders for a climb, you would not shift your weight to the ground to raise the ascender; rather, you would shift your weight to another ascender, which you would also move up the rope.

Creating an Ascending System

As demonstrated in the previous exercise, one ascender can hold you on the rope. However, to move up the rope effectively, you need two or more ascenders. When two or more ascenders are

worked together for traveling up a rope, the arrangement is known as an *ascending system* (Box 10-1).

Many different ascending systems are used in rope work. The differences involve the kinds of ascenders used, the combinations in which they are attached to the climber's body, and the parts of the body to which they are attached. Each ascending system has its advantages with regard to safety, ease of use, and speed and ease of movement. However, no one system offers all these advantages, and each system has at least one drawback.

When beginning your training in ascending, you should use ascending systems that combine safety and ease of use. Some hallmarks of this type of ascending system include the following:

- The system should require more use of your legs and feet and less use of your arms and hands. Your legs are stronger and have greater stamina than your arms.
- The system should hold you upright on the rope with your body weight over your legs. This requires less arm strength, encourages use of the legs, and contributes to safety.

Box 10-1	**Maintaining Three Points of Attachment in Ascending**

A commonly accepted safety guide for ascending is the *three points of attachment* rule. This means that when the climber is moving one ascender, he or she is attached to the rope by two devices. In many ascending systems, such as the ones shown in this chapter, three ascenders are used on the rope. When only two ascenders are used, it may be necessary to "tie off short" to maintain a margin of safety (see the section, Tying Off Short).

- The system should be able to support you in a sitting position while you are on the rope. Ascending is a tiring activity that often requires short periods of rest, possibly in a sitting position.
- The system should have attachments to the seat harness (and in some cases to a chest harness). Some systems have attachments only to the feet and depend on arm and body strength to hold the climber upright. These are risky systems, sometimes called *death rigs*.

Whatever system you choose, it is important that it be fine-tuned to your body height and build. With a fine-tuned system, rope ascending is no more work than climbing a ladder. Conversely, a system that is poorly fitted and out of adjustment quickly exhausts even the most physically fit individual.

Tying Off Short

Tying off short is a safety procedure that involves tying directly into the main-line rope to ensure an additional attachment. This procedure is used in certain situations during ascending when the danger exists that climber may lose attachment to the rope. For example, tying off short would be used when:

- A climber is using only two ascenders and must take one ascender from the rope to move past a knot or go over the edge of a cliff or building.
- A climber must cross a knot on the way up the rope.

- A climber must go over an edge or obstruction and does not have a quick attachment point. (A *quick attachment point*, also known as a quick attachment safety, is a short sling attached on one end to the climber's seat harness and on the other end to an ascender, which can be easily attached with one hand to a secure point.)
- A climber is using an ascending system that cannot guarantee the person will remain upright if one ascender fails. (A well-designed ascending system has at least two points of contact above the climber's center of gravity so that if either ascender fails or comes off the rope, the climber ends up sitting in his or her harness rather than hanging upside down by a heel. See the following section, Maintaining a Safety by Tying Off Short.)

The procedure for tying off short is as follows (Figure 10-6):

1. Reach beneath the lowest ascender to the slack rope hanging below you (Figure 10-6, *A*).
2. Take a large bight of that rope and pull it up.
3. Tie a figure 8 on a bight in the bight of rope (Figure 10-6, *B*).
4. Clip the figure 8 on a bight into a spare carabiner that is clipped into the seat harness (Figure 10-6, *C*).
5. Complete the move past the obstacle (Figure 10-6, *D*).
6. When finished with this safety, unclip the figure 8 on a bight from the carabiner, untie the knot, and allow the rope to drop back down below you (Figure 10-6, *E* and *F*).

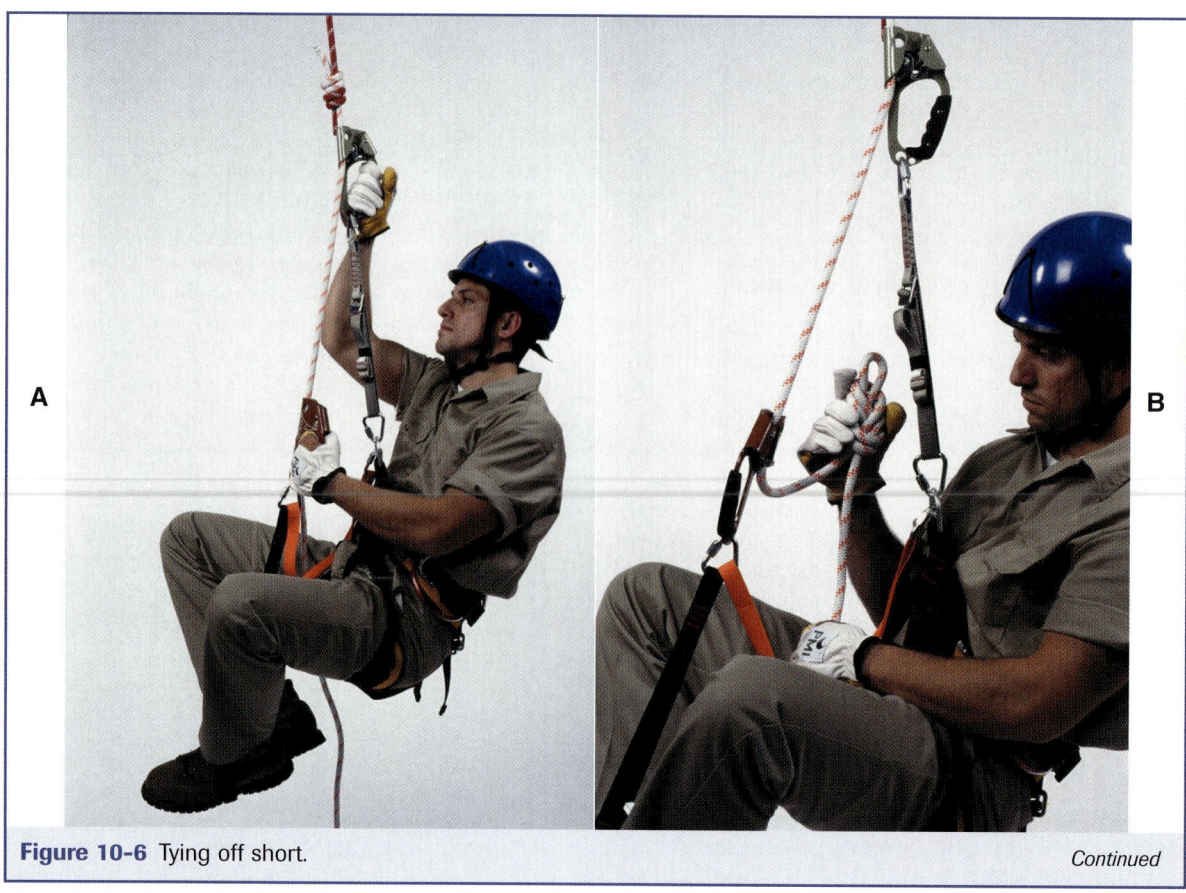

Figure 10-6 Tying off short.

Continued

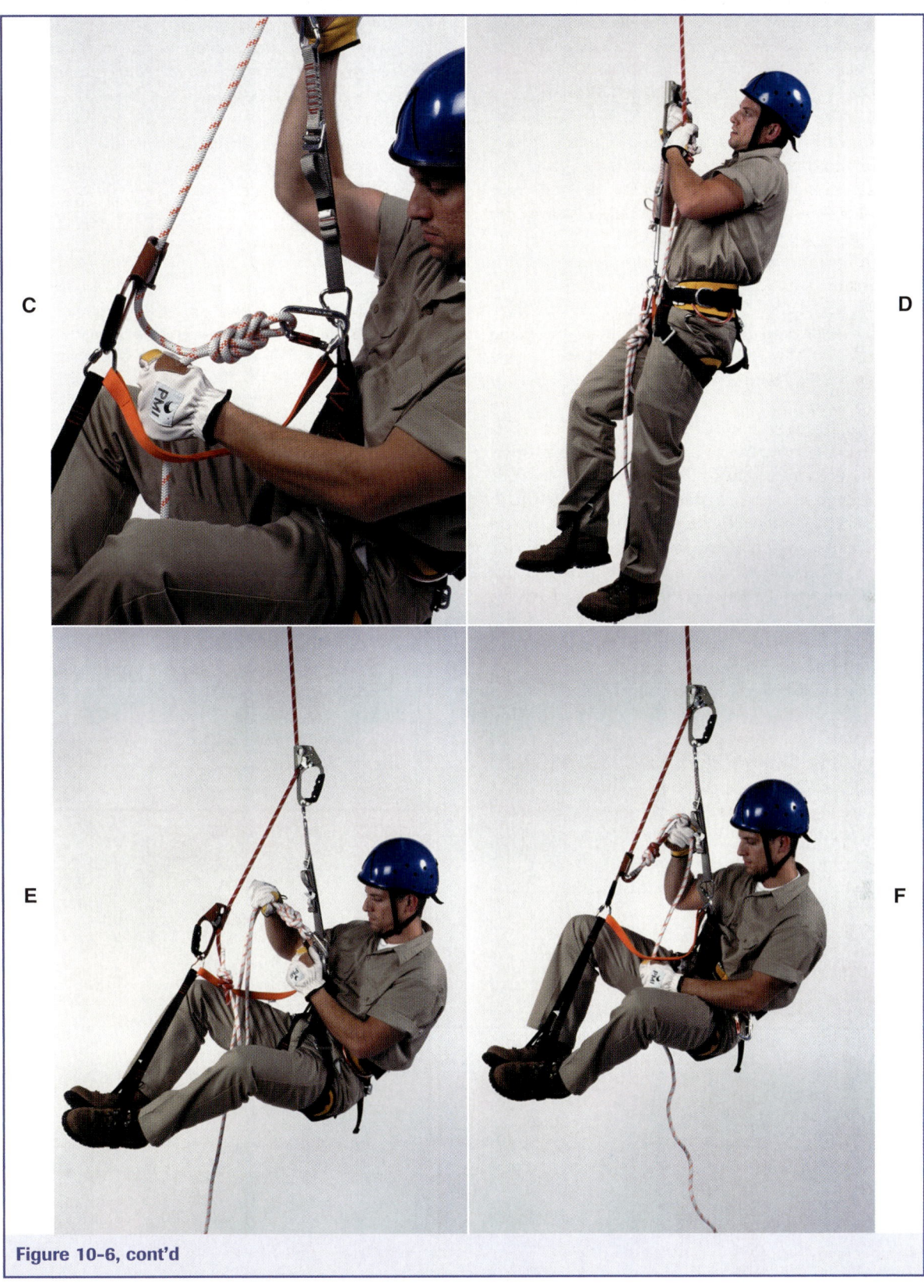

Figure 10-6, cont'd

Maintaining a Safety by Tying Off Short

If you are using an ascending system that ensures you will remain upright if an ascender fails, you can create a continuous safety by tying off short.

1. Tie off short as soon as you have ascended high enough that a fall would injure you.
2. Leave the figure 8 on a bight knot clipped into your seat harness carabiner as you continue to ascend.
3. Ascend until you have enough slack in the main-line rope that it no longer offers adequate protection from a fall (i.e., usually about 10 feet [3 m] or one story).
4. Tie a second knot closer to you and put it in the carabiner above the first knot.
5. Take the first knot out of the carabiner, close the carabiner, untie the old knot, and drop the slack out of the main-line rope.
6. Repeat this procedure until you have finished the climb.

Chicken Loops

A device that should be used when climbing with ascenders that are attached to the foot is the *chicken loop* (Figure 10-7). In ascending systems in which the feet are used, ascenders frequently are attached to the feet by foot stirrups, which often are simple loops of webbing or rope sling. With these systems, chicken loops should be used around the ankles to serve the following purposes:

- Chicken loops help prevent the feet from slipping out of the stirrups while the climber is ascending.
- If the climber loses all upper-body attachments and falls backward, chicken loops help keep the feet in the stirrups, preventing a fall to the ground.

Chicken loops are constructed of webbing usually 1 inch (25 mm) or larger. The webbing is stitched or securely tied into a loop that is larger than the ankle but smaller than the boot. *A chicken loop must be able to hold a person's weight without failing.*

Examples of Ascending Systems

The following sections of this chapter explore ascending techniques that use some example systems. These systems may be used with Prusik hitches (or other comparable friction hitches), general-use ascenders, or light-use ascenders. The following example systems incorporate light-use ascenders, which are more easily manipulated by a person learning ascending techniques.

Warning

Ascending is a strenuous activity, which should be attempted only by individuals known to be in good physical condition. People with preexisting cardiac or pulmonary conditions, obesity, or other medical conditions that might be exacerbated by exertion should consult a physician before attempting ascending.

Ascending Practice System

Ascending is a new and unique activity for most people. An ascending practice system can help individuals learn the technique in a controlled environment. The practice system consists of the following elements (Figure 10-8):

1. A main-line static kernmantle rope on the practice takes place. The rope runs over a directional pulley that is securely attached to a beam in the ceiling of a building (or a very strong tree limb outside) and down to a securely anchored lowering device, such as a brake bar rack or a figure 8 descender.

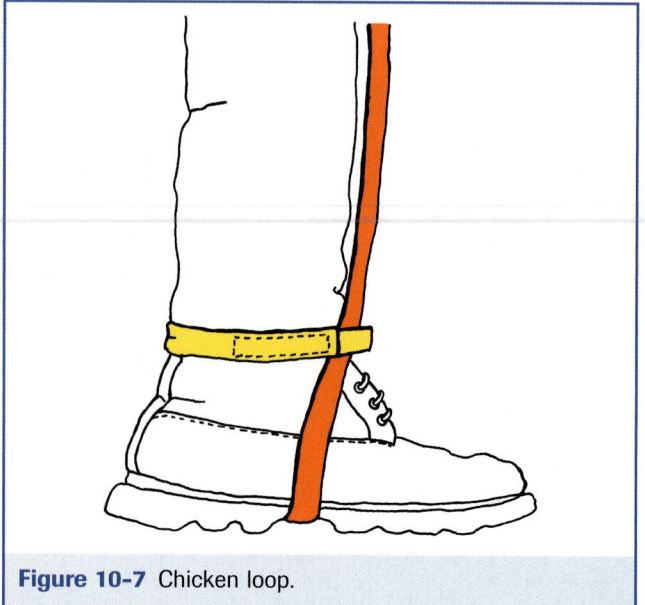

Figure 10-7 Chicken loop.

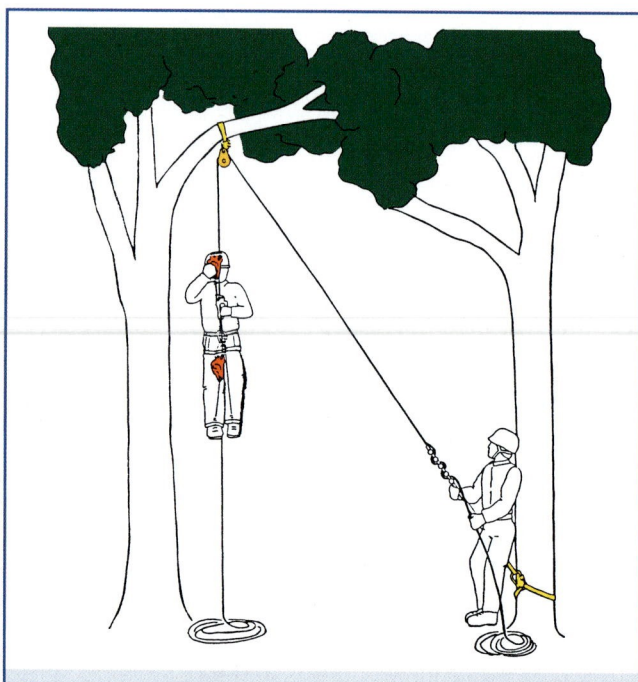

Figure 10-8 Ascending practice system.

2. In preparation for the practice, only enough rope hangs vertically to allow the person to get onto the rope.

3. The lowering device (brake bar rack or figure 8 descender) is locked off until the person begins to ascend. The person operating the braking device allows enough rope through to keep the student high enough off the deck to use the ascender but low enough that a fall will not cause injury.

4. In addition to the person operating the braking system, an assistant can help by holding the rope below the student in order to help the person as he or she begins the ascent.

5. When the student has completed the ascending cycle, the trainer operating the braking device lowers the student back to the deck so that he or she can get off the rope. The student always must stop ascending while there is still enough rope to lower him or her to the ground.

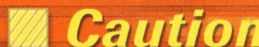

⚠️ Caution

The operator of the braking device must be thoroughly experienced in its use as a lowering device. The floor under the practice rope should be covered with a mat.

Three-Ascender System

Figure 10-9 shows a basic three-ascender system using light-use ascenders. Because the proportions of individual bodies differ, no specific dimensions for the sling attachments can be shown. You should tailor the slings for your own use, using the following guidelines:

- The system should be designed such that should the highest or next highest ascender come off rope, you will be sitting in the seat harness.
- The seat attachment (with an optional chest harness) should be the top ascender on the rope when you are resting your weight on it. *The ascender must never extend out of your reach up the rope while you are standing upright in your foot loops or sitting in your harness.*
- The ascender for your dominant foot (e.g., right foot for right-handed people) should come next on the rope. Its sling should be long enough to allow the ascender to be attached about midthigh when you are standing.
- The ascender for the nondominant foot (e.g., left foot for right-handed people) should be the last one on the rope. Its sling should be just enough shorter than the second sling to allow the third ascender to be immediately below the second ascender when both ascenders' slings are tight.
- All the knots must be contoured well, dressed, and pulled down tightly.

Using the Three-Ascender System (Figure 10-10)

For this exercise, use the ascending practice system as described earlier.

1. Before you start, make sure that someone is attending the lowering device and that initially it is locked off tight (Figure 10-10, *A*).

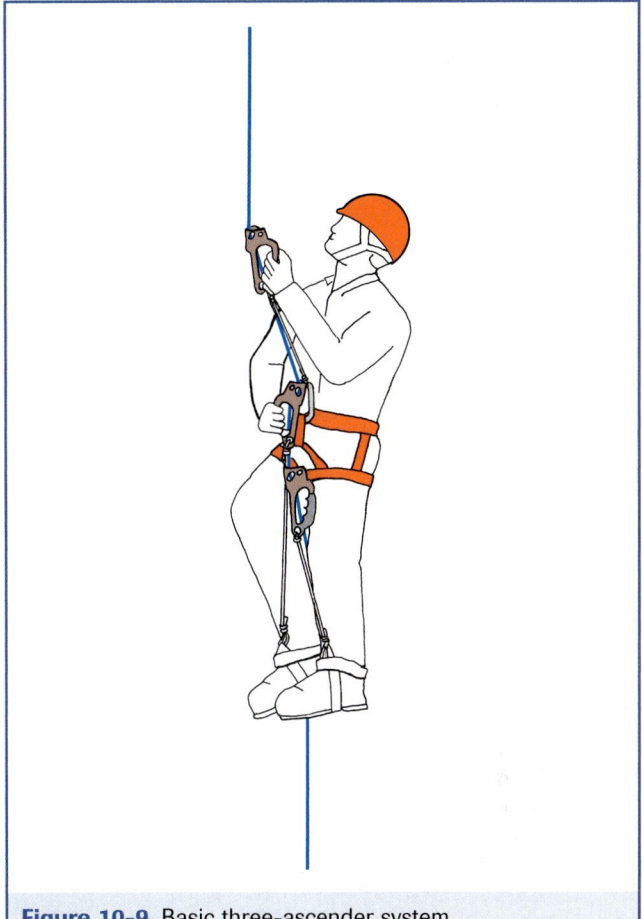

Figure 10-9 Basic three-ascender system.

2. With one hand, reach up and pull the main-line rope taut. Attach the ascender for the seat harness as high up as you can get it on the tensioned rope (Figure 10-10, *B*).

3. Attach the next ascender down (the one to your dominant foot) under the seat harness ascender (Figure 10-10, *C*).

4. Attach the third ascender under the second one (Figure 10-10, *D*).

5. To pretest the system, alternately load the seat ascender and each foot ascender to make sure they hold (Figure 10-10, *E*).

6. If possible, have another person help you get started by holding the rope down close to the ground. Otherwise, you may have to hold the rope down yourself. This is necessary in getting started because there may not be enough rope weight initially to cause the rope to slide through the ascenders as they are pushed up. Once you have gotten far enough off the ground, the rope weight will cause the rope to slide through the ascenders automatically as they are pushed up.

7. Shift your weight onto the foot stirrups and off the top ascender. Push the top ascender up as far as you can (Figure 10-10, *F*).

NOTE: When maneuvering your body up in order to raise an ascender, use your leg muscles as much as possible. The more you use your legs and feet, and the less you use your arms and hands, the less fatigued you will become.

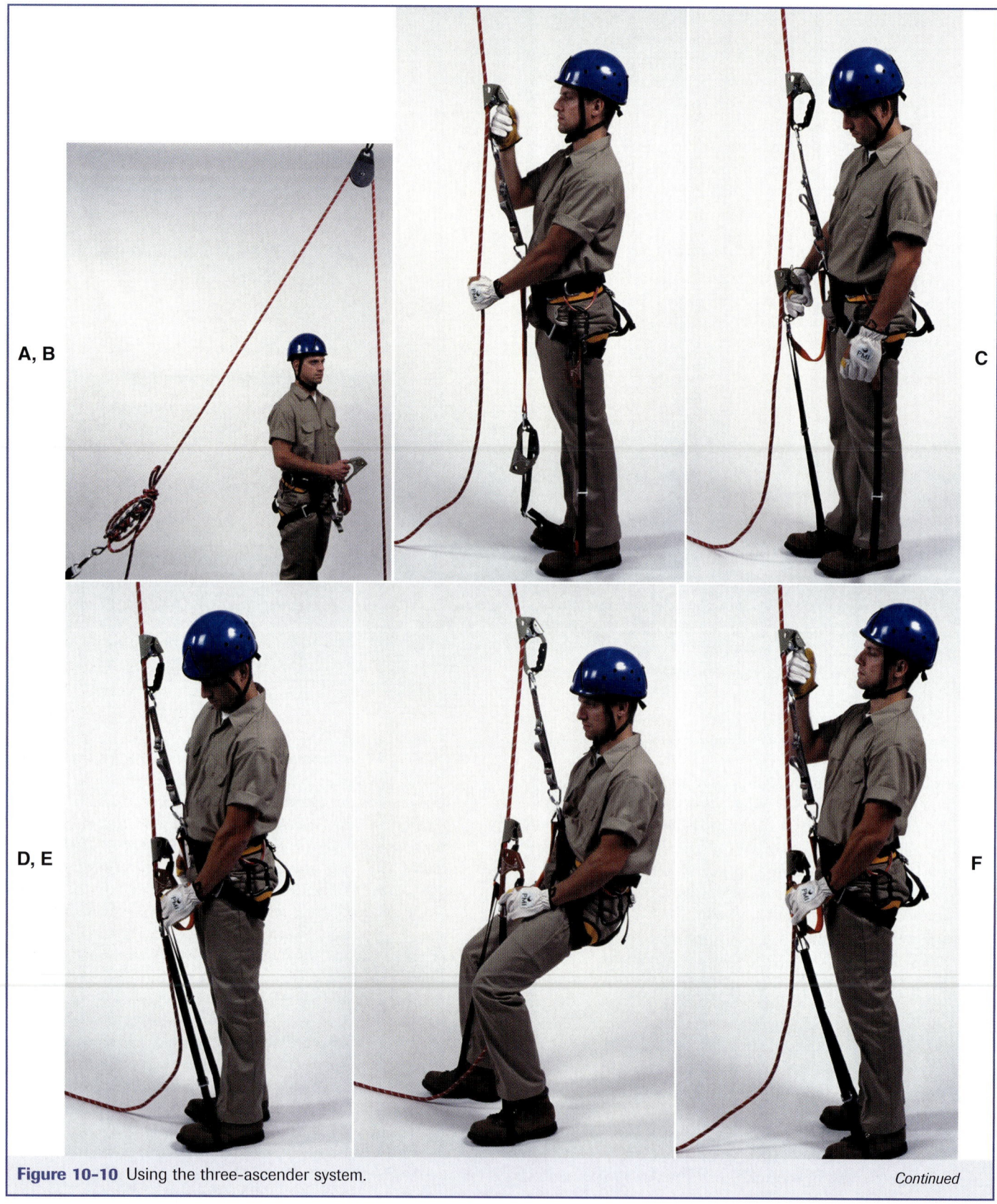

A, B

C

D, E

F

Figure 10-10 Using the three-ascender system.

Continued

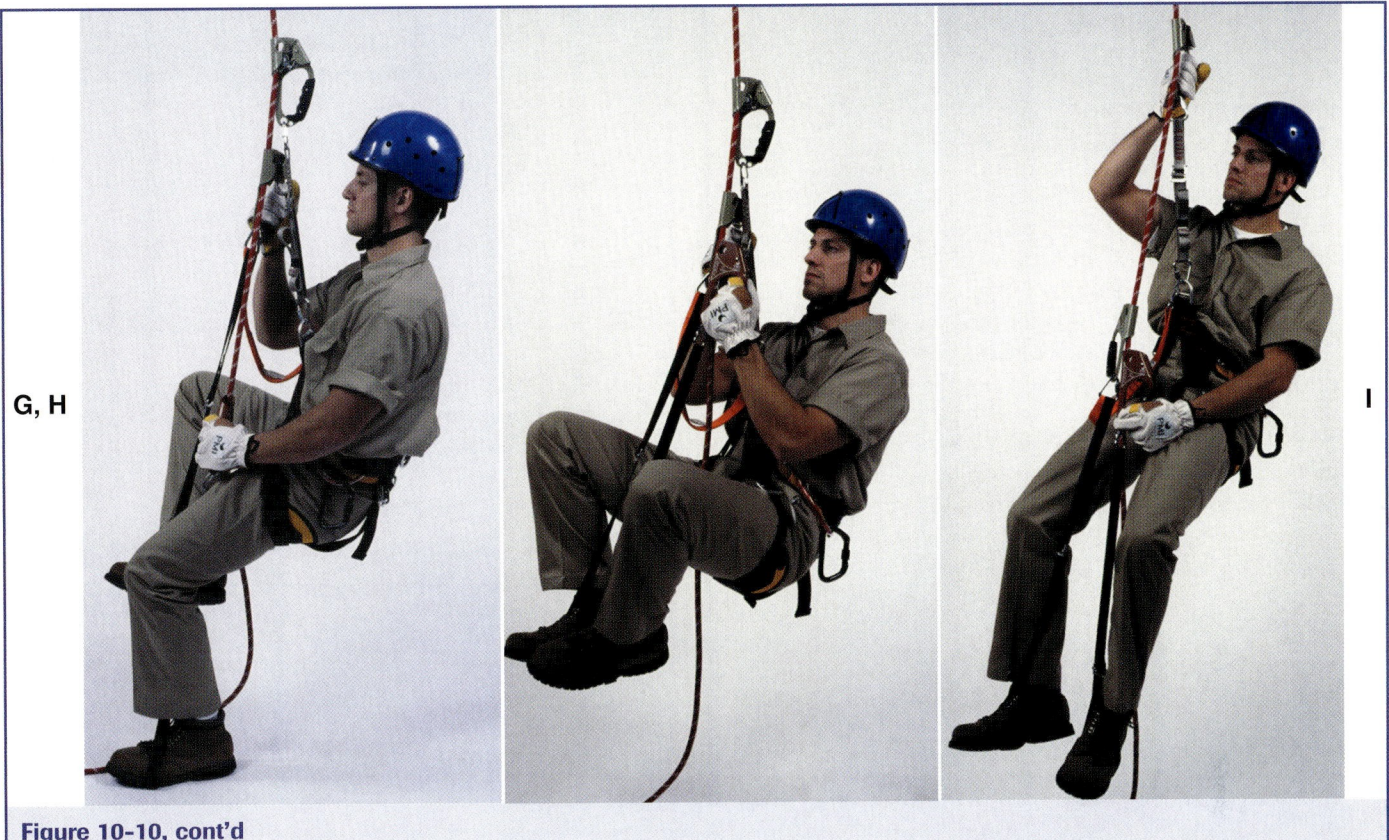

Figure 10-10, cont'd

8. Sit down so that you are supported by the top ascender. Take the weight off the next ascender in line by lifting the foot attached to it. Raise this foot ascender as far as it will easily go (Figure 10-10, *G*).

9. Take your weight off the remaining foot ascender by lifting the foot attached to it and raise the ascender as far as it will go (Figure 10-10, *H*).

NOTE: As you progress up the rope, the person attending the lowering device should slowly let rope out so that you remain a safe distance off the ground. However, you should be up high enough so that the rope pulls through the ascenders by its own weight as you raise the ascenders.

10. Continue the cycle by repeating steps 7, 8, and 9 until you start running out of rope or you become fatigued. Have the operator of the lowering device lower you back to the ground (Figure 10-10, *I*).

11. Remove all the ascenders from the rope.

Other Ascending Systems

The three-ascender system is just one example of an ascending system. There are dozens of different ascending systems, from which one can be chosen based on specific factors, such as:

The distance that must be traveled up the rope
- The climber's physical strength
- The stamina of the user
- Differences in physique (e.g., a body that is apple or pear shaped, thin or fat)
- The speed required for the climb

With proper research and experimentation, each person can find the type of ascending system that is just right for him or her. A good place to begin the search is the book, *On Rope: North American Vertical Rope Techniques,* by Bruce Smith and Allen Padgett (1996, National Speleological Society) (see Appendix A).

Ascending Over an Edge

Usually the most difficult maneuver in ascending is going over the edge at the top of a cliff or building. As a general rule, and just as in rappelling, the higher up the rope is anchored, the easier it is to go over an edge.

The specific technique for getting over an edge depends on the particular nature of the edge.

Edge with a Gradual Rollover

1. Ascend until the top ascender is about to make contact with the wall.
2. Push yourself away from the wall using one hand and your feet.
3. Raise the top ascender above the contact point.
4. Take care not to get your fingers caught between the hardware or rope and the wall.
5. As you move upward and your weight is on the ascender above the contact point, the other ascenders should follow more easily.

Undercut Edge

1. Ascend until the top ascender is about to make contact with the wall.
2. Bring the lower ascenders up as far as it is comfortable to do so.
3. Try to work the top ascender over the edge by pushing away from the wall with one hand and with your feet or knees.
4. If this is impossible and you have a quick attachment safety (QAS), place the QAS above the edge and place your weight on the QAS while moving the top ascender over. If you don't have a QAS, tie off short into the main-line rope.
5. Remove the top ascender from the rope and move it up and over the edge and immediately clip it into the rope.
6. Begin ascending again. The two remaining ascenders probably can be eased over the edge once your weight is on the main-line rope above the edge. If this is not the case, follow the same procedure as you did with the top ascender. *Until you are in a safe, secure position and in no danger of falling, never have fewer than two ascenders securing you to the rope.*

Changing Over

Changing over means switching from an ascending mode to a rappelling mode or from a rappelling mode to an ascending mode while still on the rope. It is a skill that adds to vertical

Box 10-2	**Equipment Needed for Changing Over**

- ❑ Two locking carabiners in the seat harness tie-in point: the one currently in use and a spare to be used when changing over.
- ❑ Harness gear loops or a gear sling. The equipment not currently in use is attached to the loops or sling (e.g., the rappel device while you are ascending, the ascenders while you are rappelling).
- ❑ Equipment for ascending and for rappelling.

competency and is particularly useful in emergencies, such as when you rappel to the end of a rope and find that it does not reach the bottom. Box 10-2 lists the equipment required for a changeover.

Procedures for Changeovers

Changing Over from Ascending to Rappelling (Figure 10-11)

For this exercise, use the ascending practice system described earlier.

1. Before you start, make sure a responsible, experienced person is attending the lowering device, which initially must be locked down tight.

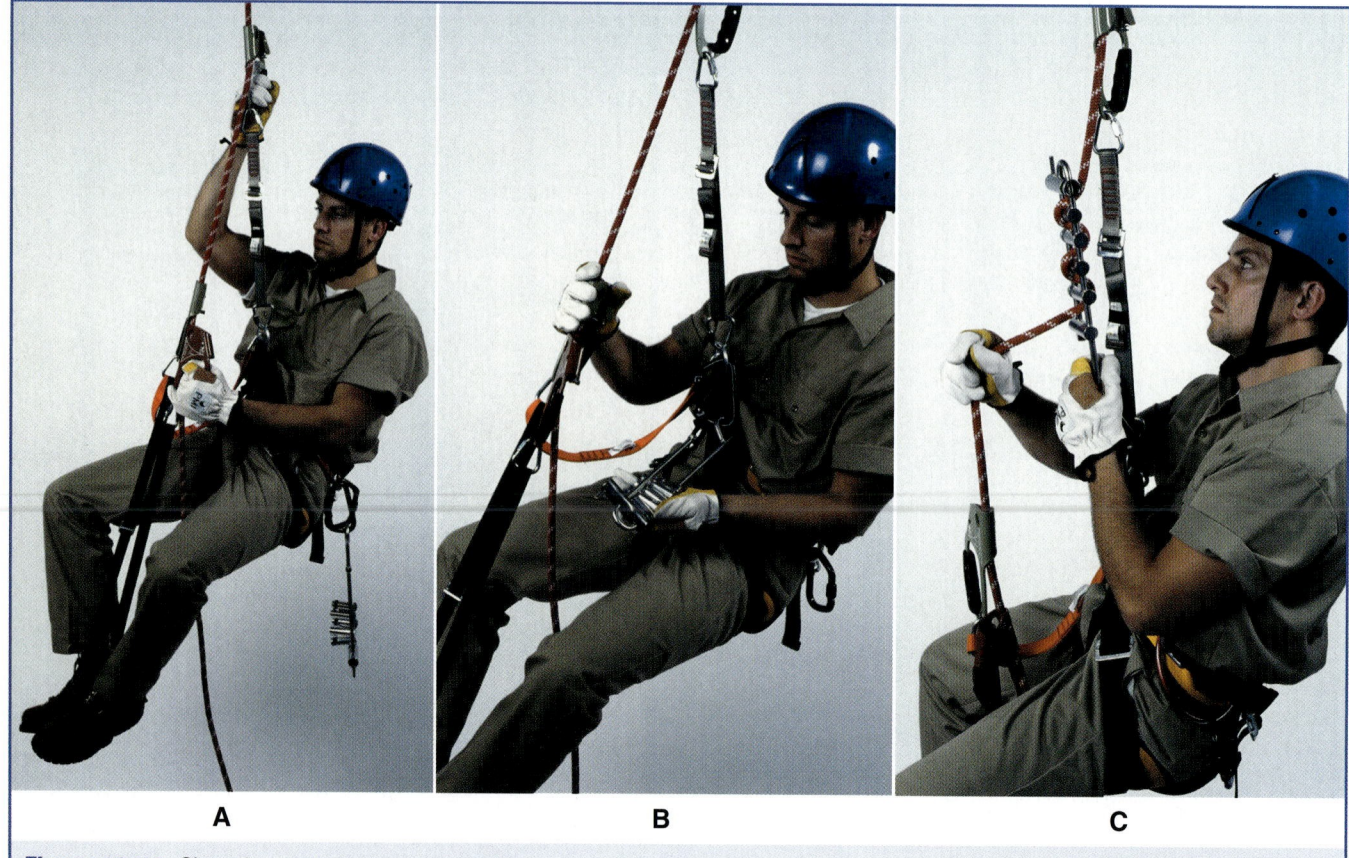

| A | B | C |

Figure 10-11 Changing over (ascend to rappel).

Continued

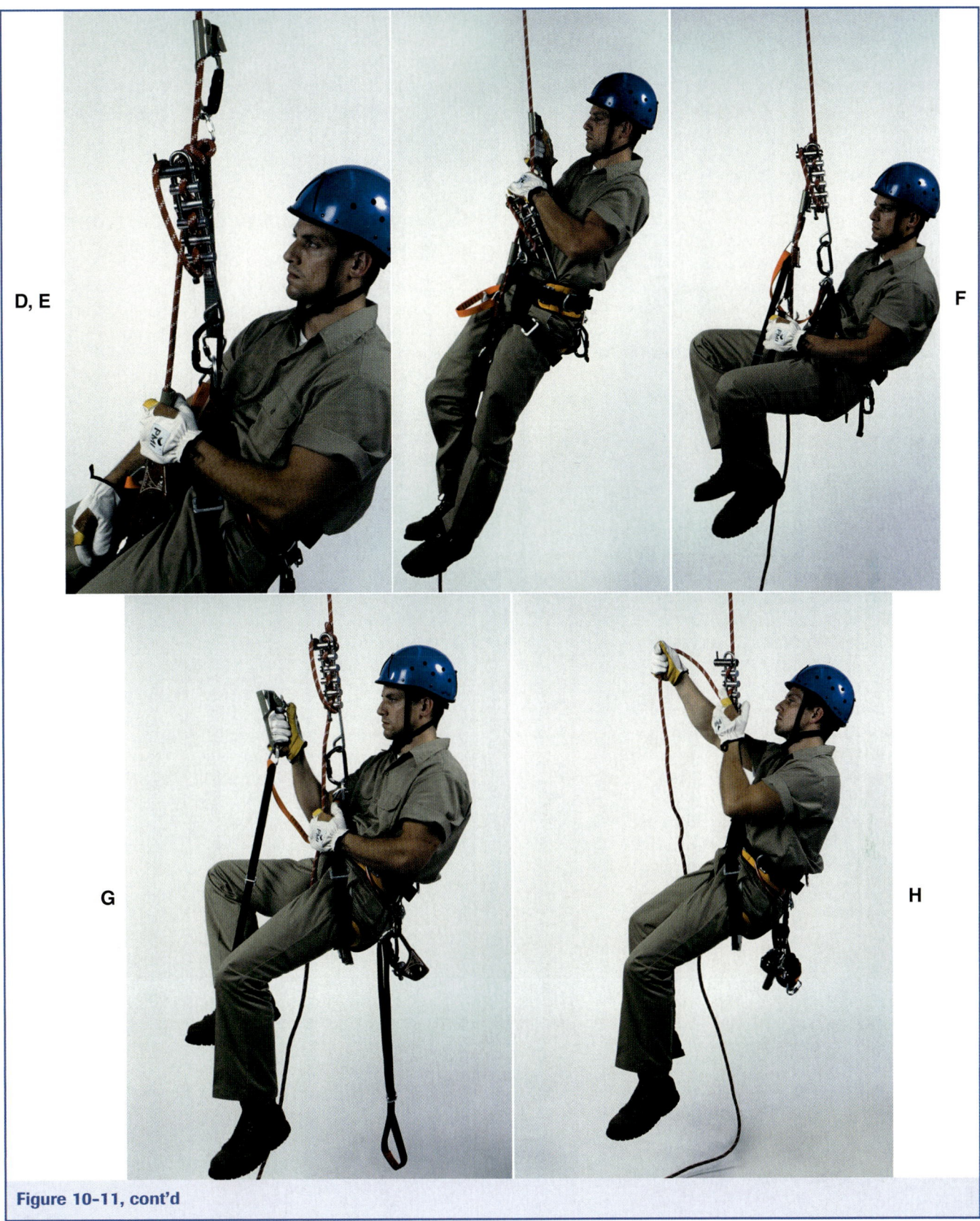

D, E

F

G

H

Figure 10-11, cont'd

2. Using a three-ascender system, begin ascending the rope.

3. When you reach the point where you want to changeover, stop your ascent (Figure 10-11, *A*).

4. Remove your rappel device from your equipment sling and clip it into the second locking carabiner that is attached to your seat harness tie-in point and that currently is not in use in the ascending system. If the rappel device is a brake bar rack, lock the carabiner (Figure 10-11, *B*).

5. Sit down on your seat harness ascender (the top one) so that your weight is on it.

6. Take your weight off the foot ascenders. Move these ascenders back down the rope so that there is slack in the rope between the foot ascenders and the seat ascender. *Do not touch the cam safety levers and do not remove the ascenders from the rope at this time.*

7. Attach the rappel device to the slack rope between the foot ascenders and the seat ascender. Remove all slack in the main-line rope between the rappel device and the top ascender (Figure 10-11, *C*).

8. Securely lock off the rappel device. Make sure there is no slack between the rappel device and the top ascender. If you have not done so already, lock the seat harness carabiner that attaches the rappel device to the seat harness (Figure 10-11, *D*).

9. Move a foot ascender back up the main-line rope only far enough so that when you put your weight on it, it removes the weight from the seat harness (top) ascender.

10. Shift your weight to the foot ascender and remove the weight from the seat harness ascender.

11. Remove the seat harness ascender from the rope (Figure 10-11, *E*).

12. Sit down so that the rappel device takes your weight. Remove weight from your foot ascender by lifting your foot (Figure 10-11, *F*).

13. Remove all remaining ascenders from the rope (Figure 10-11, *G*).

14. One by one, remove the ascender slings from your body. To secure them, wrap them around the ascender to which they are attached and clip them into your equipment sling.

15. Unlock the rappel device and proceed with the rappel (Figure 10-11, *H*).

Changing Over from Rappelling to Ascending (Figure 10-12)

16. Stop the rappel at the point where you want to begin the changeover. Lock off the rappel device securely, following the guidelines given in Chapter 9 on p. 131 (Figure 10-12, *A*).

17. Remove the seat harness (top) ascender from the equipment sling. Clip the sling into the spare carabiner in seat harness's front tie-in point (the one currently not in use). Lock the carabiner (Figure 10-12, *B*).

18. Place the top ascender on the rope as far up as you can push it. It is important that there be no slack in this ascender sling. (One way to ensure this is to let slack through the descender until the top ascender sling comes taut.)

19. Place the other ascenders on the rope connected to the proper slings via the feet. If any of these interfere with

the position of the rappel device, back them off down the rope a short distance below the rappel device (Figure 10-12, *C*).

20. When all the ascenders are securely attached, unlock the rappel device and slowly let rope through it. When your weight is off the rappel device, remove the device from the rope and clip it back into the harness gear loop (Figure 10-12, *D-F*).

Extricating an Obstruction from a Jammed Rappel Device

For the high angle technician, the ability to extricate hair or clothing from a jammed rappel device without using a knife is an essential skill. The skills and equipment required for this procedure are similar to those used in changing over.

Because of the real possibility of a jammed rappel device or similar emergency, it is wise to carry the following spare equipment when rappelling:

- Two ascenders, any type with connecting slings, or two Prusik loops (the length of the Prusik loops will vary, depending on the rappeller's body proportion)
- A large locking carabiner

Using Ascenders to Extricate an Obstruction from a Jammed Rappel Device (Figure 10-13)

1. Using the ascending practice system, begin a rappel.

2. Assume that the rappel device is jammed (Figure 10-13, *A*). Simulate this by locking off the rappel device securely (Figure 10-13, *B*).

3. Remove the seat (top) ascender from your equipment loop and clip the end of the sling into a spare locking carabiner. Clip the carabiner into the seat harness front tie-in point. Lock the carabiner (Figure 10-13, *C*).

4. Place the ascender on the rope above the rappel device. Slide it up as far as it will go.

5. Remove a foot ascender from your equipment sling and attach the end of the sling to your foot. Put the ascender on the rope above the rappel device (Figure 10-13, *D*).

6. Put your weight on the ascenders and remove the weight from the rappel device.

7. Remove the obstruction (e.g., hair, clothing) from the rappel device. Simulate this by unlocking the rappel device and causing it to go slack on the rope (Figure 10-13, *E*).

8. Replace the rappel device on the rope and lock it off so that there is no slack in the main-line rope between the rappel device and the next ascender up.

9. Put your weight on the foot ascender and remove the weight from the seat ascender.

10. Remove the seat ascender from the rope (Figure 10-13, *F*).

11. Shift your weight off the foot ascender and onto your rappel device (Figure 10-13, *G*).

12. Remove the foot ascender from the rope (Figure 10-13, *H*).

13. Remove both ascenders and slings connecting your body, secure them, and clip them into the equipment sling.

14. Unlock the rappel device and continue the rappel (Figure 10-13, *I*).

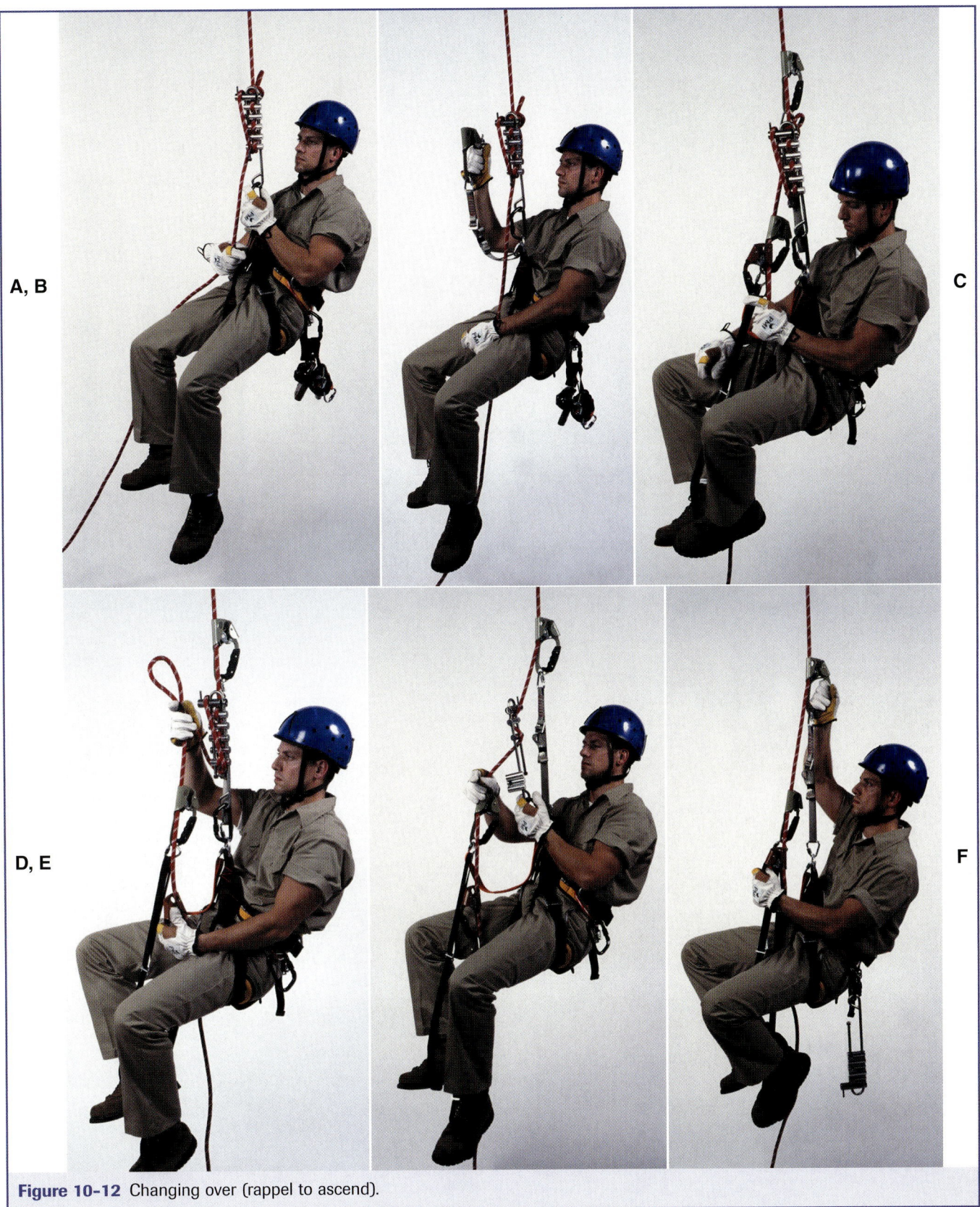

Figure 10-12 Changing over (rappel to ascend).

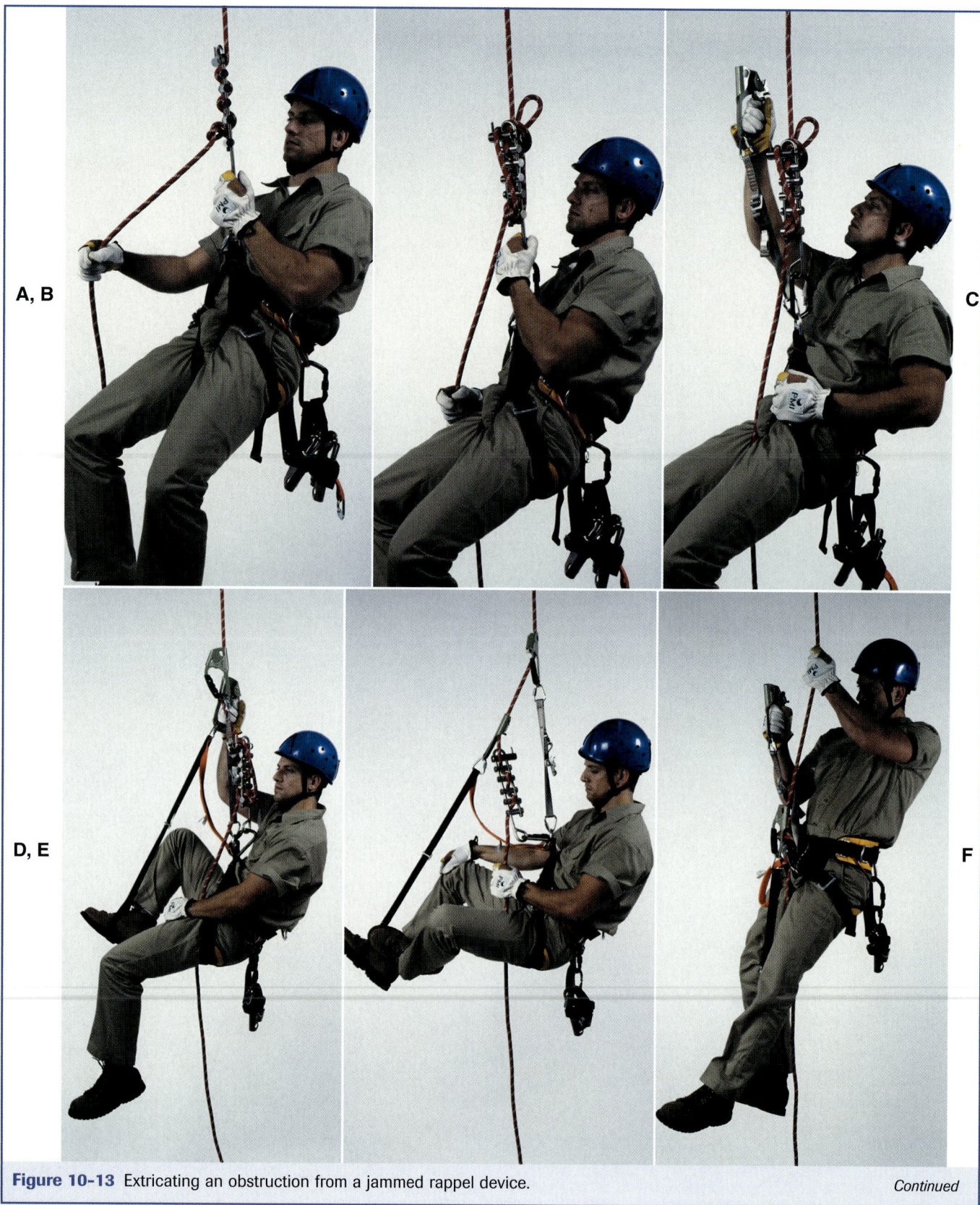

A, B

C

D, E

F

Figure 10-13 Extricating an obstruction from a jammed rappel device.

Continued

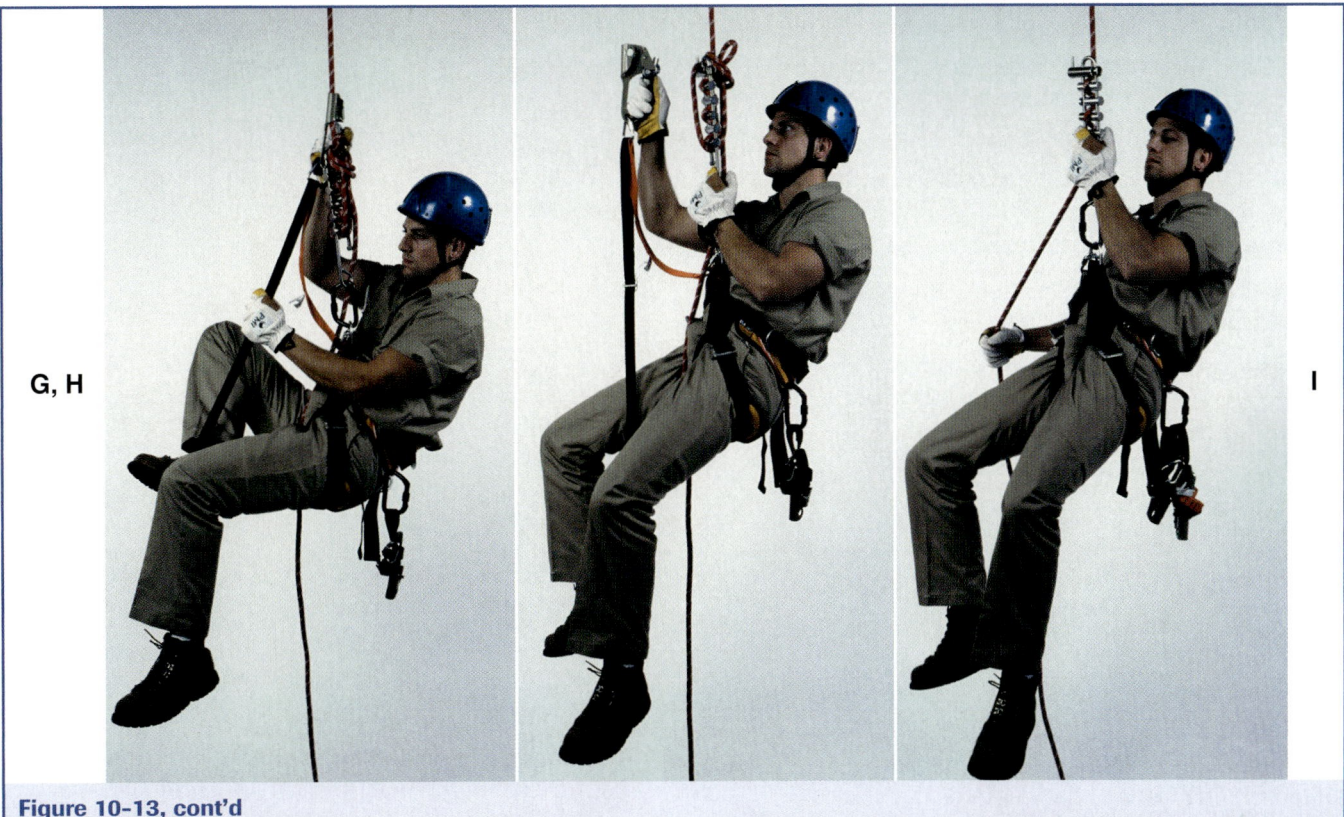

G, H

I

Figure 10-13, cont'd

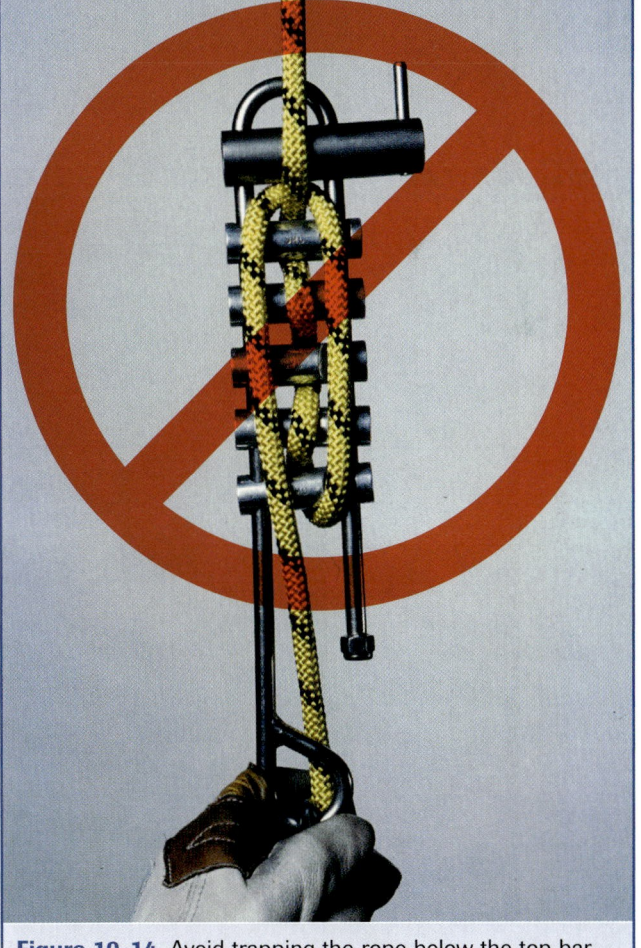

Figure 10-14 Avoid trapping the rope below the top bar.

Evaluation Exercises

Cognitive and Affective Exercises

1. What are the two basic types of ascenders?

2. What are the differences between general-use and light-use ascenders?

3. Ascenders are attached to the climber's body with _____, connectors made either of _____ or _____.

4. What is the minimum number of ascenders required for ascending?

5. _____ _____ were the first type of rope grab devices used in ascending.

6. The Prusik hitch operates more efficiently if the cord of which it is made is _____ in diameter than the main-line rope to which it is attached.

7. Name three possible modes of failure that could occur when using light-use ascenders.

8. When you are ascending with a light-use ascender, you must never touch the _____ _____ unless you intend the ascender to come off the rope.

9. List at least three characteristics of a good ascending system.

10. _____ _____ _____ is the safety procedure of tying directly into the main-line rope.

11. What safety feature is used to prevent the feet from slipping out of an ascender sling?

12. To conserve strength during ascending, what parts of the body should be used more than other parts?

13. Usually the most difficult maneuver in ascending occurs when a person has to _____.

14. What kind of procedure would be appropriate if you rappelled to the bottom of a rope and found that the rope did not reach the bottom?

11

Rescue Preplanning and Response: Rescuer Safety and Situational Awareness

Ken Phillips, Tom Vines, Steve Hudson

The material in this chapter conforms to guidelines published by the National Fire Protection Association (NFPA), specifically standard 1006, *Professional Qualifications for Rescue Technicians* (2002). NFPA standards are revised regularly, and readers are advised to review the latest version of this standard.

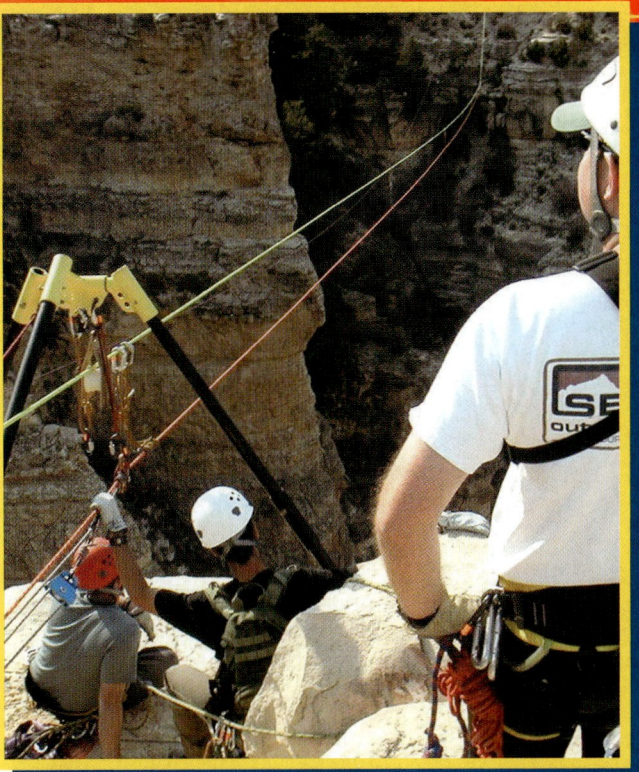

Objectives

On completion of this chapter, you should be able to:

1. Explain the role of preplanning in a rescue operation.
2. Describe the application of the incident command system (incident management system) during a rescue.
3. Explain the meaning of span of control during an emergency response.
4. Detail the functions of the Incident Safety Officer.
5. Explain the techniques used to maintain effective communications during a rescue.
6. Describe situational awareness and its application during an emergency response.
7. List techniques for effective risk management during rescue operations.
8. Detail an effective means of briefing personnel during a rescue.
9. Describe the importance of conducting a hot debrief (operational after-action review).

Key Terms

Clear Text Spoken communication style that avoids the use of any abbreviated codes in order to facilitate understanding by all emergency personnel.

Hot Debrief (After-Action Review) Immediate review after an emergency response operation, conducted with involved personnel, to identify operational deficiencies and planned corrective actions.

Incident Command System (ICS) A standardized emergency management system (also referred to as the incident management system [IMS]) that was developed to organize all functions needed to manage and support the response to an emergency situation.

Incident Safety Officer (ISO) The person responsible for monitoring current and projected hazards associated with dangerous conditions affecting rescuers and others.

Initial Incident Commander First emergency responder to arrive at the scene; this individual assumes the role of incident commander until he or she is relieved.

National Fire Protection Association (NFPA) A national organization that sets standards and fire service guidelines for rope and related equipment, along with performance standards for rope rescuers in the fire service.

Preplan Written or mental contingency preparation for potential emergency operations.

Rope Rescue Rescue in a high angle, steep, or extreme environment where the use of rope and related equipment is necessary.

Situational Awareness The ability to "know what is going on around you." During emergency operations, responders' ability to maintain situational awareness is diminished by stress, poor communications, and overtasking.

Span of Control The ratio of subordinate personnel to one supervisor during an emergency incident. The optimum span of control is considered to be 5:1; this may be increased to a maximum of 7:1.

Subject The person being rescued, or one who is in harm's way; also called the victim.

Unified Command Management of an emergency incident through the incident command system in which multiple agencies or jurisdictions are involved, each one having an incident commander assigned to the operation.

Organization and Management: the Crucial Elements in Rescue Success or Failure

Failure of rope rescue personnel to complete a task successfully in an efficient manner often can be traced to failure in the organization and management of the rescue team. The first step in organization is the preplan.

Preplan

A *preplan* is the organization and preparation done before any rescue situation arises. Thus, when such an event does occur, preplanning ensures that the response is timely and effective.

Evaluation of Local Needs and Capabilities

The preplan begins with evaluation of local needs and capabilities in rescue situations. The following determinations are important in this evaluation:

- *Local rescue needs:* This determination includes assessing the kinds of rescues that have occurred in the past and their severity, as well as the kinds of rescue situations that could possibly arise.
- *Locations that generate incidents or have existing hazards:* Thorough preplanning can include obtaining area guidebooks and aerial photographs and preparing hazard identification maps through local geographic information systems (GIS) resources.

- *Jurisdictional and operational responsibility for rescue in a local area.*

The next decision to be made is the nature of the team and under whose authority it will operate.

Operational Aspects of the Preplan (Figure 11-1)

A written preplan should be prepared to guide responders through the operational aspects of a rescue operation. This preplan should specify the following:

- How requests for emergency assistance are handled.
- Who initiates an operational response for rescue incidents.
- Notification procedures for team leaders and members.
- Contacts for backup resources and outside agencies.
- How a rescue team fits in and to whom the team reports.
- The command structure on scene.
- The communications setup, including radio frequencies.
- Medical control contacts and protocols.
- Standardized operating procedures and techniques used by the team during rescue operations.
- Established landing zones and known aerial hazards.
- How the rescue team conforms to regulations and standards.
- Established protocols and guidelines for recovery operations.

The preplan can also provide essential legal documentation to show compliance with regulations and can assist with documentation in case of liability. If a group has written operating

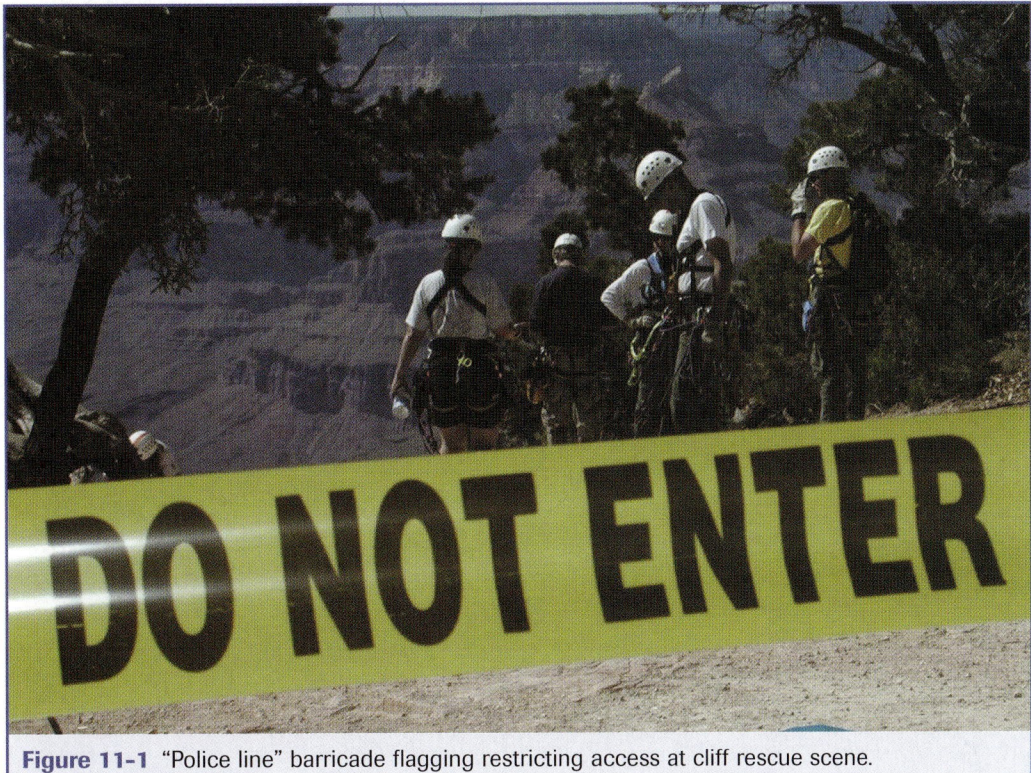

Figure 11-1 "Police line" barricade flagging restricting access at cliff rescue scene.

guidelines, however, it is important that the team closely adhere to those guidelines. Even the best-written guideline may not provide for all possible situations during an emergency response. If an incident commander encounters a situation for which deviation from a guideline is necessary, he or she should carefully consider whether the deviation is ultimately *in the best interest of rescuer and patient safety*.

Two important elements of the preplan are a review of rescue tactics used and identification of training deficiencies. To meet these requirements, those preparing the preplan should do the following:

- Inventory available equipment and human resources, including skill levels.
- Strengthen joint agency operational responses by conducting regular training sessions with cooperating agencies to facilitate teamwork.
- If incidents recur in certain areas, survey emergency access points and train at identified target sites. Preestablish anchors at sites where incidents occur repeatedly.
- Decide if your team is ready for the potentially most difficult rescue in your response area (e.g., foul weather/night operations, joint agency responses, multipitch lowerings).
- Prepare as much as possible for a "worst case rescue." It may not be realistic actually to use a complex worst case rescue as a training exercise. A more realistic objective may be to break the training into smaller segments that address operational deficiencies of the rescue organization. Develop written standard operating procedures and guidelines that identify organizational structure, communications setups, rescue techniques, safety practices, and other important information.

Guidelines and Procedures

Rescue teams can enhance their efficiency and safety by following established procedures; team members already know the actions expected of them and can anticipate a team leader's instructions. If there are no established operating procedures in place, field personnel must make significantly more operational decisions. This reduces efficiency and increases the likelihood of an incorrect decision.

Rescue groups should decide if their procedures should adhere to appropriate national standards. A fire rescue organization, for instance, may adhere to **National Fire Protection Association (NFPA)** standards. However, guidelines and procedures must be realistic and must be followed. If a group has written guidelines but does not adhere to them, and something goes wrong, the group could be in as much legal trouble as if it did not have the guidelines. For this reason, *it is essential that guidelines be realistic and appropriate to the group's rescue demands and team personnel.*

For example, it may seem ideal to have the most stringent qualifications for members allowed on rescue operations. However, if only a few team members can pass these qualifications, the criteria are counterproductive. Or, if the operating guidelines are too specific about the techniques to be used, rescuers may be restricted in dealing with unexpected and changing situations.

Guidelines should be written with the intent of providing rescuers with realistic information on goals, procedures, and safety, yet leave as much flexibility as possible on the techniques used to achieve those goals. Most of all, guidelines must be written as briefly and clearly as possible so that they can be read and understood quickly and easily.

Rescue Cache Preplanning

One way to shorten response time and increase the efficiency of rigging is to organize the location (or locations) and *mobility* of your equipment (Figure 11-2):

- Store rescue equipment in one or more central locations or rescue vehicles, ready for rapid response.

- Assemble *hasty packs,* with the goal of rapid deployment. Assemble equipment packs by function to meet both initial medical and technical rescue functions. (For example, packs or assembled modules can be organized for hauling rigging, lowering, anchoring, or other technical functions.) Label packs with secure tags or markings on the outside of

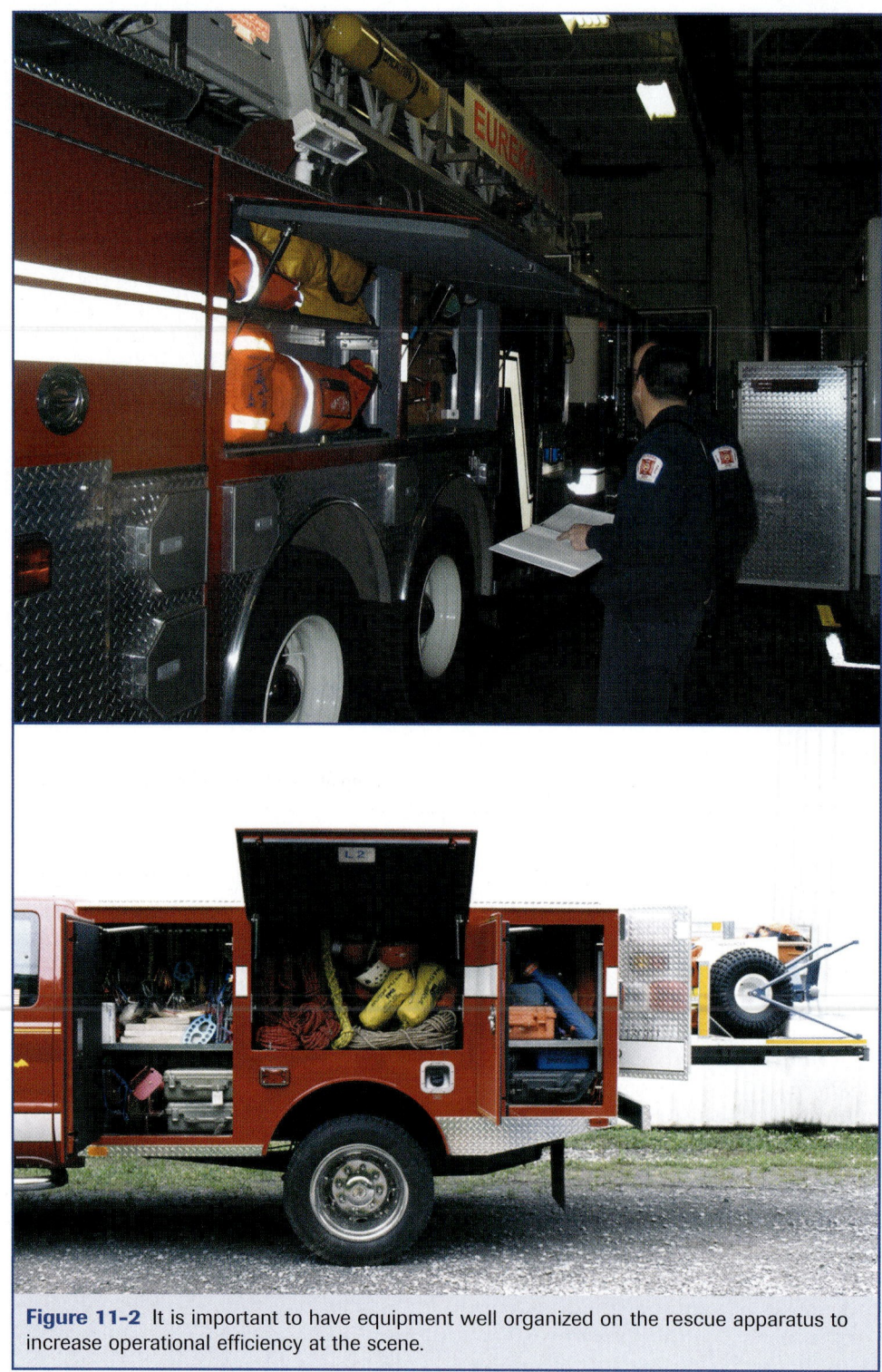

Figure 11-2 It is important to have equipment well organized on the rescue apparatus to increase operational efficiency at the scene.

the pack. Include a current inventory tag so that the contents can be checked after a rescue or practice. If helicopter operations are a possibility, include the weight on each pack.

■ Protect gear from harmful ultraviolet damage by bagging ropes and storing equipment away from direct sunlight. When storing rope on a vehicle, avoid proximity to batteries, because ropes can be damaged by acids or acid fumes.

Incident Command System

In the chaos of an emergency scene, it is essential that rescue personnel be able to rely on a common organizational structure that permits them to manage an incident efficiently and safely.

In North America, the **incident command system (ICS)** is used for the management of emergency situations. In the fire service, ICS is also known as the *incident management system (IMS)*. NFPA guideline 1561, *Standard on Emergency Services Incident Management System,* addresses incident scene management and its importance in reducing firefighter fatalities. Rescue accidents and failures repeatedly can be traced to a lack of adequate scene management or command. This single critical factor has a greater likelihood of affecting operational efficiency and safety than tactile skills, such as rigging speed or proficiency with knots. Using ICS for rescue operations permits efficient use of resources, ensures personnel accountability, and promotes improved mutual aid responses. The modular nature of ICS allows it to grow with the complexity and scope of the incident. ICS permits multiple agencies to join forces in a seamless manner and to produce a coordinated effort during an emergency incident.

The incident command system starts with the arrival of the first emergency responder with jurisdictional responsibility. This person immediately becomes the **initial incident commander**. As additional personnel arrive, the initial incident commander may be relieved of this role or may continue in it, depending on the needs created by the emergency and the qualifications of the individual. *Ultimately, there should be no question of who is in command.*

The incident commander needs to be in the most advantageous position possible and must be able to hear all radio communications. This may involve working from a site where the incident commander can directly observe the rescue operations from a vehicle; in a wilderness situation, the commander may be stationed at a trailhead. **Clear text**, a spoken communication style that avoids the use of abbreviated codes, should be used for radio transmissions. This optimizes interagency communication.

Distinctive identification (e.g., helmet, vest, or clip-on tag) helps in making assignments known as additional emergency personnel arrive. Assignments should also be identified on the radio to enhance incident-wide understanding of who is in command.

The incident commander develops an incident action plan, which may be verbal or, for incidents of longer duration, is put in writing. This plan establishes the overall strategic decisions and assigned tactical objectives for the incident, such as a decision to raise or lower a subject.

Box 11-1	**Example of the Incident Command System at Work**

A rescue operation organized under the incident command system (ICS) can be expanded as the operation becomes more complex and as more resources and jurisdictions become involved, as shown in Figure 11-3. An example of this flexibility can be seen in the initial ICS organization of a response to a multivehicle traffic incident (Figure 11-3, *A*). Upon arriving on the scene, the first responders realize that rope rescue is required and that the site involves multiple jurisdictions (Figure 11-3, *B*). As the situation develops, the plan shows an expanded ICS organization for this rescue, including an aviation component to meet the need for a helicopter (Figure 11-3, *C*).

Most rescue activities occur under the "operations" function of ICS. One of the most important advantages of the incident command function is its flexibility. The ICS framework can be expanded or contracted, depending on the size and nature of the incident. This is particularly important when the response to an incident grows, involving many more people. The organization adapts so that no one is overtasked in his or her span of control.

Span of Control

One problem encountered during incident management arises when leaders are placed in charge of too many people. The leaders consequently become overwhelmed trying to make sure that each person completes his or her assigned task; in other words, these leaders do not have a manageable **span of control**. The optimum span of control is considered to be a ratio of one supervisor to five subordinate personnel. If necessary, this may be increased to seven subordinates. Beyond that number, a supervisor may become overtasked. If the number of assigned personnel increases, the group should be divided into subgroups or a smaller tactical level management component (TLMC), such as teams, groups, divisions, or sectors, each with its own leader.

Supervisors must maintain a constant awareness of the position and function of all personnel assigned to them during an emergency incident. They should provide for rest and rehabilitation of emergency personnel by rotating crews on long duration incidents. Personnel accountability should be accomplished through tactical worksheets, command boards, or apparatus riding lists. This tracking of resources also provides for efficient use of incident personnel.

Multijurisdictional/Multiagency Operations

Rescue operations may involve more than one jurisdiction or agency. This can lead to conflicts over who is in charge and can complicate the development of unified strategies and tactics. ICS works to solve these conflicts through the use of **unified command**. Under unified command, each agency or jurisdiction involved has an incident commander assigned to the operation. The incident commanders jointly decide the incident objectives and appoint a single operations chief to carry them out. The key to unified command is the use of a *single* operations chief. The different agencies involved may easily maintain the integrity of

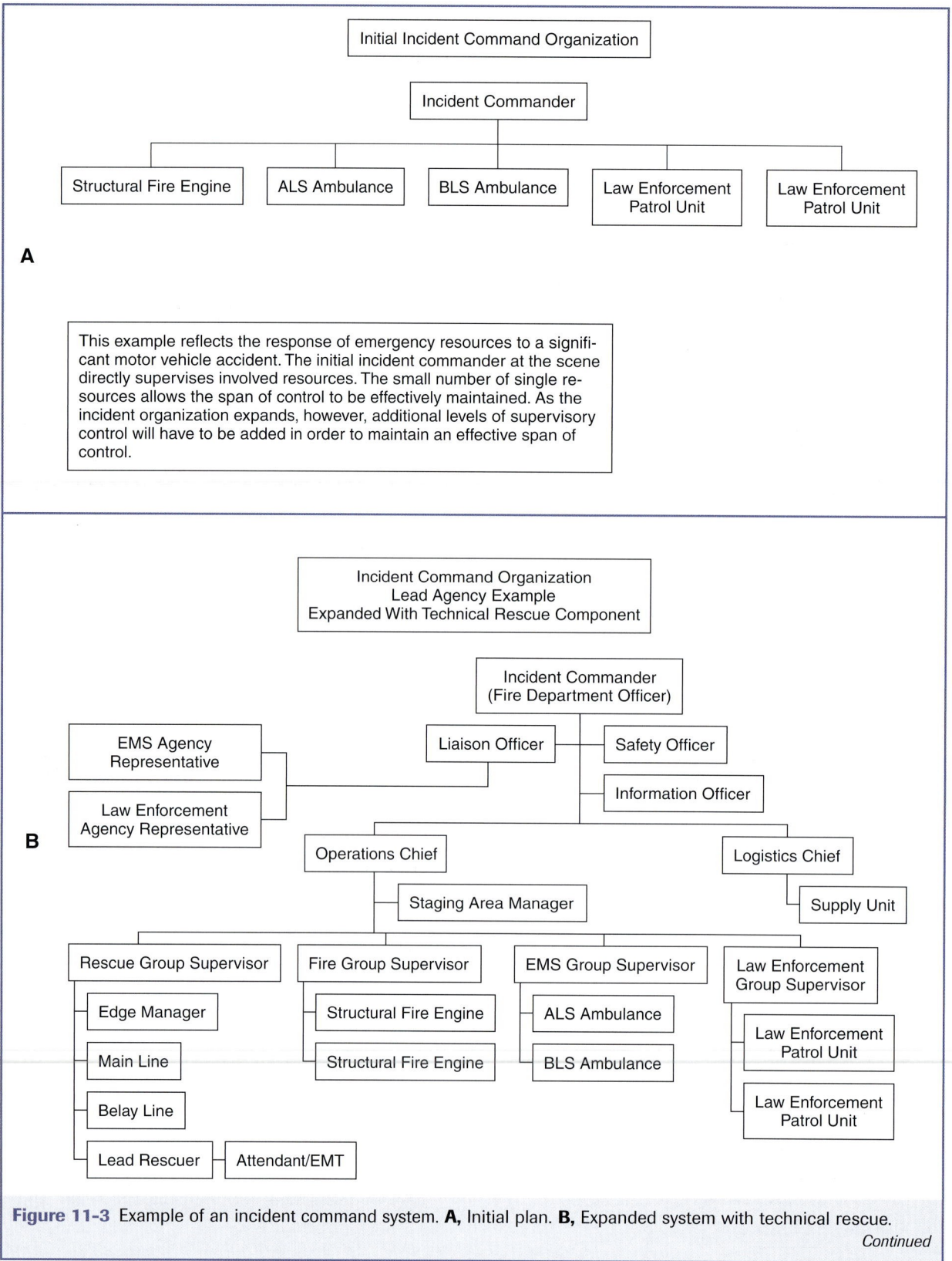

This example reflects the response of emergency resources to a significant motor vehicle accident. The initial incident commander at the scene directly supervises involved resources. The small number of single resources allows the span of control to be effectively maintained. As the incident organization expands, however, additional levels of supervisory control will have to be added in order to maintain an effective span of control.

Figure 11-3 Example of an incident command system. **A,** Initial plan. **B,** Expanded system with technical rescue.

Continued

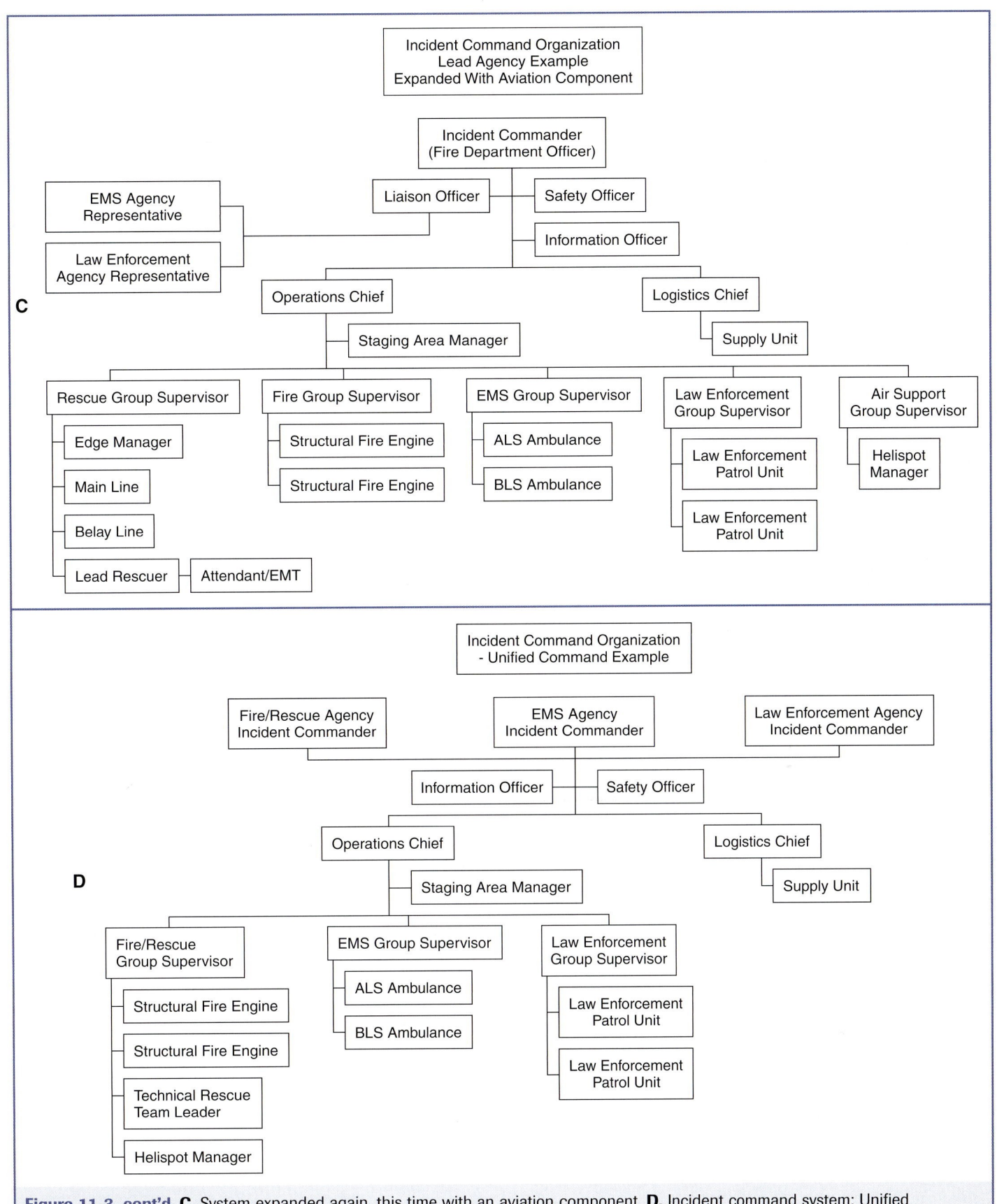

Figure 11-3, cont'd C, System expanded again, this time with an aviation component. **D,** Incident command system: Unified Command structure.

their established teams by keeping their personnel together in functional units, such as sectors, groups or divisions, without any loss or team efficiency (Figure 11-3, *D*).

With a multiagency response format, the lead agency with primary jurisdiction over the scene (e.g., the fire department) has a single incident commander in charge of the incident. Each involved agency with personnel assigned to the incident has an *agency representative,* who reports to a *liaison officer.* Personnel from the separate agencies may also be kept together in functional units for operational efficiency.

Command Staff

Command staff functions include positions that directly support the incident commander and contribute to the overall management of the incident. Command staff includes the incident safety officer, the liaison officer, and the information officer.

Incident Safety Officer

An *incident safety officer (ISO)* is an operational necessity during a potentially hazardous activity. Rope rescue, by its nature, is hazardous, therefore every rope rescue operation should have an assigned ISO. The ISO immediately performs a reconnaissance of the incident for hazards and provides the incident commander with a risk assessment by evaluating the scene conditions, rescuer activities, and incident operations. The ISO can initiate actions to mitigate possible hazards, for example, through apparatus placement or use of personal protective equipment. The ISO is responsible for making sure that all rescuers at a scene know the established safety zones and hazards and has the authority to stop any operation he or she sees as a threat to safety. The ISO must also be alert to transmission barriers that could result in missed, unclear, or incomplete communication. Selection of an incident safety officer during a high angle rescue should be based on the individual's technical expertise in rope rescue procedures.

In the incident command system, the incident safety officer is at the level of the incident commander. Optimally this means that the ISO does not get involved in other activities, such as operations, so that he or she can stand back and be objective about any threats to safety. An ISO should be present at every geographic location or sector where a potentially hazardous operation is taking place.

Some teams rotate the position of ISO among their members on scene. However, it is essential that the ISO be an individual experienced in rescue who thoroughly understands equipment, rigging, and rescue techniques. If possible, he or she should not be pulled into the operation itself. With a small team response, however, the position of incident safety officer may have to be a collateral duty for a team member.

The incident safety officer monitors the following:

- Hazards, including hazardous atmospheres and falling debris
- Personal safety equipment, including helmets, gloves, and breathing apparatus
- Safe work practices for specialized equipment, such as helicopters, watercraft, and so on
- Rescue rigging, including belays, anchors, rope padding, and unlocked carabiners

- Personal rigging, including seat harnesses, locked carabiners, and correct tying of knots
- Fatigue, hydration levels, and environmental exposure

Effective ways to reduce the risk to rescue personnel include the following:

- Effective training that simulates conditions encountered in emergencies
- Rest and rehabilitation of emergency personnel
- Continuous evaluation of changing conditions
- Reliance on the accumulated experience of team members

Finally, the incident command system should also be applied to training drills and exercises that involve hazards similar to those encountered at actual emergencies.

Notification

An accurate initial report must be obtained, and a standardized format should be used to collect appropriate information. Size-up information should include the following:

- Accident location and access route
- Number of victims
- Suspected injuries
- Distances involved
- Anticipated hazards
- Callback numbers for additional information

Response

In organizing the response, the consecutive elements of a search and rescue (SAR) incident should be used. Using the National Association for Search and Rescue (NASAR) *LAST* principle (Box 11-2), incident commanders should project events during the response and manage resources so as to maintain the highest level of operational efficiency. Put into effect, this translates into making sure that if the operation is in the *access* phase, adequate emergency medical service (EMS) equipment and personnel are available to stabilize the patient's condition and that transport has been arranged.

Investigation

Incident commanders must decide whether law enforcement investigation is required because of an associated crime or possible tort liability. Thorough documentation of the scene and of factors relating to an accident is important. In the event of a fatality from a fall, steps must be taken immediately to preserve the accident scene. Remember that the point from which the

Box 11-2	The *LAST* Principle

The consecutive elements of a search and rescue incident can be memorized according to the National Association for Search and Rescue (NASAR) *LAST* principle:

- ❏ Locate
- ❏ Access
- ❏ Stabilize
- ❏ Transport

subject fell, and its surrounding area, are an important part of the crime scene. If law enforcement personnel are significantly delayed in reaching the scene, identification of any witnesses should be completed and, if practical, some immediate photographs of the accident should be taken.

Critical Incident Stress Management

Critical incident stress management (CISM) provisions should be in place to meet the needs of personnel involved in the call. Immediate defusing sessions should be conducted when appropriate to support the mental health of emergency responders.

Leadership

In a rope rescue operation, there should be only one rescue team leader. However, the team should include several individuals capable of serving as leader when needed. The team leader does not have to be a person who can do everything better than everyone else. However, he or she must be knowledgeable about what is required to get the job done and what elements must be put together to make sure things happen in a timely manner.

The rescue leader is not a dictator. A single person is fallible, therefore the leader must be able to solicit opinions from other experienced members and use their advice. It is a good idea for the leader actively to solicit input from team members. This helps the leader to see any elements he or she may have missed and helps define the problem for the rest of the team.

The team leader must also be flexible. A rescue situation may change, it may not be what the first call reported it to be, or the first plan may not work. The leader, therefore, must be able to develop alternative plans.

The leader must make sure that team members clearly understand their assignments. One good practice is to have the captain of each group repeat their assignment to the leader.

Goals and Direction

Often, a **rope rescue** is, in effect, the solving of a puzzle: how does the team rescue the subject using its rope, hardware, skills, and ingenuity? To arrive at the answer, the team must know the question: what are we about to do? This is best presented in a briefing (Box 11-3). A briefing should always be given to the

Box 11-3	**Format for Briefing in Emergencies**

1. Here's what I think we face.
2. Here's what I think we should do.
3. Here's why.
4. Here's what we should keep an eye on.
5. Now, talk to me.

Adapted from Weick KE: South Canyon revisited: lessons from high reliability organizations, Paper presented at Decision Workshop on Improving Wildland Firefighter Performance under Stressful, Risky Conditions: Toward Better Decisions on the Fireline and More Resilient Organizations, Missoula, Montana, June 12-16, 1995.

personnel primarily involved in the operation. They should know what the problem is (e.g., a subject trapped on a ledge), what the overall solution will be (raise the subject with a hauling system), what their unit's task will be (provide an anchor system for the hauling system), and what each person's role will be (have the necessary equipment ready for the riggers).

To best move toward the goal, each leader should make sure that each task is assigned to a unit (one or more individuals) that has a person in charge who is responsible for seeing the task done and for communicating with the other leaders. Everyone involved in the rescue must have a clear understanding of his or her task.

Strategy and Allocation of Resources and Time

The focus of the rescue response must be the subject of the rescue. The role of EMS provider is delegated to a rescue team member so that the subject's medical condition can be evaluated as soon as possible.

While the subject's medical condition is assessed, all other team members should be involved in preparing for the rescue. An effective way to accomplish this preparation is to divide the job into specific tasks. Each task is assigned to a subgroup headed by individuals responsible to the group leader. Among subgroup tasks would be jobs such as rigging, anchoring, preparation of the litter, evacuation, crowd control, communications, safety equipment control, and rope management. The *operations chief* makes sure that all the actions of the various subgroups mesh in order to achieve the ultimate goal: the rescue.

During *initial attack* rescue operations involving only one operational period (8 to 12 hours), the position of *plans chief* is typically not activated. The incident action plan (IAP) is formulated from the tactical objectives by the incident commander and operations chief, who communicate it verbally to field personnel. However, during *extended attack* incidents, which involve several operational periods, the plans chief assumes the task of developing a written IAP for each operational period. This plan is based on the development of the incident and the status of resources.

Communications

In the high angle rope rescue environment, effective communication is extremely important for coordination of the operation and for the safety of all involved. However, conditions in the high angle environment often make normal communication very difficult.

Other sections of this manual describe some standard voice communications used in rope work. However, in many high angle situations, the ability to hear voices is severely restricted by distance, wind, and noise factors, such as falling water.

The solution to this problem may seem to be use of radio communications, but conventional radio systems are subject to disruption by physical conditions at the rescue site. Typical problems involve interruption of radio transmission by confined spaces, rock overhangs, structures, and intervening ridgelines. In some cases the situation can be improved by having all team members switch from *repeater* channels to *simplex* (direct car to car) communication. Simplex communication can avoid the problem of barriers between the communicators and the repeater site. However, for the simplex system to work, the communicators must be in the same area or working in line of sight of one another.

If the team will be working with more than one frequency, there must be a systematic way to keep track of radio channels. Without a system for channels, confusion arises as individuals try to find a usable channel. At the least, the result is embarrassment; at worst, it is life-threatening chaos.

If every radio has the same frequency setup, channel numbers can be used to indicate a frequency (e.g., "All units switch to channel 11."). If the frequency setup varies among the radios, the frequency name must be used ("All units switch to state law enforcement mutual aid."). In any case, either the channels must be labeled on the radio or a frequency sheet must be kept with the radios at all times.

A common problem encountered by rescue team members is management of a radio on a vertical face, an environment in which both hands tend to be occupied with other activities.

One means that some teams have used for short-range communications is the voice-activated, or VOX (voice operated exchange), headset. However, the units may not fit well with some helmet designs, and they can be put out of commission in close quarters, in which elements of the system can get snagged or torn off.

An effective solution is the radio chest harness (Figure 11-4). Only a simple, short hand motion is required to key the mike.

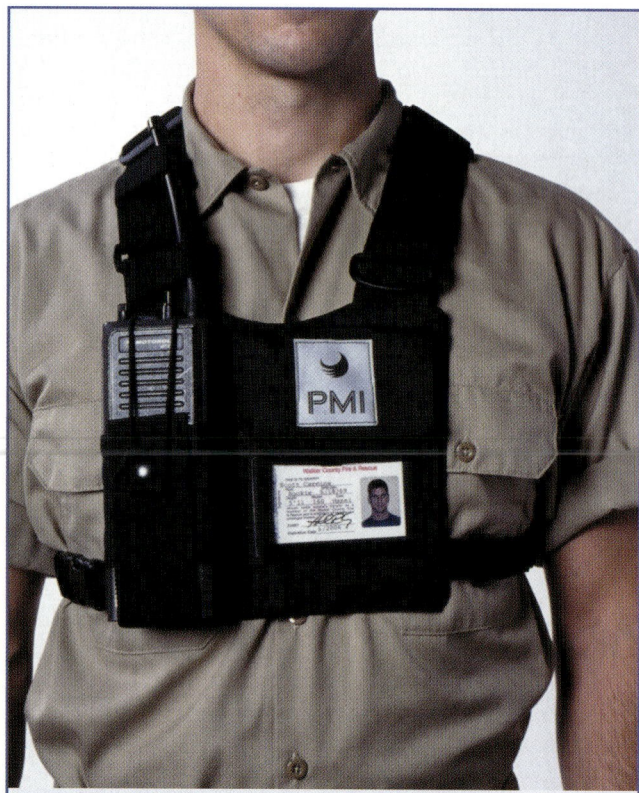

Figure 11-4 Radio chest harness.

Also, although the radio is close at hand, it is protected and out of the way of much of the activity involved in rope work. Because it is next to the body, the chest harness keeps radio batteries warm and extends their performance in cold weather. In noisier environments the addition of a remote microphone, which can be positioned at shoulder level, improves the rescuer's ability to hear transmissions.

A non-electronic alternative is the use of whistle blasts for communications. Obviously these are limited in the amount of information that can be communicated, but they often are audible where nothing else works. The exact form of these whistle communications must be worked out and practiced beforehand. *SUDOT* is a recognized whistle command system used in rope rescue:

S—Stop (one blast)
U—Up (two blasts)
D—Down (three blasts)
O—Off rope (four blasts)
T—Trouble! (continued long blast)

Another non-electronic communication system that is even more primitive than whistle blasts but that might be necessary in certain critical situations is a technique that might be called digital communication or use of a yes-or-no signal.

This type of system might be necessary when a subject is high on a cliff or far across a valley. In such situations normal two-way communication is impossible, and the subject does not have a radio.

For this system, the rescuers use a loud hailer to ask questions that allow a "yes" or "no" answer. The subject replies with a flashlight blink or a raised arm.

Positioning a lookout across a canyon or at the bottom of a cliff face provides an operational advantage for a rescue. The lookout is able to observe the rescue efforts and relay information that rescue personnel on the cliff face cannot readily acquire.

Human Side of Communications

Often the greatest detriment to good communication is not electronic or mechanical failure but the communicators themselves. In high angle situations, it is imperative to communicate in a clear, concise, and specific manner. For example, does "right" or "left" mean as you face the cliff or as you face away from it? On a cliff face, directions are oriented to a climber or rescuer facing the rock. Therefore, to the right of the rescuer would be *face right*, and to the left of the rescuer, *face left*. In river and stream operations, *river right* is on the rescuer's right as he or she faces downstream, and *river left* is on the left facing downstream.

It is important to reduce the command vocabulary to as few words as possible and to use only words that are clear, concise, and have few syllables. Also, the same words should be used for specific actions. As noted in the sections on lowering and hauling systems, the only word for cessation of action is "Stop!" Another word should never be substituted; "whoa," for example, could easily be mistaken for "slow," or even worse, for "go."

It is imperative that all rescue team personnel immediately speak up with critical information. Assuming that someone else on the team sees a hazard may result in a needless tragedy.

Key Points for Maintaining an Organized Rescue (Figure 11-5)

The following steps can help keep a rescue operation organized and on target:

- Initiate a quick size-up of the incident, to verify the initial report and scope of the incident, by sending the closest available resource directly to the scene.
- Organize an immediate initial response to reach and stabilize the victim. Medically stabilize the subject by treating any life-threatening injuries; physically stabilize the individual so that he or she cannot fall farther; and psychologically stabilize the person with professional reassurance.
- Use ICS and IMS and identify positions (verbally on the radio and through the use of vests).
- Establish an accessible staging area for equipment that does not block or interfere with the area used for operational rigging.
- Limit communications with the rescuer or rescuers in technical terrain to the edge manager or the operations chief. Working in the vertical realm is an awkward task.

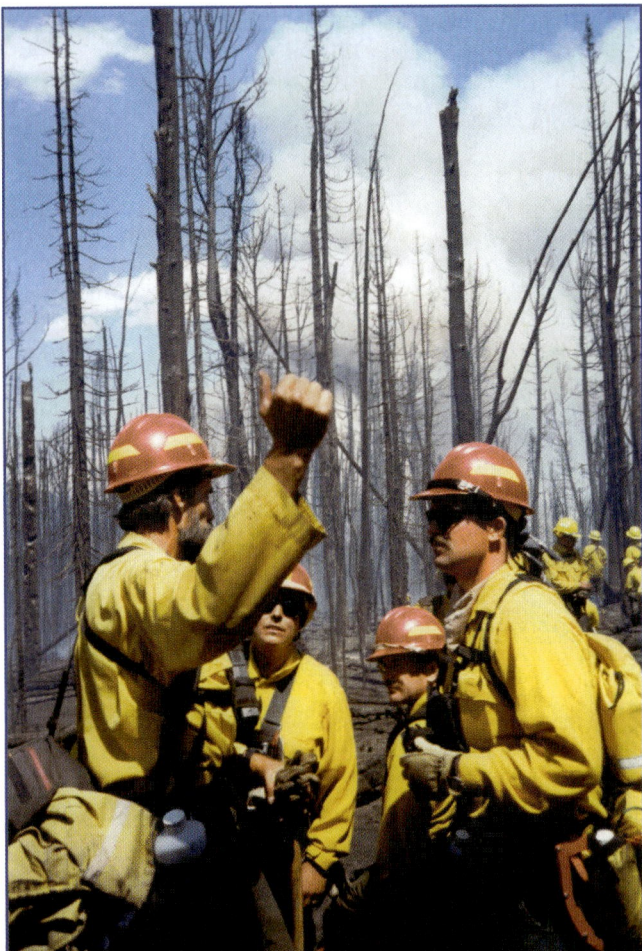

Figure 11-5 Incident commander giving instructions to a small group of firefighters. Instructions preferably are given face to face at the scene of the rescue operation for the most effective means of communication.

Rescuers' efficiency is compromised if they are overtasked with too many instructions.

- Stay ahead of the logistics curve. Plan and act now. Be prepared for a rescue to take longer than expected. Request additional resources, supplies, and equipment well in advance so that efficiency does not suffer.
- Keep rescue systems simple and safe. An overly complex system may compromise efficiency.

Important Safety Reminders

The following guidelines can help ensure the safety of those participating in the rescue operation:

- Do not rush! Maintain a sense of "controlled urgency."
- Choose well-trained, experienced rescuers for the core of the team. The most highly skilled rescuers should be used in decision-making roles and where technical competence is absolutely essential. Less experienced or less skilled personnel can easily function as low angle litter bearers, hauling team personnel, or equipment runners.
- Make sure rescuers are prepared for contingencies and have adequate personal gear to stay warm, dry, fed, and well hydrated.
- Establish a well-marked safety perimeter. Consider using flagging or a chalk-line, as well as chemical lightsticks at night, to identify this line.
- Make sure that rescuers are tied in when working within 10 feet (3 m) of an exposed edge. Establish a marked safety perimeter with flagging, chalk, or chemical lightsticks.
- Minimize the number of personnel working near an exposed edge.
- Designate an ISO (this might be a collateral role for a rescuer).
- Perform a safety check before using a system; recheck equipment when in use.
- Engineer a *redundant* system; rescue systems have backups.
- Use standard communications terminology and techniques.
- *Aggressively* use appropriate personal protective equipment (PPE) (e.g., gloves, footwear, helmet, harness, personal flotation device, hearing protection, Nomex clothing, safety goggles, sunscreen) for *all* incident hazards, environments, and tasks. Have spare equipment available. Wear helmets in the rock fall zone.
- Use edge protection to protect lines from sharp rock edges.
- Establish safety lines where exposure places personnel at significant risk of injury (Figure 11-6).
- Make a point of not standing inside a bight under tension during a raising operation. Take steps to prevent personal injury in case a change of direction fails in a hauling system. Stand to the outside of the rope bight.
- Never get on a rope without adequate gear to go up the rope and down the rope. If you are rappelling, make sure you have ascenders with you.
- Secure loose gear in a cache adjacent to the rescue operations area.
- Keep a Prusik and trauma scissors with you to handle a self-rescue situation.

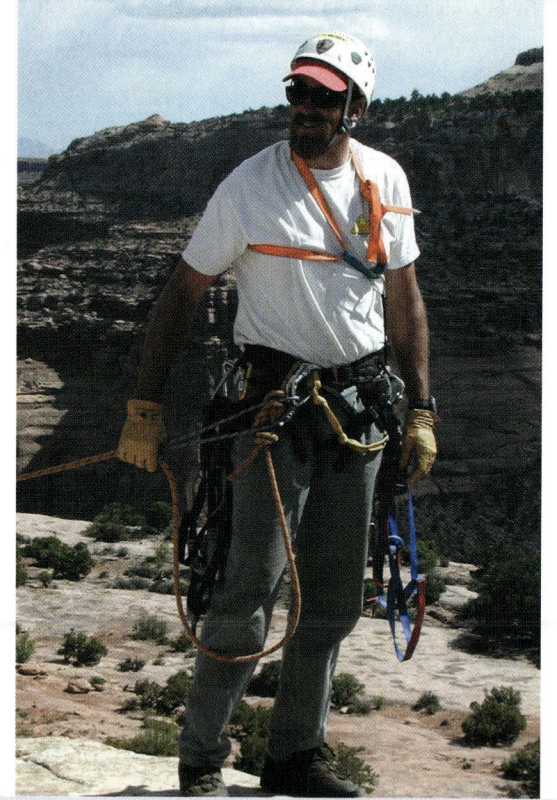

Figure 11-6 A rescuer uses an edge safety line with two separate points of attachment to the harness. The rigging reduces the likelihood of accidental detachment.

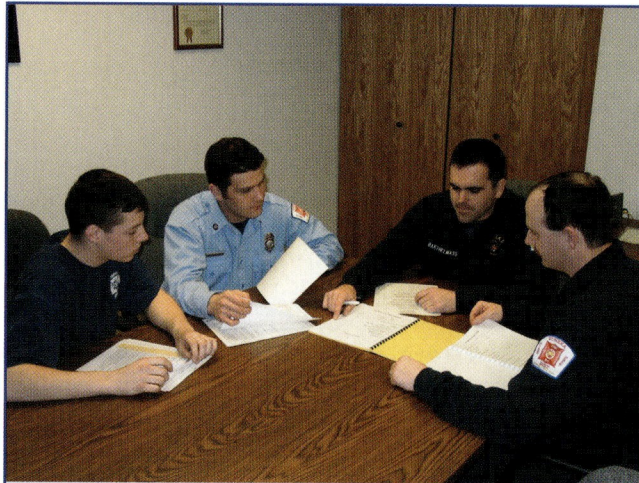

Figure 11-7 Small group of rescuers conducting a "hot debrief."

▨ *Caution*

Safety Considerations

Remember your priorities for operational safety:
- ❑ YOU ARE **NUMBER ONE!**
- ❑ Your fellow rescuers are your SECOND concern.
- ❑ The subject is your THIRD priority.

Safety is of paramount importance at all times. If you see any action that is unsafe, your responsibility is to **speak up!**

Remember that no one is infallible, including you. The worst case scenario is having a rescuer injured, resulting in two patients. Plan and execute a safe response so that you don't create an incident within an incident.

- ■ Make sure to avoid cross-gate forces and three-way forces on carabiners.
- ■ Derig gear after the rescue, starting at a cliff edge and working away from it.

After-Action Review: Hot Debrief (Figure 11-7)

When the operation is finished, immediately conduct an after-action review to evaluate operational efficiency with involved

---

Box 11-4	**Hot Debrief Agenda**

Basic items to be covered in a hot debrief include the following:

1. **What was planned?**
   - ❑ List the objectives and expected actions.

2. **What actually happened?**
   - ❑ Review any actions that were not standard operating procedure for safety concerns.

3. **Why did it happen?**
   - ❑ Discuss the reasons for ineffective or unsafe performance.
   - ❑ Concentrate on *what*, not *who*, is right.

4. **What can we do next time?**
   - ❑ Identify effective and ineffective performance.
   - ❑ Determine how to apply the lessons learned from this operation to the next rescue operation.

Adapted from Incident Response Guide (NFES #1077), NIFC, Boise, ID.

---

rescuers and to focus on possible improvements for the next response. This review is known as a ***hot debrief*** (Box 11-4).

One obvious value of a hot debrief is that details are fresh in the minds of the rescuers. Personnel also are less prone to be defensive and often are more open to comments about their performance. Discussion of performance issues during a hot debrief is more likely to lead to permanent self-improvement than such a discussion held during a delayed debrief, because individuals have had time to develop mental justifications for deficiencies in their performance.

NOTE: Documentation of a hot debrief, without focusing on individuals, is useful for team personnel who were not present at the operation. This allows any important lessons learned to be communicated to everyone.

Incident Review

With more complicated rescue operations, a more detailed, formal incident review often is scheduled to allow an *honest* evaluation involving all the responding agencies.

A moderator, who preferably was not involved in the incident, leads the review, which includes a posted agenda, to evaluate operational safety, effectiveness, and efficiency. A structured format helps keep the procedure on track and productive.

All participants should be reminded at the outset that the overall objective is to improve future operational responses.

In the incident review, actions that require follow-up and the individuals responsible for accomplishing this task must be documented.

Situational Awareness

Most high angle and rescue operation accidents are not related to equipment failure but to human error. The question, then, is how to engineer and plan for the human factor on all rescue operations.

Military air crash investigators often cite a loss of **situational awareness** as a contributing factor in serious accidents (Box 11-5). An aviator's ability to maintain an accurate perception of the external environment and to detect and act on any problems encountered is also a valuable asset for technical rescue personnel.

Communicating for Safety

Emergency responders often see operational hazards during an incident but fail to speak up and get them corrected. In situations involving critical communication, it is most effective to *use direct statements*. Although they appear rude, direct statements are difficult to ignore and are very productive.

The following are the six components of direct statements:
1. Address the person to whom you are talking by name.
2. Begin with, "I," "I think," "I believe," or "I feel."
3. State your message as clearly as possible.
4. Use the appropriate emotion for your message so that it is delivered as you intended.
5. Require a response by using such statements as "What do you think?" or "Don't you agree?"
6. Don't let the matter go. Don't disengage with the other person until you have achieved an understanding.

An example of a direct statement might be, "John, I think we need additional personnel for this rescue. Don't you agree?"

It may sound elementary, but this technique is very effective. A direct statement gets the person's attention and forces the individual to deal with your concern rather than allowing him or her to ignore your message.

Incident Risk Management Process

The following five steps comprise the incident risk management process.
Step 1: Situation awareness
- Gather information.
  - Incident objectives
  - Weather forecast
  - Communications
  - Local factors/terrain/hazards
  - Incident organization
Step 2: Hazard assessment
- Identify all possible tactical hazards.
Step 3: Hazard control
- Mitigate potential hazards through the use of safety procedures and protective equipment.
Step 4: Decision point
- Issue a "Go" or "No go" on the planned course of action.
Step 5: Evaluation
- Self
  - Inadequate experience for the activity?
  - Distracted from primary task?
  - Fatigue or stress reaction a problem?
  - Hazardous attitude?
- Situation
  - What is changing?

| Box 11-5 | Maintaining Situational Awareness in Emergencies |

Situational awareness refers to the emergency responder's ability to do the following:
- Maintain an accurate perception of the external environment.
- Identify the source and nature of problems.
- Detect a situation requiring action.

Factors that Diminish Situational Awareness

- Insufficient communication
- Fatigue and stress
- Task overload
- Task underload and boredom
- Group mindset
- A philosophy of "press on regardless"
- Degraded operating conditions
- Rapidly changing and unplanned operational conditions

Ways to Prevent Loss of Situational Awareness

- Actively question and evaluate the progress of the mission.
- Analyze his or her individual situation.
- Update and revise his or her image of the mission.
- Use assertive behavior when necessary.
  - Make suggestions.
  - Provide relevant information without being asked.
  - Ask questions as necessary.
  - Confront ambiguities.
  - State opinion on decisions and procedures.
  - Refuse unreasonable requests.
- **Remember: It is OK to say NO!**

Adapted from U.S. Navy Situational Awareness Training Program. Prepared by Grand Canyon National Park SAR.

Table 11-1	Common Hazards in Rescue Work: Technical Rescue Tactical "Watch Outs"
Hazard	**Corrective Action**
Ineffective communications.	Give briefings in person and aggressively maintain incident communications with all personnel.
Failure to protect against sharp edges.	Aggressively use edge protection.
"Weld abrasion" caused by nylon rubbing against nylon.	Carefully engineer rigging to prevent this condition.
Misuse and inattention to equipment; improperly tied rigging.	Continually recheck gear during the rescue operation.
Cross-gate forces on carabiners.	Rig correctly and recheck rigging frequently.
Carabiner gates unlocked or held open by webbing or rocks.	Check rigging frequently.
Loose Prusiks.	Inspect Prusiks visually and by feel.
Failure to wear helmets or to be tied in.	Keep an eye on one another.
Rescuer fatigue, thirst, boredom, and distraction.	Change out belayer, rehydrate often, and encourage disciplined behavior.

Evaluation Exercises

Cognitive and Affective Exercises

1. List seven things that should be included in a preplan.

2. Name three essential considerations for which rescue and medical personnel should plan before an incident.

3. What is the standardized management system commonly used for all types of emergencies?

4. The optimum span of control is considered to be a ratio of _____ subordinate personnel to one supervisor.

5. In the incident command system, the incident safety officer operates at what level?

6. Name three things in rope rescue that the incident safety officer is responsible for monitoring.

7. Which NFPA guideline specifically addresses incident management?

8. Unified command of an emergency incident is executed using how many operations chiefs?

9. List the statements included in the five-step format for briefing in emergencies.

10. Describe situational awareness.

11. List four actions rescuers can take to prevent loss of situational awareness during an emergency response.

APPENDIX

Operational Search and Rescue Response Safety

Steps for Achieving Precision in Search and Rescue

This reference is designed as a job aid to promote effective decision making and risk management during search and rescue (SAR) operations. It highlights numerous operational red flags for which rescuers must be on the alert. Use of this aid should not delay your decision making; rather, this guide should be consulted as a reference on a recurring basis. Preplan by studying these principles *before an emergency response is required*.

5M Model of Systematic Risk Management

The five Ms are: *mission, method, management, man* (a generic reference to incident personnel), and *medium*.

Mission (Incident Assignment)

- Have you obtained all available initial mission information?
- Are your mission image and plan accurate?
- What is the operational tempo?

- Be vigilant for "go fever" in personnel.
- Watch out for personnel running or shouting.
- Don't allow the level of urgency to drive the mission.
■ Is a response appropriate at this time?
  - Calculate the accurate urgency of the situation.

Method (Techniques and Means of Conducting the Mission)

■ Is the level of response appropriate?
  - Overresponding is reckless and exposes management to liability.
  - Underresponding is inexcusable and exposes management to liability.
■ Have you selected the appropriate technique for the task?
■ Are the correct initial actions being implemented immediately?
■ Have alternative techniques been adequately evaluated?
  - Consider the time, hazards, personnel exposure, and overall efficiency involved for alternatives.
■ Are operations within equipment performance capabilities?
■ Are adequate systems of communication in place?
  - Actively prevent the loss of incident communications.
  - Use relays, cellular, satellite phone, or an adjacent agency frequency.
  - Use brevity, radio etiquette, clear text, and dedicated frequencies.
■ Has a thorough briefing of the mission at hand been provided for all involved personnel?
  - In-person briefings are the most effective.
  - Give clear instructions and make sure there is no misunderstanding.
■ Can you identify any omissions or deficiencies in the plan?
■ Are you staying ahead of the "power curve"?
  - Anticipate and take action to prevent possible delays in the mission.
  - Ensure sufficient timeliness of logistical support.
■ Are any apparent shortcuts being taken by involved personnel?
■ Is there disagreement over the correct technique to be used?
  - Solidly review the conservative method/approach/technique.
■ Are the dynamics of the mission being observed?
  - Reevaluate and update your mission image.
  - Are you making false assumptions?
  - Gather and consider all the field intelligence you can.
■ Have you considered outside resources?
■ Have you accounted for failure of the plan?
  - Have a backup plan available and be prepared to initiate it.

Management (Controls, Procedures, Oversight, and Supervision)

■ Has "command" been identified to all involved personnel?
■ Is an adequate incident command system (ICS) organization in place?

■ Is compliance with policy and operating procedures being shown?
■ Is safety being *openly promoted?*
■ Are established policies and procedures known by involved personnel?
■ Are adequate oversight and supervision in place?
■ Has staging of additional resources been identified, and is it in use?
■ Is a personnel accountability system in place?
■ Have plans been made for rest and rehabilitation of involved personnel?
  - Fatigue, stress, and dehydration profoundly affect performance.
  - Rotate rested personnel.
  - Provide for critical incident stress management (CISM) support.
■ Is a hot debrief and/or mission review planned?
  - Actively seek out and implement mission feedback.

Man (Incident Personnel)

■ Are personnel being overtasked?
  - Increase the number of personnel and delegate tasks.
  - Encourage personnel to request assistance.
■ Is an adequate number of trained personnel being deployed?
  - Make sure rescuers' qualifications are current.
  - Select personnel on the basis of skills and proficiency.
■ Has the personal preparedness of all personnel been assessed?
  - Mental preparedness
  - Physical preparedness
  - Personal survival equipment (is the person prepared to remain overnight?)
  - Personal protective equipment (PPE)
■ Is situational awareness being maintained?
  - Constantly revise the mental image of the mission and incident conditions.

Medium (Environmental Forces)

■ Have all environmental hazards been *openly identified?*
■ Are mitigation efforts being used where possible?
■ Has an accurate weather forecast been obtained?
■ Is the mission operating within safe environmental parameters for personnel and machines?

12

Medical Considerations in High Angle Rescue

Michael V. Callahan

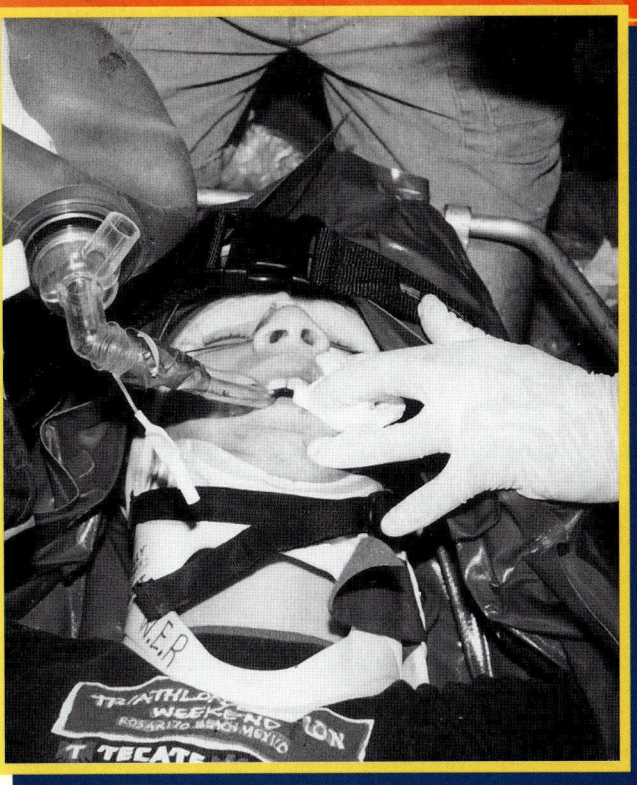

The material in this chapter conforms to guidelines published by the National Fire Protection Association (NFPA), specifically standard 1006, *Professional Qualifications for Rescue Technicians* (2002), and standard 1670, *Operations and Training for Technical Rescue Incidents* (2004). NFPA standards are revised regularly, and readers are advised to review the latest version of these standards.

Objectives

On completion of this chapter, you should be able to:

1. List four factors that affect medical preplanning for high angle rescue.
2. List five qualities involved in choosing medical equipment to be used in high angle rescue.
3. Describe the composition of a litter medical kit.
4. Describe how a rescue for a subject who is uninjured or has minor injuries or illness would differ from a subject whose medical problems cannot wait until rope rescue is completed.

Key Terms

Litter Medical Kit (LMK) A smaller version of the rescue team medical kit that is designed for the management of emergency problems that may arise while the rescue subject is on rope or restrained in a litter or when the larger rescue medical kit is unavailable.

Medical Preplanning The prediction of conflicts that may arise between patient care and rescue operations as well as the prognostic adaptation of medical and rescue systems.

Medical Care during a High Angle Rescue Operation

The rope rescue and helicopter short haul patient often needs both technical rescue and urgent medical care (for example, a rescue involving a subject whose medical condition may be critical, and medical care cannot be delayed until the rescue is completed). Members of the rescue team, therefore, should expect to use both technical rescue skills and medical skills during high angle and helicopter rescues. Ideally, the team will be able to attend to the patient's immediate medical needs before the litter is transported. Many rescue teams understand the limitations of providing care during the technical stages of rope rescue and go to great lengths to reduce the amount of time the patient is confined to the technical rescue system. However, with unconscious, critically injured, or deteriorating patients, medical care must be continuous during the rescue. Interventions that may be required during rescue include simple supervision of the patient's airway (which is done for all litter patients); routine emergency medical procedures, such as oropharyngeal suction and management of intravenous (IV) lines; and more complicated techniques, such as intubation, emergency IV access, and resuscitation.

This chapter provides a general outline to help the rescue team develop a specific approach to the medical care of the patient during helicopter and high angle rescue. The chapter is not an instruction handbook for medical care of the patient. Rather, it serves as a guide to the integration of the two operational arms of high angle rescue: management of rescue systems and medical care of the patient.

The chapter covers the integration of patient care and high angle rescue by focusing on the following areas:

- Medical preplanning
- Medical equipment
- Training

More detailed information on medical care of the rescue patient is available through organizations that include education on rescue medicine and prolonged and delayed patient transportation in their medical programs.

Medical Preplanning

Providing quality medical care within the constraints of the rope rescue system is a challenge further is complicated by the wide variety of medical problems that can arise during rescue operations. It is no surprise, then, that many rescue courses attempt to separate rescue operations into different disciplines: technical rescue and patient care. This separation may make sense from an organizational standpoint, but it does not reflect real-life conditions, in which medical care and rescue functions must be performed simultaneously. Managing a rescue and concurrently providing medical care requires careful preparation and realistic training scenarios. One method of preparation focuses on *medical preplanning*, which helps prevent conflicts that may arise between the delivery of medical care and rescue operations. Specifically, medical preplanning helps minimize problems by identifying them in advance and adapting either the medical or the rescue system accordingly.

Medical preplans will depend on the availability and composition of personnel, equipment, and financial resources and therefore vary among teams and agencies. Table 12-1 lists common factors that influence medical preplanning for high angle rescue.

Medical Personnel

A common problem during high angle rescue arises from the division of rescuers into either medical or technical rescue personnel. It makes good sense to give the most highly qualified medical personnel responsibility for patient care. However, it is unwise and impractical to assume that that person will always be present, able-bodied, and focused on the patient. The realities of rescue require that teams respond regardless of whether all resources or personnel are present. Under these conditions, patient care should not be overly compromised because of the absence of key team members.

Medical preplanning helps minimize this problem. Preplanning allows categorization of medical skill among the team members in advance and the development of a contingency plan for shortcomings in on-scene medical care. One method of increasing medical capability is to increase the number of medically skilled team members. This helps ensure that quality medical care is always available during rescue. The number of medical personnel can be increased by prioritizing medical care, by providing incentives for team members to seek higher levels of medical training, by rotating personnel into the role of litter attendant or manager of the medical kit, and by challenging the team with a variety of medical or trauma problems during training exercises.

Table 12-1	Factors Affecting Medical Preplanning for High Angle Rescue
Factor	**Effect on Medical Preplanning**
Medical personnel	Teams with several medical personnel are resilient and more responsive to challenges and maintain effective operations despite shortages in personnel.
Medical skill	Effective medical capability allows medical care to be initiated before the patient reaches the ground, a period of time that may last hours (such as with a tower or big wall rescue) or days (such as in caving or a mass disaster).
Medical control	Medical control supports medical preplanning by identifying resources, developing effective protocols, and providing feedback.
Financial resources	Medical preplanning is affected by financial constraints. However, effective medical preplanning may prevent wasteful spending on resources that are inappropriate for high angle rescue.

Medical Skill Level

There is no universally recognized standard for medical care during high angle or helicopter rescue. Similarly, there is no minimum level of medical training or certification required of the rescuer. The level of medical care delivered during rescue may influence the selection of rescue systems. For example, the litter bridle of a paramedic-attended litter may be configured to permit endotracheal intubation and allow the litter attendant to compress the Ambu bag. In contrast, the bridle system of the first responder, who is less likely to attend to an intubated patient, may be less complex and more adaptable to different litter configurations (Figure 12-1).

The litter attendant should be selected based on the technical and medical needs unique to an individual rescue situation. The most appropriately experienced medical personnel—*who are also qualified for litter operations*—should attend to critical patients. High angle rescue, in which a patient's life may hang in the balance, is a poor environment for attempting unfamiliar and dangerous medical procedures. For this reason, all rescuers who may care for the patient should practice medical procedures using realistic simulations.

Higher levels of medical training do not necessarily ensure that the patient will receive better medical care. For example, an experienced litter attendant certified at the first responder level will have less difficulty managing both the litter and the patient than a paramedic who is inexperienced with maneuvering the litter over obstructions, managing the litter attendant lines, and reaching between loaded lines to care for the patient. Each team must decide independently the correct guidelines for balancing of rescue and medical skills in the litter attendant and then revise them for each rescue. The team should also remain focused on increasing medical training for their best rescuers and increasing rescue training of their best medical personnel.

Special Cases

In exceptional circumstances, the patient may require both the most advanced medical care and the most proficient litter handling skills a rescue team has to offer. Even if these skills are found in a single team member, both medical care and litter handling are likely to be improved by the addition of a second litter attendant. In such cases, the medical attendant should be placed in a position that allows access to the patient regardless of the litter's orientation. The second attendant serves as a dedicated litter handler. He or she should be placed centrally on the litter and provided with a personal protection rope system with mechanical ascenders, which would allow the rescuer to adjust his or her position to better control the litter and to negotiate maneuvers over vertical obstructions and overhung roofs.

Medical Control

The majority of modern rescue teams find it either necessary or beneficial to operate under some form of medical control. Advantages of medical control include immediate assistance with the care of difficult patients, constructive feedback on past rescues, help with evaluation and adaptation of promising new medical protocols or devices for the high angle rescue system, and a visible medical backstop to support field medical operations. By assisting rescue teams in this way, medical control serves as a key resource for improving the medical capability of the high angle rescue team.

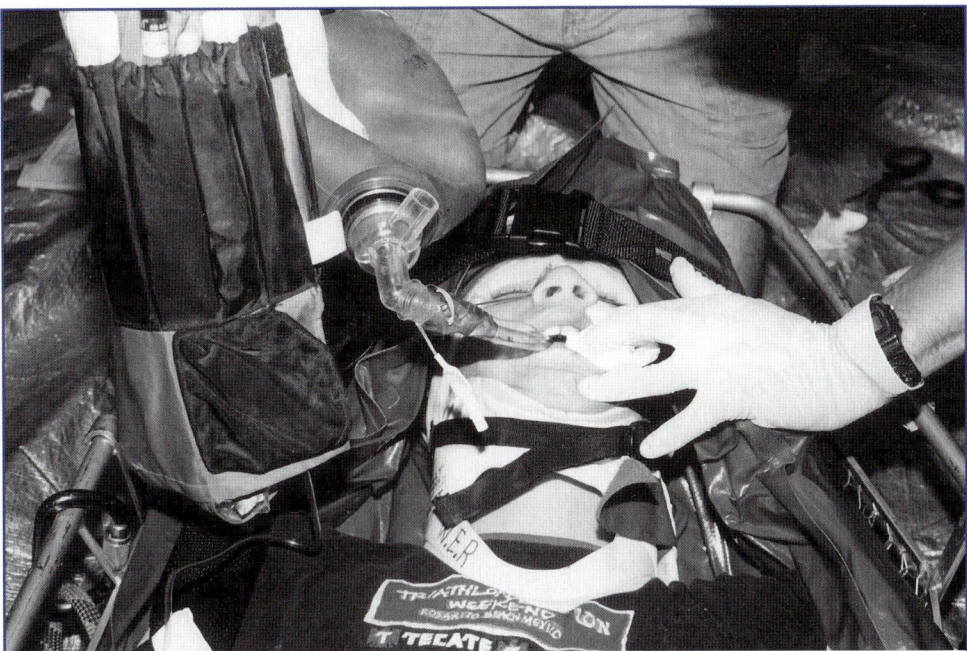

Figure 12-1 The litter bridle for vertical litter systems must not interfere with medical care such as airway management, vital sign assessment, emergency drug treatment, or the rescuer's view of the patient's head and neck region. Note the litter medical kit, which partially obscures the rescuer's right hand.

Medical control may consist of on-scene control, usually provided by a qualified member of the rescue team, or remotely delivered medical control, such as that provided by a physician at a nearby hospital. Many medical control officers are physicians recruited by the team, and many of these are unfamiliar with high angle rescue operations. This unfamiliarity may lead the medical director to recommend methods for stabilization, packaging, and extrication that are not ideal for high angle rescue. Examples of improperly adopted medical protocols include recommendations that all unconscious, free-hanging patients undergo spinal immobilization before lowering and that rigid femur traction devices be used for all suspect leg injuries, regardless of the rescue setting.

Problems such as these may be reduced if medical control personnel are familiarized with the unique and dangerous treatment environment of high angle rescue and if medical control and rescue teams work together to develop appropriate medical protocols for each team and each rescue scenario. Many teams have found it helpful to include hospital-based medical control officers in field training exercises, because this helps increase awareness about the rescue environment. Medical control officers who are familiar with the rescue environment are more likely to make appropriate recommendations regarding patient care.

After identifying an appropriate medical control source, the team must adopt protocols for treating both frequent (e.g., lower leg fracture), and high-risk (e.g., head trauma) medical problems. Qualified personnel need to review the team's medical capability to make sure that it has an appropriate balance between the patient's prehospital needs and the rescue team's abilities.

Financial Resources

Working within a budget is a necessary skill for maintaining high quality rescue teams. Many team leaders find it necessary to consider the cost of medical equipment, supplies, and training along with the cost of other resources such as helicopters, response vehicles, and rope rescue equipment. For this reason, financial considerations are an important part of medical preplanning.

The links between preplanning and funding vary among teams. For example, rescue teams that extricate hypothermic patients or the victims of industrial chemical exposures may find that the benefits of providing thermal or environmental protection to the patient justify the increased cost of specialty litters and mattresses. In contrast, rescue teams operating in warmer areas and those with few occupational exposure patients may choose less expensive spinal immobilization equipment and direct funds into other areas.

A limited financial budget does not mean that quality medical care is impossible. In fact, monitoring changes in the annual cost of rescues, as well as continuing evaluation of the service life, repair potential, and replacement cost of equipment, may allow teams to maintain rescue operations throughout busy seasons and during disaster response operations, which may consume team resources at an accelerated rate.

Medical Equipment

Few pieces of medical equipment are specifically designed for high angle rescue. Most equipment is adapted from that used in prehospital emergency medical service (EMS), in which patient care is delivered in the back of ambulances rather than on an elevated platform or within a rescue litter. Prehospital (street) EMS equipment is also designed to clamp to rolling stretchers or to be slung from the backs of EMS personnel, functions either impossible or unwise for the high angle rescuer.

A second important distinction is the difference in the severity of the user's environment. High angle rescue exposes equipment to inclement weather, extremes of temperature, and physical damage caused by impact against elevated platforms or rock faces. Teams should understand, therefore, that destruction of valuable equipment is likely. The use of expensive equipment should be carefully reviewed to determine the risk-benefit ratio for each rescue.

Medical equipment often lacks the durability required for high angle rescue and thus may represent an unacceptable capital expenditure. Many patient monitoring devices designed for prehospital "street" EMS are too large, heavy, or complex for use in short haul and high angle rope rescue. Dependence on fragile, expensive, and potentially unreliable equipment may prove to be a disservice to patients. For example, medical equipment designed for other environments such as the emergency department may interfere with the rope rescue system.

One example of this is the use of rigid femur traction splints, which become entangled with litter bridles and hang up on overhanging obstructions during raising or lowering operations. However, foregoing stabilization of a potentially fractured femur should not be delayed until the patient is transferred to the ground team, because the severity of damage to adjacent muscle and neurovascular structures increases with the length of time the femur remains unaligned. A reasonable low-cost alternative to rigid femur splints exists, such as the compact Sager traction device or equivalent equipment produced by European or Australian manufacturers.

This is just one example of the ways equipment selection plays an important role in the quality of medical care during rescue. Virtually all rescue teams have found it necessary to alter the rescue system to reduce interference with the care of the patient or to change the manner in which medical care is provided to allow for certain rope rescue configurations. Either way, it is important to remember that rescue of the patient and medical care of the patient are not conflicting priorities.

The choice of medical equipment should also vary with the patient population served. For example, metropolitan fire departments and rescue teams that perform high angle rescue at amusement parks and in metropolitan areas may expect to encounter a higher percentage of medical problems than a mountain rescue team that mainly responds to climbing accidents. General considerations for medical equipment are provided in Table 12-2.

Benefit to Patients

High angle rescue is a treatment environment that imposes limitations on the ability to deliver medical care. Some teams,

Table 12-2	General Considerations for Medical Equipment Used in High Angle Rescue
Factor	**Important Aspects**
Benefit	Medical equipment should be worth the weight, risk, special attention, and expense and should not compromise the safety of high angle rescue.
Weight	The weight of the kit increases with the duration, level, and range of medical care provided. Equipment should be selected based on the likelihood that a specific problem will be encountered and the probability that the equipment will improve the quality of care.
Durability	The use of electronic patient monitoring equipment in high angle rescue should be carefully evaluated, because the risk of damage is high, and the value to the patient may be minimal. Durability is also critical for stored equipment and pharmaceuticals. Expensive medical consumables (e.g., sterile gloves) may start to degrade in as little as 9 months.
Training	Rescue teams and their patients both benefit when realistic medical simulations and challenges are used to train rescuers. Training with medical and rescue equipment must be integrated.
Adaptability	Medical equipment should be adaptable to a variety of rescue systems, including those used by neighboring teams that participate in mutual aid operations.

therefore, may find it impossible to provide certain levels of patient care. Consequently, the rescue team should critically review each piece of medical equipment to judge its benefit to the patient. The advantages of specific medical devices should be weighed against alternative methods of performing the task required of the device. For example, patient monitors, which record cardiac rhythm, capnography (exhaled carbon dioxide), oximetry (oxygen saturation), and blood pressure, are usually too expensive, cumbersome, and heavy for rescue. More important, the data provided by these devices can be acquired through a combination of skilled manual assessment of vital signs and the use of small, cost-effective devices such as fingertip oxygen saturation monitors.

Also, it is unwise to rely entirely on electronics in the rescue environment, be it communications gear, global positioning system (GPS) units, or medical telemetry equipment. Eventually, such equipment will be unavailable or inoperable, endangering mission readiness and patient care. For this reason, teams should depend primarily on the assessment skills of the medical providers rather than on the electronic readout of patient monitoring devices. Rescue medicine must emphasize the importance of quality medical assessment. Despite these shortcomings, electronic monitors can be useful to teams called to rescue patients with a history of cardiac disturbances or complex medical illnesses.

Weight and Durability

For teams that use helicopters or that manually transport equipment to staging sites at higher elevations, the weight of medical equipment is critically important. All equipment should be reviewed to ensure that it is the lightest and most durable of available options. Common areas where weight is reduced include spinal immobilization devices, stretchers, medical consumables (in particular oxygen delivery systems and IV fluids), and patient monitors.

Most of the medical equipment used in rescue has been made more rugged in an attempt to increase durability. Making equipment more durable has obvious benefits; however, it also increases weight, bulk, and cost and may still be insufficient to

protect equipment during rescue operations. In recent years the increased visibility of specialized rescue teams in the military, industrial, and civil service sectors has prompted the development of lighter, more appropriate equipment, which increasingly is becoming available (Table 12-3).

Litter Medical Kit

The *litter medical kit (LMK)*, a smaller version of the rescue team medical kit, is designed for the management of emergencies that may arise when the patient is on a rope or restrained in the litter or when the larger rescue medical kit is unavailable. The LMK is designed to be light, portable, and easily accessible and to provide resources for a short period. Many well-designed LMKs can be replenished in the field from the team medical kit. For example, an LMK used for extended cave or big wall rescues may contain 1 L of spare crystalloid IV fluid, which can be replaced from the 4 to 6 L that may be carried in the larger kit. Under field conditions, the best LMK has the following characteristics:

- It is small and durable.
- It is cylindrical rather than square or bulky.
- It is constructed of waterproof durable fabric (e.g., PVC nylon).
- It has a durable tie-in at the top.
- It is top loading and has few side zippers.
- It has several large chambers.
- It has internal fasteners for tying in equipment (e.g., IV bags).
- It has a light internal color to improve the visibility of its contents.
- It is easy to use while hanging in vertical situations, in the darkness, or in poor weather.
- It contains drugs and equipment appropriate for treating high-probability injuries.
- It is appropriate to the provider's level of certification.

Improving on the LMK requires careful preplanning, preparation and evaluation. Adapting the LMK to the skills and needs

Table 12-3	Recommendations for Selected Medical Equipment Used in High Angle Rescue
Category	**Comment**
Litter	*Wire baskets (e.g., Traverse, Junkin):* The new-generation wire baskets are extremely durable and less prone to litter spin under helicopter rotor wash. Patients in wire stretchers require increased protection from the elements and separate spinal immobilization. *Soft litters (e.g., SKED):* Stretchers are light, provide excellent protection from the elements, and are easily configured for a variety of rescue applications. Disadvantages include possible instability when used in rotor wash and continued need for spinal immobilization. European and some North American agencies use Jenny bags, which require special harness systems and careful selection of patients.
Spinal immobilization	*Full spine splints (e.g., MDS, Germa, Thompson):* Vacuum splints are the gold standard for preserving neutral spine position, immobilizing against movement, and protecting against the elements. Excellent results are achieved by combining vacuum splints with nonrigid litters. *Half spine splints (e.g., Oregon Spine Splint, Kendrick Extrication Device):* These splints stabilize the axial spine. They are lightweight and durable and provide acceptable resistance to lateral forces. However, they do not adequately stabilize pelvic and lower extremity fractures.
Cervical immobilization	Cervical spine devices are similar in size and weight but vary in performance. Several models (e.g., Necklock) take up little space. Improvised cervical immobilization (e.g., using SAM splints) requires considerable practice to be effective.
Suction	Suction devices are mandatory for litter transport. Suction devices must be designed for the purpose and must have adequate reservoirs to allow for multiple aspirations.
Extremity splints	Ladder splints are light and inexpensive. Malleable splints (e.g., SAM splints) provide excellent versatility and protection.
Bag mask	Soft masks occupy less volume and provide a better seal for patients with maxillofacial trauma and facial hair. Ambu bags should be made of cold-resistant synthetic compounds and may be compressed for storage.
Medical consumables	The amount of intravenous (IV) fluids and oxygen should be appropriate for each rescue, and excess supplies should be removed. Bulky equipment should be stored in the main medical kit and not in the litter medical kit.

of the teams is an important first step. LMKs for the first responder likely will contain basic trauma dressings, oropharyngeal airways, and suction devices. The paramedic LMK likely will contain a few appropriate injectable medications, IV fluids, and ultraportable monitoring devices, such as fingertip oxygen monitors (e.g., Nelcor). LMKs are unlikely to contain splints, oxygen masks, or IV start kits, because these interventions most likely will have been applied when the litter and the patient were stationary; addition of this equipment increases the weight and bulk of the LMK.

In cases in which advanced life support (ALS) personnel initially treat the patient and then transfer the individual to a litter attendant for raising, lowering, or short haul operations, the litter attendant must understand how to support the medical therapy or equipment and know what to do in the event of an emergency. This skill is particularly critical with intubated patients transferred to litter attendants for lowering operations. In this situation, the attendant must know what to do if the BVM (e.g., Ambu) bag becomes disconnected, the patient expels the endotracheal (ET) tube, or the artificial airway becomes compromised.

Practical Points for the Litter Medical Kit

The ideal LMK is streamlined to allow for easy handling and access while suspended from the litter. Simplicity of patient care and avoidance of unnecessary risks are key points. For example, patients requiring IV support or injectable drugs should have an IV line placed with a saline lock. Continuous IVs are rarely needed and pose a risk, because tubing and IV bags may become entangled in the litter bridle or may be inadvertently pulled out by rescue activities.

Medical equipment in the LMK may include numerous small items that are not easily secured. Dropping of medical equipment such as IV bags, oral airways, and intubation tubes is common but potentially disastrous in high angle rescue. The LMK should be kept with the stretcher at all times to prevent the two from being separated during transport.

Weight and volume limitations require that the LMK be adapted for each rescue by exchanging supplies with prepackaged, swappable units. For example, an oil platform worker exposed to hazardous materials requires oxygen supplementation, possibly even manual ventilation. However, for a dehydrated mountain climber, the priority is prompt administration of IV fluids. In cases such as these, the LMK is adapted to support either oxygen delivery or maintenance of IV resuscitation. The amount of each resource stored in the LMK should be kept to a minimum to maintain a slim profile and reduce weight. In exceptional circumstances, such as deep cave rescue and extreme big wall rescue, in which the patient may remain in a technical rope system for many hours, additional resources may need to be either included or be ferried to the litter attendant.

Medications for the Litter Medical Kit

The value of drug treatment during the rescue phase of patient evacuation is the subject of debate. Many teams include small quantities of all medications found in the large team medical kits, including oral medications such as nonsteroidal analgesics. However, when medication use during rescue is retrospectively reviewed, it becomes evident that only a few medications are used with any frequency. This observation, combined with insight into the difficulties facing the litter attendant attempting to provide care while free hanging and managing the litter, raises several points about the benefit of LMK medications:

1. Whenever possible, pharmaceutical treatment should be initiated before the technical phases of the rescue (e.g., before the stretcher leaves the elevated platform).
2. Any drug administered during lowing or raising is given in response to an emergency situation; therefore immediate circulating drug levels are necessary. For this reason, the LMK should contain only injectable medications. Non-emergency medications can wait until the litter reaches the ground.
3. Injectable drugs must be compatible with the route of administration and with the IV fluid. This is a common problem with intravenously administered lorazepam (Ativan), which can precipitate in IV tubing when mixed with incompatible fluids.
4. Medications that exert their effect over a period of hours (e.g., dexamethasone given for neurotrauma) are unlikely to produce measurable benefit when administered during the rescue unless the litter operation lasts several hours.
5. The medications in the LMK should address the needs of high probability injuries. For example, most high angle rescue patients have traumatic or exposure injuries and are unlikely to need emergency medications for diabetic or cardiac patients.
6. The number of drugs in the LMK increases with the level of medical care provided. For example, LMKs that accompany an intubated patient must have additional paralytic agents, narcotic analgesics, and sedatives for retreatment of a patient who begins to fight manual ventilation or who expels the ET tube.
7. The injectable medications in the LMK should be easy to access and are packaged in single-dose vials.

8. The drugs in the LMK must be inventoried and rotated to prevent degradation caused by prolonged storage or extremes of temperature.
9. Each of the medications in the LMK should be partnered with a drug that will counter the side effects of therapy. This is particularly important for kits that contain narcotic sedatives and benzodiazepines (i.e., Valium).

Preparation and Training

Rescue teams may encounter problems when they transport patients with particularly severe injuries or complex medical problems. In a minority of cases, the patient requires both urgent rescue and continuous high-level medical attendance. Preparing in advance for the range of medical possibilities has important advantages both to the rescue team and to the patient. Preparation includes organization of team personnel, completion of the medical preplanning steps described previously, and integration of these steps into comprehensive, realistic training exercises.

Assessment and Interventions

The following sections review the medical needs that most often arise in a high angle rescue.

Airway and Breathing

Airway and breathing are primary concerns in all emergency medical cases. In a high angle rescue, assessment and management of airway and breathing are more complex than in other types of rescue. Airway emergencies that occur during rescue operations, such as an airway becoming blocked by blood, bone fragments, or vomit, require immediate action under difficult circumstances.

If the patient is unconscious, the airway must be under constant supervision to prevent occlusion that can occur secondary to improper positioning, deterioration of the patient's condition, or accumulation of body fluids. Current standards of medical practice in the United States require that a medical

Table 12-4	Injectable Medications Used in High Angle Rescue
Condition	**Appropriate Drug**
Analgesia	Morphine sulfate (note: naloxone)
	Ketorolac tromethamine given intravenously (IV) or intramuscularly (IM)
Ventilation	Albuterol (as metered dose inhalant [MDI])
Central nervous system (CNS) sedation	Dextrose 50%
	Haloperidol (IM or IV)
	Decadron injectable (extended care rescue teams, such as military and National Park rescue teams)
	Diazepam (note: flumazenil)
	Flumazenil
	Naloxone
Nausea	Prochlorperazine
Shock or allergy	Epinephrine 1:10,000 (1:1,000 IM)
Maintenance of IV lines	IV saline flushes, heparin flushes

attendant be with any patient at risk for airway or breathing difficulties, including unconscious patients and any patient with altered mental status. In addition, any patient with spinal immobilization must have a litter attendant available to intervene in case of airway or breathing compromise. By these criteria, the overwhelming majority of high angle rescue patients will require a litter attendant.

Questions about the airway and breathing that should be answered before packaging and moving the patient include the following:

- Does the patient have a clear airway and normal mental status?
- Could the injuries or illness result in the onset of airway difficulties during high angle rescue?
- Is the mouth free of tooth fragments, blood clots, gum, tobacco, and dentures?
- Is the patient at risk of vomiting (e.g., faint, nauseous, hypotensive)?
  NOTE: Vomiting often occurs suddenly and sometimes regardless of the individual's medical or trauma status.
- How will the attendant clear the airway during lowering or raising operations?
- Can respiration be monitored while the attendant directs the litter over obstacles?
- How will the attendant perform rescue breathing if the patient develops respiratory failure?

Airway and Breathing Interventions
Basic Life Support

1. Open the airway with a jaw thrust while maintaining neutral cervical position.
2. Maintain the airway with an airway adjunct (oral or nasal pharyngeal airway).
3. Provide mouth-to-mask ventilation or ventilation using a bag-valve-mask (BVM) or flow-restricted oxygen powered (FROP) ventilatory device (these devices consume oxygen at a high rate). Note that BVMs require two rescuers – one rescuer to maintain an effective mask seal while the other compresses the Ambu bag. For this reason, the team leader should consider controlled intubation, which allows one rescuer to perform manual ventilation while the other manages litter operations.
4. Administer oxygen. Make sure the mask has been stabilized to prevent displacement from the face.
5. Pre-position a manual suction device close to the patient's mouth (author's preference is V-VAC or equivalent).

Emergency Medical Technician Basic Level Interventions

1. Provide ventilations via BVM.

Advanced Life Support

1. If necessary, maintain an open airway with a pharyngeal/esophageal airway device (PEAD), Combi-Tube, or ET intubation. Prevent mistakes in obtaining surgical and alternative invasive airway access (e.g., retrograde intubation or cricothyrotomy) by practicing on difficult cases in a controlled setting, such as the operating room or emergency department. All invasive airway procedures should be completed before the patient is transported.
2. All intubations should be controlled. Rapid-sequence intubation protocols are acceptable providing the rescuer can ventilate the paralyzed patient if intubation fails.
3. Endotracheal suctioning must be performed on all patients in the first few minutes after intubation. Suctioning can never wait until the patient has been transferred to the ground team.
4. Administer antinausea drug (antiemetic) to prevent vomiting.

Circulation

The term circulation refers to adequate tissue perfusion, with an intact vascular system, no blood loss, and adequate cardiac output. The ability to control major internal or external hemorrhage in the rescue environment is limited. For this reason, patients with major hemorrhage are an evacuation priority. Prehospital treatment of hemorrhage is palliative and at best results in stabilization of the patient's condition. Priority response measures include (1) prompt reduction of the rate of blood loss; (2) aggressive replacement of intravascular volume, typically with crystalloid IV fluid; and (3) prevention of hypothermia and end-organ damage caused by prolonged hypotension.

The transition from hypotension to hypovolemic shock often is sudden, and many teams have been caught unprepared, with the patient poorly positioned for emergency measures (e.g., hanging far above ground without IV access or IV fluids).

Patients must be continuously assessed for the onset of shock. Signs of shock include the following:

- Increased pulse rate
- Poor pulses in the extremities
- Mottled, discolored, cool and clammy skin
- Reduced urine output
- Altered mental status

The earliest evidence of shock includes an increased heart rate, a drop in diastolic pressure, and anxiety.

Questions regarding the circulatory status that should be answered before packaging and moving the patient include the following:

- Does the patient have a pulse? (Check the pulses in both injured and uninjured extremities.)
- Can the pulse be accurately monitored during the rescue operation? (Consider adjusting clothing and padding to allow for convenient pulse checks.)
- Will cardiopulmonary resuscitation be possible during the rescue operation? (Effective CPR can be performed only when the patient is lying supine on a rigid surface.)
- Does the patient show signs of shock? (Remember, the onset of shock is not instantaneous; it appears over time. Trends in blood pressure, pulse, respiration, urine output, and level of consciousness must be monitored.)
- What must be done immediately to treat for shock? (Consider adjusting the height of the litter bridles to allow the patient to be positioned correctly.)
- What rescue procedures will increase or reduce the possibility of shock? (Make sure the procedures are appropriate for the rescue system.)

- Is control of hemorrhage effective, and is internal bleeding being missed? (This requires close attention to the patient's vital signs and level of discomfort, as well as the ability to monitor locations of insidious blood loss.)

Circulatory Interventions

Basic Life Support

1. Administer high-flow oxygen. Whenever possible, use small, streamlined oxygen tanks that are firmly attached to the litter. Note: New generation carbon fiber oxygen tanks are expensive but save as much as 30% more than conventional aluminum cylinders.
2. Elevate the patient's feet to a 15-degree incline.
3. Apply direct pressure, pressure points, and tourniquets for external bleeding control.
4. If necessary, perform CPR.
5. Assess oxygenation with a pulse oximeter.
6. Apply traction splints to control blood loss from a femur fracture (blood loss often is insidious).

Advanced Life Support

1. Administer crystalloid IV fluid through a large-bore peripheral IV catheter. (Make sure to stabilize the IV line against movement; whenever possible, a second IV line should be placed as a precaution against loss of access.)
2. Administer crystalloid, colloid, or blood products through peripheral, interosseous, or central venous lines.
3. Administer antishock medication for hypotension only after completion of IV hydration.

Head and Spine Considerations

Indications of spinal injury include the mechanism of injury, numbness and tingling, inability to move an extremity, flaccid muscle tone, shock, absent or difficulty breathing, incontinences, and back or neck pain. If the mechanism of injury is consistent with spinal injury, the spine must be immobilized from the head to the hips. A cervical collar used alone is not effective.

Ambulance personnel traditionally use rigid backboards, but these are very uncomfortable for long periods and may cause the patient to squirm, which counteracts the purpose of immobilization. For prolonged evacuation, a "conforming backboard," such as a vacuum mattress or a spinal extrication device (e.g., Kendrick extraction device [KED] or OSS), are more comfortable and in the long run provide better immobilization. Conforming backboards must be properly secured with the patient in the litter so that no lateral or longitudinal movement occurs. Any patient suffering from trauma above the clavicles, trauma with periods of unconsciousness, or serious orthopedic injury (e.g., a fracture of the femur, pelvis, or humerus) or who has fallen 15 feet (5 m) or farther must have full spinal immobilization.

Head trauma patients are prone to nausea, vomiting, altered mental status and, with more critical injuries, hypertension and bradycardia. Bleeding from head wounds may be considerable and if not controlled may result in shock. Head trauma should be considered in patients with alterations in consciousness; inadequate or chaotic respirations; skull fracture; bloody fluid from the ears, nares (nostrils), or mouth; facial injury; head cuts; lacerations or bruises; amnesia; or ataxia (vertigo/dizziness).

Questions about the status of the head and spine that should be answered before packaging and moving the patient include the following:

- Is there a possibility of head or spinal injury?
- Should spinal precautions be performed before the patient is moved?
- Should the patient be secured to a spinal immobilization device before being immobilized in a litter? (Virtually all trauma patients are treated in this manner.)
- Can the litter attendant support the patient's breathing and circulation during evacuation?

Head and Spine Interventions

Basic Life Support

1. Treat the patient with full spinal precautions.
2. Administer oxygen via a nasal cannula or nonrebreather mask.
3. Apply traction splints and full spinal immobilization.

Advanced Life Support

1. Administer a balanced salt solution through a large-bore peripheral IV catheter.
2. If indicated, administer colloid or blood products through peripheral or central venous lines.
3. Consider use of osmotic stabilizers or antiinflammatory agents for patients with head trauma. (Head trauma patients transported by litter should be treated with a potent antiemetic, because emesis may prove disastrous in this setting.)

Nonmedical Patients

A nonmedical rescue involves a patient who either is not injured or who has a mild illness or minor injuries that do not require urgent medical attention. Examples of non-medical rescues include retrieval of stranded window washers on a commercial high-rise building, single rescue pickoff of a patient in a burning building, or lowering an exhausted big wall climber. During nonmedical rescues, the rescuer need only ensure that the patient is transported safely, and no specialty medical care is required.

Medical (Trauma) Patients

A rescue in which medical care is required poses a markedly different challenge to the rescue team because stabilizing medical care should not be delayed until the rope rescue has been completed. Common examples of rescues requiring medical treatment and monitoring during rope operations include raising unconscious patients from toxic environments, rescue of utility linesman electrocuted while working on power lines, and lowering a climber with an extremity fracture or head trauma.

Rescue and Medicine: Putting It Together

The following guidelines can help in the process of integrating efforts and techniques in order to meet both the rescue and medical needs of the patient:

- Care must be taken to protect patients from injury during rope rescue.
- Not all injuries require treatment before rescue (e.g., sprains, dehydration).
- A type 1 rescue can become a type 2 rescue if the patient deteriorates, suffers from exposure, or receives additional injuries, such as from an overhead rock fall.
- Advanced medical capabilities are more likely to conflict with high angle rescue systems and may also delay completion of the rescue.

- Advanced medical procedures (e.g., intubation, insertion of IV lines) are difficult to perform while suspended from a rescue litter and should be done before rope rescue or helicopter short haul operations are begun.
- Well-performed basic medical care is safer and more effective than improperly performed advanced medical care. ALS medical personnel and resources should be chosen with care, and medical care should be prioritized in training sessions.
- Alternative methods to rope rescue (e.g., litter carry-out) should be considered for all critical or deteriorating patients.
- The rope rescuer should anticipate and prepare in advance for medical problems that may arise during rescue operations. Table 12-5 presents a summary of the advantages to be gained with proper preparation.

Integration of patient care and rescue procedures is a difficult challenge, but one that cannot be neglected.

Table 12-5	Advantages of Preparation and Training
Outcome	**Reason**
Improved patient care	Preparation and training, along with ongoing review of cases, allow the team to focus their training on high yield, frequently used medical skills that have the greatest benefit for patients.
Reduced anxiety (the rescuer)	Rescuers unprepared to meet the medical needs of patients may be anxious and uncertain. Preplanning, together with training and critical review, helps prepare rescuers for problems both expected and unexpected.
Reduced anxiety (the patient)	An unprepared rescuer is easily identified by patients and bystanders. Lack of patient confidence may result in the rescuer losing control of the patient, which may in turn result in desperate "grabs" at the rescue equipment, jeopardizing patients and personnel and delaying rescue. Preplanning increases rescuer confidence, allowing for more effective control of a terrified patient.
Contingency planning	Cross-training all team members in patient care ensures that medical capability is always available during a rescue.
Medical kits	As teams become more familiar with the local patient population and patterns of accidents, medical kits become more streamlined and efficient, as well as easier to use.
Efficient rescue operations	Preplanning improves the integration of rescue and medical operations, saves time, and reduces payload.

Evaluation Exercises

1. Determine which of the rescue patients below are non-medical rescues and which are medical rescues:
   - A dehydrated patient with nausea and mental status changes who is stranded on a mountain ledge
   - A teenage boy unable to walk out from the backcountry because of fatigue
   - A highline technician who lost consciousness after a fall but who is now alert and oriented to person, place, and time
   - A healthy oil platform worker with a right mild ankle fracture and no pulse in the right foot
   - A patient overcome by noxious fumes while working on an industrial catwalk

2. List four factors that affect medical preplanning for high angle rescue.

3. Identify three advantages of having a medical control officer affiliated with your rescue team.

4. List five important qualities that must be considered when choosing medical equipment to be used in high angle rescue.

5. Describe five ways in which the litter medical kit differs from the team medical kit.

13

Rescue Belaying

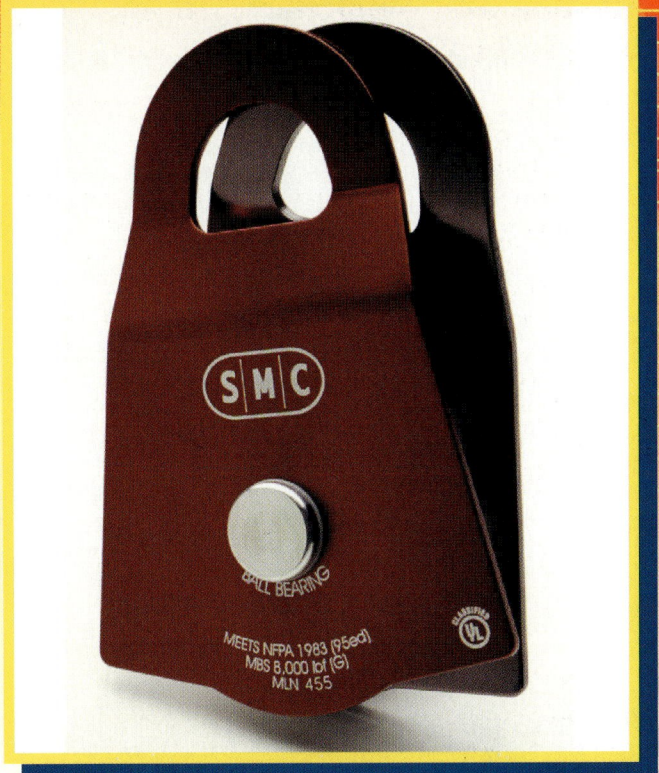

Prerequisites

Before attempting the activities described in this chapter, you must have demonstrated that you can properly:

1. Use and care for rope.
2. Use and care for other equipment needed in the high angle environment.
3. Tie correctly and without hesitation the knots described in Chapter 6.
4. Apply the principles of anchoring and rig a safe and secure anchor.
5. Apply the principles of belaying and safely and confidently belay another person using either a Münter hitch or a personal belay device.

Objectives

On completion of this chapter, you should be able to:

1. Tie a load-releasing hitch.
2. Rig a tandem Prusik belay system.
3. Operate a tandem Prusik belay system.
4. Rig a Prusik minding pulley.
5. Operate a Prusik minding pulley.
6. Operate a 540° Rescue Belay in a belay system.

The material in this chapter conforms to guidelines published by the National Fire Protection Association (NFPA), specifically standard 1006, *Professional Qualifications for Rescue Technicians* (2002), and standard 1670, *Operations and Training for Technical Rescue Incidents* (2004). NFPA standards are revised regularly, and readers are advised to review the latest version of this standard.

Key Terms

Automatic Belay A belay that locks off the belayed rope automatically when a sudden force is applied. Such belays do not depend on the belayer to activate the device to arrest a sudden fall, but they may require the device to be fed rope to operate correctly.

Conditional Belay A belay that does not lock automatically when sudden force is applied; also known as a *manual belay or brake belay*. A traditional one-person belay (as discussed in Chapter 8) is considered a conditional belay, because most arrest the falling load only if properly activated by the belayer.

Load-Releasing (LR) Hitch A type of hitch usually tied in webbing or accessory cord in such a way that it can sustain major loads and, with tension still on it, can be used as a mechanism to release the tension in the system into which it is inserted. Well-constructed load-release hitches allow the load to be let out several meters under control.

Prusik Minding Pulley (PMP) A pulley with specially shaped side plates that help manage Prusik hitches.

Tandem Prusik Belay System Two triple-wrap Prusik hitches of differing lengths set a few inches apart in a series on a belay rope, used to grab the rope in case of main-line failure or to hold the load while the lowering and raising systems are adjusted.

Rescue Belays

When more than a one-person load must be belayed, greater control is needed than is available with one-person belay devices.

Some one-person belay systems may work for more than one person if conditions are just right. For example, when a rope runs over an edge, the added friction can help control the load. However, many varying conditions are involved, such as the belayer's grip strength, that make it difficult to predict the reliability of the belay. Consequently, some of these devices and techniques will not reliably catch the load if more than one person's weight is on it. In addition, most one-person belay devices are not designed by the manufacturer to catch more than one person's body weight.

Brake Belays

A variety of belay systems can be used for rescue loads, but each system has disadvantages. Some rope rescue systems use two ropes running through a braking device, such as a brake tube. Other systems use two brakes, each controlling a rope attached to the rescue load, such as a litter (see Chapter 16). Two commonly used braking devices in these two rope systems are the brake bar rack and the brake tube. These two brake systems are designed so that each lowering device backs up the other. In essence, each braking device belays for the other one. A brake belay often is referred to as a **conditional belay** because it arrests a falling load only if the brake device is operated properly.

Use of a brake belay has distinct disadvantages. For example, in a two-brake system, the individuals operating the brakes must be well coordinated and alert for failure of the other system. Difficulty with reversibility is another drawback. With most brake systems, changing direction suddenly from lowering to hauling is not easy. For example, it is very difficult to pull rope back through a brake bar rack with most bars engaged. With a brake

tube, it is possible to reverse direction, although it may be somewhat difficult in some conditions. However, if the operation is to involve only a straight lowering, reversibility may not be a concern.

On the other hand, brake belays offer several advantages in certain situations. For example, they do not require special equipment solely for the belay, and the roles of brakeman and belayer require the same skills and can be interchanged easily. Also, brake belays usually do not accidentally engage and hang up; they do not require load-releasing hitches; they provide a soft catch; and they are predictable in the way they will perform.

The dilemma for rescue belaying is that no system is guaranteed to work every time and under all conditions.

Tandem Prusik Belay System

A system that has been shown to work under many rescue belay conditions is the **tandem Prusik belay system**. It consists of two triple-wrapped Prusiks anchored securely and placed in line on the belay rope (Figure 13-1). The system is designed such that in case of failure, the Prusiks, if rigged correctly, exert a clutching action and grab the rope. This means that instead of an abrupt shock load occurring, such as might happen with metal camming devices, the load is stopped gradually.

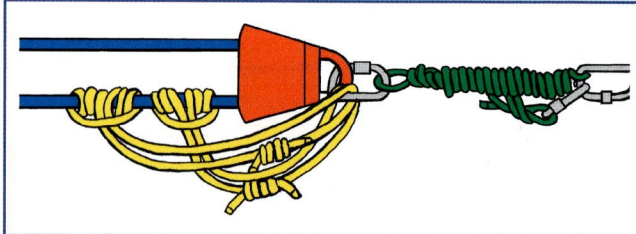

Figure 13-1 Tandem Prusik belay system with load-releasing hitch.

Under certain conditions, the Prusiks may not catch. For example, if the equipment is icy or muddy, if Prusik cord of the wrong diameter or material is used, or if the hitches are not tied tightly enough, the belay rope may slip through the Prusiks.

Tandem Prusiks can fail under other conditions. In high-impact situations, for example, tandem Prusiks can cause the belay line to fail by pinching it until the rope separates. Also, the Prusik material itself can fail, particularly if the wrong size or type of Prusik cord is used to build the tandem three-wrap Prusik belay system.

The success of a tandem Prusik belay very much depends on the interaction of the Prusik cord material with the rope material. To make sure the system will work when needed, you should test your Prusik cord with the rope you will be using in a rescue situation.

It is very important to have a knowledgeable, alert person tend the Prusiks, because if they are not tended correctly, they may not catch when needed.

Load-Releasing Hitches

A properly constructed Prusik belay system requires some means of releasing the Prusiks should they jam. There are several ways to release the load, and these techniques usually involve a **load-releasing (LR) hitch**. The type of LR hitch described in this text is the *radium releasing hitch* (see discussion later in the chapter), which was chosen because it can withstand high shock loads and can lower the arrested load under control.

The LR hitch serves two primary purposes:

1. If the belay line becomes loaded accidentally, the LR hitch can be used to shift the load back to the main line.
2. The LR hitch has some shock absorbing capacity.

In addition, the LR hitch can be used for some purposes other than belaying, such as changing over from a raising system to a lowering system or from a lowering system to a raising system.

Constructing the Tandem Prusik Belay System

To ensure that the tandem Prusik belay system works as intended, you must follow the steps in the right column closely.

> ### ▨ **Warning**
>
> Tandem Prusik belays do not work in all rescue conditions. Prusiks can slip on ropes that are muddy or icy. A Prusik-type belay may not be appropriate in a hazardous environment in which a hang up could cause severe injury or death.
>
> The success of a tandem Prusik belay very much depends on the interaction of the material in the Prusik hitch with the rope material. Before relying on a tandem Prusik belay, test the materials you are using for their holding power.
>
> A tandem Prusik belay must be tended by a person who is knowledgeable in its operation and remains alert at all times during its use.

Tandem Prusiks

The following procedure assumes that a ½-inch (12.7 mm) rope is used for the belay line.

1. Use about 10 feet (3 m) of 8- or 9-mm nylon climber's accessory cord cut into two lengths:
   - 65 inches (1.65 m)
   - 53 inches (1.35 m)
2. Using a grapevine (double fisherman's) knot, tie the ends of the longer length together to form a loop. Then, using the same knot, tie the ends of the shorter length together to form a second loop. You should now have two separate loops.
3. Tension both loops to snug down the knots. There should be ¼-inch (6 mm) of tail after tensioning.
4. Place the longer loop across the rope; approximately one third of the loop should be on one side of the rope and two thirds on the other side. Bring the longer section of the loop around the rope and through the bight formed on the other side of the rope by the one-third portion. Repeat this two more times, forming a Prusik with three wraps on the rope.
5. Position this longer Prusik on the rope nearest the load.
6. Using the shorter loop, tie a second three-wrap Prusik as described in step 4 above. Position this second Prusik between the first Prusik and the anchor.
7. Be sure to wrap the two Prusiks in the same direction on the rope. Position them so that the double fisherman's knots are between the Prusiks and the anchor carabiner.
8. Dress the Prusik hitches (see Chapter 6, p. 69). There should be about 4 inches (10 cm) of space between them when both are fully extended from their anchor.
9. At the anchor, clip the Prusiks into a large locking carabiner. Clip the long Prusik in first, then the short one.

Radium Releasing Hitch

The materials needed for a radium releasing hitch (Figure 13-2) include the following:

- Two locking carabiners of suitable strength for rescue loads
- 33 feet (10 m) of 8-mm nylon static kernmantle rope or 8-mm nylon accessory cord

1. Tie a compact figure 8 on a bight in one end of the cord.
2. Clip the loop (bight) of the knot into the load-side carabiner with the loop close to the carabiner's spine. This load-end carabiner is where the tandem Prusiks or other load is attached to the LR hitch. (Figure 13-2, *A*).
3. Bring the standing part of the cord up through the anchor-end carabiner close to the carabiner's spine and back down and through the load-end carabiner next to the previously tied figure 8 on a bight (Figure 13-2, *B*).
   NOTE: The anchor-end carabiner must be attached to an anchor system capable of sustaining the full load of the system during and after a main-line failure.
4. Once again bring the cord back up to the anchor carabiner. However, this time tie a Münter hitch onto the anchor carabiner next to the previous wraps on the gate side of the end. Make sure to tie the Münter hitch in its release position with the loose (standing) end toward the gate side of the anchor carabiner. At this point, you should have a 3:1 mechanical advantage system built between the two carabiners with a Münter hitch to control release of the load (Figure 13-2, *C*).

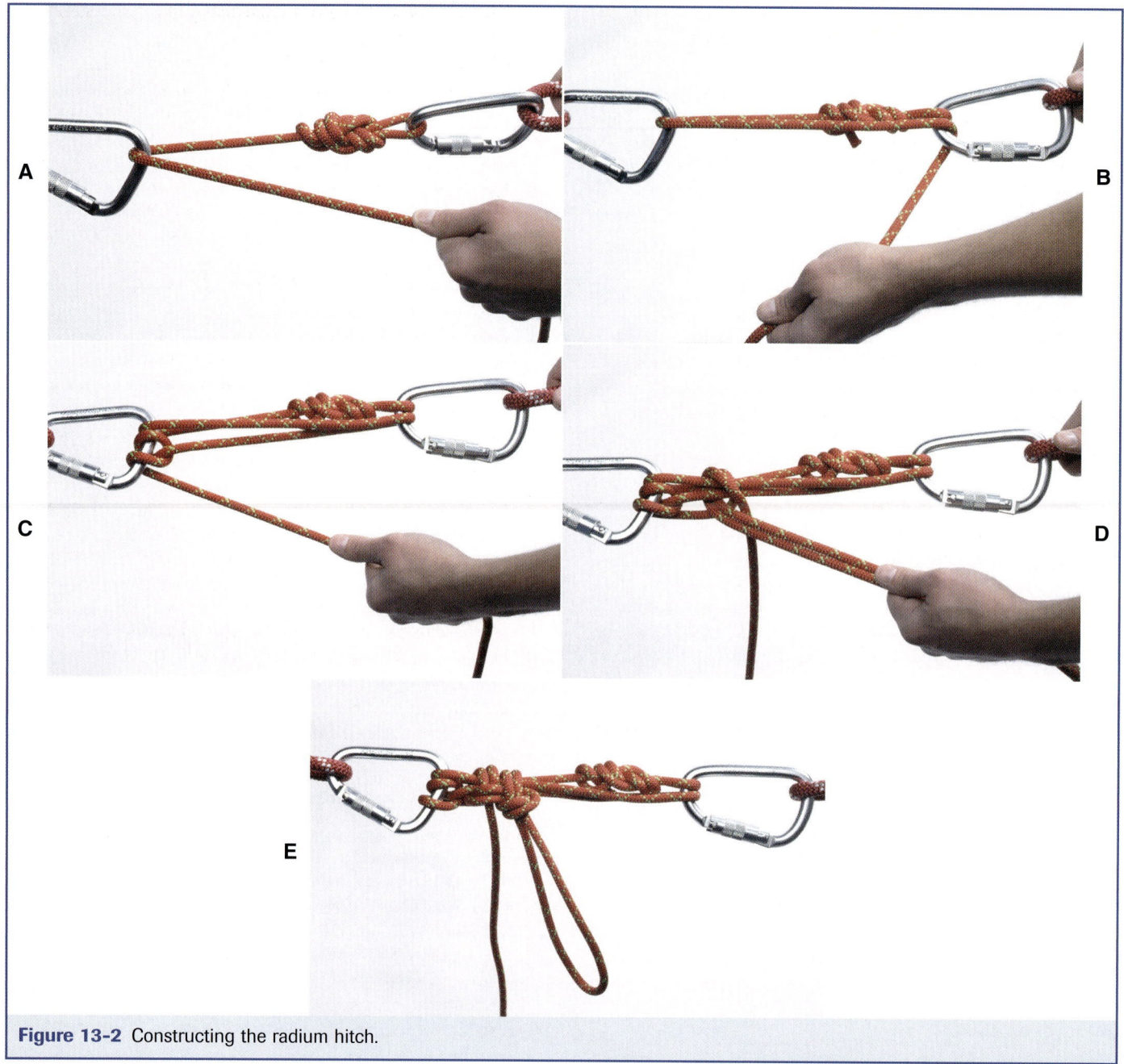

Figure 13-2 Constructing the radium hitch.

5. Secure the hitch by taking a bight in the standing end of the rope and tying a half hitch around the three parallel cords just below the Münter hitch. Back it up with an overhand-on-a-bight knot around the bundle (Figure 13-2, *D, E*).

6. As final security, tie a figure 8 on a bight in the standing end of the cord and clip it into an anchor as a backup, so that the system is secure even in the event of an unintended complete release by the operator when the hitch is released under load.

7. Check to make sure the gates of both carabiners are locked.

Releasing the Radium Releasing Hitch

If the Prusiks jam or become loaded, the following procedure will release them (Figure 13-3).

1. Untie the overhand-on-a-bight knot. Leave the figure 8 on a bight in the loose end of the hitch attached to the anchor for now (Figure 13-3, A).

2. Maintaining tension on the Münter hitch, carefully untie the half hitch below the Münter hitch (Figure 13-3, B).

3. Slowly ease the tension on the Münter hitch, allowing the radium hitch to lengthen as the Münter hitch controls the load using the 3:1 part of the release hitch under the control of the 3:1 mechanical advantage and the Münter hitch.

4. If the load is insufficient to pull slack through the hitch, slowly feed cord into the Münter hitch (Figure 13-3, C).

become loose, the belayer immediately must call "Stop!" to halt the operation.

- To check for tightness, the belayer should listen for the sound caused by the rubbing of the sheath of the belay rope against the inside of the Prusik as the rope slides through. If no sound is heard, the Prusiks must be retightened.

The basic technique to Prusik tending is to keep one hand cupped on the Prusiks as the rope is pulled in or let out. Use your other hand to take up or pull out the belay slack and to feel the tension so that you can decide if more or less rope is needed.

Giving Slack or Feeding Out the Belay in a Lowering Operation

1. Start with your hands together (Figure 13-4, *A*).
2. Keep one hand cupped on the Prusiks to hold them in place and to prevent them from coming tight when you don't want them to do so. This is the *Prusik hand*.
3. With a twist of the wrist of the other hand (the *feeling hand*), pull out about 18 to 24 inches (45 to 60 cm) of the rope through the Prusiks (Figure 13-4, *B*).
4. You should now have a shallow S curve in your feeling hand between the Prusik hand and the belayed load.
5. As the belay begins to come tight, the S curve will flatten out, thus straightening out the wrist of your feeling hand (Figure 13-4, *C*).
6. This is the signal to slide the feeling hand back up against the Prusik hand and again pull out another 1 to 2 feet (0.3 to

5. Once slack has been obtained at the load-end carabiner and tandem Prusiks, resecure the Münter hitch or rerig the system as needed.

Operating (Tending) the Tandem Prusiks (Figure 13-4)

The tandem Prusiks should be tended by a belayer wearing gloves. The belayer should keep the following points in mind:

- Before a lowering or raising operation, the belayer must inspect the Prusiks to make sure they have been tied correctly, they are neat and dressed, and they are the appropriate distance apart.
- The belayer must make sure the Prusiks are snug on the rope. If at any time during the operation the Prusiks

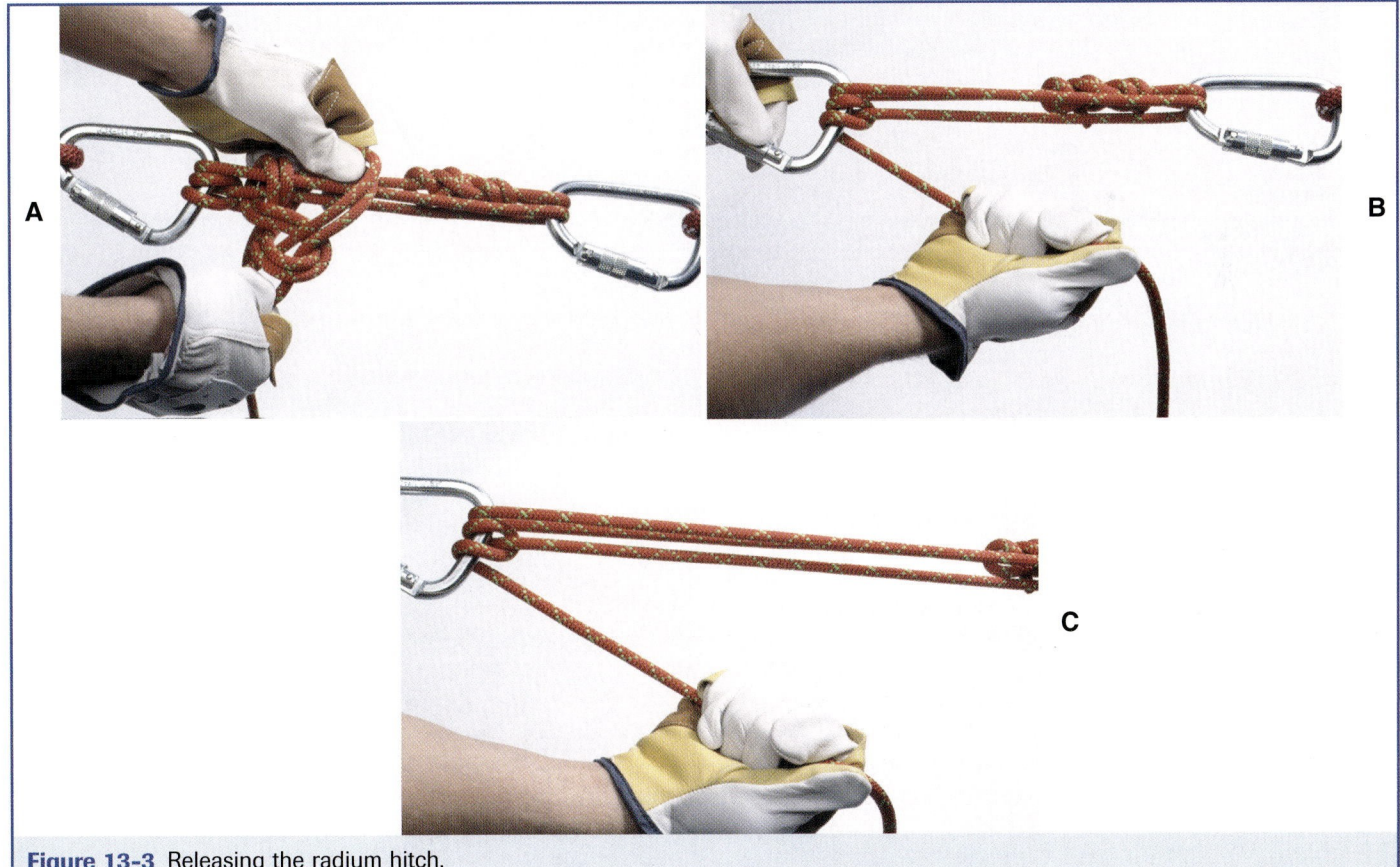

Figure 13-3 Releasing the radium hitch.

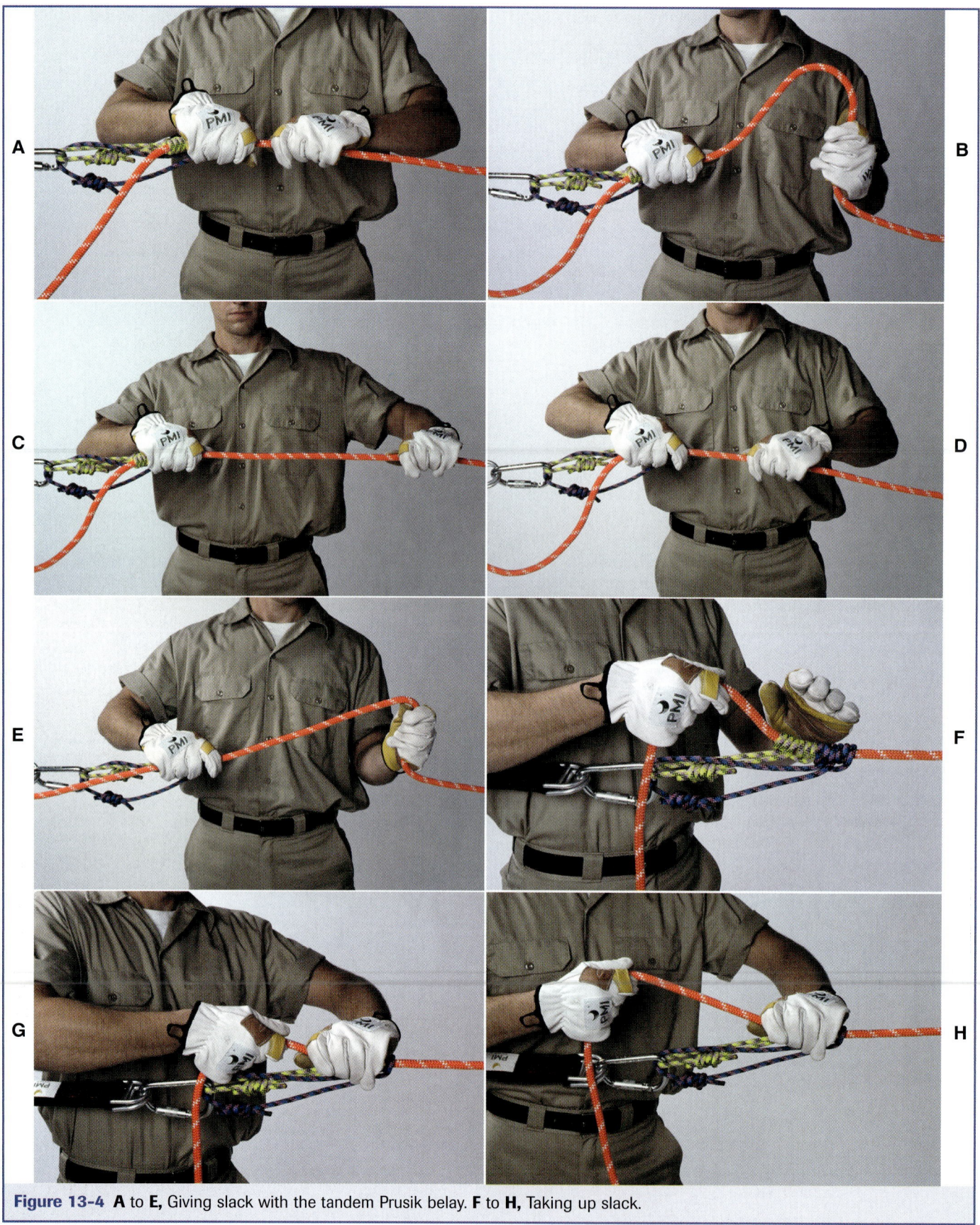

Figure 13-4 **A** to **E,** Giving slack with the tandem Prusik belay. **F** to **H,** Taking up slack.

0.6 m) of slack, forming the S again in your feeling hand (Figure 13-4, *D*).

7. Make sure the Prusiks remain snug during the operation. You should be able to hear the Prusiks sliding on the rope.

Taking in Slack or Belaying a Raising Operation

1. Hold the Prusiks in your Prusik hand in a way that keeps them almost but not completely snug against their anchor (Figure 13-4, *F*).
2. Pull any available slack through the Prusiks by applying tension to the belay line with the feeling hand (Figure 13-4, *G*).
3. As slack develops, remove it by sliding the Prusiks forward toward the load with the Prusik hand and keeping tension behind the hitch with the feeling hand (Figure 13-4, *H*).
4. Take care not to run the Prusiks too tight, because the load may suddenly change direction, and the Prusiks would quickly jam. Should that happen, the LR hitch or some other means of unloading the Prusiks would be needed if the load direction could not be changed back to a raise.

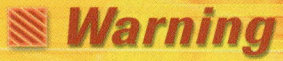
Warning

- ❏ Belayers must be alert at all times. Failures often occur with no warning.
- ❏ While belaying with tandem Prusiks, do not allow the rope to contact any part of your body other than your hands. You could be injured if the belay activates.

Prusik Minding Pulley

The ***Prusik minding pulley (PMP)*** is sometimes used in raising operations to help operate the Prusiks (Figure 13-5). The tandem Prusiks, when rigged correctly, catch on the edge of the pulley side plates as the rope enters the pulley. The side plates of the PMP are designed to keep the Prusik knots sliding on the rope and to prevent them from binding in the pulley. The PMP is designed such that should a failure occur, the tandem Prusiks will grasp the rope and catch the load.

As with any Prusik safety system, the Prusiks must be tight enough to grasp the rope automatically if the rope should start to slip through them. The rescuer who tends the Prusik minding pulley must make sure the Prusiks remain tight and properly dressed.

Rigging the Prusik Minding Pulley (Figure 13-6)

1. Rig the PMP to a load-releasing hitch on a suitable anchor.
2. Run one end of the belay rope through the pulley and tie the Prusiks to the belay rope on what will be the load side of the pulley.
3. Secure the Prusiks in the load-end carabiner of the LR hitch with the PMP next to them.
4. The shorter Prusik loop should be only a finger width or so below the side plate when the Prusik is attached to the pulley's carabiner and slightly snugged up.
5. The longer Prusik loop should be about four finger widths below the shorter one. More distance than that makes the

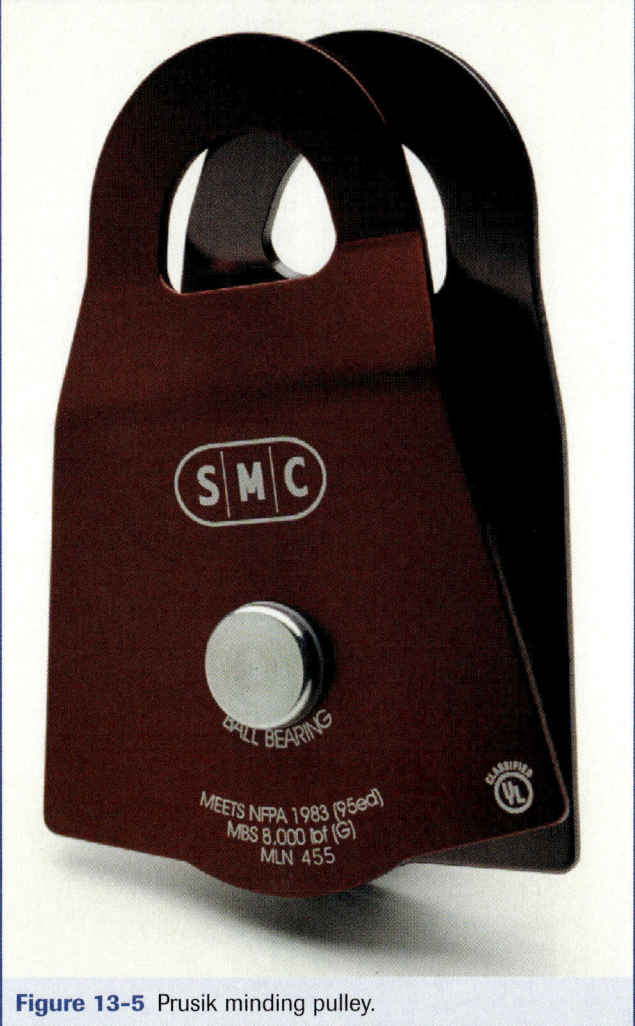
Figure 13-5 Prusik minding pulley.

system very inefficient, and the belay system could fail to arrest the load in a sudden emergency.

Operating the Prusik Minding Pulley (Figure 13-7)

1. As the load is hauled, pull the belay rope through the PMP. Do this by keeping one hand on the rope feeding into the pulley (the load side) as you pull the rope on the opposite side with your other hand. The Prusiks should "tend" themselves.
2. When the hauling operation is at rest and the slack is out of the belay, the hand grasping the rope on the load side should move toward the Prusiks and snug them back towards the load to limit excess slack should the belay be suddenly loaded.
3. If the Prusiks have been tied so that the cord is very loose and the Prusiks must travel a distance before setting, shock loading of the system may occur.
4. Any time the opportunity arises (e.g., during pauses in hauling), retighten the Prusiks.
5. For the best efficiency, keep the angle between the ropes going in and out of the PMP as close to 0 degrees as possible.
6. The belayer must remain within reach of the PMP whenever it is in operation.

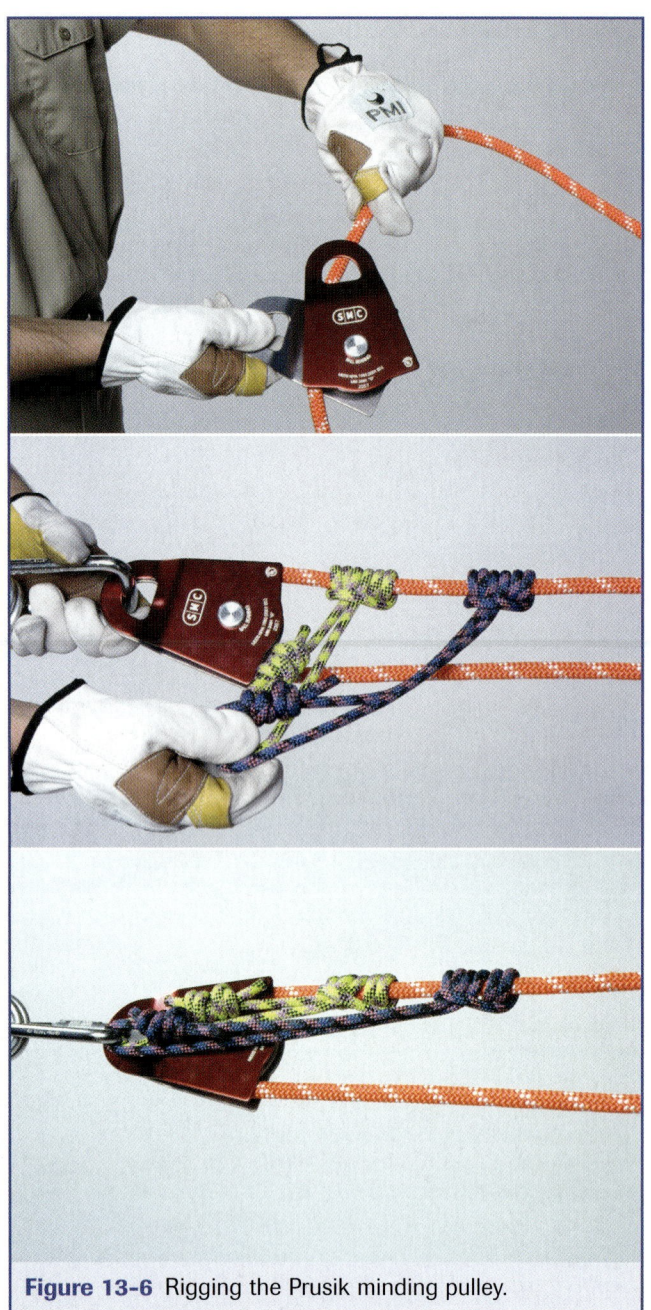

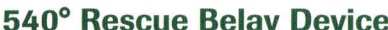

Figure 13-6 Rigging the Prusik minding pulley.

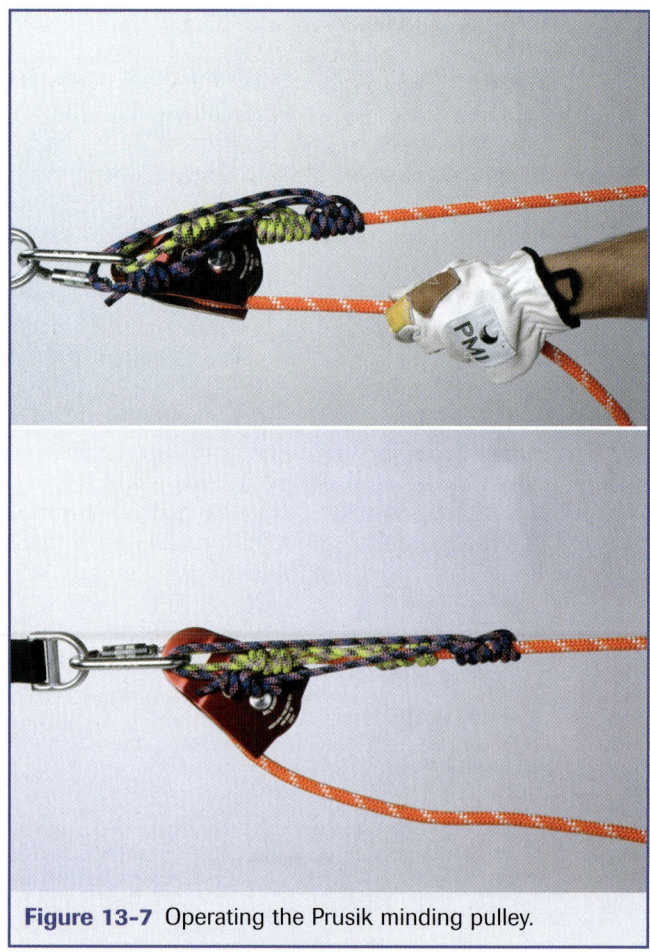

Figure 13-7 Operating the Prusik minding pulley.

540° Rescue Belay Device

The 540° Rescue Belay (Traverse Rescue, Kelowa, British Columbia) is a relatively new device (Figure 13-8). It works as an *automatic belay* for rescue loads, meaning that it can safely arrest the load and lock itself onto the rope when necessary, yet it easily lets rope in and out when it is unloaded. The unique design allows the device to operate properly when loaded with rope wrapped in either direction. A built-in lever resets the locking mechanism to quickly release an arrested load, eliminating the need for a separate LR hitch or device. Two models of the 540° Rescue Belay are available, one for 10.6- to 11.6-mm static ropes and one for 11.5- to 13-mm static ropes.

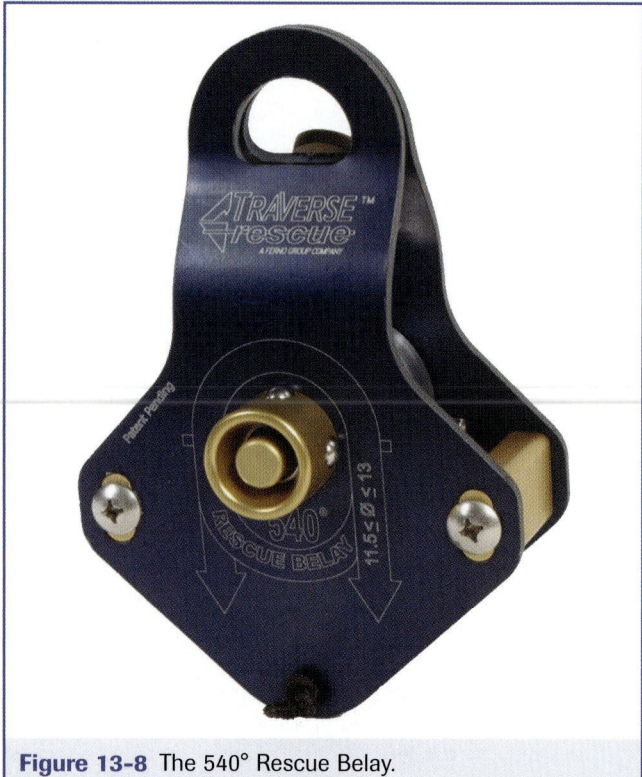

Figure 13-8 The 540° Rescue Belay.

The 540° Rescue Belay meets the criteria of the Belay Competence Drop Test of the British Columbia Council of Technical Rescue. This means that it can catch a 3.3-foot (1 m) drop of a 617-pound (280 kg) rescue-sized load onto 10 feet (3 m) of 12.7-mm kernmantle rescue rope within 3.3 feet (1 m) of additional travel (prerebound) and with less than 15 kN of peak force.

Advantages

- It allows bidirectional loading.
- It does not require an LR hitch.
- It is self-locking.

Disadvantages

- It is specific to a narrow range of rope diameters.
- It is heavy (the device weighs 1 pound, 6 ounces [624 g]).
- It works best with a new, clean rope; old, dirty, fuzzy ropes can cause it to lock up frequently.

Rigging the 540° Rescue Belay

Use a suitable locking carabiner to attach the 540° Rescue Belay to the belay anchor system.

Loading the Rope (Figure 13-9)

1. Remove the front plate of the 540° Rescue Belay by depressing the push-pin.

2. Wrap the rope around the oval pulley one and one-half times, or 540 degrees. Because the 540° Rescue Belay is symmetric and bidirectional in design, the wraps may start from either side of the pulley.
3. Make sure the one and one-half wraps are divided by the rope guide pins on each side of the pulley. The device will not work if only half a wrap is placed over the pulley.
4. Replace the front plate and confirm that the push-pin balls have completely returned to their locked position. Also make sure that both the running end (free or loose end) and the standing part (load-side rope) lie between the two stationary wedges and exit below the pulley. The keeper cord connecting the front and back plates must lie between the two ropes exiting the device.

NOTE: Because the 540° Rescue Belay is symmetric, it can be loaded either from the left or the right side, and either rope exiting the device can be used as the load rope. The 540° Rescue Belay is best used with a kernmantle rescue belay rope with lower stretch properties.

Belaying while Lowering or Raising (Figure 13-10)

Keep all parts of the 540° Rescue Belay, including the release lever, completely unimpeded by any obstruction or obstacle that could interfere with proper belay technique, locking or releasing of the device, or release capability. Wear gloves to protect your hands, and stay a sufficient distance from the device to keep your

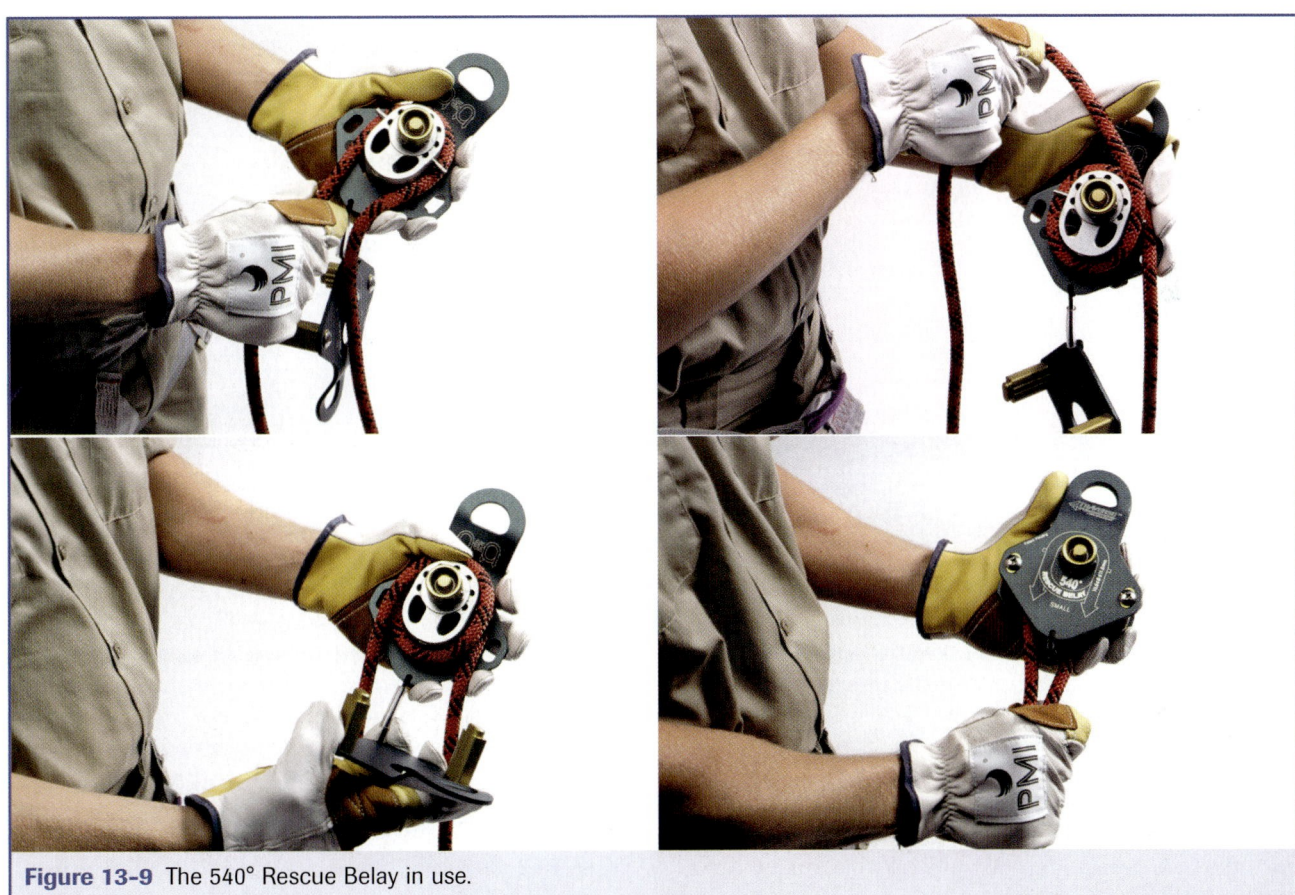

Figure 13-9 The 540° Rescue Belay in use.

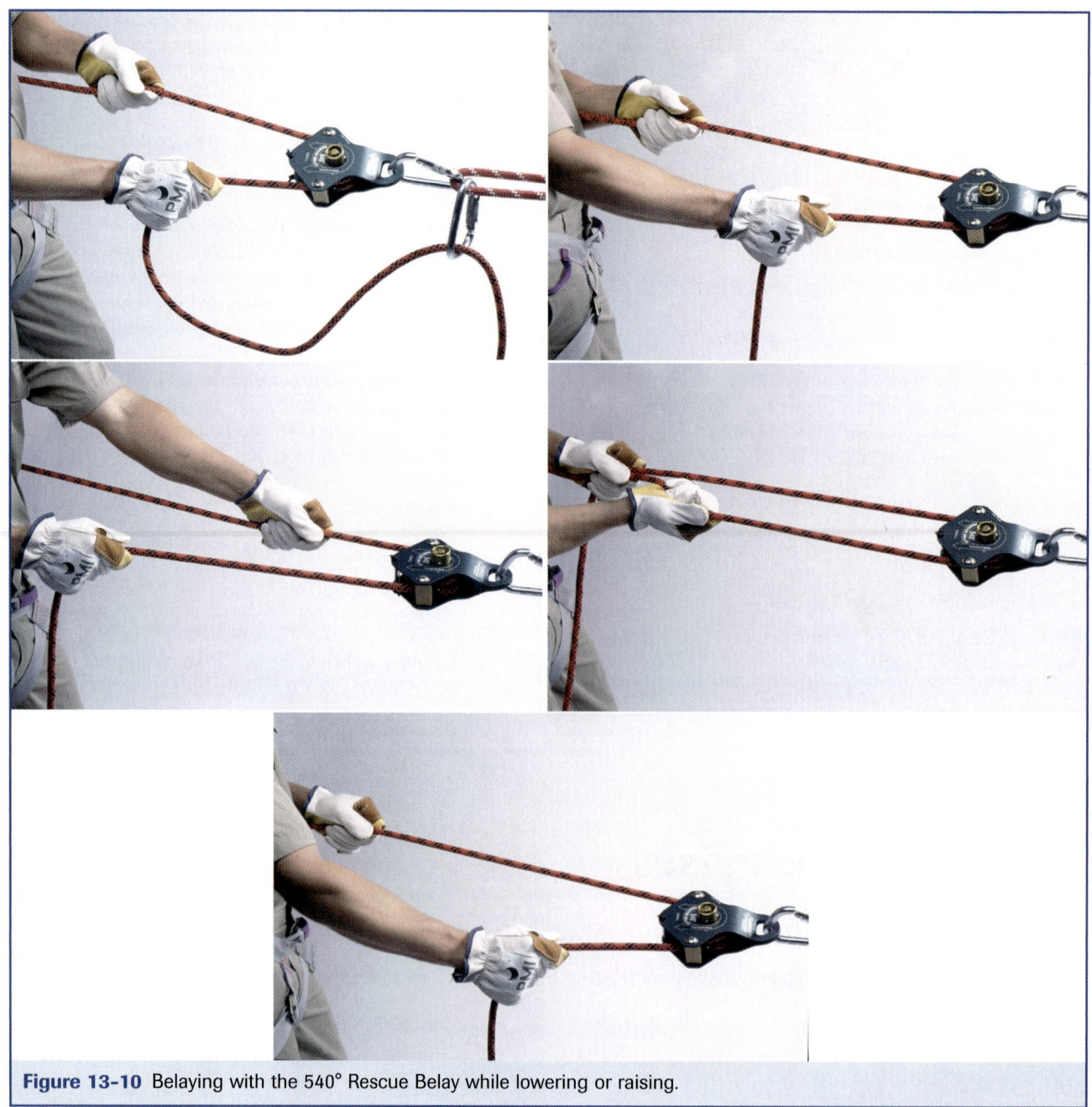

Figure 13-10 Belaying with the 540° Rescue Belay while lowering or raising.

hands free of moving parts. Always keep a firm grip on the running end of the belay rope; this ensures that the rope will lock if the load suddenly drops.

IMPORTANT: Self-locking occurs with sudden drops. However, with a slow fall and/or a supple or smaller diameter rope, resistance must be applied to the running end of the rope to ensure rope locking. Self-locking for slow falls can be improved by clipping the running end of the rope through a separate carabiner attached to the anchor, behind the 540° Rescue Belay. Never belay the load using the release lever to manage the feed, because this may prevent rope locking if the load drops suddenly.

To prevent accidental rope locking while lowering or raising, feed rope straight into the 540° Rescue Belay. This is especially important with wet, dirty, muddy, fuzzy, or stiff ropes. While lowering, with a gloved hand, provide resistance to the standing part (load-side) and with the other hand simultaneously feed running-end rope into the device. While raising, pull up on the standing part and feed it into the device and then pull on the running end.

Manually Locking Off the Belay Rope

To lock off the belay, manually trigger the 540° Rescue Belay by firmly holding the running end of the rope and sharply tugging

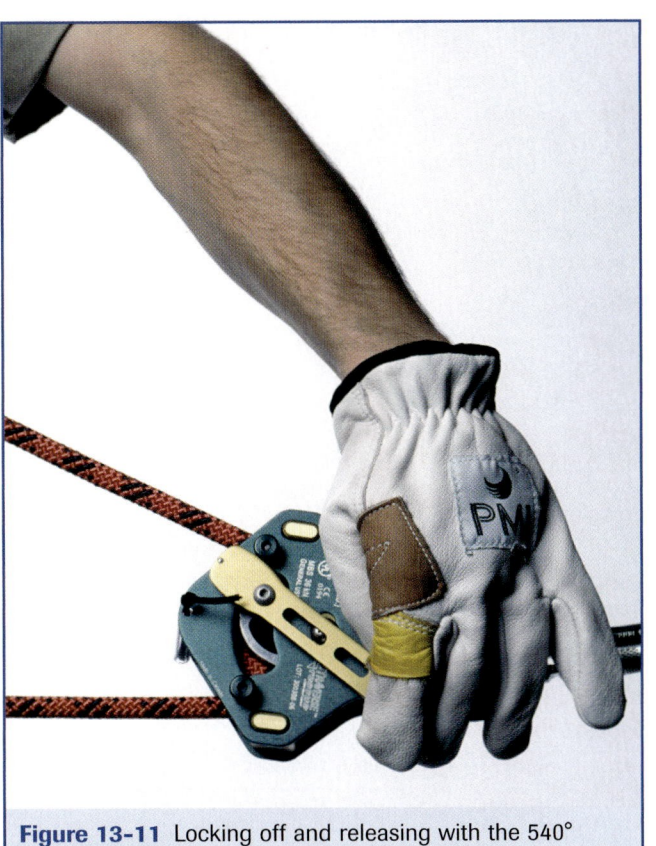

Figure 13-11 Locking off and releasing with the 540° Rescue Belay.

the standing part. The lock-off can be made more secure by tying the running end of the belay rope around the standing part with an overhand-on-a-bight knot. If the belay must be left unattended, the device first must be locked off.

Releasing a Locked Belay Rope (Figure 13-11)

The 540° Rescue Belay is not to be used as a general descent-control device. If the belay rope is only lightly locked, quickly reversing the direction of feed can return the pulley to its neutral or centered position. If this cannot be done, make sure the main line is locked off, then use the release lever slowly to transfer the tension back to the main line, maintaining a firm grip on the running end of the rope. Make sure the pulley has returned to its neutral position before continuing.

If the 540° Rescue Belay receives a significant shock force (e.g., catches a rescue-sized load), the rope in the device may stiffen while arresting the fall; it therefore may be more difficult to release the load until that portion of the rope has passed through the device. *If releasing the load is difficult, a webbing sling may be threaded **temporarily** through the top of the release lever to make the pulling easier; remove the webbing as soon as the load has been released.*

Evaluation Exercises

Cognitive and Affective Exercises

1. What are the two primary problems in using a two-line braking system, such as brake bar racks or brake tubes, in a belay situation?

2. What are two advantages of using a two-line braking system, such as brake bar racks or brake tubes, in a belay situation?

3. What are the primary components of a tandem Prusik belay system?

4. Name three conditions under which a Prusik belay system might fail.

5. What is the main purpose of the load-releasing hitch?

6. What four things should you check when inspecting a Prusik belay system?

Psychomotor Exercises

7. Correctly tie a radium load-releasing hitch.

8. Correctly rig a tandem Prusik belay system.

9. Correctly operate a tandem Prusik belay system.

10. Correctly rig a Prusik minding pulley.

11. Correctly operate a Prusik minding pulley.

14

Pickoff Rescue Techniques

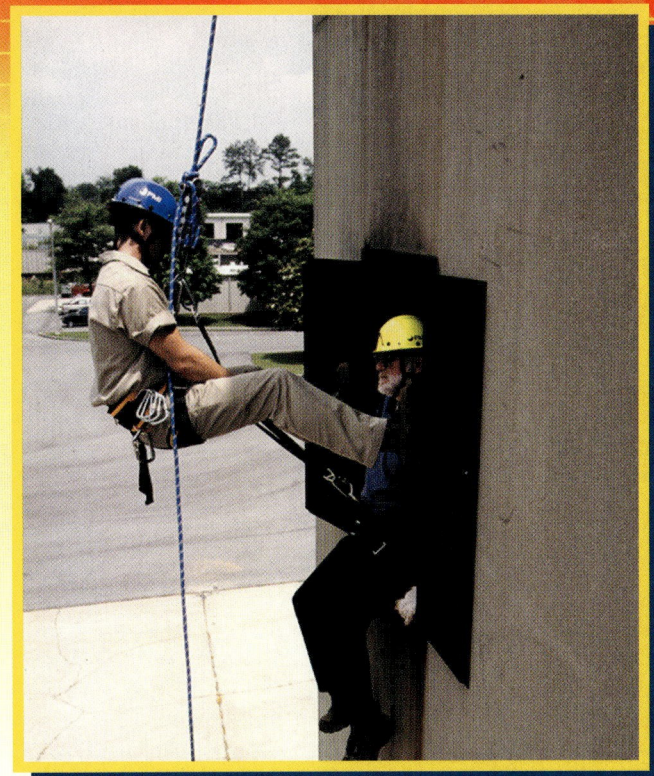

Prerequisites

Before attempting the activities described in this chapter, you must have demonstrated that you can properly:

1. Use and care for rope.
2. Use and care for other equipment needed in the high angle environment.
3. Tie correctly and without hesitation the knots necessary for safe, effective work in the vertical environment (see Chapter 6).
4. Apply the principles of anchoring and rig a safe and secure anchor.
5. Apply the principles of belaying and safely and confidently belay another person using either a Münter hitch or a personal belay device.
6. Apply the principles of rappelling: rappel safely and under control, tie off the rappel device to operate hands free of the rappel device and rope, and then return to a safe and controlled rappel.
7. Apply the principles of ascending: tie correctly and without hesitation a Prusik hitch and know how to use it; comprehend the uses and limitations of mechanical ascenders; confidently and safely ascend a fixed rope using either friction hitches or mechanical ascenders; confidently and safely change over from rappelling to ascending and ascending to rappelling; and extricate yourself from a jammed rappel device or similar problem.

Objectives

On completion of this chapter, you should be able to:

1. Describe the kinds of conditions in which pickoff rescue techniques might be appropriate.
2. List the skills and equipment required for a pickoff rescue.
3. Discuss the rescue considerations and priorities in the following pickoff rescue situations: (1) subject wearing a seat harness, (2) subject not wearing a seat harness, (3) unconscious subject, and (4) hostile, combative subject.
4. Discuss the medical concerns and priorities in a pickoff rescue.
5. Safely and efficiently perform a pickoff rescue of a person wearing a seat harness.
6. Securely tie a hasty seat onto a subject with either a hasty seat harness or a combination hasty seat with tied chest harness.
7. Safely and efficiently perform a pickoff rescue of a person not wearing a seat harness.

The material in this chapter conforms to guidelines published by the National Fire Protection Association (NFPA), specifically standard 1983-01, *Standard for Fire Service Life Safety Rope and System Components* (2001), standard 1670, *Standard on Operations and Training for Technical Rescue Incidents 2004 edition*, and standard 1006, *Professional Qualifications for Rescue Technicians (2002)*. NFPA standards are revised regularly, and readers are advised to review the latest version of this standard.

Key Terms

Pickoff Rescue A rescue in the high angle environment involving an uninjured or slightly injured subject in which a single rescuer usually has direct physical contact with the subject and in which a litter is not initially used in the rescue operation.

Using the Pickoff Rescue

A **pickoff rescue** in the high angle environment involves a single rescuer who has direct physical contact with a rescue subject to remove the person from a hazardous situation. Other individuals may be involved in the rescue in support capacities or to perform vital tasks such as belaying. Teamwork and good communication are essential in a pickoff rescue.

Pickoff rescue techniques do not usually involve the use of a litter. Rather, the subject often is attached directly to the rescuer's rappel system, and the rescuer then rappels or is lowered so that control of the body weights of both rescuer and subject is maintained.

Although this chapter does not cover advanced techniques, two such procedures are worth mentioning here. In one such technique, a rescuer might ascend the rope with the subject attached to the rescuer's ascending system. In another advanced technique, the subject may be lowered by means of a braking device suspended on rope or attached to midface anchors while the rescuer remains in position on the rope.

Pickoff rescue generally is performed only when the subject is uninjured or only slightly injured. It is extremely difficult for only one person without a litter to rescue a seriously injured subject without complicating the injuries. It is essential, therefore, that pickoff rescuers evaluate and stabilize the subject's injuries before moving the individual. The only exception to this rule might be the existence of an immediate threat to life, such as a hazardous atmosphere, explosion, or fire.

To be able to evaluate a subject competently and treat injuries, pickoff rescuers should have emergency medical training at least to the level of DOT first responder and preferably to the level of emergency medical technician (EMT) or higher.

Most pickoff techniques require that the rescuer begin the procedure above the subject and rappel or be lowered to the subject's area. When access is available only from below, the rescuer begins below the subject and ascends a rope to the area.

Pickoff Rescue Situations

Pickoff rescue techniques might be used when:
- It is appropriate for only one person to perform the rescue
- There is a shortage of personnel or resources (or both)
- The urgency of the situation is such that there is no time to await additional personnel
- The benefits of a pickoff rescue outweigh the risks involved

A need for a pickoff rescue might arise in any of the following situations:
- A firefighter's interior exit is blocked during a fireground operation, and there is no time to set up a ladder and no opportunity for self-rescue.

- An equipment malfunction has stranded a high-rise window cleaner on the side of a building, out of reach of ladders.
- A construction worker has become stranded on scaffolding.
- A potential suicide has climbed to an exposed area to jump but is hesitating.
- A rock climber has fallen and is only slightly injured but needs assistance in getting off the face.
- A sightseer or picnicker has slipped onto a ledge and cannot go up or down.
- A hiker has blundered into dangerously steep terrain and is unable to move because of the danger of falling.

Teamwork and Communication

Pickoff rescue usually involves only one rescuer in direct contact with the person in distress. However, this does not mean that other rescuers will be kept from the operation. The rescue process will proceed more safely and efficiently if other skilled and knowledgeable people are involved in essential tasks, such as belaying, lowering or raising, spotting, and communications.

Also, if the rescue subject is to be rappelled or lowered to the ground and has injuries, personnel are needed at the arrival spot to attend to the individual's medical needs. Several people may be needed to perform a litter evacuation to an ambulance or to provide other medical care.

Skills and Equipment Required for a Pickoff Rescue

In a pickoff rescue, several sets of rope-work skills often are performed at the same time, and several different kinds of equipment are used simultaneously.

The success or failure of the operation hinges on whether the appropriate system was chosen for the rescue. The pickoff rescuer must have an absolute knowledge of the equipment and the ability to perform the necessary skills. This capability comes only with constant practice of the skills required for efficient use of the equipment.

Pickoff rescue procedures can involve multiple ropes in use together, along with more connecting lines, slings, and equipment. This poses a greater challenge in rope and equipment management. The rescuer must have the experience and knowledge to remain aware of all the rope, equipment, and webbing in use. He or she must prevent the damage that can occur when one rope runs across another (see p. 39), must keep the lines from tangling, and must be able to manipulate the required line without hesitation.

Anchors and other equipment used in a pickoff rescue must be able to withstand the potential load (such as the combined weight of two people) plus an appropriate system safety factor.

Before lowering the rappel line, the rescuer must size up the situation. If the subject is barely hanging on, hitting the person with the rope could knock him or her off the face. Also, if the rope is close to a panicky subject, the person could grab it, stopping the rappel or causing injury or death both to himself or herself and the rescuer.

A possible solution is to keep the rope in a bag and rappel with the bagged rope (see Protecting the Rappel Rope Below You, p. 139, along with the warning about rappelling with a bagged rope). The rescuer must always make sure there is enough rope in the bag to reach the bottom of the rappel.

As a rescuer, your choice of rappel device and the way you use it are critical to your ability to perform a pickoff rescue safely. The weight of two people is very difficult to control using, for example, a single wrapped figure 8. If you decide to use a large figure 8, you must increase friction by double wrapping the figure 8.

Another problem with using a figure 8 is that it tends to twist the rappel rope, aggravating your rope control problems. For greater control, consider using devices, such as the brake bar rack, that allow you to vary control according to the load.

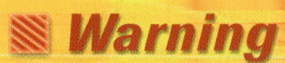

Warning

Pickoff rescues should be performed only by rescuers who have been trained in the technique and who have demonstrated the required skills.

The Belay Question

In some pickoff rescues, a belay may be desirable. However, it may not always be feasible. In fact, in some situations a belay could impede the operation or even endanger the individuals involved.

Consider, for example, a situation in which the rescuer and the subject each has his or her own rope. What would happen if both individuals were also belayed with additional separate ropes? *Four* ropes would now be involved. Rope tangle and possible damage from rope cross would be possible. The problem of rope management would increase as rescuers tried to decide which line went to specific harness tie-in points and how each line would affect other lines as angles changed with the positions of the people involved.

Situations in which a belay might be required include the following:

- Training and practice
- Prolonged operations, in which fatigue is a factor
- Exposure to objective hazards, such as falling debris

The question of whether to use a belay must be answered with decision making based on training, experience, and the specific situation.

Medical Considerations

Assessment is the most important aspect of medical considerations for the pickoff subject. A subject suitable for pickoff rescue has minor injuries and faces no risk of disability or life-threatening injuries.

The assessment of the subject should be thorough and as complete as possible considering the environment and precarious situation. Until this assessment has been completed, the rescuer should maintain spinal precautions as much as possible (see Chapter 12).

Assessment of the subject follows a simple format, which is presented in Box 14-1.

If the answer to any of the questions in Box 14-1 indicates that the subject has a problem in this area of patient assessment, consider whether it would be preferable to begin treatment and move the person with a litter evacuation rather than a pickoff rescue.

If the subject has very minor injuries (e.g., small lacerations, minor musculoskeletal injuries), it may be advisable to move the person with a pickoff rescue.

If no immediate threat to life exists, it may be wise to use an organized rescue team and follow proper spinal precautions with a litter. Erring on the side of patient care is always the best approach. For many groups, it takes just as long to perform a safe pickoff rescue as it does to perform a litter evacuation, because the latter procedure is practiced most.

Unless immediate, life-threatening environmental factors prevent it, at a minimum, the medical assessments just described must be made before a subject is moved and must continue during the course of the rescue.

Rescue of a Person Wearing a Seat Harness

Use of the technique for rescuing a person wearing a seat harness assumes that the subject is wearing a secure seat harness that will keep him or her relatively upright during the procedure. Box 14-2 lists the equipment needed for this procedure.

Pickoff Rescue Practice System

For a practice session for pickoff rescue techniques, the practice rescue subject should be in a stable position and only a short distance off the ground to minimize the possibility of injury from a fall.

As the training sessions move farther off the ground, practice subjects initially should be either tethered or belayed until the rescuers secure them.

Procedure for Pickoff Rescue of a Subject Wearing a Seat Harness (Figure 14-1)

1. Station a practice rescue subject wearing a seat harness in a position of minimum fall potential. Examples would be a low cliff ledge, a first-floor window of a practice building, or a low beam.
2. At the top you, as rescuer, rig one or more anchors for your main-line rope. Your rope should be off to the side of the rescue subject so that it does not knock rocks or other debris onto the person, but close enough so that you can easily pendulum over to the subject.

Box 14-1 — Format for the Medical Assessment of a Pickoff Rescue Subject

The parameters checked first include the following:
- ❑ Level of consciousness (e.g., alert, verbal, painful, unconscious [AVPU])
- ❑ General appearance
- ❑ Airway

Airway

- ❑ Does the subject have a clear airway?
- ❑ Do you need to maintain the airway during the rescue?
- ❑ Does the subject have objects in his or her mouth (e.g., gum, tobacco, dentures) that need to be removed?
- ❑ Is the subject vomiting or likely to vomit?
- ❑ How will you clear the vomitus during the course of the rescue so that the subject does not aspirate it?

Breathing

- ❑ Is the subject breathing spontaneously?
- ❑ Will you be able to monitor breathing during the course of the rescue?
- ❑ Will you need to perform rescue breathing before and during the rescue?

Circulation

- ❑ Does the subject have a pulse?
- ❑ Will you be able to monitor the pulse during the rescue operation?
- ❑ Is cardiopulmonary resuscitation (CPR) necessary and will it be possible during the rescue operation?
- ❑ Does the subject show signs of shock?
- ❑ What must be done immediately to treat for shock?
- ❑ What rescue procedures will increase or diminish the likelihood of shock?
- ❑ Is life-threatening bleeding a factor? If so, how can you stop it?
- ❑ Does the potential exist for life-threatening bleeding?

Spinal Injury

- ❑ Is spinal injury a possibility?
- ❑ Do you need to maintain spinal precautions while moving the patient?
- ❑ Should you secure the subject to a spinal immobilization device before moving the individual?

Box 14-2 — Equipment Needed for Rescue of a Person Wearing a Seat Harness

- ❑ One main-line rope with an adequate safety factor for a two-person load.
- ❑ One sewn, manufactured seat harness with thigh and leg supports for the rescuer.
- ❑ One rappel device with enough friction to handle the weight of two people and, preferably, with variable friction.
- ❑ Two large, locking carabiners (in addition to the locking carabiner already in the rescuer's seat harness tie-in point).
- ❑ One short sling (approximately 2 feet [0.6 m]) with a loop in both ends or an adjustable rescue pickoff strap that will support one person's weight with an adequate safety factor.

▨ Warning

During a pickoff rescue, anchors, rope, hardware, and personnel are subjected to suddenly increased loads, shock loading, and loads that may come from directions other than those anticipated. For these reasons, the following rules apply:

1. Anchors must be rigged for increased and multidirectional loading.
2. Carabiners must be locked, aligned in manner of function, and monitored so that they remain in manner of function.
3. The rescue system must have an adequate safety factor.
4. Rescuers must be prepared to handle sudden increases in weight and to provide extra friction on rappel devices.

3. Don a harness with leg and thigh supports. Clip a locking carabiner into the seat harness's front tie-in point.
4. Attach to the seat harness carabiner a rappel device that has both variable friction and enough control to handle the weight of two people. Lock the carabiner on the rappel device.

NOTE: The brake bar rack qualifies on both points. If one is not available, double wrap a large figure 8 with ears. Use the figure 8 only if you know from experience that you can control the combined weight of yourself and the rescue subject (see Gaining Extra Friction from the Figure 8 Descender, p. 125). Be aware, however, that this will complicate your personal rigging. If you plan to use this technique in pickoff rescue, practice it beforehand.

5. Clip a large locking carabiner onto one end of the rescue sling or adjustable rescue pickoff strap. For the moment, leave this first carabiner unlocked. With a second large locking carabiner, attach the other end of the sling into the rappel device tie-in point so that the weight of the rescue subject will be taken directly on the rappel device. *Do not clip this rescue sling directly into your seat harness* (Figure 14-2).

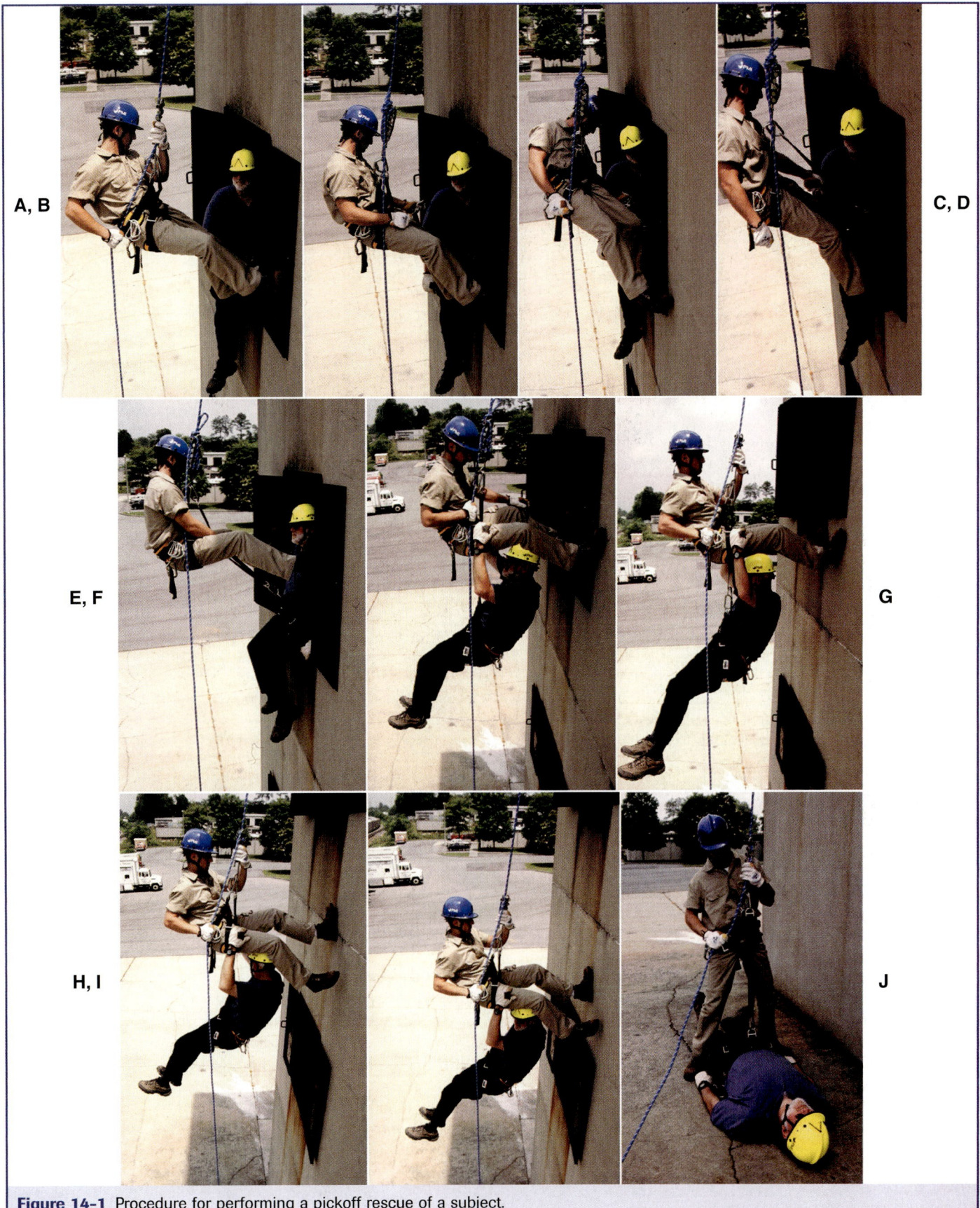

Figure 14-1 Procedure for performing a pickoff rescue of a subject.

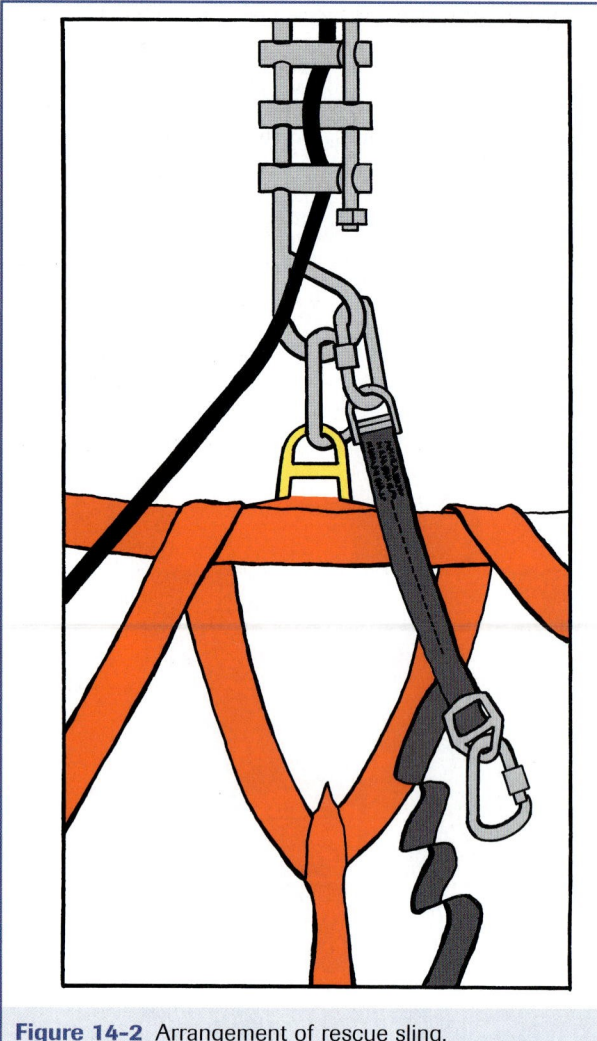

Figure 14-2 Arrangement of rescue sling.

Physical Situation

❑ Is the subject secure or in immediate danger of falling?
❑ Is there loose debris above the subject that your rope could dislodge?

Emotional Situation

❑ Is the subject hostile to you?
❑ Is the subject about to grab you?
❑ Will the subject follow directions?
❑ Is the subject comfortable in the high angle environment?
❑ Is the subject experienced in high angle work so that he or she can assist in the procedure?

Initial Assessment of the Subject's Medical Needs

❑ Is the subject conscious and alert?
❑ Is the subject breathing?
❑ Is uncontrolled bleeding present?
❑ Is spinal injury a possibility?
❑ What are the obvious injuries?
❑ What are the subject's physical complaints?

| Box 14-4 | **Communicating with the Rescue Subject** |

❑ Reassure the subject.
❑ Tell the subject who you are.
❑ Tell the subject exactly what you plan to do.
❑ Ask if the subject is injured.
❑ Describe in detail how you will perform the rescue.
❑ Tell the subject how he or she can help:
   1. Do not move until told to do so.
   2. Do not grab anything unless told to do so.

6. Lock the carabiner that connects the rescue sling to the rappel device tie-in point.

7. Rappel to the rescue subject (see Figure 14-1, *A*). Slow your rappel as you approach the subject. Simultaneously size up the situation (Box 14-3) and communicate with the subject (Box 14-4).

8. Stop and tie off your rappel device when you are about 2 feet (0.6 m) above the level of the subject (see Figure 14-1, *B*). *Always stop above the subject.* If initially you are too high to reach the subject, you can always unlock and rappel down; if you are too low, you may have problems completing the rescue technique.

9. Have the subject stay put, if possible in a sitting position. While you are talking with the person, begin your initial medical evaluation.

10. Take the large locking carabiner at the bottom of the sling attached to your rappel system, lean over and clip it directly into the subject's seat harness tie-in point. *Do not clip into any parts of the harness not meant to support the load of the wearer.* Eliminate as much slack in the sling as possible. *Avoid slack in the rescue sling* (see Figure 14-1, *C*).

11. After clipping the rescue sling into the main part of the subject's harness, immediately lock the carabiner. You now have the subject secured to your system. If you are using an adjustable pickoff sling, take up all the slack in the sling (see Figure 14-1, *D*).

12. Brace with your legs spread wide and your feet against the wall (see Figure 14-1, *E*).

13. Tell the subject to do the following:
   ▪ If the person is not sitting but is able to do so, tell him or her to get into a sitting position.
   ▪ Have the subject place his or her legs together between yours.
   ▪ Have the subject place his or her hands on your legs for support.
   ▪ As the subject holds onto your legs, have the person very slowly swing down between your legs until his or her weight comes onto the sling. While the subject is doing this, direct the person, reassure him or her, and brace so that you and the subject do not slip (see Figure 14-1, *F*).

- Tell the subject that he or she can hold onto the sling to feel more steady. For balance, keep the weighted sling between your legs during the remainder of the procedure.

14. When the subject's full weight is on the sling and the person has stabilized, unlock your rappel device and begin to rappel very slowly (Figure 14-1, *G*).
15. If you are close enough to the cliff or building face, fend away from it with your feet.
16. As you approach the ground, tell the subject to lie down as his or her body touches the ground. You will straddle the subject.
17. When the subject is in a stable position, with his or her weight off the rescue sling, disconnect the person from your system by unclipping the individual from the short sling.
18. Remove your rappel device from the rope.

Removing the Subject's Weight on Rope

Note that in the above procedure, the stranded subject is not hanging on rope. A stranded subject hanging on a rope may create additional challenges. If the subject is attached to a tied-off rappel device, then after the subject has been secured to the rescuer's system, the rescuer may be able to slowly free the subject from the rappel device and bring the person's weight onto the rescuer's system.

However, if the subject is tied directly to the end of a rope, such as may occur with a fallen climber, the problem becomes lifting the climber up a short distance to free him or her from that rope. The rescuer may have to construct a miniature hauling system to use when on rope. (See Chapter 18 for possible approaches to this problem.)

![Warning]

⚠ **Warning**

When performing pickoff rescue techniques, do not clip any attachments supporting the weight of the rescue subject directly into your own seat harness, for the following reasons:
1. Painful and possibly damaging pressure may be exerted on the rescuer's body, particularly in the groin area.
2. The seat harness will be stressed in an unnatural manner, which creates the potential for damage and failure.

Rescue of a Subject Not Wearing a Seat Harness
Placing a Manufactured Seat Harness on the Subject

There is a good chance that the subject of a pickoff rescue will not be wearing a seat harness. In such cases the rescue procedures essentially are the same except that the rescuer must either put a sewn, manufactured harness on the subject or tie a hasty harness onto him or her.

Placing the harness for rescue can be a very difficult process. The rescuer probably will be hanging on a rope at a difficult angle (perhaps even upside down), dealing with a frightened and perhaps injured subject, in difficult environmental conditions.

Because of these difficulties, the student rescuer first should practice a pickoff rescue on a subject wearing a seat harness and then try a pickoff that requires placing a seat harness on the subject.

Some manufactured pickoff devices are easy to apply while the rescuer is hanging from a rope and are designed specifically so that the subject does not have to step in or through them. Some of these are designed like a diaper (Figure 14-3), and others are easily applied harnesses. If available, a manufactured pickoff harness usually is preferable to an improvised, tied one. The following points should be considered when purchasing such devices:

- The harness should be designed so that it can be placed on the subject with as little disruption as possible. In particular, it should be able to be donned without the subject becoming unbalanced by having to step into the harness.
- The harness must be easy to figure out and quick to put on. It should not have a multitude of buckles, snaps, or adjustments.

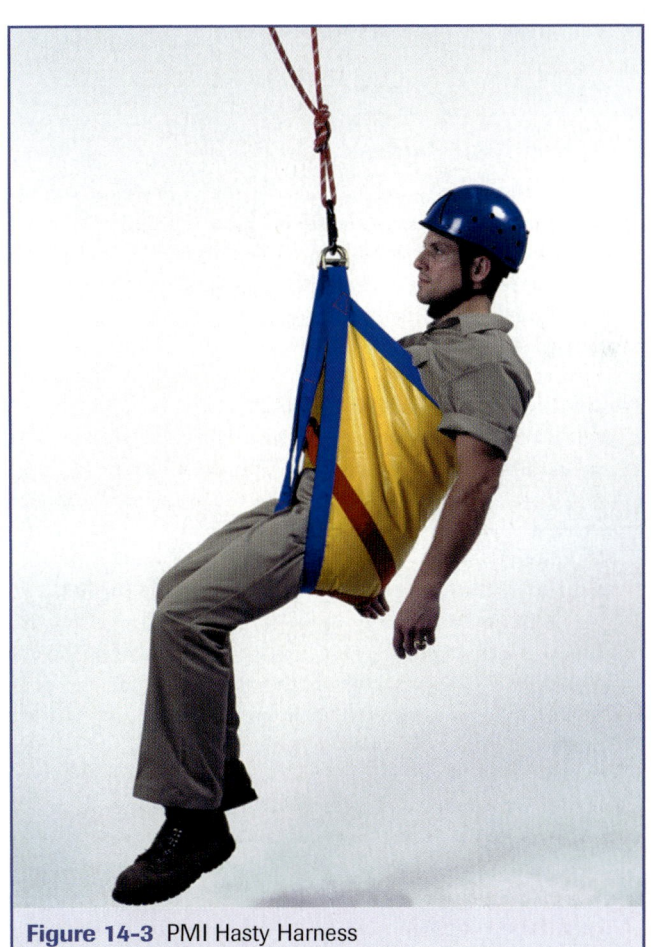

Figure 14-3 PMI Hasty Harness

Placing a Tied Seat Harness on the Subject

A variety of tied harnesses can be used for a pickoff rescue. Some points to consider when choosing one include the following:

- The rescuer should be able to tie the harness with a minimum of physical disruption to the subject.
- The harness should be quick and easy to tie under difficult conditions.
- The harness should be self-adjusting.

⬛ *Warning*

1. Before you go over the edge in a rappel, particularly in a rescue, check for loose personal items or vertical gear. All items and gear must be secured so that they do not fall out of pockets, packs, or gear slings. In addition to possibly injuring the rescue subject or other rescuers, you may lose an essential piece of equipment just when you need it the most.
2. Always perform a last-minute safety check:
   - ❏ Make sure harness buckles are correctly secured and all carabiners are locked and aligned in the correct manner of function.
   - ❏ Make sure knots are tied correctly and anchors are secure.
   - ❏ Check for any loose clothing or hair that might be drawn into the descender.
   - ❏ Make sure your helmet is secure.

Tied Hasty Seat Harness

The hasty seat harness can be placed on a subject with a minimum of disruption. It is created from a piece of tubular webbing 10 to 15 feet (3 to 4.6 m) long, depending on the size of the subject. Before the rescuer begins the rappel, the webbing is tied in a continuous loop using a ring bend (water knot) that is backed up.

Tying a Hasty Seat Harness (Figure 14-4)

1. If possible, approach the subject from behind. Place the loop across the subject's shoulder so that the sides of the loop hang down along his or her side and the top of the loop runs across the back of the subject's neck.
2. With both hands, reach around the sides and under the arms of the subject and the vertically hanging sides of the loop.
3. Reach down with either or both hands, go between the subject's legs *from the front,* and grasp the bottom of the loop. Take the loop firmly in both hands.
4. Pull the loop back through the subject's legs and up toward the front of his or her waist.
5. As you pull the loop up through the subject's legs, let the top section of the loop running across the subject's shoulders fall down the back. If necessary, you can help this along with your chin or head.
6. Continue pulling on the lower end of the loop. As you pull the slack out of the loop from behind, the webbing will slide down your arms and past your hands to form the harness.

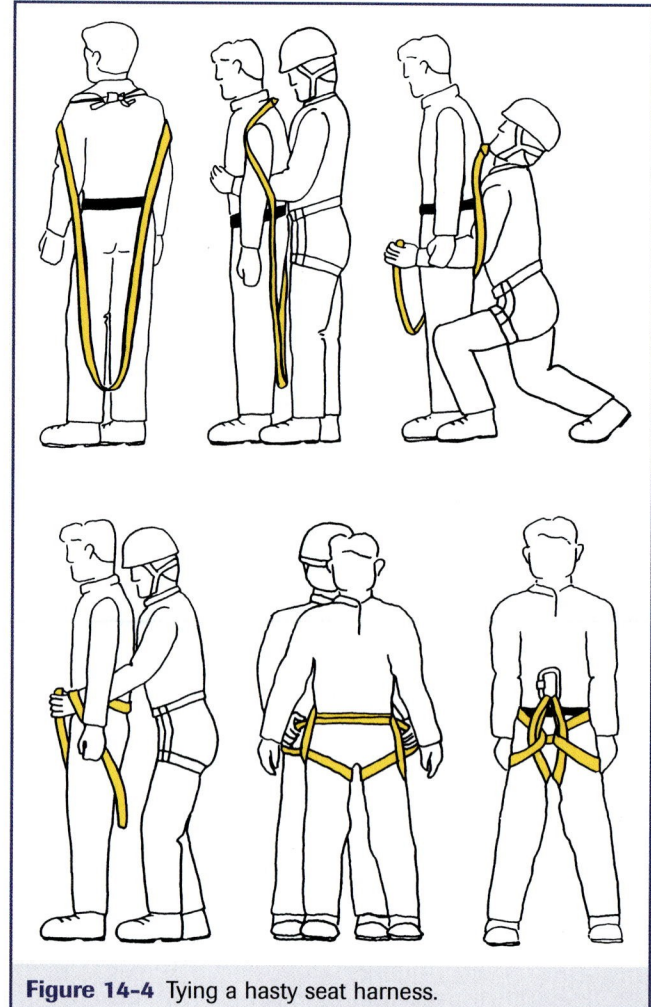

Figure 14-4 Tying a hasty seat harness.

7. To cinch down the webbing, take a loop in each hand and pull each one to an opposite side so that the webbing is contoured around the subject's body. Make sure the webbing remains taut.
8. Bring the two loops back to the center and clip them together with a locking carabiner.

Rescue Chest Harness

A rescue chest harness is used for subjects who have trouble remaining upright in a seat harness. Such individuals include people with large upper body size in relation to the lower body or with "spare tires." They tend to lean back or even fall over backward when positioned only in a harness. Placing a chest harness on a rescue subject can help hold the person upright. Figure 14-5 shows a rescue chest harness. This chest harness *must not be used by itself in pickoff rescue;* it must be used together with a rescue seat harness, such as the hasty seat harness or a sewn, manufactured seat harness.

Tying the Rescue Chest Harness

Figure 14-6 shows the procedure for tying a quick chest harness, which can be used together with a seat harness for a pickoff rescue.

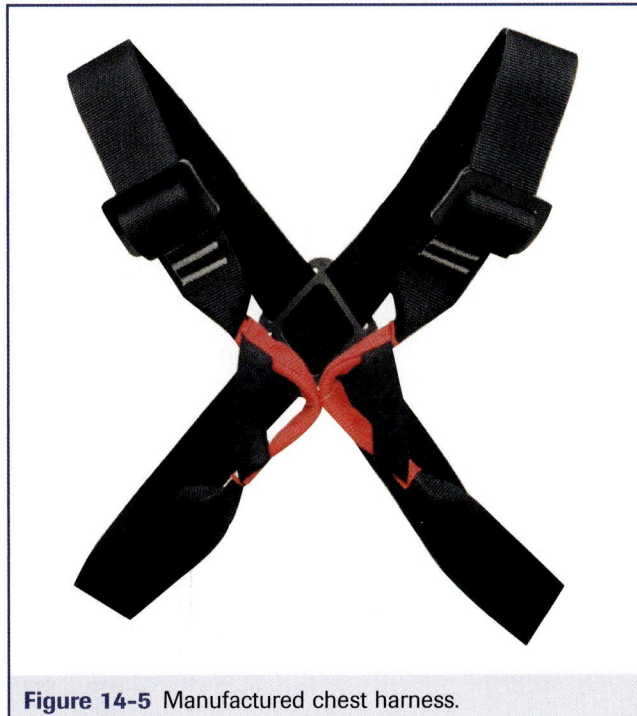

Figure 14-5 Manufactured chest harness.

1. Take a continuous loop of webbing tied with a ring bend (water knot) backed up with an overhand knot, or use a sewn continuous loop.
2. Twist the loop into a figure **8**.
3. Lay the loop across the subject's back with the loop crossing on the back at armpit height.
4. One at a time, put the subject's arms through each loop.
5. Bring each loop to the center of the chest.
6. Clip the loops together with a carabiner. Or, if the harness is too loose, pull one loop through the other and clench it down. Clip a carabiner through the long loop.
7. Make sure the seat and chest system is equalized. Neither the seat harness nor the chest harness should take the full load. They should be stable so that the subject does not "accordion" when the load is applied at acute angles.

Combining the Chest Harness with the Rescue System

8. Clip the carabiner from the chest harness into the end of the rescue sling (where you have previously clipped the carabiner for the seat harness). Do not clip the two carabiners together, so that you can adjust either the seat harness or the chest harness.

Alternative Approach: Lowering/ Raising Pickoff

One approach to a rappel pickoff is the lowering and possible raising of the rescuer from the top. In this procedure, a lowering team at the top lowers a rescuer to the subject. The procedure usually involves two ropes: a main-line rope for the rescuer and subject and a separate belay line.

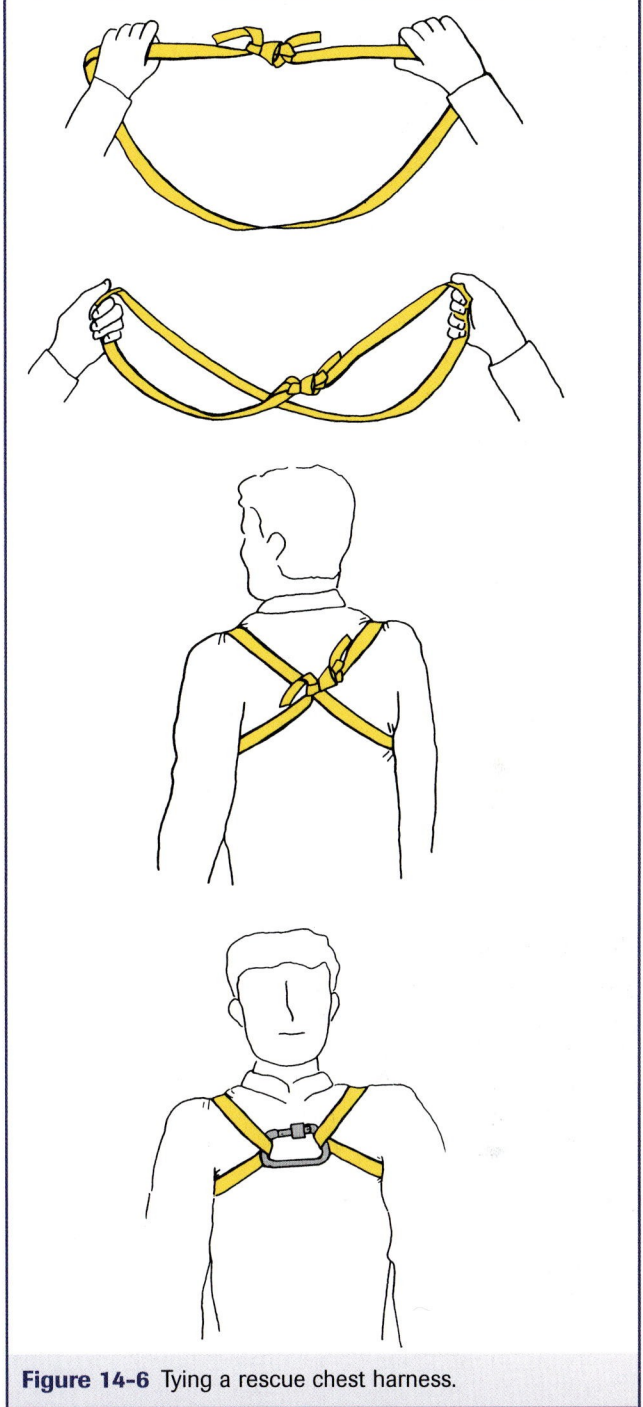

Figure 14-6 Tying a rescue chest harness.

The lowering team lowers the rescuer to the subject. The rescuer attaches the subject to the main-line system and to the separate belay system. The team at the top then either lowers both individuals to the ground or attaches a haul system and hauls both to the top.

Advantages

- Allows the rescuer greater use of the hand that would be used for rappelling
- May ensure greater control of the lowering; includes a belay

Disadvantages

- Requires more personnel
- Requires more complete communication
- Requires team practice to coordinate the procedure

See Chapters 17 and 18 for additional information on lowering and hauling for rescue.

Rescue of an Unconscious Subject
Medical Considerations

An unconscious subject should be rescued using a litter unless there are overriding considerations, such as an immediate threat to life. If a litter cannot be used for an unconscious subject, special pickoff rescue techniques may be required.

In addition to the primary survey for *airway, breathing, and circulation (ABCs)*, an unconscious subject poses particular medical considerations:

- If a particular threat of airway blockage exists, continuous attention must be paid to keeping it clear.

- If unconsciousness is the result of trauma (e.g., from a fall) or if the cause is unknown, it must be assumed that the subject has a spinal cord injury and spinal immobilization is required.
- Because the subject may not be able to describe his or her injuries, hidden injuries (e.g., fractures) may be present.

When a person becomes unconscious, hearing is the last sense to go. Therefore always talk positively with an unconscious subject, even though you suspect he or she is unable to hear you. This communication eventually may elicit a response and may prevent the person from becoming combative.

An unconscious subject is unable to hold himself or herself upright or to fend off from the face of a building or cliff. Consequently, the unconscious subject should be in a full-body harness or combination seat/chest harness, whether manufactured or tied.

Evaluation Exercises

Cognitive and Affective Exercises

1. Describe the general medical condition of the subject in most pickoff rescues.

2. Unless an immediate threat to life exists (e.g., hazardous atmosphere, explosion, or fire), what should a pickoff rescuer do before moving the subject?

3. Name three general circumstances in which a pickoff rescue technique might be appropriate.

4. Give two reasons why you must size up the situation before dropping your rope to rappel for a pickoff rescue.

5. What is one possible way to keep your rappel rope secure in a pickoff situation?

6. Regarding medical considerations, what is the most important factor for the pickoff subject?

7. List the minimum equipment required for the rescue of a subject wearing a seat harness.

8. In a pickoff rescue, where should the end of the pickoff strap closest to the rescuer be attached?

9. After you have assembled the gear and rigged for a pickoff rescue, what is the one thing you should always do before going over the edge?

10. What should be your position in relationship to the subject when you stop and tie off your rappel device to perform a pickoff rescue?

11. In addition to the primary survey for airway, breathing, and circulation (the ABCs), what are two major medical considerations associated with an unconscious subject in a pickoff rescue?

12. Name three requirements for a full-body combination seat and chest harness used for the subject in a pickoff rescue.

15

Use of Litters in High Angle Rescue

Michael V. Callahan, Tom Vines, Steve Hudson

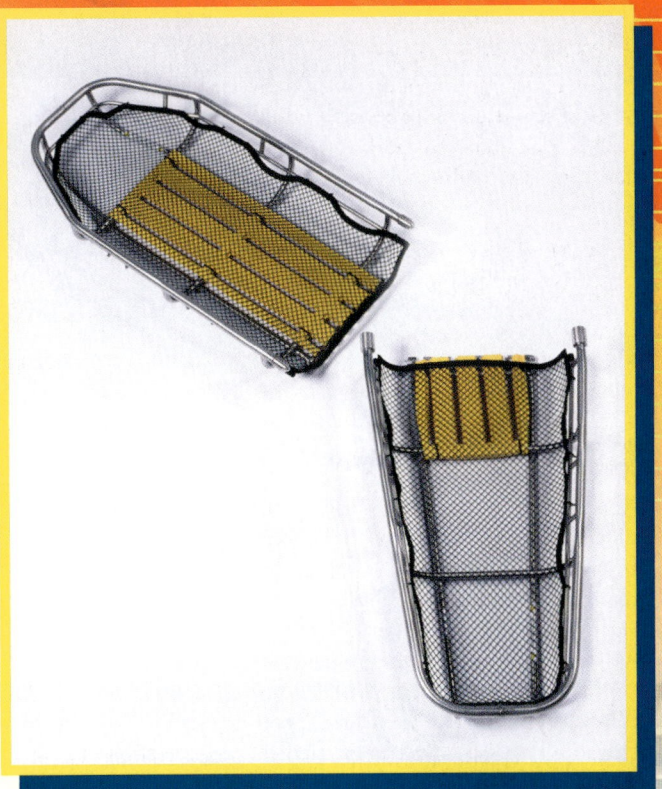

The material in this chapter conforms to guidelines published by the National Fire Protection Association (NFPA), specifically standard 1006, *Professional Qualifications for Rescue Technicians* (2002), and standard 1670, *Operations and Training for Technical Rescue Incidents* (2004). NFPA standards are revised regularly, and readers are advised to review the latest version of this standard.

Objectives

On completion of this chapter, you should be able to:

1. Describe the requirements for litters used in rope rescue.
2. List the advantages and disadvantages of plastic litters.
3. List the advantages and disadvantages of break-apart litters.
4. List the advantages and disadvantages of flexible litters, such as the Sked litter.
5. List the major concerns for packaging a subject in a litter.
6. List the requirements for a spine board to be used in a litter.
7. Package a subject in a litter so as to protect the person from major environmental effects.
8. Use webbing to tie a subject into a litter in a manner that addresses concerns about physical stabilization and prevention of injury.

Basket Litter A litter with a rigid structure that is shaped to hold a rescue subject. It is constructed of rugged materials so as to protect the subject and to resist damage when used in the rescue environment.

Break-Apart Litter A litter designed to be separated into sections so that it can be transported to the rescue site more easily and can be stored in smaller spaces.

Flexible Litter A litter that does not have an inherent rigid structure, but rather is made of a flexible material, usually plastic, that can be wrapped closely around the subject.

Litters in Rescue Operations

Rope rescue often means dealing with an injured or ill individual. Transportation of the injured or sick person from the rescue environment to an ambulance or helicopter usually requires a litter. Knowing how to package the subject in the litter and how to move the litter holding a subject are essential skills for the rope rescue technician. This chapter reviews the common types of litters used for rescue, how to package the subject in commonly used litters, comfort and protection for a subject in a litter, some basic medical considerations for litter subjects, and some basic suggestions for moving the litter.

Attaching the litter to a rope rescue system requires additional rigging not detailed in this chapter. Rigging of litters is discussed in Chapter 16 (for low angle evacuation) and Chapter 17 (for high angle lowering).

Litter Functions

Litters provide the following basic functions in the rescue environment:

- They serve as a means of transporting a sick or injured subject.
- They help to physically stabilize the subject during transport.
- They protect the subject from physical and environmental hazards and from further injury.
- They provide a means of attaching the subject to the rescue system.
- They provide a platform for medical interventions and equipment

Types of Litters
Metal Basket Litters

The litter traditionally used in rescue operations is the *basket litter*, sometimes called a *Stokes litter*. At one time, the term *Stokes* referred to a specific design of wire basket litter, but it now often is used as a generic term for a basket litter. The word *basket* suggests that the litter contains the subject to help keep him or her from falling out. When rescuers use a basket litter, they are said to place the subject *in* it as opposed to placing the subject *on* the type of stretcher commonly used in ambulances or hospitals.

Basket litters for rescue are constructed of rugged materials that help protect the subject and resist damage in the rescue environment. Basket litters may be constructed of a wire frame and covered either with a metal or plastic mesh (Figure 15-1). The stronger metal litters have support members constructed of tubular stainless steel. Lighter weight litters made of conventional steel tubing and metal strap are not as strong and do not provide as much subject protection.

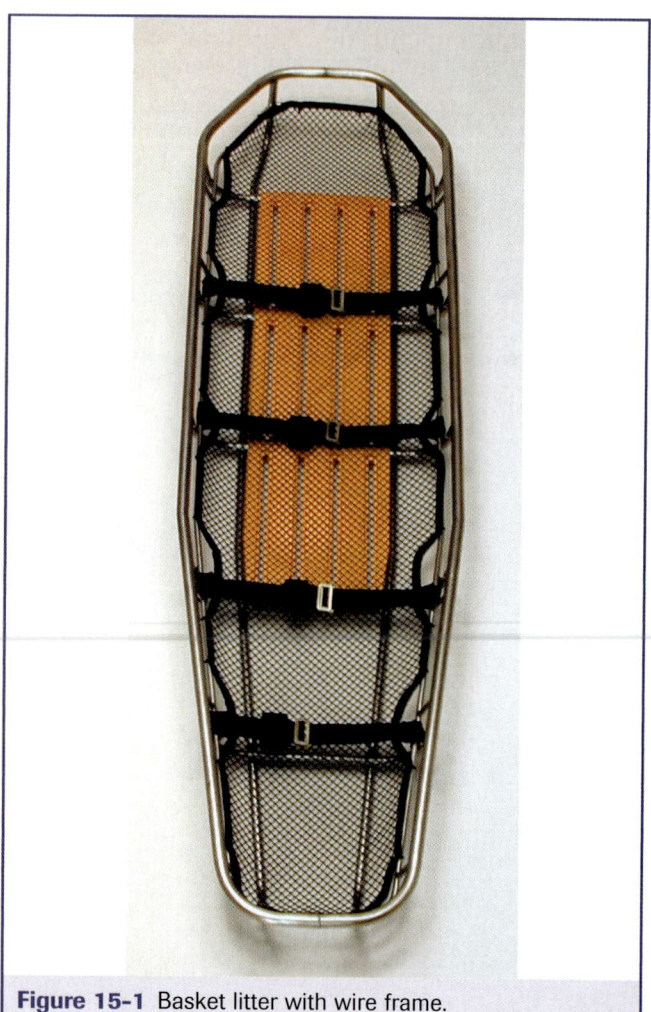

Figure 15-1 Basket litter with wire frame.

Older litters may have been abused, may suffer from rust damage, or litter welds may have degraded — three factors that together weaken the litter. Plastic-coated steel models may appear to be in good condition, but corrosion may be present under the coating.

The titanium tubing litter is a recent innovation that provides an extremely lightweight and strong basket. Titanium models cost more than traditional metal basket litters.

Some models of basket litters have a leg divider. These litters cannot accommodate a standard spine board. Basket litters have either a rectangular shape or are tapered at the foot end. The rectangular shape allows the subject to be loaded with the head at either end and permits use of wider spine boards.

Basket litters in the traditional shape may be difficult to maneuver through confined spaces. Some of the newer basket litters have a narrow profile, allowing them to be moved more easily through confined spaces.

Fabric inserts sometimes are used to replace the mesh of basket litters. The inserts are designed with solid or mesh fabric and are attached with straps to the bottom litter rail. Pulled tight, an insert forms a flat, raised surface above the bottom of the litter. The insert adds to the subject's comfort and makes it easier to slide the subject into the litter. However, because an insert raises the subject higher in the litter, it changes the loading dynamics of a litter.

Among the most popular basket litters are those manufactured by Ferno and its subsidiary, Traverse Rescue, Cascade Toboggan, and by Junkin Safety Appliance Co. (Louisville, Kentucky).

Plastic Basket Litters

Plastic basket litters are available in two basic designs. One type is all plastic except for a metal top rail (Figure 15-2). The other type has a stainless steel frame, similar to that of a metal basket litter, with a plastic shell (Figure 15-3). The second type is stronger, maintaining strength even if the plastic is fractured, and has more metal attachment points, allowing for a variety of rigging options.

Plastic litters are not as strong and usually do not last as long as the better (stainless steel or titanium) metal basket litters. Plastic litters should not be exposed to sunlight for extended periods, because ultraviolet radiation degrades the plastic, causing it to fade and become brittle. Older models of plastic litters are particularly susceptible to this type of deterioration, and the plastic may fracture when stressed under extremely cold conditions.

Advantages of Plastic Litters

- Usually weigh less than most metal litters
- Slide easily along rough surfaces and snow
- More protection for subject

Disadvantages of Plastic Litters

- May degrade with time (plastic parts)
- May retain water and snow if not properly drained
- May be blown about in high winds and helicopter rotor wash

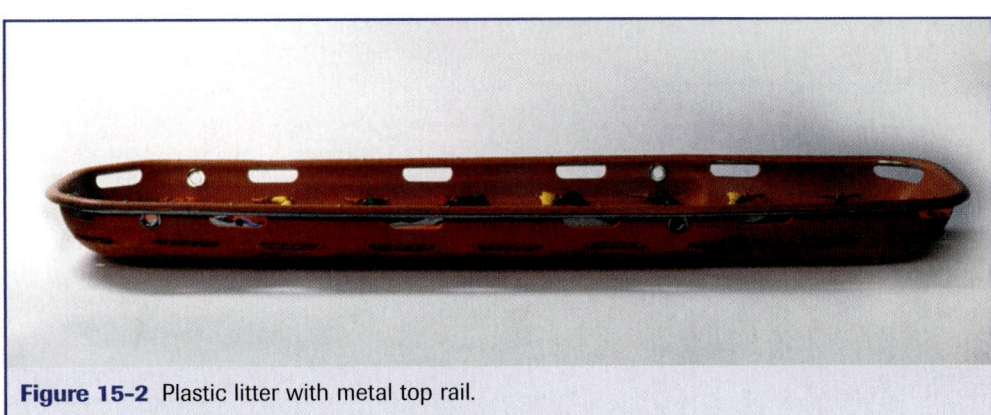

Figure 15-2 Plastic litter with metal top rail.

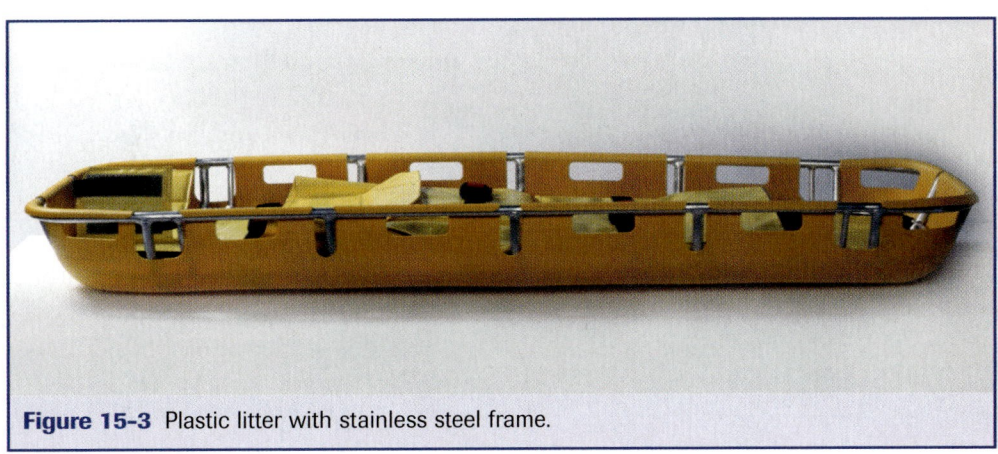

Figure 15-3 Plastic litter with stainless steel frame.

The two most popular models of plastic litters used in rescue operations are the Ferno-Washington 71 and the Junkin JSA-200.

Break-Apart Litters

A *break-apart litter* can be broken down into sections for easier transportation to the rescue site (Figure 15-4). When separated into sections, it can be lashed to a pack frame or packed into a vehicle space smaller than that required for one-piece litters.

Before a break-apart litter is used for high angle rescue, the way the portions are connected and the strength of the litter once the sections have been joined must be taken into consideration. Some break-apart designs are joined by quick-release pins, which may be a weak point in a litter rigged for high angle work. To account for possible failure of the break-apart joint, some rescue teams back up the joint with webbing.

Another problem is that the pins for the litter can easily be lost and may be more difficult to manipulate in certain conditions, such as cold weather. The Traverse break-apart litter connects on the bottom with two bars with interlocking teeth that act as a hinge, and the top rails connect with a locking sleeve.

Although break-apart litters are more compact when broken down, they are slightly heavier than the one-piece designs. They also are more expensive than one-piece litters.

Choosing a Litter for Rescue Operations

If the litter is to be used for rescue operations, only those designed and constructed for this purpose should be purchased.

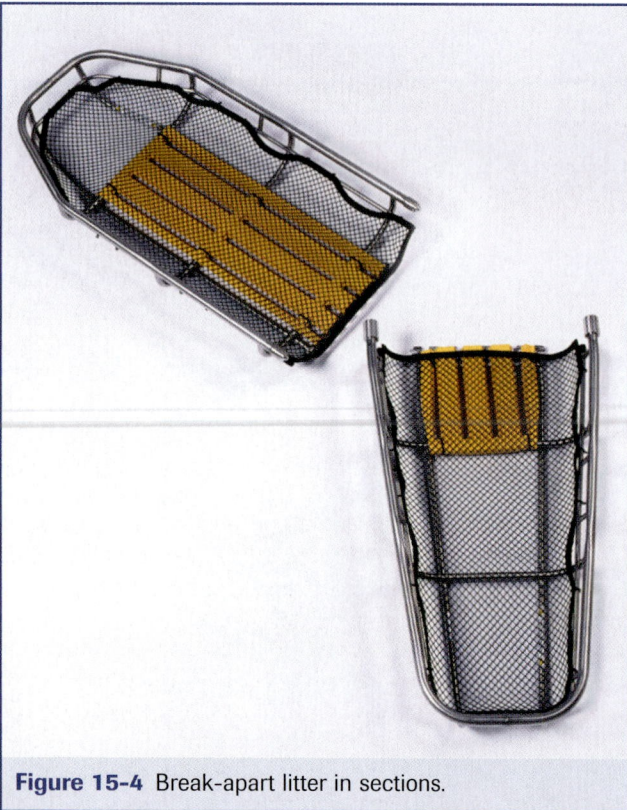

Figure 15-4 Break-apart litter in sections.

Litters for high angle rescue must be strong enough to allow rigging for rescue and to support the weight of the subject and litter attendant. Litters for rope rescue need strong, convenient tie-in points to which rescuers can attach rigging. The litters must be durable enough to resist damage and to protect subjects against the effects of impacts with rocks, walls, trees, and debris, which often occur with handling of a litter in the rescue environment. Rescue litters should have at least three handholds on each side and two at each end that rescuers can easily and comfortably grip while transporting a subject.

Cheaper litters, which are sold for the first aid and mass casualty markets, are not designed for the potential loads found in high angle rope rescue. The so-called chicken wire metal mesh found in some cheaper litters should be avoided, because it has sharp ends that can cut skin, tear fabric, and puncture vacuum splints. Also if a secondhand litter is used, its history must be known. Litters may have corrosion or a history of abuse, which means they could fail under the stress of rescue.

Flexible Litters

Unlike a basket litter, a *flexible litter* does not have an inherent rigid structure; rather, it wraps closely around the subject. Because of their flexibility, these litters often are easier to work through confined spaces.

Sked Litter

The Sked litter (Skedco, Portland, Oregon) (Figure 15-5) is a commonly used flexible litter. It consists of a heavy sheet of polyethylene plastic about 3×8 feet (0.9×2.6 m) when laid out flat. When the Sked is conformed around the subject like a cocoon, the litter becomes more rigid (Figure 15-6). The litter has built-in straps and buckles to help form the Sked around the subject. Because it conforms to the subject's size, thus creating a relatively small additional cross-sectional area, the Sked often is easier to move through confined spaces than are basket litters. Most Sked litters have an adaptable harness system that allows the subject to be transported either in the horizontal or the vertical position. The Sked can be rolled into a compact shape that is stored or transported in its own backpack, which is 9 inches (22.9 cm) in diameter and 36 inches (91.4 cm) long. Accessories for the Sked, such as rigging straps and the Oregon Spine Splint half spine board, can be stored in this package.

Advantages of Flexible Litters

- Lightweight
- Can be stored or carried in a compact backpack
- Adaptable
- Drag easily over rough surfaces even when pulled only from one end.
- Reasonable cost

Disadvantages of Flexible Litters

- Require additional spine immobilization
- Not rigid enough to be carried by two people at either end
- Not as convenient as basket litters for litter teams to carry when loaded with a subject

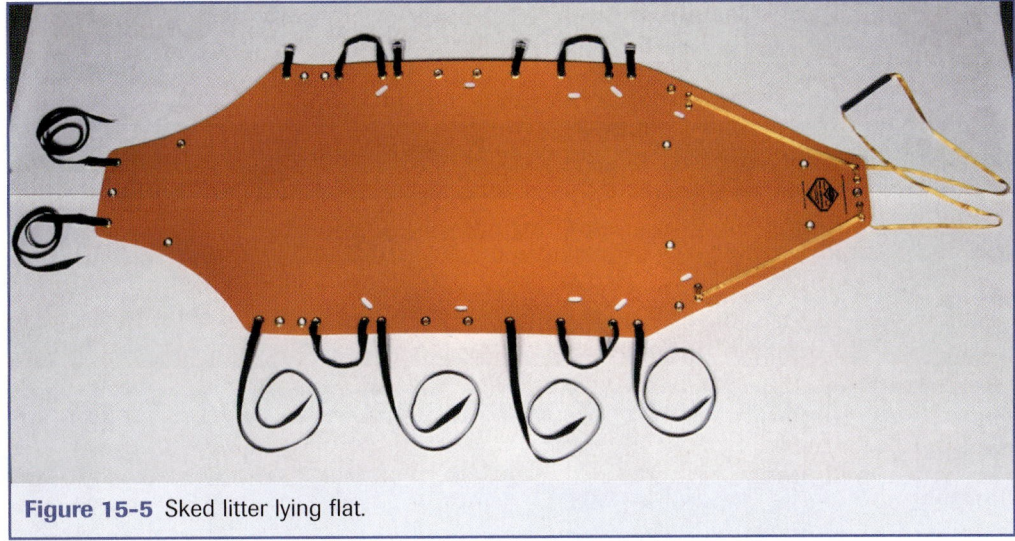

Figure 15-5 Sked litter lying flat.

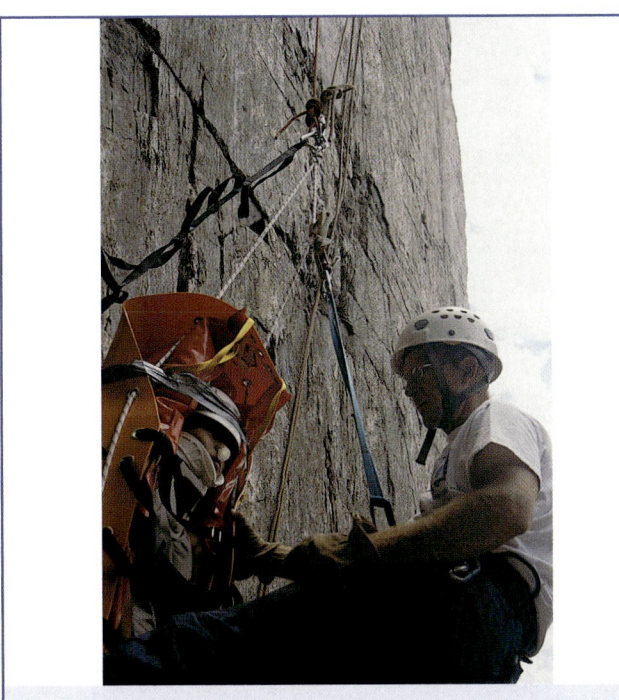

Figure 15-6 Sked litter conformed around a subject.

- Catch wind and rotor wash
- Cannot be used with most litter wheels

Protecting Spinal Injuries in Flexible Litters

Subjects suspected of having spinal injuries who are transported in flexible litters, such as the Sked, also require spinal immobilization. The method used to immobilize the spine in flexible litters varies with the model of litter. For example, the Oregon Spine Splint (Skedco, Portland, Oregon) was designed to be used in the Sked, but it also can be used in other types of litters. The rescue team should practice their spinal immobilization technique with the litter to determine in advance the best system.

Packaging the Subject in the Litter

Packaging is the term used for placing the injured or ill subject in a litter and securing the individual for evacuation. Packaging concerns include the following:

- Protecting the subject from physical and environmental hazards
- Providing for the subject's comfort
- Physically stabilizing the subject to prevent harmful movement
- Protecting medical equipment, such as intravenous (IV) access sites or bandages

Protecting the Subject in the Litter
Protecting the Subject's Underside

Protecting the underside of the subject is a particular concern in a wire basket litter. This type of litter is uncomfortable and offers little protection on the bottom from protruding objects such as twigs, branches, or stones. To protect the bottom and make the litter more comfortable, line the litter with material such as a closed-cell foam pad and/or blankets. Make sure to pad hollow spaces along the body, such as behind the knees and in the small of the back.

Protecting the Subject from Environmental Effects

The subject should be protected from wind, cold, and rain with a waterproof and windproof outer layer. If the environment is cold, line the bottom with a foam pad or blankets for extra insulation. A waterproof layer can be provided with a large, plastic tarp about 15 feet (4.5 m) square. Lay out the tarp on the litter before placing the subject in the litter (Figure 15-7).

When providing insulation for subject warmth, use material that allows access to all sides of the subject. Sleeping bags should have zippers or Velcro closures that open all around the subject's torso. The commercially made hypothermia bags used in hospital transport work well. If such sleeping bags or hypothermia bags are not available, blankets can be used.

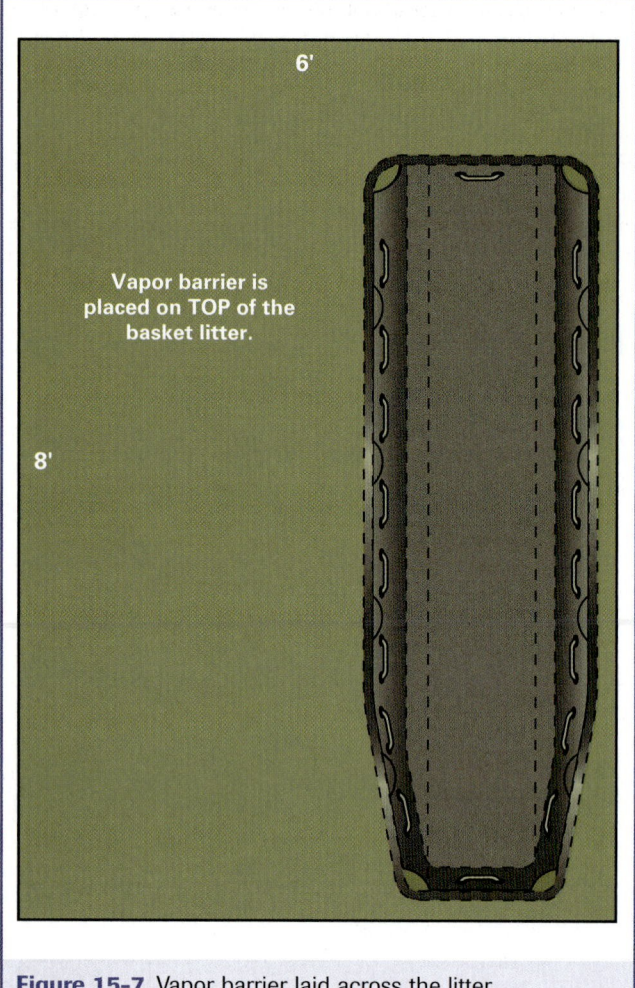

Figure 15-7 Vapor barrier laid across the litter.

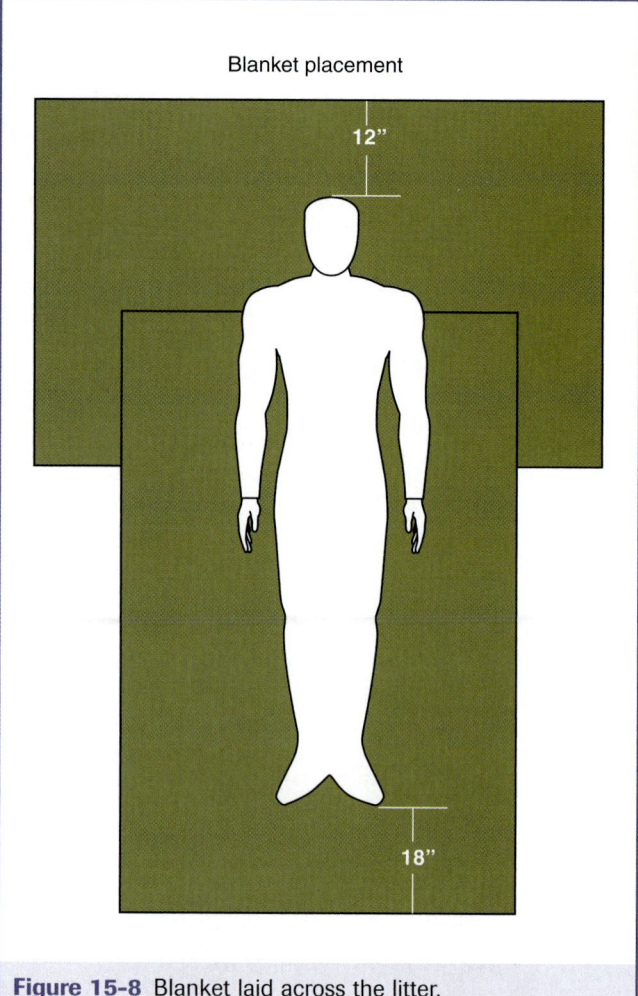

Figure 15-8 Blanket laid across the litter.

The following method works well for improving environmental protection:

1. Lay a blanket across the litter (Figure 15-8). The blanket should be made of a nonabsorbent layer, such as polyester, to help keep the patient's skin dry.
2. Place the subject in the litter and wrap the blanket around the person.
3. Fold the waterproof tarp over the subject (Figure 15-9).

Remember that subjects may saturate the insulation with blood, spilled IV fluids, and waste, and this increases heat loss. Wet insulation should be removed and replaced at the first opportunity.

Protecting the Subject's Face and Eyes

Litter subjects usually cannot shield their faces from branches or their eyes from falling debris or rain. Face and eye protection may include a litter shield (Figure 15-10) (which can produce claustrophobia in some subjects), a face shield or, at the least, goggles. Many a subject has complained that rescuers dropped debris into the person's face as they worked near or stepped over the litter.

Airway Management

As with other forms of emergency medical care, the subject must be packaged with concern for airway management. Package the individual so that you can roll the subject package in case of vomiting or other airway threats. The litter bridle (see p. 261) must be rigged such that the subject can be turned on his or her side to allow the airway to be cleared. A suction device should be placed near the head. If a mask or pharyngeal airway (endotracheal or nasotracheal tube) is required, it should be placed before the litter is moved. Airways should be stabilized to prevent displacement during movement. The suction device should be placed where it can be reached quickly.

As a practical matter, it is difficult to clear the airway effectively while wearing protective leather gloves. Litter attendants should wear rubber gloves underneath the rope rescue gloves and should practice quick glove removal during training.

Cervical Spine Considerations

Subjects suspected of having cervical spine injuries (which are most rescue subjects) require cervical immobilization regardless of the type of litter used. The method of cervical spine immo-

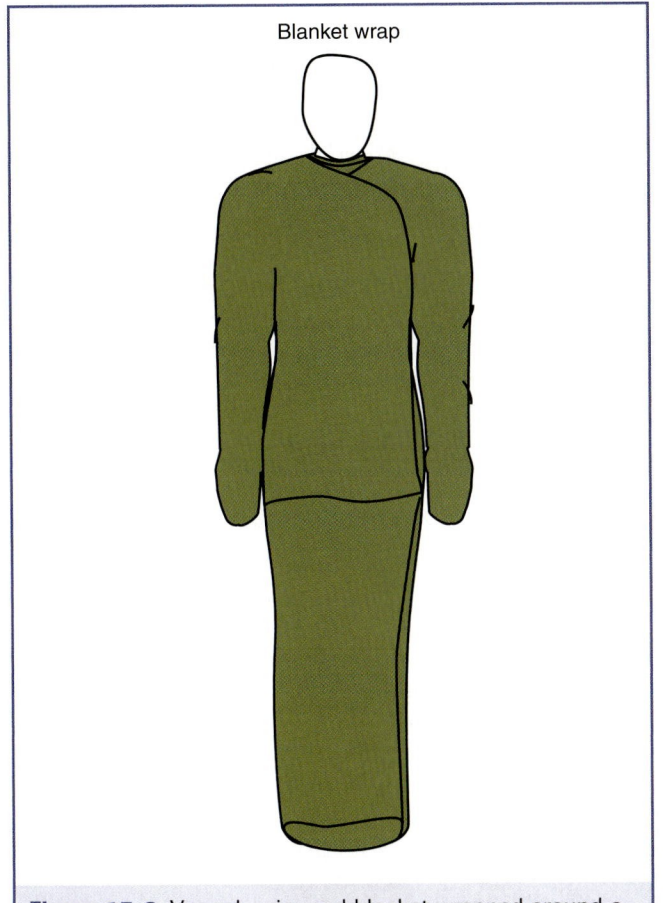

Figure 15-9 Vapor barrier and blanket wrapped around a subject.

bilization selected should not interfere with the operation of the litter and should allow the litter attendant access to the subject.

Spine boards offer convenience and safety for subjects who need cervical spine precautions. If necessary, it is easier and quicker to move a subject on a spine board from the litter to an ambulance or helicopter stretcher or an x-ray table. To prevent additional pain and possible tissue damage in areas of tissue pressure, any rigid splint used on the subject should be padded where the splint comes in contact with pressure points, such as the back of the heel, the hip, shoulder blade, and back of the head.

Packaging the Subject with Possible Spinal Injuries

For all subjects suspected of having spinal injuries, the spine must be immobilized, even if a rigid stretcher is used. A full spine board is not always required. Effective stabilization can be accomplished using spinal immobilization devices such as a Kendrick Extrication Device (K.E.D.) (Ferno) or the Oregon Spine Splint (OSS) (Skedco).

Commercial Devices for Spinal Immobilization

Spine Boards
A full spine board (Figure 15-11) must meet certain requirements. It should:

- Be appropriately shaped and narrow enough to allow placement inside the litter
- Be rigid, to prevent movement of the spine
- Be made of strong, easily cleaned material
- Have attachment points to allow attachment to the litter
- Have handles for lifting
- Allow insulation of the subject

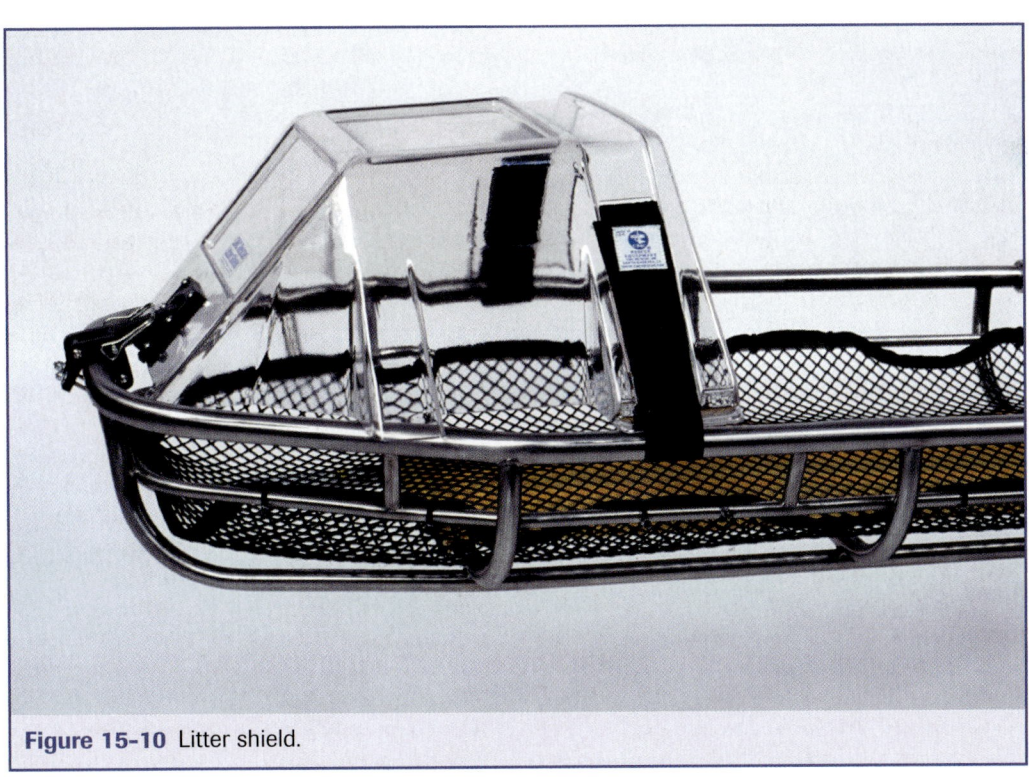

Figure 15-10 Litter shield.

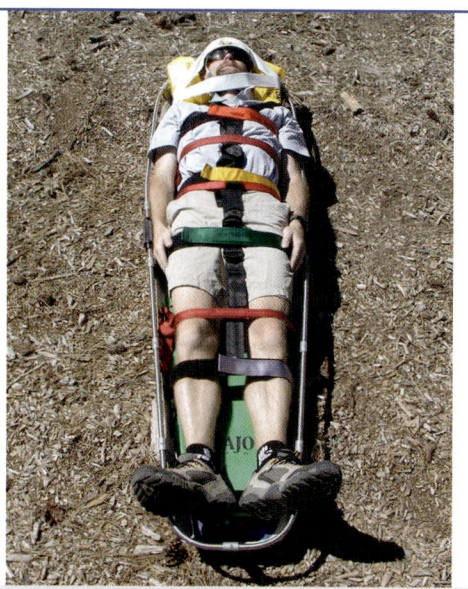

Figure 15-11 Subject on a spine board in the litter. (Courtesy Ken Phillips.)

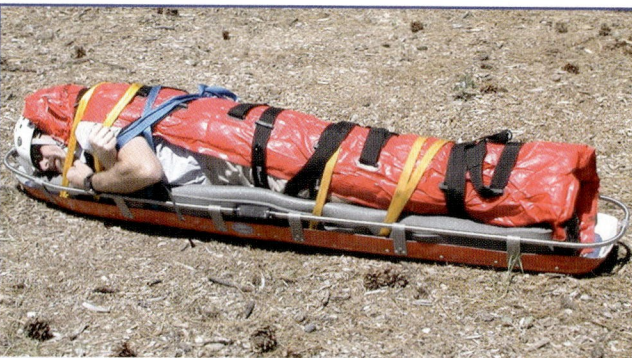

Figure 15-12 Subject on a vacuum mattress in the litter. The vacuum mattress can assist in supporting a subject in a lateral recumbent position to assist airway drainage. (Courtesy Ken Phillips.)

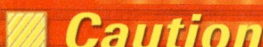

> **Caution**
>
> Before placing the subject on a spine board, always make sure the spine board meets the following criteria:
> - It fits in the bottom of the litter you will be using in the rescue.
> - It fits in the helicopter if air evacuation is a possibility.

Half Boards

THE KENDRICK EXTRICATION DEVICE AND THE OREGON SPINE SPLINT (OSS II)

The K.E.D. and the OSS II are integrated, half-length spine boards constructed from artificial materials. These devices are highly adaptable, provide effective stabilization under most circumstances, and allow rapid immobilization of the spine.

Vacuum Mattresses

A common spine board is flat, without contours, and hard. Immobilization of subjects on rigid spine boards can be painful for the subject even for a short period of time. Immobilization on rigid spine boards for longer periods can result in what is known as *tissue interface pressure*, or *pressure points*. Over time, sufficient pressure at these points can result in *pressure necrosis*, or *bedsores*. Recent advances in the use of vacuum mattresses have provided new and improved methods of spinal immobilization. Vacuum mattresses provide the same degree of immobilization as traditional methods while conforming comfortably to the subject. Because they contour to the body curves, they are less likely to cause pain and tissue damage from pressure.

One problem in the packaging of subjects in litters is providing sufficient packing of body voids to reduce subject movement during rescue. *Vacuum mattresses* are airtight mattress splint devices filled with polystyrene beads that become

interlocked when air is sucked out of the vacuum mattress (Figure 15-12).

Vacuum mattresses have the same overall weight as full spine boards, but they offer some advantages:

- Insulation from the cold
- Protection from water and snow
- The ability to conform to the individual subject
- Greater subject comfort in the extended transport environment (e.g., greater than 1 hour to the emergency department).

Vacuum splints also have some disadvantages, although many of these have been improved upon in recent years. The disadvantages include:

- Higher cost
- Risk of puncture (although the splints can be repaired in the field)
- Retention of water and snow
- Possible restriction of access to some areas of the subject, particularly the posterior aspects

Packaging the Subject with Long Bone Fractures

All suspected fractures must be protected with rigid splints and protective bandages. Basket stretchers with hard shells provide the best protection for a subject suspected of having long bone fractures. Subjects transported by flexible litters require more precautions to prevent further damage to the splinted extremity. All splints and dressings should allow the extremity to be examined by the litter attendant to make sure the nerves and blood vessels are intact.

Some femur traction splints commonly used in urban ambulance transport (e.g., the Hare splint) are too bulky and long to use in rescue litters. When applied to a subject, they often extend above the litter top rail and beyond the foot end of the rescue litter. This can cause additional subject discomfort, can expose the affected limb to further injury, and can complicate rescue rigging and handling. Consequently, rescuers should plan to use and practice with more compact, portable femur traction devices, such as the Sager traction splint (Minto Research and Development, Redding, California) and the Kendrick traction device (KTD).

Packaging the Subject for Rope Rescue

The section Medical Considerations for Patients in High Angle Rescue, Chapter 12, should be reviewed at this point.

Before packaging the subject, make sure the litter is secure from falling down slope or over an edge. If possible, package the subject in a level area. If on a slope, package the subject with the head up slope unless medical conditions prevent this. Having the subject's head higher on a slope helps keep the person more comfortable and oriented. If the litter is near an edge or if the possibility exists that the litter could slide down slope, secure it with a safety line or belay lines.

Package the subject so that the person will not fall out whatever the angle of the litter. The subject also must not shift inside the litter.

The litter attendants should be constantly assessing the subject's airway and breathing. If a threat to the subject's airway develops, such as vomiting, the attendants must be ready to tip the litter and clear the airway.

Packaging the Subject in the Litter

The major concerns when packaging a subject for rope rescue include the following:

- Transporting the subject in the litter must not cause additional harm. Packaging for the litter should not impede the airway and circulation.
- Packaging should allow monitoring of the subject's medical condition, including level of consciousness, airway, breathing, circulation, and vital signs.
- The subject must be protected from environmental factors (e.g., cold, wetness, and falling debris).
- The subject must be packaged so that the person is as comfortable as possible and will remain so in case the evacuation is a lengthy process. Subjects should be packaged without being painfully restrained while avoiding excessive pressure on restraints.
- Before packaging, the subject's pockets must be checked for hard objects that could create pressure points.
- The subject must be physically stabilized so that he or she does not fall out whatever the angle or direction of litter movement.

Physically Stabilizing the Subject in the Litter

During an evacuation, the litter will be lifted, tilted, and carried at various angles. The subject must be packaged so that he or she does not slip lengthwise in the litter, slide from side to side, or come out of the litter. Any tie-in system must allow access to the subject for periodic assessment and treatment, in case the subject's condition changes; it also must allow for breathing and circulation and for subject movement for comfort.

Litters often come equipped with tie-in straps, but these may be inadequate for any of the following reasons:

- The buckles may not fasten securely or may not be strong enough.
- The straps may be old and worn.
- The straps may be missing.

Materials for Litter Packaging

Equipment for litter packaging, subject protection, and medical gear, as well as other litter equipment, should be stored in their own bags and kept with the litter. This helps ensure that the right amount of gear is available for subject packaging and care when needed and that it is not being used in other parts of the rescue system.

Litter Subject Tie-Ins (Box 15-1)
Commercial Subject Tie-In Systems

Manufactured subject restraint systems for litters are available. These can save time and effort (Figure 15-13).

Improvised Litter Subject Tie-In

Rescuers commonly use 1-inch wide (25 mm) webbing to secure a subject in the litter. The following litter subject tie-in system is one example of a number of different systems used to secure a subject in a litter. Rescuers need to practice tie-in systems to find the best one for their needs and to prepare for actual rescues. The following system has two parts—an upper torso component

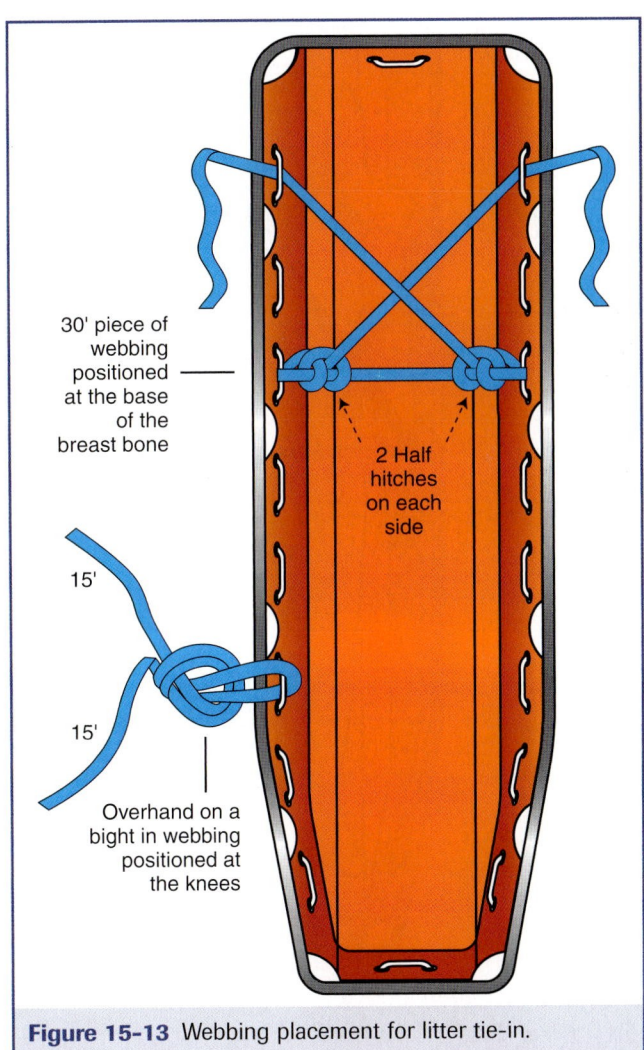

30' piece of webbing positioned at the base of the breast bone

2 Half hitches on each side

15'

15'

Overhand on a bight in webbing positioned at the knees

Figure 15-13 Webbing placement for litter tie-in.

Box 15-1	Anchoring Subject Tie-Ins to the Litter

- ❏ Avoid running tie-in webbing over the top rail of the litter. Webbing over the top rail is subject to abrasion and cutting, which could weaken the subject tie-in. Also, tie-in webbing on the top rail could interfere with rescue rigging (e.g., bridles or spiders) that may need to be attached there.
- ❏ If the next lowest (second down) rail is accessible, attach the tie-in webbing to it. If the second rail is not accessible, anchor the webbing to a vertical support member, the structural tubing that runs under the litter to the opposite side. The lower the tie-in points, the more downward pull is exerted on the subject and the more secure the person will be.
- ❏ Some litters, such as the Ferno-Washington 71, have a rope laced around the lower perimeter of the basket. This is designed as an anchor for the subject tie-in.

and a lower torso component. The upper torso component uses two pieces of 1-inch (25 mm) wide tubular webbing, each 30 feet (10 m) long. The lower torso component uses one piece of 1-inch (25 mm) tubular webbing that is 30 feet (10 m) long.

Upper Torso Component (Figure 15-14)

1. Using two half hitches, tie one end of each 30-foot (10 m) length of webbing at each side of the litter, positioned at the base of the subject's sternum.
2. Using a horseshoe blanket roll, pad around the subject's head and shoulders. The blanket roll must cover down to the edge of the shoulders.
3. Starting from the subject's right side, bring the webbing under the subject's right shoulder (this works best if this section of webbing is placed in the bottom of the litter before the subject is placed in it). Then bring the webbing around the subject's left shoulder where it is padded by the blanket roll and diagonally across the chest and right arm.

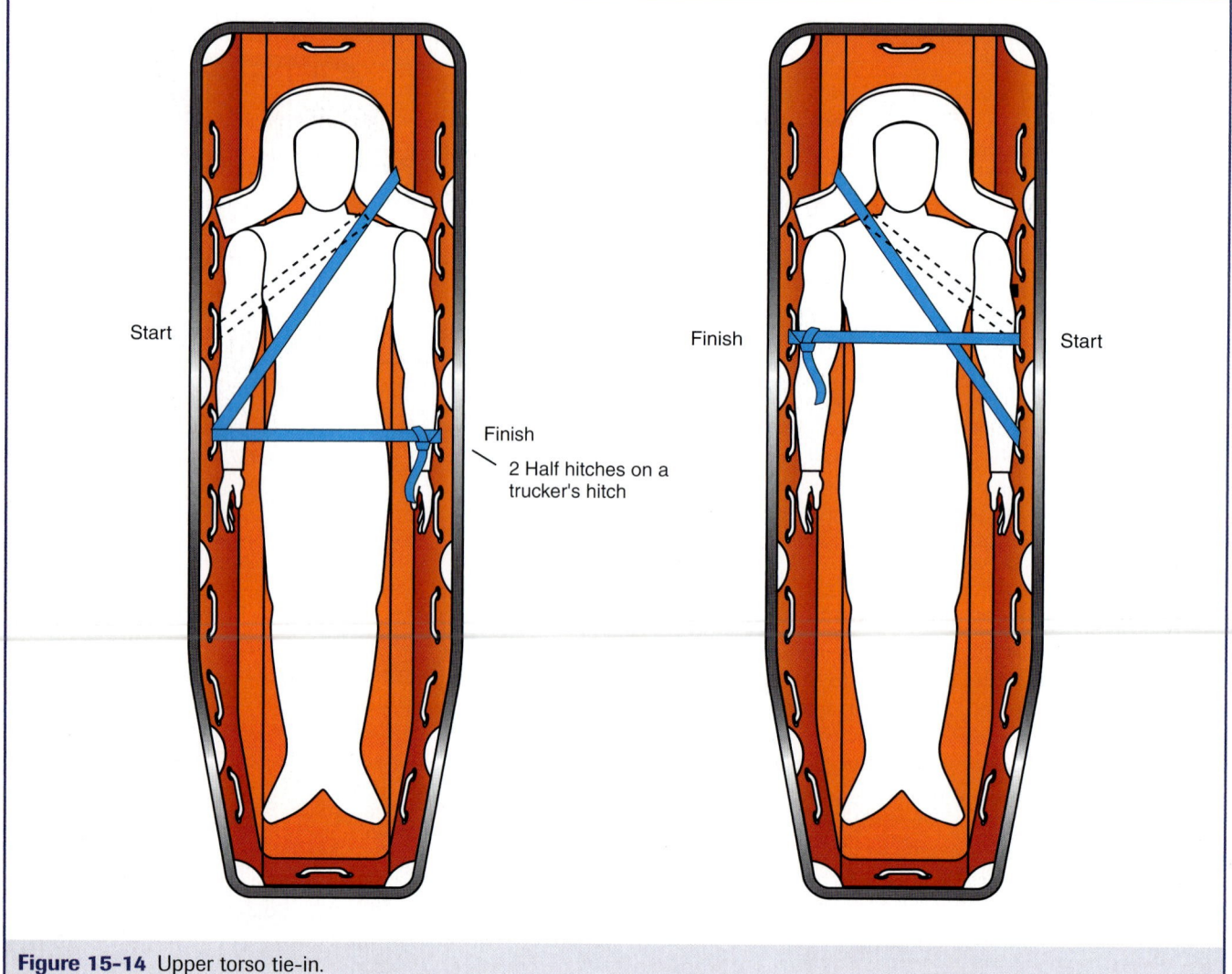

Figure 15-14 Upper torso tie-in.

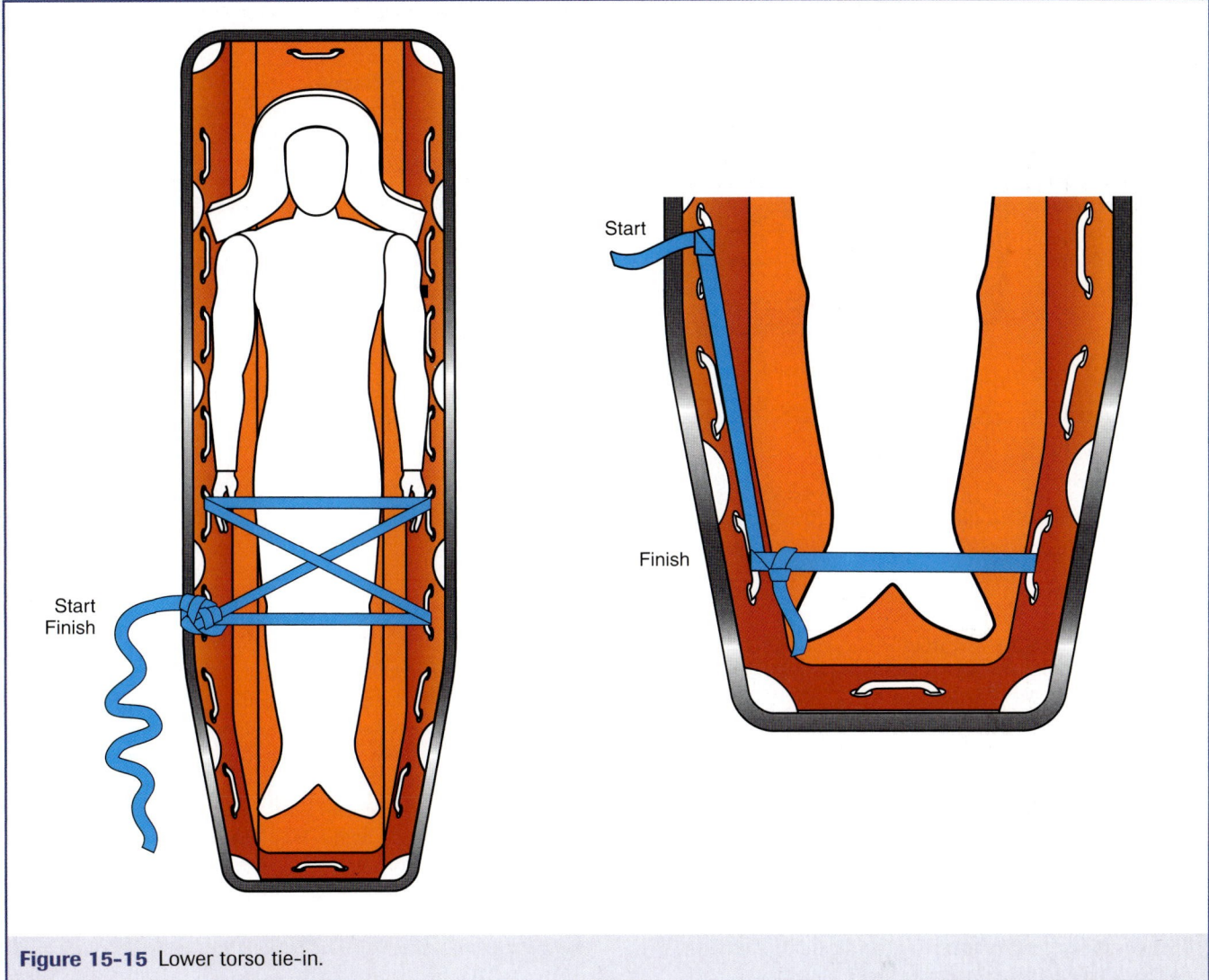

Figure 15-15 Lower torso tie-in.

4. Run the webbing through a litter tie-in point on the right side by the hips, bring it across the subject's hips, and tie it off at the opposite tie-in point at the subject's left side.
5. Now, using the webbing tied off on the subject's left side of the litter, bring the webbing under the subject's left shoulder, around the subject's right shoulder where it is padded by the blanket roll, and diagonally across the chest and left arm.
6. Run the webbing through a litter tie-in point on the left side, bring it across the subject's chest and tie it off at the opposite tie-in point at the subject's right side.

Lower Torso Component (Figure 15-15)

1. Find the middle of each of the remaining pieces of 30-foot (10 m) webbing.
2. At the middle of the webbing piece, use an overhand-on-a-bight knot to attach the webbing to a litter tie-in point at the level of knees at the subject's right side.

> ### ▨ *Warning*
>
> 1. *Do not* lash webbing horizontally across the upper chest or neck. If the subject slides down in the litter, a line of webbing across this area could strangle the subject.
> 2. If the webbing is too tight, prolonged loss of circulation could result in serious medical problems, such as compartment syndrome. In extreme cold, reduced circulation can increase the potential for frostbite or for burns from rewarming sources such as hot water bottles or heating pads. Pad the pressure points created by tie-ins. Check the subject's circulation after completing the tie-in. Recheck circulation at regular intervals.
> 3. Litter tie-ins can work loose. Rescuers must constantly monitor the litter lashing.

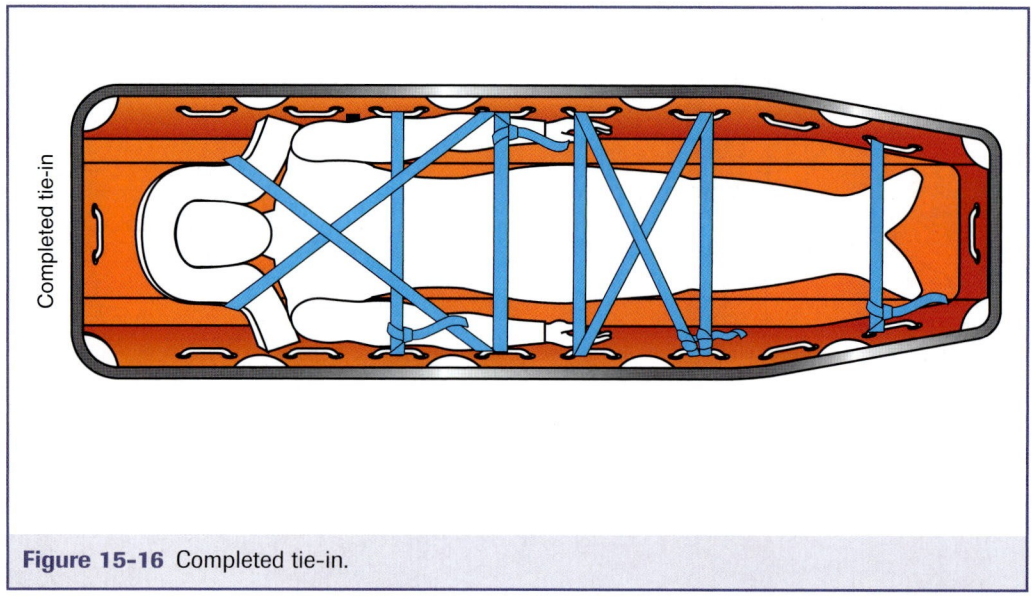

Completed tie-in

Figure 15-16 Completed tie-in.

3. Using one side of the length of webbing, run the webbing to the opposite side of the litter and run it through the next tie-in point up toward the head.

4. Bring the webbing across the litter and run it through a tie-in point at the same level on the opposite side.

5. Bring the webbing across the litter diagonally to a tie-in point that is the next one down toward the knees.

6. Now bring the webbing across the litter to the tie-in point where you started and tie it off with an overhand-on-a-bight knot.

7. Take the second half of the piece of webbing, bring it down below the feet and up to a litter tie-in point opposite the tie-in point where you started.

8. Run the webbing through this tie-in point and back to a tie-in point at the side of the ankles.

9. Run the webbing through this tie-in point and across the ankles and tie it off at the opposite tie-in point (Figure 15-16).

Alternative to Foot Stabilization

An alternative to tying in the subject's feet (starting with step 7 above) is to place a seat harness on the subject and use it for lengthwise stabilization. This may be necessary if, for example, the litter subject has a fracture of the lower extremity. See Chapter 21 for examples of improvised harnesses that can be used for litter subjects.

Immobilization of the Head

Suspected cervical injuries must be immobilized according to accepted medical protocols. If the rescuer is certain the subject has no cervical injuries, the area around the head should be padded, but the padding should allow for head movement. If there are no injuries to the neck or head, the subject can be allowed enough space to raise or roll the head. This will allow subjects to orient themselves as the litter is moved.

Helmet Considerations for the Subject

Many subjects are wearing a helmet at the time of the rescue. If the subject is wearing a helmet and a spine injury is possible, the helmet must be removed or it will interfere both with proper spinal immobilization and with the subject's airway and breathing status (Box 15-2). The head should be examined for injury if none is present, and if the possibility of C-spine injury has been ruled out, the helmet may be left in place. Subjects with head injuries should be treated with dressings, and the area should be protected against additional injury. A subject without a head injury who is not wearing a helmet should be given a helmet before the rescue. The rescuer is reminded that the back of the helmet will often lift the subject's head off the stretcher, leading to forward flexion of the neck. Unintended flexion of the neck can be prevented by slight elevation of the shoulder and neck using a thin layer of padding behind the neck.

If no helmets are available, the head area can be packed with blankets, packs, clothing, or other soft material and the head taped in place with duct tape across the forehead only. Sweat, moisture, and blood all weaken the adhesive ability of duct tape. Rescuers should not rely on duct tape alone to hold the subject's head in position. Remember that spinal immobilization straps and duct tape can get repositioned on the subject, increasing the risk of the subject choking.

Padding the Subject

If the litter has a leg divider, the top of the divider must be sufficiently padded to protect the subject's groin. To prevent side-to-side movement of the trunk, pad the spaces along the sides of the subject with soft material such as blankets or clothing. For the comfort of the subject, pad under the hollows of the body, such as behind the knees, in the small of the back and (unless cervical immobilization is a factor), behind the neck. Also pad bony parts such as the occiput, the back of the skull.

Box 15-2 | Helmet Removal

Two rescuers are needed for this procedure.

Step 1

First rescuer: Take position above the subject's head. With your palms pressed on the sides of the helmet and your fingertips curled over the lower margin, stabilize the helmet, head, and neck in as close to a neutral in-line position as the helmet allows.

Second rescuer: Kneel at the subject's side, open or remove the face shield if needed, and undo or cut the chin strap.

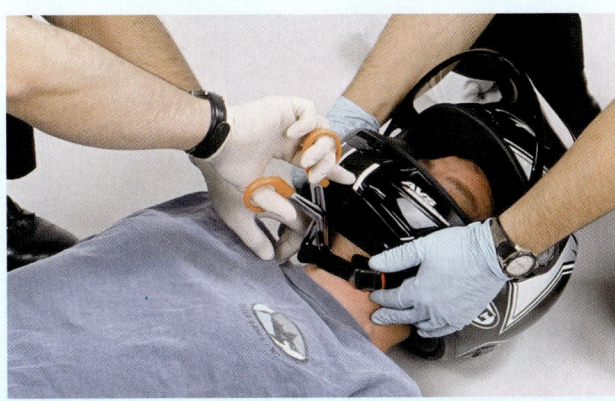

Step 2

Second rescuer: Grasp the subject's mandible between your thumb and first two fingers at the angle of the mandible. Place your other hand under the subject's neck on the occiput of the skull to take control of manual stabilization. Your forearms should be resting on the floor or ground or on your thighs for additional support.

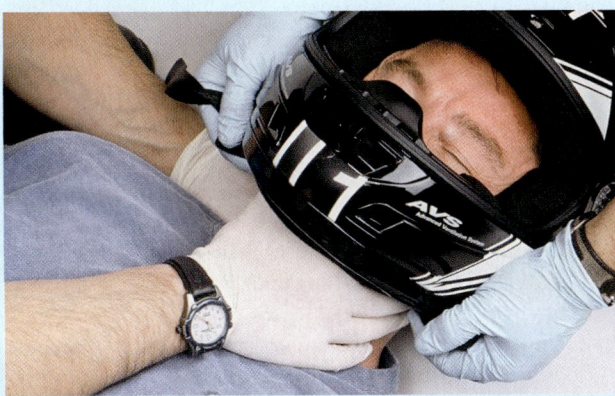

Step 3

First rescuer: Pull the sides of the helmet slightly apart, away from the subject's head, and rotate the helmet with up-and-down rocking motions while pulling it off the subject's head. Move the helmet slowly and deliberately. Take care as the helmet clears the subject's nose.

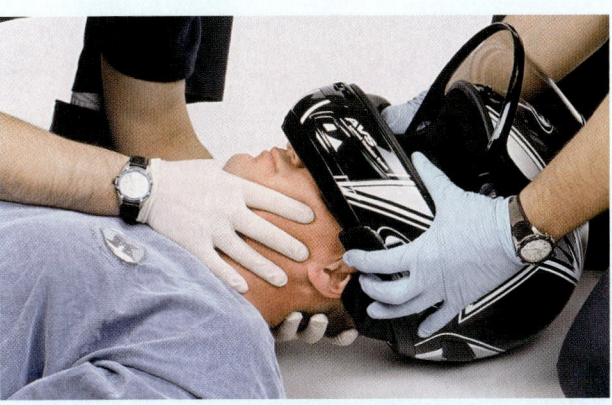

Step 4

Once the helmet has been removed, place padding behind the subject's head to maintain a neutral in-line position. Maintain manual stabilization and place an appropriate-size cervical collar on the subject.

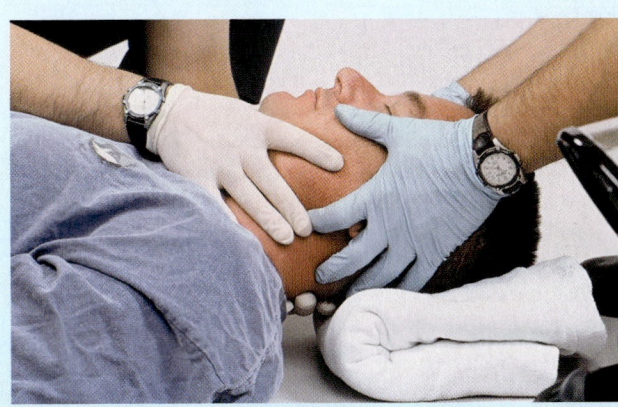

Modified from McSwain NE, Salomone JP, editors: *Prehospital trauma life support,* ed 5, St Louis, 2003, Mosby.

Carrying the Litter
Litter Slings

Rescuers often must carry a litter with a subject from the rescue site to a vehicle or helicopter. Carrying a litter with one hand on the litter rail can be extremely tiring. A littler sling can help relieve the load by spreading it to the shoulder (Figure 15-17).

Depending on the size of the litter bearer, a litter sling can be made with a 14- to 18-foot (4.5 to 6 m) length of tubular webbing. Using a ring bend (water) knot, create a continuous loop in the webbing. Attach the loop to the litter rail with a large carabiner or by cinching it onto the rail. Run the line over the shoulder and grasp the other end of the web with the hand away from the litter.

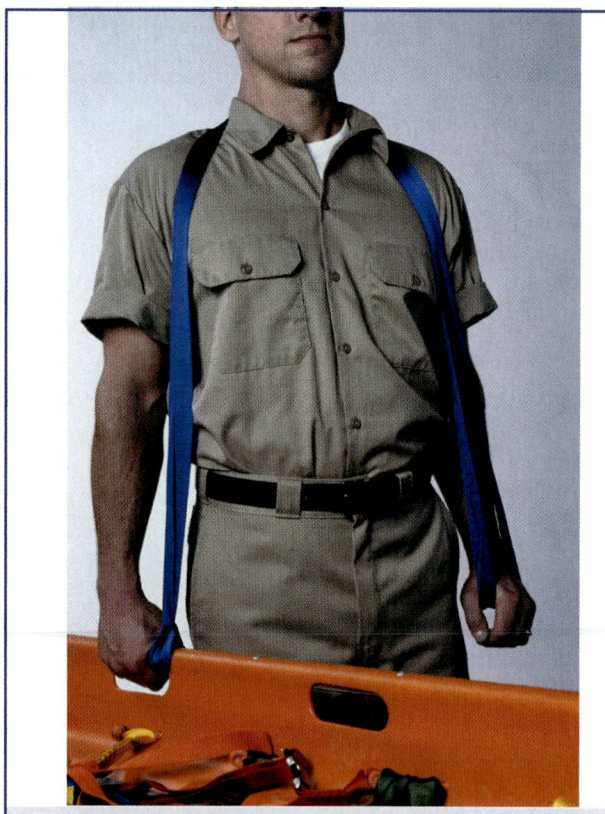

Figure 15-17 Litter sling.

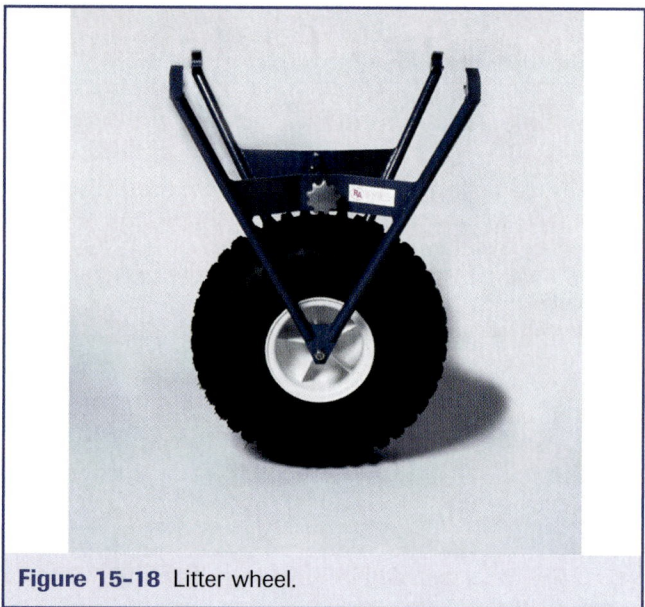

Figure 15-18 Litter wheel.

Even with litter slings, carrying a litter with an adult subject can be an exhausting process. This usually requires six litter bearers at one time. If possible, at least two additional bearers should be available to relieve other bearers. This relief often is accomplished by a process of rotation, with the two relief bearers approaching the rear of the litter to take up the position of the two rear bearers. The bearers then move forward on the litter until the two front bearers move off the litter and go on ahead. In this position they serve as scouts, looking for obstacles and alerting the other bearers to hazards. At the next rotation, the two scouts move to the rear, and the process continues.

Litter Wheels

A device that can help save rescuers' energy and speed up an evacuation is the litter wheel. Litter wheels are available in a variety of designs, but the one most commonly used in the United States is the single wheel design, which uses a recreational vehicle tire (Figure 15-18). The litter is attached to the wheel with either a clamping device or straps. When using the wheel, rescuers walk beside or at the ends of the litter (or in both places), holding and balancing the litter, because the wheel supports most of the weight. When rescuers encounter a minor obstacle, such as a rock or log, they lift the litter with the wheel attached and set it down on the other side.

If a wheeled litter is to be used on a flat, smooth surface to transport a subject who requires only a minimum amount of care, only two litter tenders may be needed, one at each end. However, handling a wheeled litter in more rugged terrain usually requires a minimum of four rescuers, two on each side. More difficult terrain may require additional attendants.

Rescuers should practice using the wheel before using it for a rescue. Such practice can help rescuers understand aspects of wheeled litter handling, including how to find the center of gravity for proper balance.

Other tips for using litter wheels include the following:

- Litter slings can help rescuers manage and control the litter
- In rugged and steep terrain, place a rescuer in front of and behind the wheeled litter, each wearing a chest harness with slings attached to the litter. This helps in pulling the litter and braking it on slopes.
- Clip or tape a bicycle pump to the wheel frame. Depending on the terrain, the tire may have to be deflated slightly for subject comfort. These tires often have slow leaks, and the pump can be used to reinflate them.
- In steep terrain, the wheeled litter may require a belay.

Evaluation Exercises

Cognitive and Affective Exercises

1. List three important qualities of a litter that will be used in rope rescue.

2. List two advantages and two disadvantages of plastic litters.

3. List an advantage and a disadvantage of break-apart litters.

4. List three advantages and three disadvantages of flexible litters, such as the Sked litter.

5. List three major concerns when packaging a subject in a litter.

6. List three requirements for a spine board to be used in a litter.

Psychomotor Exercises

7. Using a tarp and blanket, package a subject in a litter to protect the person from cold weather environmental effects.

8. Use webbing to tie a subject into a litter, bearing in mind concerns about physical stabilization and prevention of injury.

16

Low Angle Evacuation

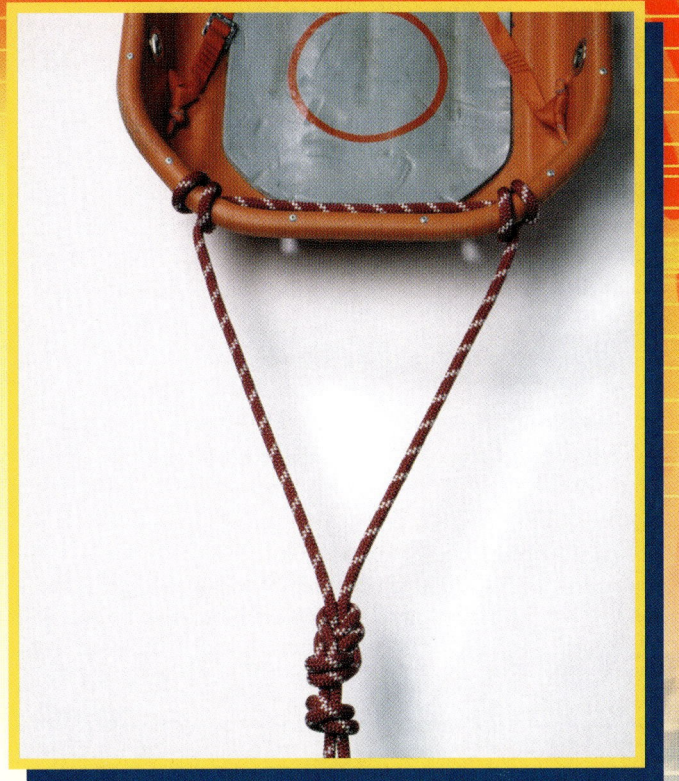

Objectives

On completion of this chapter, you should be able to:

1. Describe the steps involved in a low angle evacuation and list some examples of areas in which low angle evacuation may be needed.
2. Given a selection of equipment, choose what would be used in a low angle evacuation system.
3. Describe the medical and packaging considerations for a subject during a low angle evacuation in both summer and winter conditions.
4. Discuss the functions of and be able to assume the following roles in low angle evacuations: litter tender, litter captain, brakeman, and haul team.
5. Discuss the functions of rope, braking systems, the progress capture device (PCD), the haul cam, and pulleys in a low angle evacuation.
6. List several examples of communications concerns during an evacuation.
7. Identify the elements of a hauling system in a low angle evacuation.
8. Explain the principles and application of a 1:1 haul system, a counterbalance haul system, and a 2:1 haul system.
9. Package a rescue subject for low angle evacuation, following local protocol or the guidelines set forth in this text.
10. Construct the rigging for a litter in a low angle evacuation.
11. Rig the braking and belay systems and the PCD for low angle evacuation.
12. Repeat from memory the voice communications used in low angle evacuation.
13. Construct a 1:1 or a counterbalance hauling system for low angle evacuation.

Prerequisites

Before attempting the activities described in this chapter, you must have demonstrated that you can properly:

1. Use and care for rope.
2. Use and care for other equipment needed in the high angle environment.
3. Tie correctly and without hesitation the knots necessary for safe, effective work in the vertical environment (see Chapter 6).
4. Apply the principles of anchoring and rig a safe and secure anchor.
5. Apply the principles of rescue belaying and safely belay a rescue load using the techniques described in Chapter 13.

The material in this chapter conforms to guidelines published by the National Fire Protection Association (NFPA), specifically standard 1006, *Professional Qualifications for Rescue Technicians* (2002), standard 1670, *Operations and Training for Technical Rescue Incidents* (2004), and standard 1983, *Standard on Life Safety Rope and System Components* (2001). NFPA standards are revised regularly, and readers are advised to review the latest version of this standard.

Key Terms

Brakeman The person who operates the braking device that controls the rate of descent of a litter in a low angle evacuation.

Counterbalance Haul System A procedure for hauling that uses a 1:1 ratio and a haul team that moves in a direction opposite to the load.

Haul Team The group of individuals who provide the power to raise the load.

Litter Attendant An individual who helps control the litter or attends to a subject's medical needs during a low angle evacuation rescue. Also known as a *litter tender*.

Litter Captain In low angle evacuation, the person who manages the litter team and coordinates the litter movement with other members of the rescue team.

Low Angle Evacuation Movement of a rescue subject in an environment in which the load is supported primarily by itself rather than the rope rescue system (e.g., flat land or mild sloping surface). The litter is attached to a rope for safety and control. Also known as *slope evacuation* or *scree evacuation*.

Packaging Proper placement of a rescue subject in a litter for transport; it takes into consideration the subject's primary medical problems and physical stabilization of the individual in the litter.

Progress Capture Device (PCD) A rope grab device, general-use ascender, or hitch placed on the rope in a hauling system to prevent the rope (and the load) from slipping back down as the haul system is reset. Also commonly referred to as the *ratchet*.

Rope Handler The person in a lowering operation who assists the brakeman with rope management.

Tree Wrap A technique for running a rope around a tree trunk to create friction for a braking effect in litter lowering.

The Need for Low Angle Evacuation

The term *low angle evacuation* may not evoke the sense of excitement or challenge that comes with vertical, or high angle, rescue. However, in many areas, low angle evacuation is the most common type of rope rescue performed by emergency service personnel.

Often, low angle evacuation also is the type of rescue that poses the most problems for emergency service personnel. Many people are inexperienced with low angle evacuation and are unaware of the potential problems. Consequently, many rescuers may be poorly equipped and trained for the problems and hazards encountered in low angle rescue.

The point where low angle evacuation ends and high angle evacuation begins is not always easily defined. The essential differences concern the way the litter and the rescue personnel are used (Box 16-1).

Examples of Low Angle (Slope) Evacuation

Low angle evacuation involves any inclined or rugged area over which a litter must be carried and where it is difficult or dangerous to do so without the assistance of a rope (Box 16-2). Under some conditions, low angle evacuation is also called *broken ground evacuation*.

Elements of Low Angle Evacuation

The elements of a low angle evacuation usually comprise a litter, a rope, and an anchor system (Figure 16-1).

Box 16-1	Differences between Low Angle and High Angle Evacuation

Low Angle Evacuation
- ❏ Most of the weight of the litter tenders is supported by the ground.
- ❏ The litter is supported by a combination of litter tenders and a rope rescue system.
- ❏ Three or more litter tenders can be used.
- ❏ A rope is attached to one end of the litter.

High Angle Evacuation
- ❏ The litter tenders' weight is supported by the rope rescue system.
- ❏ The weight of the litter and the subject is supported by the rope rescue system.
- ❏ At most, two litter attendants can be used.

Box 16-2	Examples of Low Angle Evacuation Sites

- ❏ Road cuts and fills
- ❏ Loose, rocky slopes (scree or talus)
- ❏ Hills
- ❏ Snow and icy slopes
- ❏ Rugged, broken terrain
- ❏ Urban stairs
- ❏ Industrial environments

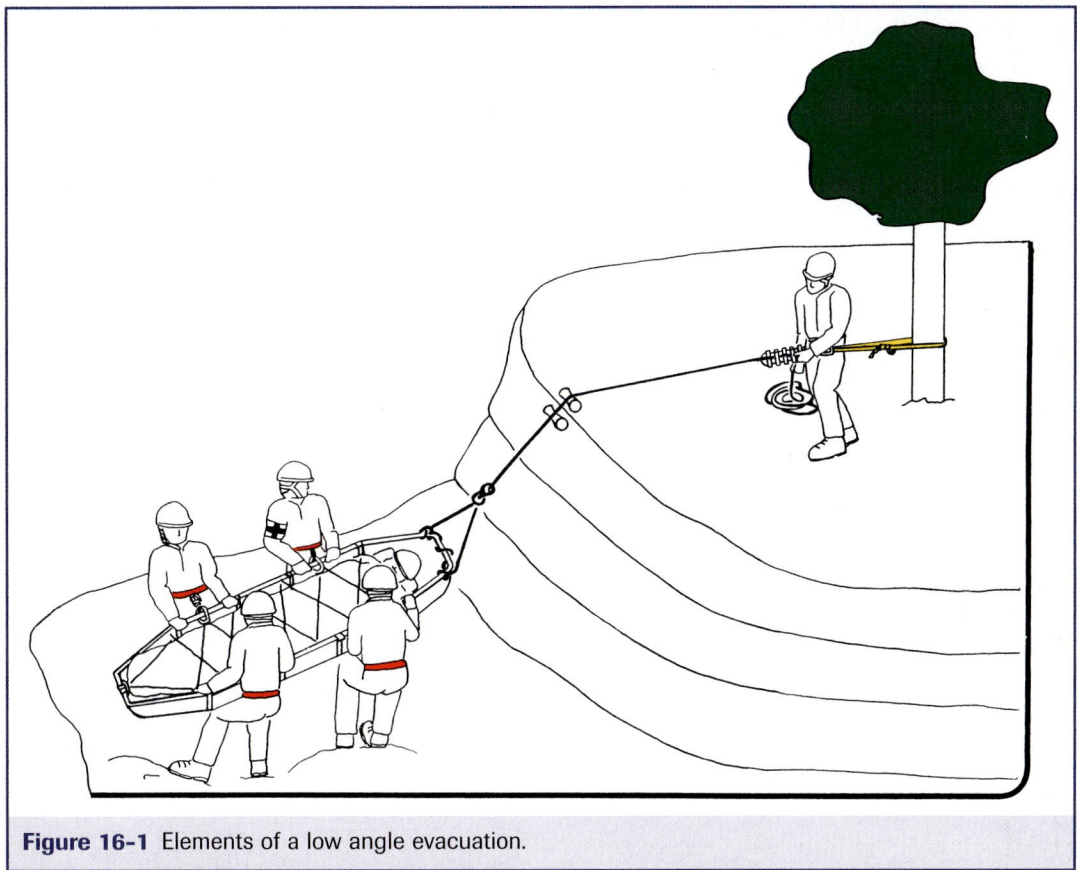

Figure 16-1 Elements of a low angle evacuation.

Litter

Requirements

Strength

The litter must be strong enough to withstand the stress of supporting the weight of the rescue subject and rescuers while being supported by rope. The litter also must be able to withstand impacts with rocks, trees, and other hard objects. It must help protect the subject.

Rigid or Semirigid Type The litter must be rigid or semirigid to protect the subject and to allow ease of handling. It must also maintain an envelope of protection for the subject despite stresses and unequal loading (see Chapter 15 for additional information on litters for use in low angle evacuation).

Tie-In Points *Tie-in points* are used to attach ropes and rescuers and to protect the subject. Tie-in points must be easily accessible and must be strong enough to withstand the stresses applied to them in low angle evacuation.

Anchor System

A safe and secure anchor system is a critical part of any low angle evacuation (see Chapter 7 for a review of the criteria for safe, secure anchors).

Rope

To maintain greater control over the operation, most rescuers prefer a rope with a minimum of stretch, such as a static kernmantle rope. The rope usually is attached to the head end of the litter.

Litter to Be Lowered Down Slope

If the litter is to be lowered down a slope, the rope runs through a braking system that creates friction, allowing the descent to be easily controlled by one person, who is known as the ***brakeman***. The brakeman controls the braking system and, in conjunction with the litter captain, the rate of descent of the litter.

Litter to Be Raised Up Slope

If the litter must be raised up slope, the rope runs through a hauling system.

Hauling System The *hauling system* allows the litter to be raised easily by the ***haul team***, the rescuers who provide the force to raise the litter up slope safely and efficiently.

PROGRESS CAPTURE DEVICE

The progress capture device (PCD) prevents the rope (and litter) from inadvertently sliding back down slope.

Standard Requirements for Slope Evacuation

Litter Attendants

Depending on the slope angle, the subject's weight, the limitations of terrain system capacity, and the overall risk-benefit, the number of litter tenders (or *litter attendants*) may range from three to six. Because the more people there are, the more they tend to get in each other's way and the more weight is added, only as many attendants should be used as are required to do the job comfortably and safely. Depending on the subject's medical condition, a medical attendant may also be present. Litter tenders connect themselves to the litter with the litter tie-ins.

Litter Tie-Ins

Litter attendants are better able to maintain their footing and stability when tied in to the litter. They lean back onto the tie-ins, putting their weight on the litter. In turn, this weight is taken by the rope, braking device, and anchors.

Medical Attendant

The medical attendant usually is the member of the team with the highest level of medical training and experience. Depending on the subject's condition, the medical attendant may be a litter tender or may need to devote his or her full attention to the subject.

Litter Rigging for Low Angle Evacuation

Two techniques are commonly used to attach the rope to the head of the litter: tying the main-line rope directly to the head of the litter or tying a closed loop directly to the head of the litter.

Tying the Main-Line Rope Directly to the Head of the Litter

If the distance of the low angle evacuation is only one rope length and the rope does not have to be detached from the litter during the operation, the main-line rope may be tied directly onto the head of the litter.

Figure 16-2 shows a typical system for attaching a main-line rope to the head of a litter for low angle evacuation. The attachment consists of a very large loop created at the end of the rope by an end knot, such as the figure 8 follow-through knot. The loop around the end rail of the litter can be made as follows:

1. At the end of the rope that is to be attached to the litter, measure off twice the distance between outspread arms (a total of approximately 12 feet [4 m]).
2. At this point in the rope, tie a simple figure 8 knot.
3. Run the rope around the head rail of the litter several times so that it evenly spreads the forces along the rail.
4. Bring the end of the rope back to the simple figure 8 knot.
5. Tie a figure 8 follow-through knot using the simple figure 8 knot. Make sure to leave several inches (centimeters) of tail past the knot.
6. Use the tail to tie a double overhand back-up knot (barrel knot).

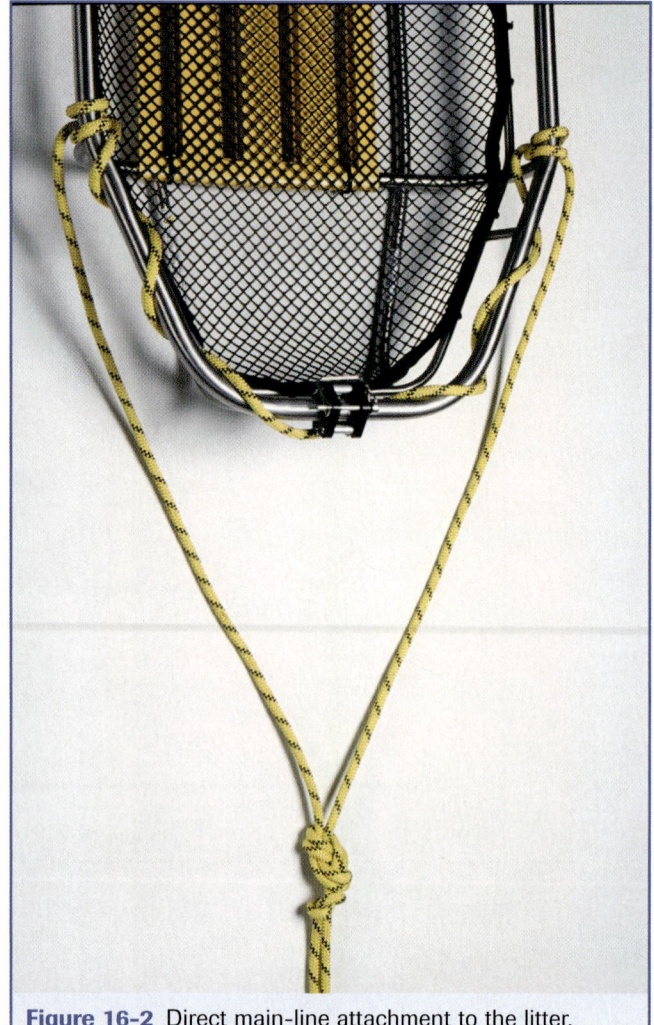

Figure 16-2 Direct main-line attachment to the litter.

7. Center the knots so that both legs of the loops pull evenly on the litter rail.
8. Be sure to dress the figure 8 follow-through knot and pull it down tightly. After doing this, make sure the back-up knot is snugged against the main knot.

NOTE: This technique cannot be used on plastic litters on which the plastic material covers the rail at both ends. Figure 16-3 shows a technique for attaching a main line to this type of litter. This technique uses clove hitches at each corner where the litter side rails meet the head end of the litter. Make sure to tie the clove hitches so that there is no slack between them in the part of the rope that is inside the litter.

9. Once the loop for the tie-in is complete, make sure it is large enough to create a safe angle on the knot (see Chapter 7, p. 92, for information on how angles that are too wide can create greater stress). The loop should still be small enough that it does not easily snag or get in the way.

Tying a Closed Loop Directly to the Head of the Litter

For low angle evacuations of more than one rope length and when the litter must be freed quickly from the system for a trail

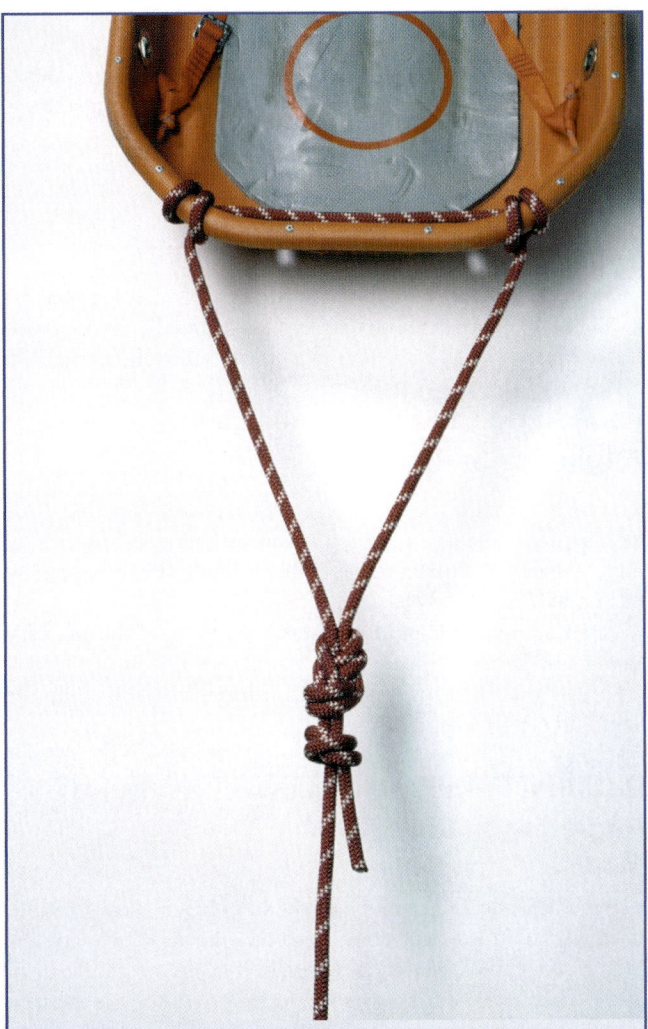

Figure 16-3 Tying the main line to a litter that has plastic-covered head and end rails.

⬛ Warning

When a main-line lowering or hauling rope is connected to the end rail of a litter, the force must be spread out evenly along the rail by weaving the attachment around the rail several times. *Never attach a main-line lowering or hauling rope to a single point on the rail of a litter.* Many litters are susceptible to failure if sudden forces pull at a single point on the rail. This is particularly true of litter rails that are butt-welded; a sudden force at such a point could break the weld, resulting in litter rail failure.

carry, the lowering rope must be removed and reattached to the litter. In such cases it is more practical to leave a closed loop of rope tied at the end of the litter. To attach the lowering and hauling line to the loop, tie a figure 8 on a bight in the end of the main-line rope and clip it to the loop with a large locking carabiner (Figure 16-4).

Suggestion

For a more stable tie-in, start the wrap of the litter rail with a clove hitch and end it with a second clove hitch on the opposite side. This prevents the bridle from slipping around as the direction of the load shifts and provides backup if one portion of the litter rail fails.

A closed loop can be created for the end of the litter as follows:

1. Take a length of rope or webbing about 6 feet (2 m) long. (Add additional rope if you will be tying a figure 8 on a bight in the loop as described in step 5 on p. 234.)
2. Run the rope or webbing around the head rail of the litter to spread the force around the rail.

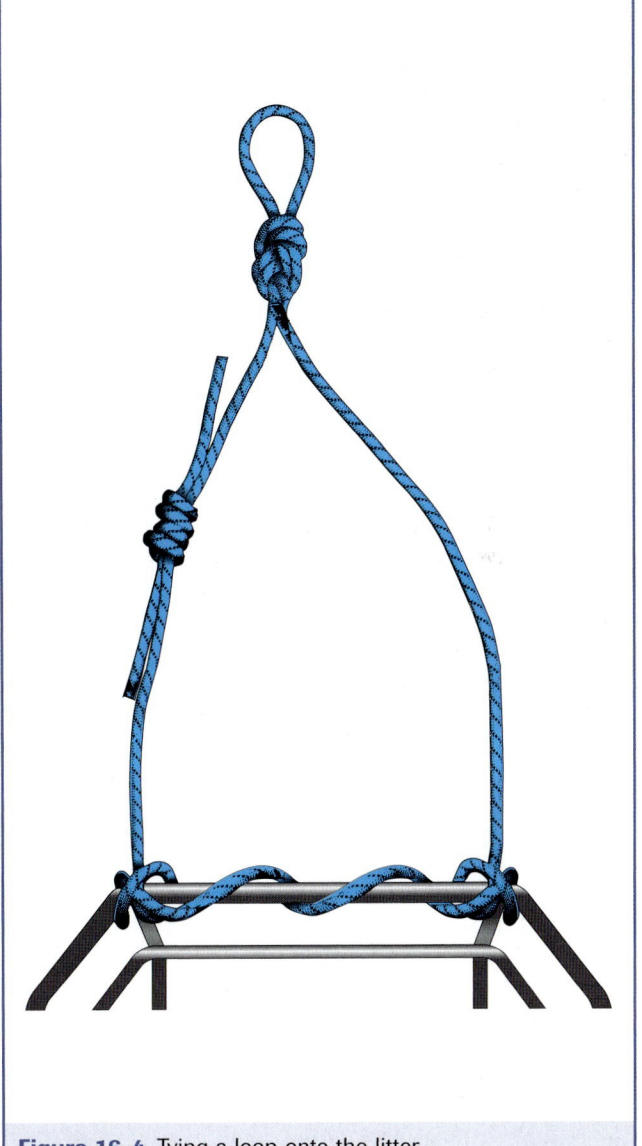

Figure 16-4 Tying a loop onto the litter.

3. Tie the two ends together with a grapevine (double fisherman's) knot, figure 8 bend knot, or some other type of joining known to have sufficient strength.
4. Adjust the grapevine knot so that it is off to the side and not in the center, where the main-line rope will attach (Boxes 16-3 and 16-4).
5. Optionally, in the center of the loop farthest from the litter, tie a figure 8 on a bight, into which the main carabiner can be clipped.

Litter Team for Low Angle Evacuation

The litter team must keep in mind that low angle litter management is very different from management of a litter on level terrain.

On level, unbroken terrain, the usual number of people carrying a litter is six (plus any additional personnel attending to the subject's medical needs). The full weight of the litter is on these individuals; they are completely supporting their own weight as they maneuver their way across the terrain.

Box 16-3	**Alternative to Rope for a Closed Loop: Webbing**

Instead of rope, webbing may be used to create the closed loop. However, care must be taken in tying such a loop with webbing, because knots tied in webbing have a tendency to work their way out. Tie the two ends of the webbing together using a ring bend (water) knot. Once the ring bend has been tied and dressed, make sure enough webbing protrudes past the knot to tie a back-up knot. Because of webbing's tendency to work out of a knot, the ring bend knot should be backed up and monitored.

Box 16-4	**Alternative Approach: Bowline Knot**

If local policy dictates that a bowline knot be used to create a loop in the end of a rope, the bowline knot may be used in place of the figure 8 follow-through knot, but with the following considerations:
- ❏ Make sure the bowline knot is tied correctly (see Figure 6-7, p. 72).
- ❏ Back up the bowline knot with a safety knot, such as the double overhand backup (barrel) knot.
- ❏ Monitor the bowline knot so that it does not "capsize" when being pulled over an obstruction such as a rock, tree, or building edge.

⚠ *Caution*

The angle made in this loop when it is attached to the main-line rope must not be greater than 90 degrees (see Chapter 7). If the angle is greater than 90 degrees, make a larger loop.

Box 16-5	**Characteristics of Litter Management on Slopes**

- ❏ The rope takes much of the litter's and the subject's weight.
- ❏ Litter movement is controlled by the rope system.
- ❏ Much of the attendants' weight is taken by the litter and the rope system.

Slopes may involve difficult and treacherous footing, making it difficult to handle the litter safely. Consequently, the approach to litter management on slopes must be different (Box 16-5}.

Packaging the Subject for Low Angle Evacuation

The sections Packaging the Subject in the Litter (pp. 217-225) in Chapter 15 and Medical Considerations for Subjects in High Angle Rescue in Chapter 12 should be reviewed at this point.

Litter attendants should be constantly aware of the subject's airway and breathing status. If a threat to the subject's airway arises, such as vomiting, the attendants must be ready to tip the litter and clear the airway.

Optional Personnel in Low Angle Evacuation
Medical Attendant

The medical attendant supervises the subject's medical care and, as it relates to medical considerations, the movement of the subject. The medical attendant usually is positioned at the head of the litter or where he or she can best monitor the subject. Where the slope is at a greater angle, the medical attendant may be safetied into the litter or main-line rope with an adjustable sling or on a separate line.

Scouts

Scouts move ahead of the litter to clear a path or to warn the team of loose debris, rocks, branches, briars, snakes, and so on.

Litter Tender Body Positions in Low Angle Evacuation

Figure 16-1 shows the body positions of the four litter attendants during low angle evacuation. Characteristically these positions are as follows:
- The tenders' bodies are turned toward the litter or slightly uphill.
- Depending on the terrain, the tender uses both hands to grip the litter rails or one hand to grip the litter rail and the other to maintain balance.
- The tenders lean back against the tie-ins, and their weight is taken by the litter and rope system.
- The litter tender's body is perpendicular to the slope.
- The tenders allow the rope system to determine the litter's rate of descent or ascent.
- Tenders space themselves out equally so that they do not bump one another.

Litter Tender Strategy for Low Angle Evacuation

The *litter captain*, in communication with the brakeman on the slope above, determines the rate of descent of the litter. The litter team members lean back into their tie-ins and allow the litter and rope system to take their weight. A litter attendant who slips continues to hold onto the litter rail and pulls his or her body taut on the tie-in. The rope system and the other team members usually can keep the litter stable and prevent the attendant from falling. The litter team, in concert with the rope, acts as a sort of self-equalizing table and provides stable transportation for the subject.

If more than one litter attendant loses footing or the terrain becomes particularly treacherous, the team captain can call "Stop" to halt the descent temporarily. This gives the team the chance to regain its stability.

Litter Tender Tie-Ins

The litter attendant tie-ins are critical for maintaining litter attendant stability and position at the litter. The litter attendant clips one end of the tie-in directly into his or her seat harness and the other end directly into the litter rail.

The simplest form of tie-in can be:

- A manufactured adjustable loop, such as a pickoff strap
- A continuous loop of webbing or small-diameter rope
- A section of small-diameter rope with a loop in each end

The tie-in can be attached to the litter top rail with a girth hitch or similar attachment. If the tenders want to be able to detach from and reattach to the rail quickly, they can clip into the litter top rail with a large locking carabiner. However, carabiners tend to slip along the rail, which can be annoying for the litter tenders. Also, not all locking carabiners have gates that will clear the rails of the basket litter. The larger rails on wire basket models and the rails on plastic litters accept only certain models of a few carabiner brands. The manufacturer's and distributor's specifications should be consulted before carabiners are purchased for this purpose.

Because each person's body proportions (e.g., trunk size and arm length) are different, the length of the tie-in will vary. However, the tie-in generally is no longer than 2 feet (0.6 m). The optimum length for the tie-in is one that holds the litter attendant in position so that he or she can have both hands on the litter rail, yet allows the attendant freedom of movement.

Adjustable Tie-In

An alternative to the fixed length attachment is the adjustable length tie-in (Figure 16-5). An adjustable length tie-in allows the attendant to change the space to adapt to varying circumstances, such as changing terrain or obstructions. It also is an advantage if different team members must use it.

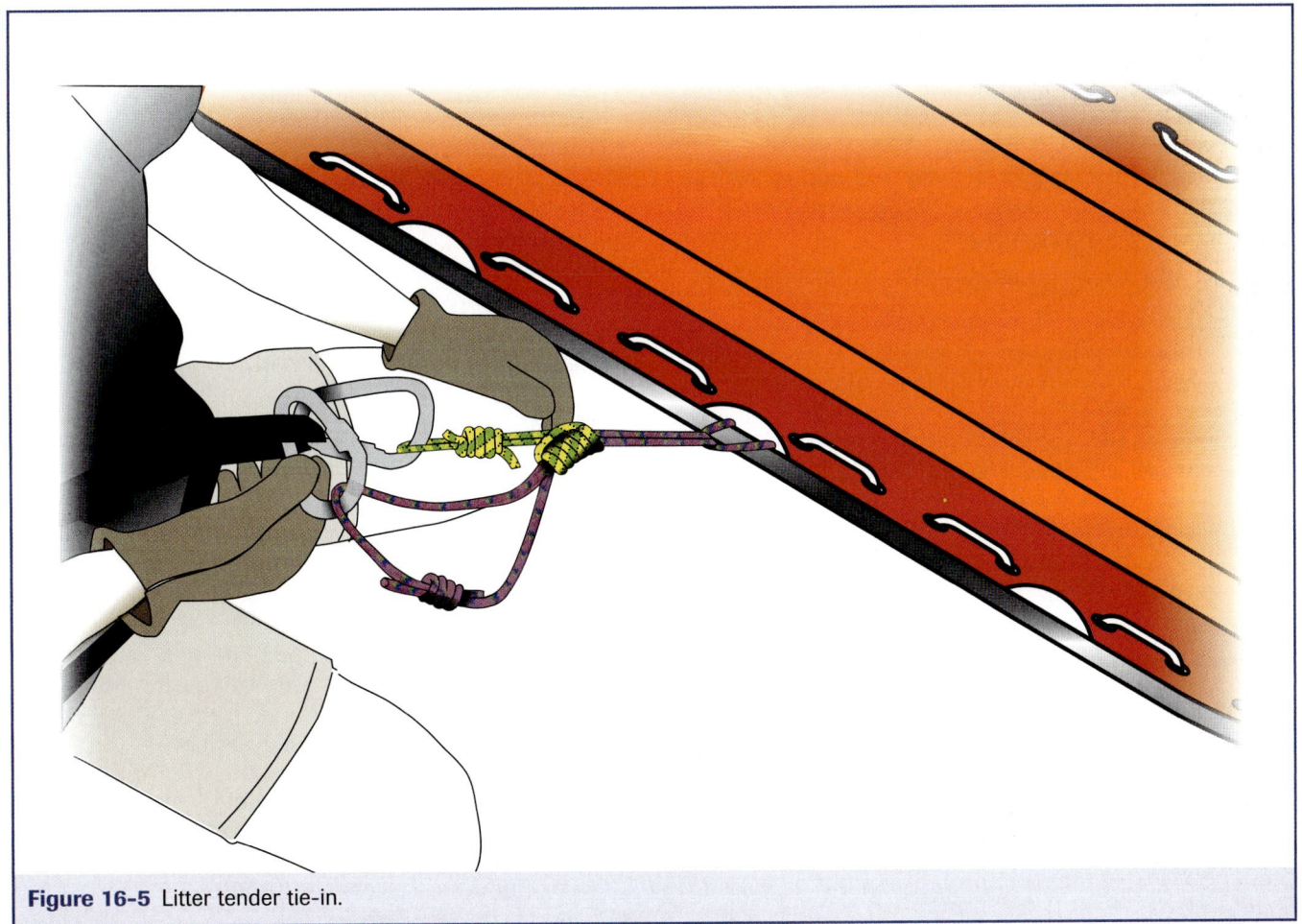

Figure 16-5 Litter tender tie-in.

An adjustable tie-in consists of two elements:

1. A fixed length safety line constructed of 8- to 9-mm accessory cord.
2. An adjustable tie-in of 7-mm accessory cord that uses a triple-wrap Prusik on the fixed line to change the distance between a litter tender and the litter. (To work properly, the Prusik cord must be of smaller diameter than the fixed safety line.)

Constructing the Adjustable Tie-In

1. To make a safety attachment, use an accessory cord 8- to 9-mm in diameter and about 6½ feet (2 m) long. Using a grapevine (double fisherman's) knot, tie the two ends together, forming a continuous loop.
2. Using a girth hitch, tie the end opposite the grapevine knot onto the litter rail.
3. Clip the end opposite the girth hitch to the litter tender's seat harness.
4. Now, take a piece of accessory cord 7 mm in diameter and about 3 feet (1 m) long and tie it into a continuous loop using a grapevine (double fisherman's) knot.
5. Attach the loop over both strands of the safety attachment with a Prusik hitch.
6. Attach the other end of the adjustable loop to the litter tender's harness using a separate locking carabiner.

Brake and Anchor Systems for Low Angle Lowering

The braking system is essential for a controlled lowering operation during low angle evacuation. It in turn depends on secure anchors (see Chapter 7 for a review of the criteria for safe and secure anchors).

The location and number of brake and anchor systems depend on whether the distance of the lowering is one rope length or more than one rope length.

Low Angle Lowering of One Rope Length

A low angle evacuation of one rope length usually means that only one brake and anchor system is needed. This system usually is placed slightly above the area where the subject is loaded into the litter.

Lowerings of one rope length usually are easier and less complicated than multilength lowerings because:

- Only one brake and anchor system is required.
- No changeover is needed to different sets of brakes and anchors.
- Fewer people are involved.

Low Angle Lowering of More than One Rope Length

Low angle lowerings of more than one rope length often are more complicated because:

- Multiple anchor and brake systems are needed.
- The rope must be changed from one anchor and brake system to another.
- More personnel are involved.
- Greater coordination is needed in the movement of personnel.

In lowerings of more than one rope length, anchor and braking systems must be rigged at strategic points down the slope. Factors that determine the placement of the anchor and brake systems along the slope include the following:

- The length of the main-line lowering rope minus the length needed on the lower end of the rope to tie into the litter, plus approximately 20 feet (6.5 m) from the top end of the rope (there must always be some spare length at the top end to avoid having the rope run out with the litter team in an awkward spot).
- The availability of anchor points.

The rigging of anchors for a braking system can be very time-consuming. In a multilength evacuation, the litter team should not be forced to stop the operation each time the rope runs out and wait for new anchors to be rigged. Two solutions to this problem are *prerigging* and *leapfrogging*.

Prerigging

If enough equipment and skilled personnel are available for anchor rigging, the anchor and brake systems can be rigged ahead of the litter team.

Leapfrogging

Leapfrogging is the practice of using two sets of rigging teams and brake teams to alternate the rigging of anchors and the operation of the brake. While the first team operates the first set of brakes, the second team rigs the second set of anchors. After the litter rope has been detached from the first set of brakes, the first team derigs the first anchors and moves them down to the position for the third anchor and brake system.

Leapfrogging can be a very effective system and can speed the evacuation of a rescue subject. However, for it to be an efficient technique, the rigging teams must be skilled at anchoring, knowledgeable about the equipment, and self-reliant. If they do not have these qualities, the entire operation may be interrupted as the litter is stopped and the rescuers wait for the riggers to finish establishing the next brake and anchor system.

Braking Systems for Low Angle Evacuation
Brake Bar Rack

The brake bar rack is useful for low angle evacuation in the following circumstances:

- Steeper slopes (the brake bar rack [six bars] usually has adequate friction).
- Terrain that varies between steep and gentle (the brake bar rack can easily vary friction) (Box 16-6).

Figure 8 Descender

The large figure 8 with ears does not provide the amount of control the brake bar rack and brake tube do, but it can be used in gentler terrain. Start with the figure 8 double wrapped to make sure there is enough friction to control the lowering.

Tree Wrap

The so-called **tree wrap** is a technique rescuers can fall back on in low angle evacuation when there is a shortage of equipment for braking systems. This technique can be used only in areas that have strong, large-diameter trees.

| Box 16-6 | **Alternative to the Brake Bar Rack: the Brake Tube** |

In low angle lowering, the brake tube can be used as an alternative to the brake bar rack (see Chapter 17, p. 272).

Advantages of the Brake Tube
- ❏ Knots can be passed through the brake tube.
- ❏ A brake tube affords good control for lowering.

Disadvantages of the Brake Tube
- ❏ A brake tube is heavier and bulkier than a brake bar rack (a concern with individual equipment rather than group equipment).
- ❏ Brake tubes are more expensive than brake bar racks.

The primary disadvantage of the tree wrap is that it tends to increase the difficulty of rope management. It also can do permanent damage to trees, and ropes can become contaminated with tree sap. For these reasons, the tree wrap should be used only when no other secure braking system is available.

Using the Tree Wrap Braking System

Figure 16-6 shows a brakeman using the tree wrap braking system.

1. Attach the main-line rope to the litter, either directly with a large loop at the end of the rope or clipped into a continuous loop attached to the litter head rail. The litter should be slightly down slope of the tree wrap location so that it does not interfere with the braking operation.
2. Stack the rope uphill of the tree.
3. Stand slightly to the side of the tree (Figure 16-6, *A*); the rope should be on your side of the tree.
4. Wrap the rope around the tree backward (Figure 16-6, *B*).
5. Make sure the rope does not cross itself on the tree (Figure 16-6, *C*).
6. The amount of friction needed depends on the following factors:
   - ■ Steepness of the slope
   - ■ Weight of the litter and team
   - ■ Circumference of the tree (a large tree, for example, rarely needs to be wrapped as much as 360 degrees)
7. Once enough friction has been obtained, have the litter team pick up the litter and take the slack out of the rope between the litter and the tree. They then lean back into the rope. If the friction is sufficient, they can begin moving down slope while you control the speed of their movement (Figure 16-6, *D*).
8. Increase friction by going farther around the tree to wrap the rope more and by gripping the rope tighter with your hands.
9. Reduce friction by moving from around the tree, to wrap the rope less, and by gripping the rope less tightly with your hands.

Rope Management in Low Angle Evacuation

Good rope management is particularly critical to smooth operation of the brake system in low angle evacuation. Without good rope management, kinks in the rope and tangles coming from the stack or bag could jam the brakes and slow the operation or bring it to a complete halt. Keeping the rope bagged helps prevent kinks and tangles.

To ensure good rope management, a *rope handler* should assist the brakeman, particularly in a tree wrap lowering. The rope handler assists by feeding the brakeman the rope and removing kinks and tangles before they reach the brakes.

The Belay Question

The question of whether to belay in a low angle evacuation must be answered on the scene by trained, experienced personnel, who will consider the following questions:
- ■ How steep is the slope?
- ■ Is the footing particularly loose or treacherous?
- ■ Is the slope icy or muddy?
- ■ What would be the consequences of a fall by the litter team?
- ■ Are the main-line brake anchors questionable?
- ■ Are plenty of anchors available?
- ■ Is thick underbrush or large boulders a factor? (The angle made by the main-line rope and the belay line in low angle evacuation is similar to an advancing wedge; this wedge could tangle in underbrush or on large boulders.)

Ultimately, in deciding whether to belay in a low angle evacuation, rescuers must answer this question: Would the potential benefit of the increased safety be worth the increased complexity in rope and system management and the increase in personnel?

Communications

Good communication in low angle evacuation is particularly critical, especially between the litter team and the brakeman. It is essential that communication be simple, to the point, and clear. For these reasons, voice communications should be limited to a few people. Among these would be the litter captain and the brakeman. If communication is a problem (for example, because of distance, wind, or a waterfall), a relay person may be necessary. Everyone else should keep quiet.

Box 16-7 presents a typical communications sequence in a low angle evacuation. Such communications may vary slightly among rescue groups. The important point is that all those

⚠ *Warning*

Before using a tree wrap brake system for low angle evacuation, consider the following points:
- ❏ The tree wrap system must be used only by those who have practiced it thoroughly under realistic conditions.
- ❏ The technique can be used only on a live, large-diameter tree that has a strong root system.

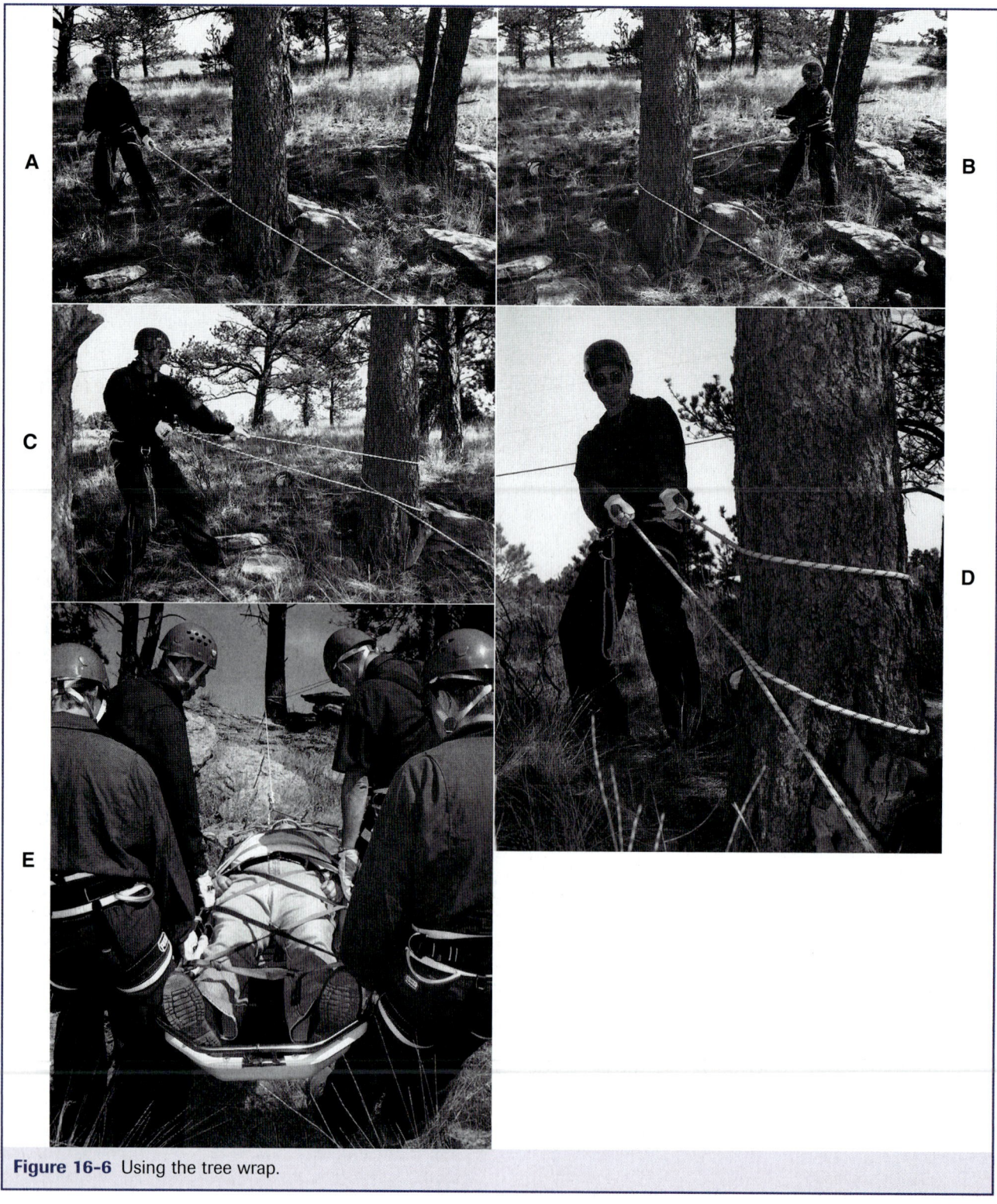

Figure 16-6 Using the tree wrap.

involved in the low angle rescue agree on the particular sequence of commands and responses.

A Typical Low Angle Lowering

The following sequence outlines the basic elements of a low angle lowering operation.

Preparation

Before movement of the litter begins, all major elements of the low angle evacuation system should be in place and prepared. Check for the following:

- The subject has been medically assessed, treated, and packaged, and his or her condition is being monitored.

Box 16-7 | Voice Communications for Low Angle Lowering

"ON ROPE?"
(Litter captain to brakeman. This indicates that the litter team is ready. The team should not proceed without a reply from the brakeman.)

"ON ROPE!"
(Brakeman to litter captain. This response indicates that the braking system is engaged and ready to be loaded.)

"DOWN SLOW."
(Litter captain to brakeman. The brakeman slowly allows rope through the brakes.)
or

"DOWN FAST."*
(The brakeman allows rope through the brake faster.)

"STOP!"
(Generally litter captain to brakeman but may be given by anyone who sees danger or a potential problem developing.)

"STOP! STOP! WHY STOP?"
(Litter captain to brakeman or vice versa. This response is given when, for an unexpected reason and without a command from the litter captain, the rope has stopped moving. The brakeman may be continuing to let out rope, but the rope may be jammed somewhere or the litter may be on a ledge. In such cases the potential for a very serious problem is obvious. This response, any "Stop" command, or any unintelligible command should result in immediate setting of the brakes (or belay if applicable.)

"ZERO!"
(Brakeman to litter captain. This response means that only about 20 feet [6.5 m] of rope is left. The litter team should set the litter down at a convenient spot so that a new brake and anchor set can be established.)

"OFF ROPE."
(Litter captain to brakeman [and belayer when used]. The litter has been set down in a secure spot, and it and the litter team are in no danger of falling.)

"OFF ROPE."
(Brakeman to litter captain. This response acknowledges the litter captain's communication.)

---

*The brakeman should repeat the "Down slow" or "Down fast" command to the litter captain so that the captain knows the brakeman understands. Otherwise, the litter may be lowered at a different rate than that desired.

- The rope has been properly attached to the litter.
- Secure anchors have been set and brakes attached to them.
- The rope is wrapped in the brakes and locked off.
- The brakeman has the rope in hand and is ready to run the brakes.
- The rope handler is ready to feed the rope to the brakeman.
- The belay line is set in the belay device (if applicable).
- The belayer is ready to belay (if applicable).
- The litter attendants are attached to the litter with tie-ins and are ready to lift the litter.

When these preparations are in place, the procedure continues as follows:

1. The litter captain directs the litter team to lift the litter. He or she says, *"One, two, three, lift."*
2. Once the captain is satisfied that all the attendants are ready, he or she says, *"Preload."* The team removes slack from the rope by holding the litter downhill against the rope and leaning into their own tie-ins. The brakeman holds the braking system fixed. This pretests the system and ensures that everything is in order and that the litter team's tie-ins are correctly set.
3. If everything is in order, the litter captain gives the voice communication, *"Down slow."* The brakeman begins to let the rope through the braking system. The rope handler feeds rope to the brakeman. The litter team leans into the system and moves downhill. (The litter captain may say, *"Down fast"* if he or she wants to move down slope faster.)

NOTE: If anything begins to go wrong (e.g., a kink slips past the rope handler and jams the brakes or a litter attendant begins to lose a boot), anyone can call, *"Stop!"*

4. The rope handler warns the brakeman that the rope is running out by calling or radioing, *"Zero!"*

5. The litter captain looks for a good place to set the litter down. When the litter has reached that place, the litter captain calls, *"Stop!"* The captain then directs the team to set the litter down. When the litter is secure and the team is in a stable position, the captain calls, *"Off rope."*

Evacuation of More than One Rope Length

6. When the litter reaches a spot convenient to the second set of brakes, the team stops and sets the litter down. The second brakeman and rope handler are already in position. Two alternatives are possible at this point:

    Alternative 1: The main-line rope now is trailing from the litter uphill to the first set of brakes but has been removed from that system. If the rope is unlikely to tangle, the brakeman can simply attach the same rope to the second set of brakes. The rope handler pulls the rope down as needed and feeds it to the brakeman.

    Alternative 2: If the main-line rope now trailing uphill is likely to snag, the brakeman detaches it from the litter. He or she then attaches a second rope, which is stacked or bagged near the second set of brakes. The team at the first set of brakes derigs the brakes and anchors, recovers the first rope as they come downhill, and then rigs the third set of brakes and anchors (leapfrogging). If belays are used, the second belayer gets ready to belay.

7. The teams repeat the cycle.
8. As soon as the litter team sets the litter down and becomes secure at the end of the first rope length, the first brakeman and rope handler (and first belayer) quickly derig the first brake anchor set. They quickly leapfrog down slope past the second brake and anchor set to rig the third brake and anchor (and belay) set. They are ready when the litter team reaches their position and detaches the rope from the

second brake and anchor set. This cycle continues until the litter safely reaches an objective, such as a road and waiting ambulance, a clearing with a helicopter, or terrain where the carryout may continue.

Hauling

Not all litter evacuations go down slope; many of them have to go up slope. Hauling techniques use many of the same principles as lowering. However, hauling systems may involve slightly more complex rope work and additional personnel.

Mechanical versus Human Power

There are two general approaches to hauling systems: mechanical power or human power. For mechanical power, some powered winches have been designed for rescue work. When rescuers practice using them and can understand their potential and limitations, these winches can help perform a low angle hauling rescue safely and efficiently. As with other types of hauling and lowering systems, the potential for human or mechanical failure always exists, therefore winches should be belayed or safetied in some other way.

One danger with winches designed for high-power applications (e.g., vehicle winches) is lack of control and too much power at the wrong time. If a litter is jammed or a hand is caught between a rock and a litter, the powered winch may not slow down until after damage has been done. This chapter focuses on simple systems that use human power efficiently to haul litters during low angle evacuations.

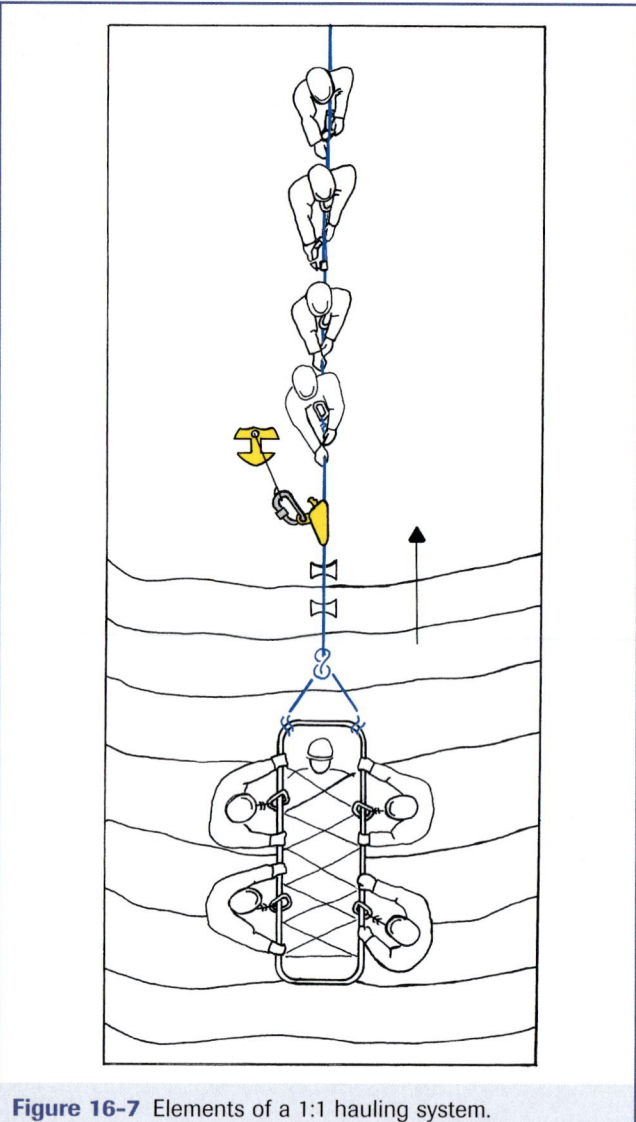

Figure 16-7 Elements of a 1:1 hauling system.

> ### ⚠ Warning
>
> - Never use a powered winch for hauling human subjects that has not been specifically designed for rescue.
> - Winches not designed for rescue lack the control needed for this purpose. Severe injuries and deaths have resulted with attempts to perform rescues with conventional powered winches.
> - Always follow the manufacturer's instructions when using a rescue winch.
> - Practice with rescue winches in realistic conditions before using them in a real rescue.

1:1 Mechanical Advantage Hauling System

One of the simplest hauling systems to be used in low angle evacuation is the *1:1 hauling system*. In essence, the 1:1 simply means that the force needed to haul the load (litter, subject, and attendants) is about the same as the weight of the load.

Figure 16-7 shows the elements of a basic 1:1 hauling system. They include the basic *litter system*, which essentially is the same as that used for lowering a subject packaged in the litter, and the litter team attached with tie-ins.

The *rope system* is attached to the head of the litter and in turn runs through a progress capture device, which is attached to a

different anchor from the *pulley*. The pulley is used to change the direction of the rope to a more convenient angle for the haul team, whose members are attached to the main-line haul rope by figure 8-on-a-bight knots in the rope or by ascenders or Prusik hitches on the rope that are attached to their seat harnesses.

Pulleys Used in 1:1 Hauling Systems

Pulleys used in 1:1 haul systems do not add any mechanical advantage (MA). In fact, some advantage is lost through the pulley's inherent friction. However, pulleys can make things more convenient for a haul team by changing the direction of the rope pull to:

- Allow the team to pull along the contour of a hill instead of straight up.
- Allow the haul to be done in a more convenient place, such as a clearing or along a road (Figure 16-8).

Chapter 5 presents more information on pulleys.

NOTE: Keep in mind that the force on the pulley and its anchor can be more than twice the load.

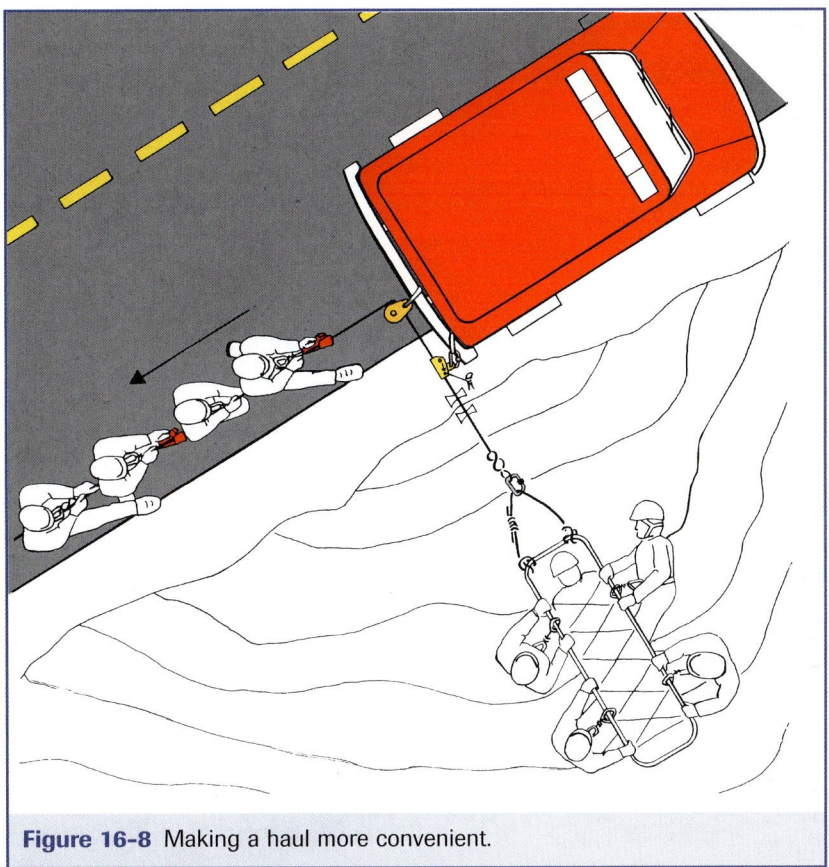

Figure 16-8 Making a haul more convenient.

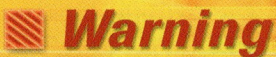

Anchors established for pulley directionals must be stronger than if they were simply supporting a weight equal to the load being hauled. The greater the angle in the rope created at the change in direction, the greater the force on the pulley and the anchor system (Figure 16-9).

The Haul Team

Haul team members should not be selected on the basis of brute force ability but according to the following criteria:
- Ability to follow commands
- Ability to react quickly
- Sensitivity to the feel of the haul rope

Communications for Hauling

The voice communications for hauling movement are initiated by the litter captain (Box 16-8). Other than one special exception, no one else initiates communications for hauling. Everyone else remains quiet.

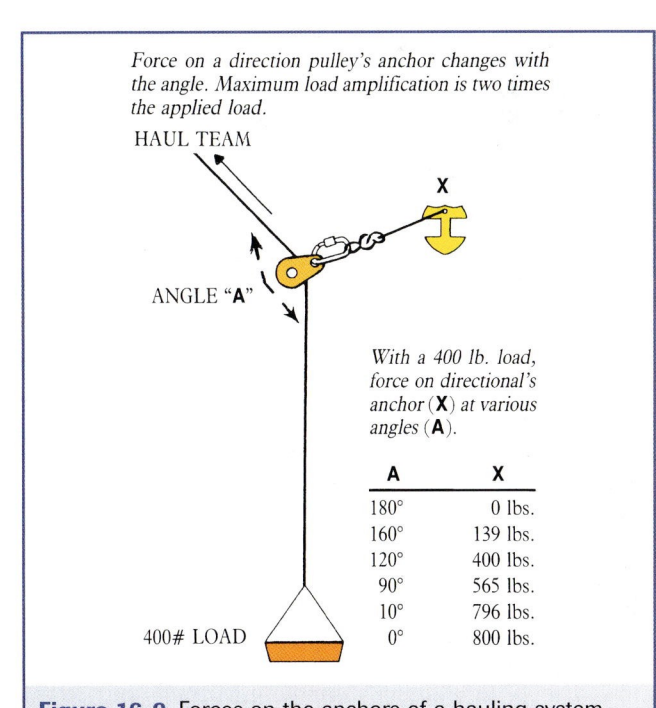

Force on a direction pulley's anchor changes with the angle. Maximum load amplification is two times the applied load.

HAUL TEAM

X

ANGLE "**A**"

*With a 400 lb. load, force on directional's anchor (**X**) at various angles (**A**).*

400# LOAD

A	X
180°	0 lbs.
160°	139 lbs.
120°	400 lbs.
90°	565 lbs.
10°	796 lbs.
0°	800 lbs.

Figure 16-9 Forces on the anchors of a hauling system.

Box 16-8 | Haul Commands

To eliminate the potential for disastrous confusion, haul commands are limited to a few standardized terms.

"HAUL."
(Begin hauling. This command needs to be given only once; the team will continue to haul until given another command.)

or

"HAUL SLOW."
(A variation used when the emphasis is on slow movement, such as when the litter is about to reach the top.)

"SET."
(The haul team immediately stops hauling and gently eases back on the load; this is done to set the progress capture device. It may be needed for safety reasons or, more commonly, to get another bite on the rope.)

"SLACK."
(The progress capture device is set, therefore the haul team slacks on the rope. This allows any part of the system to be reset, and the haul team to get another bite on the rope. [If a belay is used, the normal belay communications are also used.])

The following command may be given by anyone who sees something going wrong:

"STOP!"
(All movement stops immediately. The haul team holds tension until told to do otherwise.)

⬛ *Warning*

- ❏ Never substitute voice haul commands unless there is an overriding reason and all team members were informed before the change.
- ❏ Use only crisp, distinct terms that have no chance of being mistaken for other words. For example, do not replace "Stop" with "Whoa," which easily can be mistaken for "Slow" or, even worse, "Go."
- ❏ All commands should be given over the radio or loudly enough so that everyone—litter team, belayer, and rope handlers—can hear them.

The Important Progress Capture Device (PCD)

Whatever the type of hauling system, it is essential to have a setup that prevents the litter from falling back down slope between hauling cycles. A commonly accepted element of a haul system is the ***progress capture device (PCD)***, which uses a rope grab device such as a tandem Prusik or general-use ascender to prevent the litter from falling back.

Using PCDs in Steep Slope Evacuation

Progress capture devices should always be connected to a safe and secure anchor system that is, if possible, *separate* from the anchor system supporting the haul system (Box 16-9).

⬛ *Warning*

1. Hauling systems create enormous forces on the rope rescue system. Unnoticed problems quickly can result in catastrophic system failure. Personnel constantly must monitor for potential problems including, but not limited to:
   - ❏ Knots on moving rope that jam in cracks
   - ❏ Broken gear that causes system failure
   - ❏ Systems reaching their limit
   - ❏ Pinned arms and legs
2. Good communication must be established between team captains and the haul team.
3. The haul team must keep in mind that what seems a normal speed for them seems very fast to those being hauled (i.e., the rescue subject and the litter attendants). Therefore the haul team must:
   - ❏ Pull slowly unless told to do otherwise
   - ❏ At all times, be prepared to stop instantly

⬛ *Warning*

Never use light-use (personal) ascenders for hauling systems in which more than one person's body weight may be involved. Use of this type of ascender can result in failure in two potential ways:

1. The frame or some other portion of the ascender may fail.
2. The sharp teeth of the cam may tear the rope sheath.

Box 16-9 | Terminology

The progress capture device sometimes has been called a safety cam or a ratchet cam. However, it is not appropriate to call a PCD a "safety cam," because it does not and should not act as a belay. Using the term safety can be confusing to some individuals.

Also, although the device may act as a ratchet, the term progress capturing gives a better mental picture of its purpose, particularly for individuals without a mechanical background.

A progress capture device can be either a hard cam (general-use ascender) or a soft cam (Prusik).

Some models of general-use ascenders have an arrow with the caption, "Up"; this is the indicator for direction of use for ascending a rope. *In hauling systems, this arrow should always point along the rope toward the load (the litter and rescue subject).* Some older models of general-use ascenders do not have this arrow inscribed on the shell. However, the shell, when viewed in profile, vaguely resembles an arrowhead (see Figure 5-19,

p. 61). Again, the arrow should point in the direction of the load.

Positioning the PCD

If possible, the progress capture device should be on a separate anchor from the hauling system. However, it should be close and parallel to the main-line rope. This helps prevent shock loading and reduces the slack that interferes with haul system efficiency.

Setting the PCD

The two primary concerns in rigging a progress capture device are:

- That the device grab the rope when needed
- That the device not ride up the rope as the rope moves (this could result in dangerous shock loading)

The exact rigging of the PCD depends partly on the particular type of general-use ascender and partly on the specific circumstances of the rigging (Figures 16-10 and 16-11).

Free Running PCD Figure 16-10 and Figure 16-12, *A,* show one method of ensuring that the PCD stays in place and clamps on the rope when needed. *This technique is specific to the use of a general-use ascender as a PCD.* The technique requires the services of a person known as the *PCD tender.*

As the main-line hauling rope moves up, the PCD tender makes sure the PCD does not travel up the rope. The tender does this by holding the backside of the ascender shell with the palm and with the fingers extended out of the way of the cam. The PCD is held in this manner so that fingers and gloves do not get caught as the PCD suddenly shock loads. A finger caught by the PCD could be injured, and a glove caught in the cam could prevent it from clamping the rope.

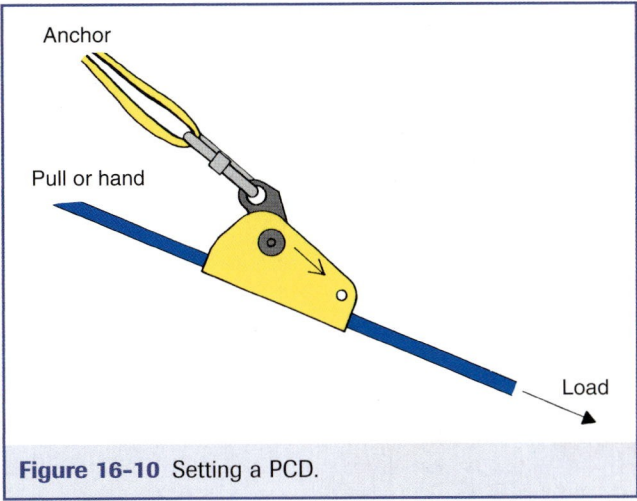

Figure 16-10 Setting a PCD.

Although use of a PCD tender can be effective, it requires extra personnel, and the potential always exists for human failure or inattention.

A second technique for using a free running, general-use ascender as a PCD is shown in Figure 16-12, *B.* A bungee (elastic) cord is clipped into the empty hole usually found toward the point of the arrowhead in some general-use ascenders. The other end of the bungee cord is anchored securely to a convenient spot toward the load. A great deal of tension is not required on the bungee cord, but there should be enough to:

- Keep the PCD from riding up the rope
- Keep the PCD closed on the rope

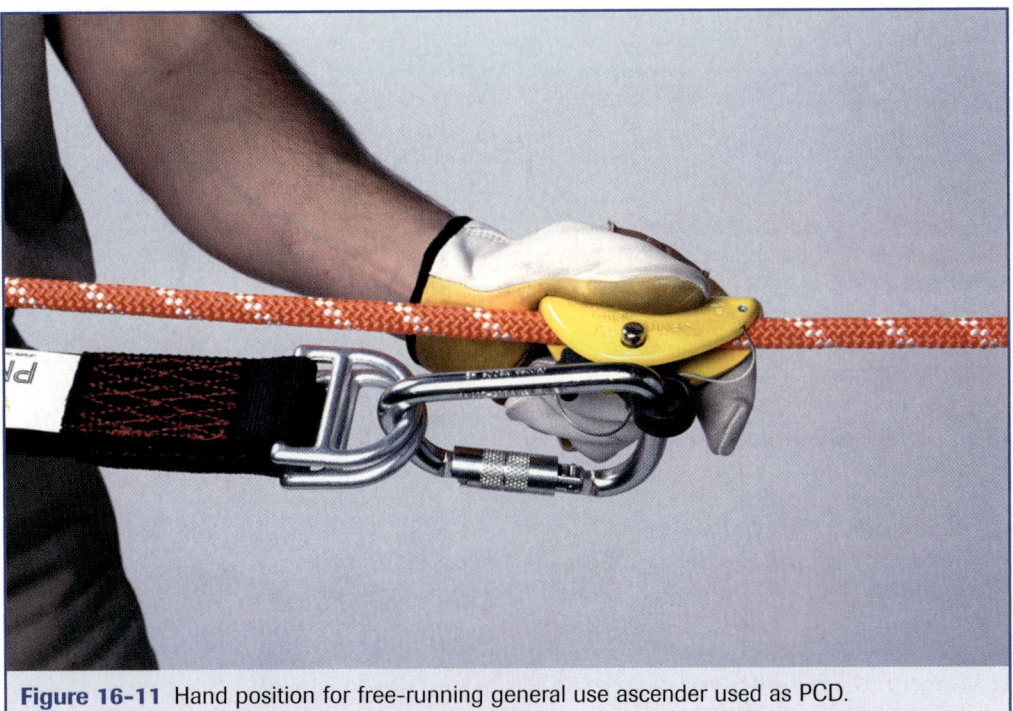

Figure 16-11 Hand position for free-running general use ascender used as PCD.

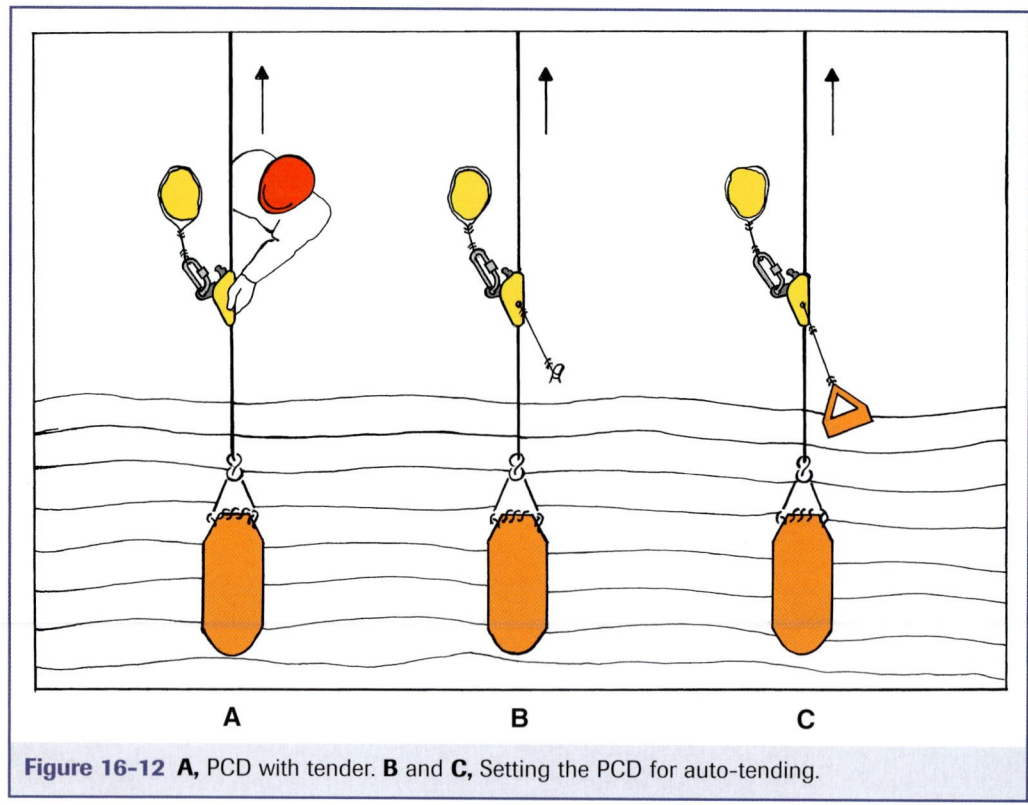

Figure 16-12 A, PCD with tender. **B** and **C,** Setting the PCD for auto-tending.

NOTE: Tie the bungee cord *only to the shell* of the general-use ascender and not to the cam itself. Otherwise, the system will not function as needed. Also, this technique of auto-tending a PCD with a bungee cord probably will not work with Prusik hitches. See Chapter 13 for information on tending Prusik hitches.

A third alternative for setting a general-use ascender PCD is shown in Figure 16-12, *C.* This method uses a short piece of cord, which is attached to a weight. The weight is hung so that it pulls the shell of the PCD toward the load.

Spring-Loaded PCD If a spring-loaded PCD has been properly rigged, the cam will close onto the rope when needed. However, the problem remains of how to keep the shell from riding up the rope as the rope moves. The solution is similar to those for the free running PCD: a cam attendant, a bungee cord, or a weighted cord.

Prusik-Type PCD Under certain conditions, a properly used Prusik system may serve as a progress capture device. For further information, see chapters 13 and 18.

Counterbalance Hauling System

In any hauling system, the major force that rescuers fight is gravity. The ***counterbalance haul system*** is a method of using gravity to fight gravity.

Strictly speaking, a counterbalance hauling system is also a 1:1 haul system. Without considering loss caused by friction and other inefficiencies, the force used to haul is the same as the weight of the load being hauled. However, the difference is this:

instead of the haul team going off to the side (as in the example on p. 241), the haul team takes advantage of gravity by going downhill. The load (i.e., the litter system) still goes uphill. Figure 16-13 shows the elements of a counterbalance haul system, which includes the litter system, the rope system, and the pulley and anchor system.

Litter System

In the litter system, the subject is medically assessed, treated, and packaged in the litter, and his or her condition is monitored. The litter team is attached to the litter by their tie-ins.

Rope System

The bottom end of the rope is attached to the head of the litter. As the litter gets to the top, the rope first runs through the PCD, which is on its own anchor system. Just above the progress capture device, the rope goes through the pulley and anchor system.

Pulley and Anchor System

In this example, two pulleys are used. The first pulley changes the rope direction 90 degrees, and the second pulley then changes the rope direction another 90 degrees, so that the rope goes back down the slope.

It may be possible to use only one pulley. However, in this situation, the use of two pulleys means a greater margin of safety and less chance of failure. Remember, *two* loads are now pulling down slope on the anchors: the weight of the load (litter system) and the force of the team's weight while also pulling downhill slightly. Consequently, two pulleys and two anchor systems share

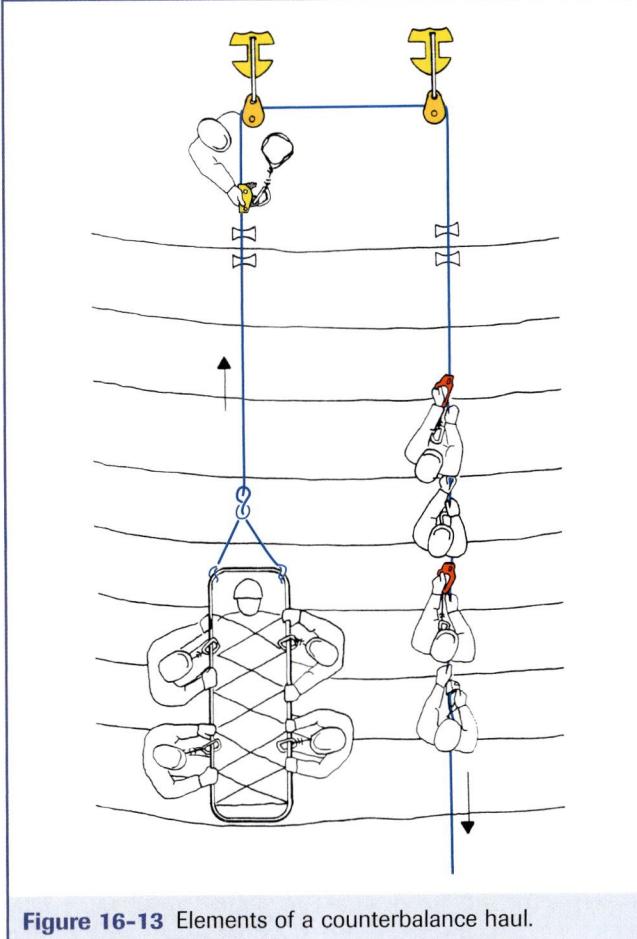

Figure 16-13 Elements of a counterbalance haul.

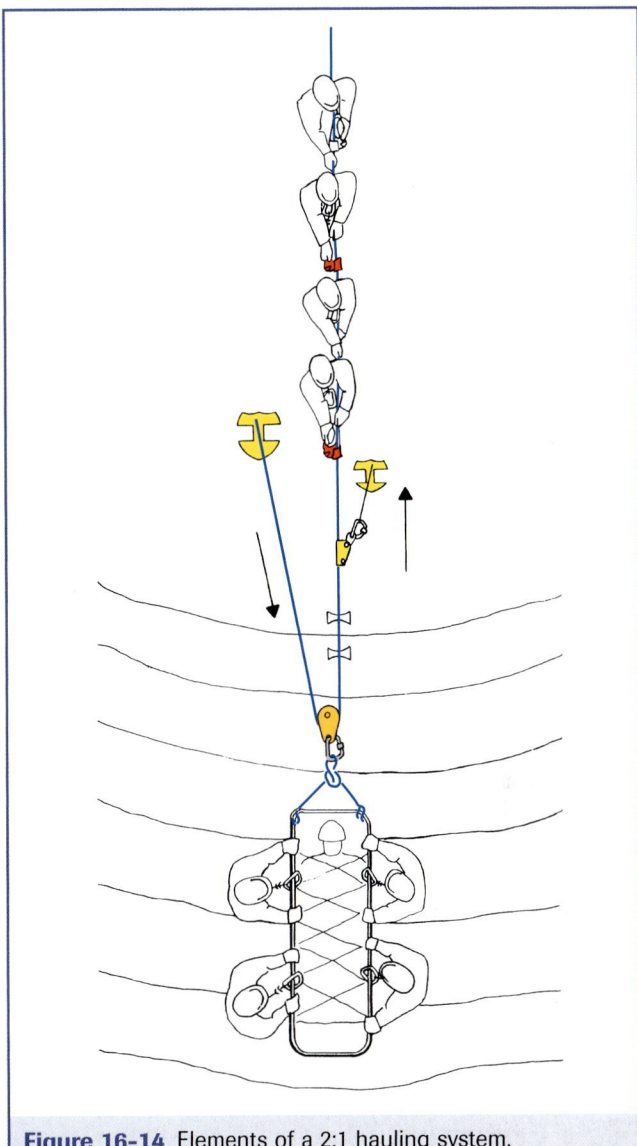

Figure 16-14 Elements of a 2:1 hauling system.

the load. Note that due to the 90 degree angle, each of the two pulleys see more than half the total load but not twice the load as in the case of a single pulley at 90 degrees (see Figure 16-9).

Having the two anchor systems and two pulleys set a distance apart means two additional advantages:

1. Less chance of the two rope strands tangling
2. Less chance for the haul team and the litter team to interfere with one another's movements

2:1 Hauling System for Low Angle Evacuation

Figure 16-14 shows a 2:1 hauling system for low angle evacuation.

In theory, with a 2:1 haul system, the force needed by the haul team to move the litter system is only half the force needed in the 1:1 haul system previously examined. However, with the 2:1 hauling system, the haul team must travel twice as far.

The 2:1 hauling system is created by anchoring a rope at the top, running it back down to the litter through a pulley that is attached to the litter yoke, and then running the rope back to the top through a PCD on a separate anchor and near the first anchor. The haul team might be able to pull uphill on the rope, but Figure 16-15 shows them going off to the side to make it a little easier on themselves. This sideways pull is made possible by running the rope over a directional pulley anchored near the anchor point of the top end of the rope.

> ### ⚠ *Warning*
>
> Although a 2:1 hauling system can make hauling easier, it increases rope management problems:
> - Two strands of rope now move along the same path.
> - A pulley is moving, which easily could become jammed on underbrush, trees, rocks, or other obstacles. Rescue personnel must be able to reach the pulley, wherever it jams, to free it. (See Chapter 18 for a possible solution to this problem.)

Other Hauling Systems

Other types of force multiplying haul systems (3:1 MA and above) may be used in low angle evacuations if:

- The slope becomes steeper.
- Fewer personnel are available for the haul team (see Chapter 18 for details on the rigging of other hauling systems).

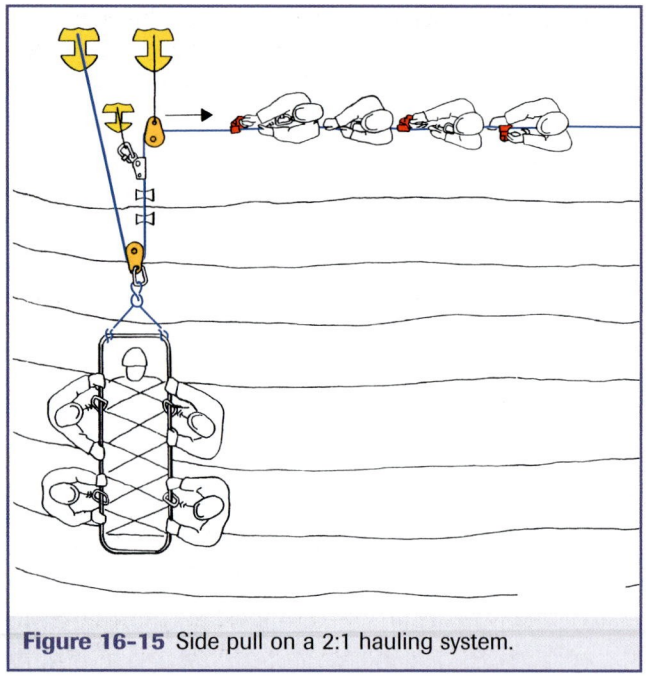

Figure 16-15 Side pull on a 2:1 hauling system.

Drawbacks to Force Multiplying Haul Systems

Remember that although force multiplying haul systems can make it easier for haul teams to move a litter, all such systems have some drawbacks, including the following:

- They are more complicated to rig.
- They take longer to rig.
- They create greater forces on elements of the system.
- They foul and perhaps fail more easily.
- The haul team must travel a longer distance than with a 1:1 system.

Safe Movement of Personnel in Low Angle Evacuation

A potential problem in low angle evacuation is the safe movement of personnel up and down the slope for rigging, medical evaluation, litter rigging, and other tasks. These individuals may have trouble with footing, thus endangering themselves. Also, they may knock rocks or other debris down onto the rescue subject and other rescuers.

To prevent this problem, one of the first actions on the scene should be immediate establishment of a restricted zone to reduce the danger to the rescuers and subject. For particularly steep areas, rescuers can establish personnel safety lines (Figure 16-16). These lines should be well anchored and established off to the side so that personnel can travel up and down them without endangering those below.

Once the safety lines have been established, personnel can move up and down either by hand or with descenders and ascenders. On steeper slopes and in high angle operations, personnel should also tie in short directly to the rope. For more information on tying in short, see p. 152 in Chapter 10.

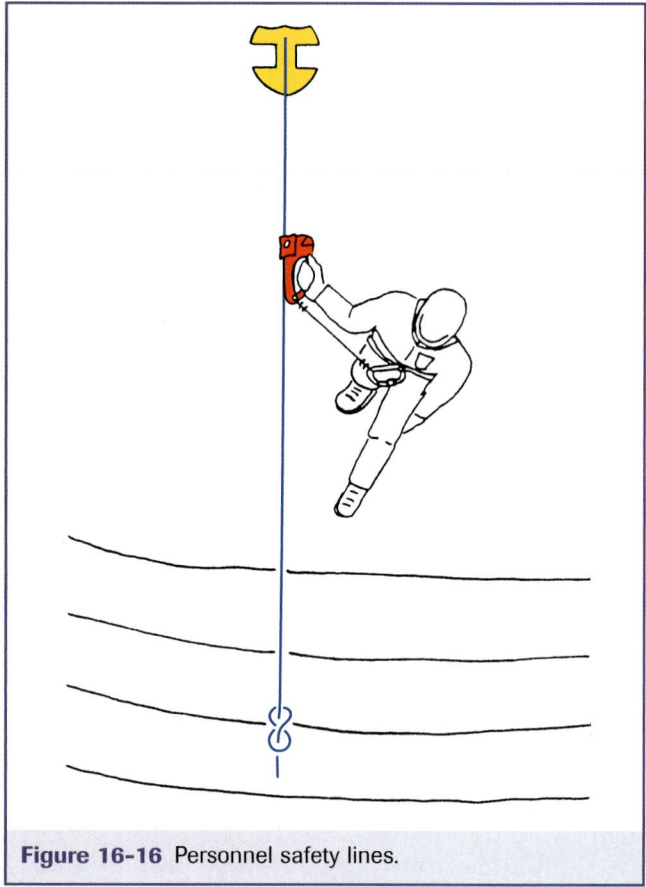

Figure 16-16 Personnel safety lines.

Evaluation Exercises

Cognitive and Affective Exercises

1. List four ways in which low angle evacuation differs from high angle evacuation.

2. Explain the consequences of using a single point of attachment to a basket litter.

3. Which of the following are not considerations in the packaging of the subject?

   A. Spinal immobilization
   B. Secure strapping
   C. Protection from the environment
   D. Availability of anchor points

4. What type of knot could be used to make a litter attendant tie-in adjustable?

    A. Ring bend
    B. Prusik
    C. Figure 8
    D. Bowline

5. If the lowering requires more than one rope length to accomplish, it is what type of lowering?

    A. Single pitch
    B. Multipitch
    C. Tandem pitch
    D. Dual pitch

6. If the lowering requires only one rope length to accomplish, it is what type of lowering?

    A. Multipitch
    B. Dual pitch
    C. Tandem pitch
    D. Single pitch

7. Name two factors that will determine the location of brake and anchor systems in a lowering of more than one rope length.

8. What are the duties of a rope handler in a low angle evacuation?

9. What are three considerations in deciding whether to have a belay in a low angle evacuation?

10. Repeat from memory and in sequence the voice communications between the litter captain and the brakeman and the litter captain and a belayer during a low angle evacuation.

11. Why should personal ascenders not be used for hauling systems involving more than one person's body weight?

12. When general-use ascenders are used in hauling systems for low angle evacuation, which way should the arrow point?

    A. Toward the anchor
    B. Toward the lateral moraine
    C. Toward the belay
    D. Toward the load

13. Name three problems that could develop in a low angle hauling system and tell which members of the team should be on the lookout for them.

14. What voice communication should be given by any member of the rescue team who sees something going wrong during a low angle evacuation?

    A. "Halt."
    B. "Belay that."
    C. "Haul slow."
    D. "Stop."

17

High Angle Lowering

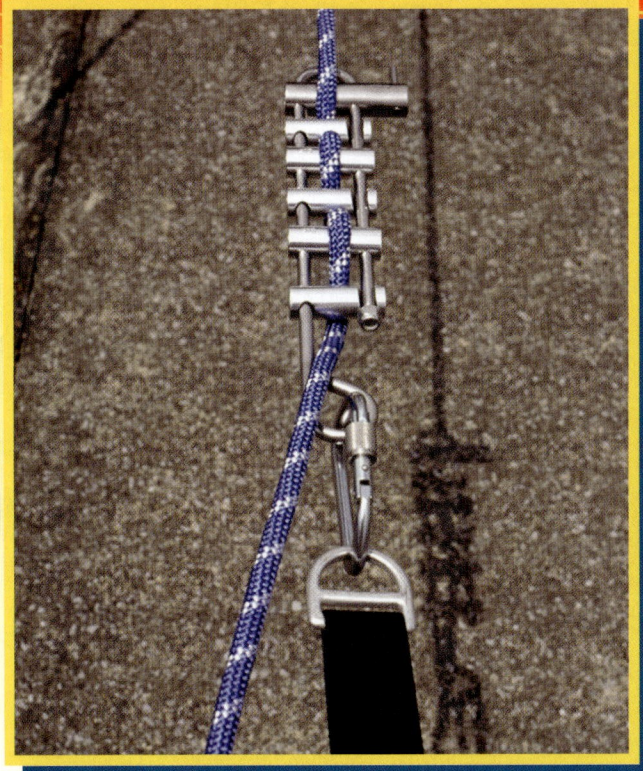

Prerequisites

Before attempting the activities described in this chapter, you must have demonstrated that you can properly:

1. Use and care for rope.
2. Use and care for other equipment needed in the high angle environment.
3. Tie correctly and without hesitation the knots necessary for safe, effective work in the vertical environment (see Chapter 6).
4. Apply the principles of anchoring and rig a safe and secure anchor.
5. Apply the principles of belaying and safely and confidently belay another person using either a Münter hitch or a personal belay device.
6. Apply the principles of rappelling: rappel safely and under control, tie off the rappel device to operate hands free of the rappel device and rope, and then return to a safe and controlled rappel.
7. Apply the principles of ascending: tie a Prusik hitch correctly and without hesitation and know how to use it; comprehend the uses and limitations of mechanical ascenders; confidently and safely ascend a fixed rope using either friction hitches or mechanical ascenders; confidently and safely change over from rappelling to ascending and ascending to rappelling; and extricate yourself from a jammed rappel device or similar problem.
8. Apply the principles of low angle evacuation: correctly set the rigging in any of the elements of slope evacuation and safely and confidently assume the role of litter tender, haul team member, rope handler, brakeman, or belayer.
9. Correctly distinguish between one-person and rescue belays; correctly tie a load-releasing hitch and demonstrate how to release it under load; correctly rig a tandem Prusik belay system and operate it; correctly rig a Prusik minding pulley and operate it.

The material in this chapter conforms to guidelines published by the National Fire Protection Association (NFPA), specifically standard 1006, *Professional Qualifications for Rescue Technicians* (2002), and standard 1670, *Operations and Training for Technical Rescue Incidents* (2004). NFPA standards are revised regularly, and readers are advised to review the latest version of this standard.

Objectives

On completion of this chapter, you should be able to:

1. Define high angle lowering and list the elements of a high angle lowering system.
2. Given a list of equipment, select the equipment needed for a high angle lowering system.
3. Discuss the medical considerations for a subject before and during a high angle lowering.
4. Describe the functions of the these positions: litter tender, brakeman, rope handler, belayer, and edge tender.
5. Describe the functions of the rope and braking systems, the belay, edge protection, spiders, and litter tender tie-ins in high angle lowering.
6. Describe the function of knot passing in a high angle lowering.
7. List the differences between single line and double line lowering systems, along with the advantages and disadvantages of each.
8. Repeat from memory the voice communications used in high angle lowering.
9. Construct rigging for a litter, braking system, and belay system and act as litter tender, brakeman, and belayer in a high angle lowering.
10. Perform a knot pass in a high angle lowering.

Key Terms

Auxiliary Tender An optional rescuer who, in order to assist the rescue, rappels or ascends alongside the litter. This person's duties may include medical assessment and/or primary treatment of the rescue subject, as well as assisting in getting the litter over the edge, in handling the litter on the vertical face, and in loading the subject into the litter.

Bridle See **Spider**.

Double Line Lowering The use of two ropes attached to the litter in a lowering; the ropes are rigged so that they may be operated independently to change the angle of the litter. Also called *scaffold lowering*.

Edge Tender The person connected to a safety attachment who works at the edge of a drop in a high angle lowering. This individual's duties include assisting in getting the litter over the edge, reducing edge abrasion to ropes, and when necessary, relaying communications between the litter tender and the brakeman.

Litter Attendant An individual who helps control the litter or attends to a subject's medical needs during a high angle evacuation rescue. Also known as a *litter attendant*.

Load The total combined objects and persons being lowered or raised by a rope in a high angle system. Some examples include a rescue subject and a rescuer, or a subject in a litter with one or two attached litter tenders.

Pigtail A short piece of rope with which the litter tender attaches to the litter system.

Single Line Lowering The use of one main lowering rope with a belay to lower a litter.

Spider The system of attaching a lowering rope to a litter. A spider usually has four or more legs that connect to various points of a litter to equalize loading. Sometimes called a *bridle* or *harness*.

The High Angle Lowering System

High angle lowering is sometimes also called vertical lowering. Both terms refer to the same principle: the controlled lowering of a rescue subject using a rope. If the subject's injuries are severe enough, the lowering is done with the subject packaged in a litter. High angle litter lowering usually is done with one or two rescuers (litter tenders) attached to the litter, and the weight of the subject, litter, and rescuers is supported by the rope.

As the rescuers lower the litter, it may run down against the side of a high angle wall, such as a cliff face or the side of a building, or it may be "free" (not touching the wall). This depends on the nature of the wall where the lowering is performed. If the top of the drop is overhung, the litter will hang out away from the wall. This might be a more difficult operation for the rescuers because they would not have the advantage of pushing

against the wall to maneuver themselves and the litter during the rescue. In some cases, when the subject is uninjured or only slightly injured, it may be possible to lower the individual without the litter, either alone or with a rescuer (see Chapter 14 for a discussion of pickoff rescue).

The following sites are some of the environments in which a high angle lowering might be used:

- Cliffs
- Buildings
- Industrial sites, either outside a structure or inside a vessel
- Construction sites, such as tower cranes
- Other structures, such as stacks, silos, or towers
- Vertical caves

Vertical lowering may take place on the outside of a structure, such as a building or stack, or on the inside, such as the interior of a silo or tank.

Lowering System

Figure 17-1 shows the basic elements of a vertical lowering system.

Load

The **load** often includes the subject packaged in a litter plus any **litter attendants**. Because of medical considerations and concern for the subject's comfort, the litter usually is lowered in a horizontal position. Also, subjects usually feel less anxious in a horizontal position because they mostly see sky or a ceiling and not the ground.

Confined space environments or obstructions, however, may require that the litter be lowered in a vertical position with the head up. The load may consist of the subject only, if the individual is uninjured or only slightly injured, or it may comprise the subject attached to a rescuer.

Litter Tenders

One or two litter tenders may be needed. Each litter tender is attached to the *master attachment point (MAP)* by at least two connections: a primary tie-in and a safety.

Attachments for the Load to the Main-Line Rope or Ropes

Litter attachments to the rope are known as **spiders** (they are also known as **bridles** or *harnesses*). Spiders are used to balance and stabilize the load. They attach at several points to the litter and come together where they attach to the rope. Spiders have at least four legs that attach to the litter, although in some systems there may be as many as six.

Main-Line or Ropes

The main-line (also called a lowering line in lowering systems) must be able to support the rescue load adequately, plus have an

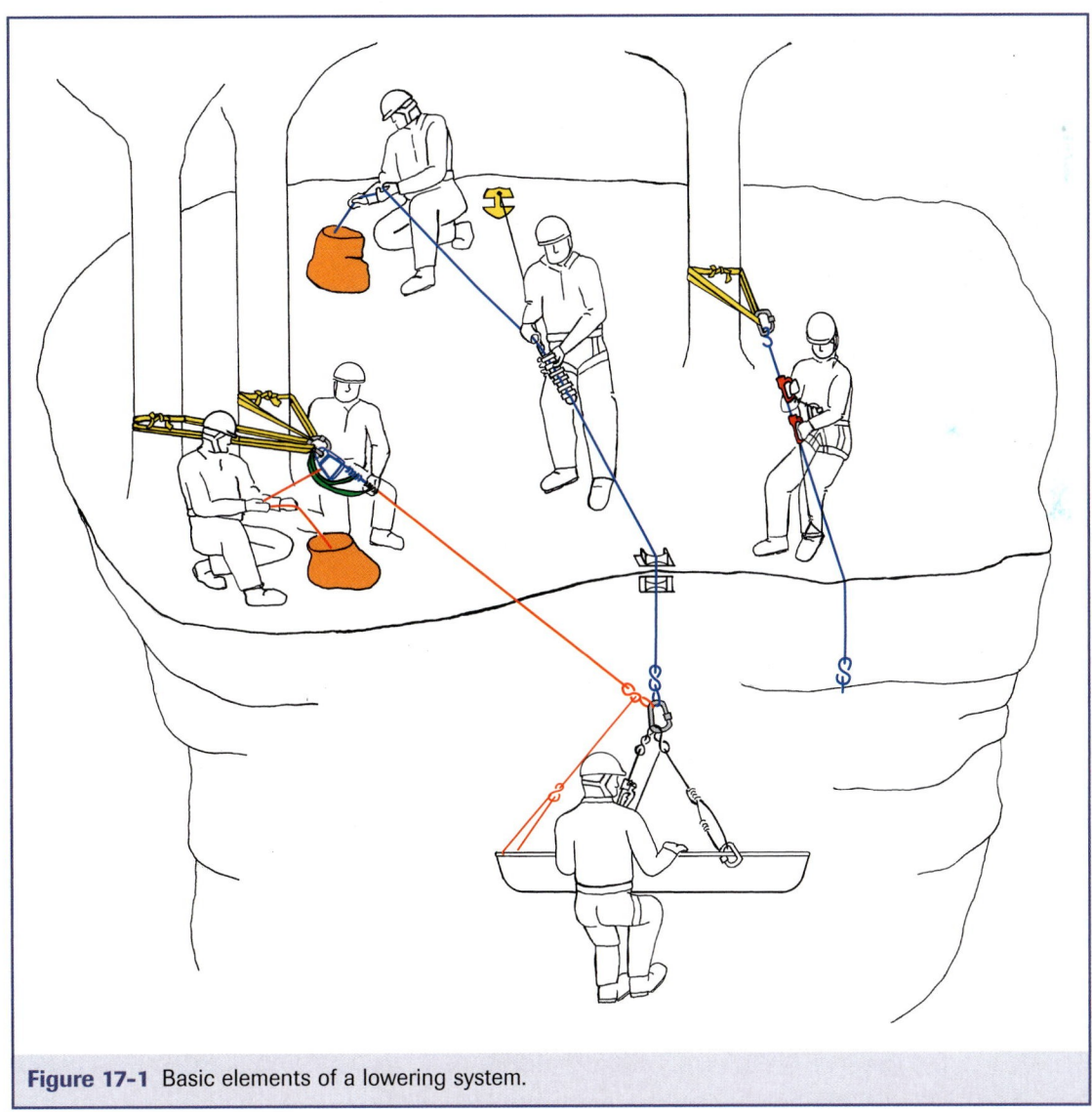

Figure 17-1 Basic elements of a lowering system.

appropriate safety factor. Some lowering systems have only one main line (lowering line) with a belay. Other systems have two main lines (lowering lines).

Belay System

The belay system is attached to the load and acts as a safety should a failure occur in the main-line lowering system.

Brake Device

Brake devices are friction devices that are the same as or similar to rappel devices. They provide friction on rope running through them to control the descent of the load.

Brakeman

The brakeman controls the speed of the load's descent by controlling the rope running through the brake device.

Rope Handler

The rope handler assists the brakeman by passing the rope to him or her, making sure there are no kinks to jam the brake device.

Belayer

The belayer controls the belay rope through the belay device and catches the load with the belay system should the main lowering system fail.

Edge Tenders

The *edge tenders* assist the litter tenders in getting the litter over the edge of the drop. They also protect the rope from abrasion on the edge and, if needed, relay voice communications between the litter tender and the brakeman.

Rescue Team Leader

The rescue team leader is the manager of the operation. In the ideal situation, the leader does not get physically involved in the actions of the rescue, such as rigging, but rather maintains an objective overall view of the operation.

Safety Officer

The safety officer does not become engrossed in other activities, such as operations, therefore he or she can stand back and be objective about any threats to safety. The safety officer must have the right to stop any operation he or she sees as a threat to safety and must be an experienced person who thoroughly under-stands equipment, rigging, and rescue techniques. The safety officer also must be able to survey a situation and know instantly if something is incorrect; he or she must always be able to stand back with an objective viewpoint and must never be sucked into the operation itself. Safety officers check for the following:

- Hazards, including hazardous atmospheres and falling debris
- Personal safety equipment, including helmets, gloves, and breathing apparatus
- Rescue rigging, including belays, anchors, rope padding, and unlocked carabiners
- Personal rigging, including seat harnesses, locked carabiners, and knots tied correctly

Braking Systems for Lowering

The principles governing the use of a braking device for high angle lowering are similar to those for rappelling. Whether used for rappelling or lowering, the device imparts friction to the rope running through it. Some devices used for lowering are the same as those used in rappelling, such as brake bar racks and figure 8 descenders.

Any braking device used in lowering must provide an adequate margin of control of the load being lowered. A figure 8 descender, for example, may provide adequate control for one person's body weight, but it may not provide enough control for loads of more than one person's body weight. To lower loads of more than one person's body weight, a device that offers greater friction is needed, such as a brake bar rack (six bars) or brake tube.

The primary difference between lowering and rappelling is that in most lowering situations, the friction device remains stationary, and the rope moves through it (this is known as a *fixed brake lower*). In rappelling, the friction device moves, and the rope remains stationary.

Belays for Lowering

Lowering systems should have redundancy so that if one line fails, another catches the load. This can mean a belay that is both apart from the main lowering system and on a separate anchor, or it can mean two separate lowering lines that back up one another.

In either situation, the systems should be rigged so that these two elements do not interfere with each other and become entangled. However, they should be close enough together to prevent a dangerous pendulum should the main-line fail and the belay be forced to catch the load.

The load caught by a belay in a rescue lowering operation may not fall as great a distance as in climbing. However, belayers must use belay devices that allow them to hold the weight of the rescue load plus any force from shock loading.

> ### ⬛ *Warning*
>
> In a rescue lowering, the belayer must never use a hip belay or any other belay technique involving rope friction around the body.
>
> Also, the belayer must never place his or her body as a link in the belay system when rescue lowering (see Chapter 8).

Communication in Rescue Lowering

As in slope evacuation, the primary exchange of communication signals in a vertical lowering takes place between the litter tender and the brakeman. If conditions permit, this should be direct communication between the two individuals. If direct communi-cation is not possible because of such factors as distance or noise from machinery, traffic, or a waterfall, a relay person might be required. If edge tenders are used, one of these individuals can be assigned as a communications relay.

Radios

Over longer distances, radios may be a necessity. They also may be required for medical control or for relaying the medical condition of the subject.

Use of the traditional hip-belt holstered radios creates some problems in high angle rescue:

- They interfere with seat harnesses and the use of equipment.
- They require extensive hand and arm movement to use the radio.
- The radios can be dropped.

One solution to these difficulties is a radio chest harness (Figure 17-2). These harnesses, which are commercially available, have the following advantages:

- The microphone is closer to the rescuer's mouth, therefore the radio does not have to be removed from a holster for use.
- The chest area usually is free of other harnesses and equipment.
- A simple hand motion can key the mike.

Another solution to communications challenges is the voice-activated radio. With the microphone positioned next to the mouth, transmission occurs whenever a person speaks. One drawback to these radios is that in high winds, the microphone may be keyed by the wind, preventing communication.

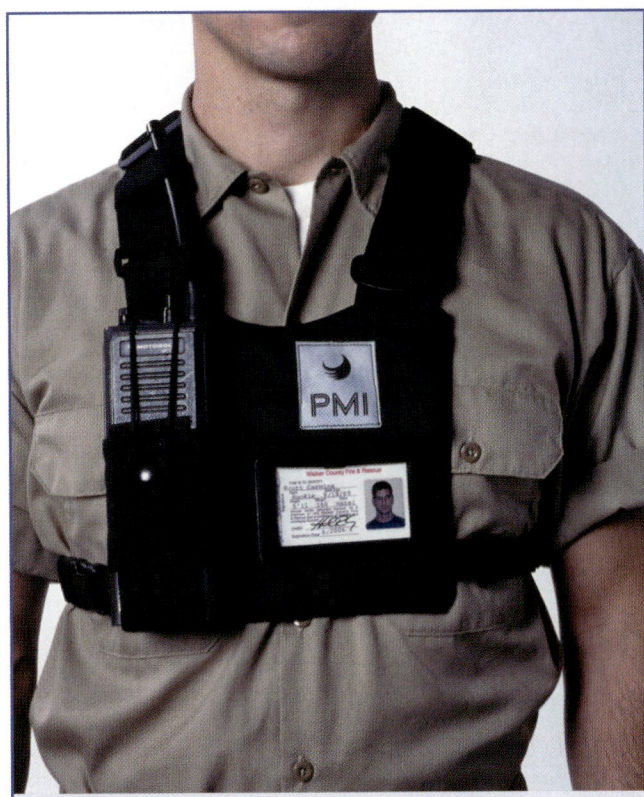

Figure 17-2 Radio chest harness.

Voice Communication

Direct and reliable communication in vertical lowering is critical to the safety of the subject and rescuers and to the success of the operation. To avoid dangerous confusion, voice communications must be limited only to a few standardized commands necessary for litter movement and for safety.

If the lowering system includes a single line plus belay, the standard belay commands are included in the lowering commands (Box 17-1).

Suggestion

When more than one rope is used for lowering, it is helpful to line management to use ropes of different colors. This is particularly true in lowering systems that use two lines, one to the head end and one to the foot end of the litter. The litter tender can maintain litter orientation, for example, by calling, "Red rope down 1 foot."

Principles of Rescue Lowering

As mentioned earlier in the chapter, any braking device used in rescue lowering must provide an adequate margin of control for the load being lowered. The first exercise presented for lowering practice uses a figure 8 descender because it is simpler to use in learning the basics of lowering loads. The figure 8 may provide adequate control for one person's body weight but should not be used for heavier loads. Lowering of loads of more than one person's body weight requires a device that offers greater friction, such as a brake bar rack (six bars) or brake tube.

This practice activity is designed to acquaint the student with the basic principles of lowering, under controlled conditions and using the weight of only one person. This lowering sequence uses a practice rescuer as a load and a figure 8 with ears as a braking device (Figure 17-3).

Lowering One Person Using a Figure 8 with Ears (Steep Slope)

1. At the top of a short slope (approximately 45 degrees), attach an anchor sling to a secure anchor. Clip a locking carabiner into it. (If a slope is not available, use a flight of stairs.)
2. At a separate secure anchor, establish a belay station with a sling and a large, locking carabiner with a belay device attached to it (see Chapter 8 for additional guidelines on belaying).
3. Have a practice rescuer clip the belay line into his or her harness with a carabiner (Figure 17-3, *A*). Attach the main lowering line to one carabiner, the belay to the other.
4. Have the brakeman lace the main-line rope onto the figure 8 as shown in Figure 17-4. The small ring should be clipped into the anchor carabiner and the carabiner gate should be locked. The large ring of the figure 8 should be pointed toward the practice rescuer and the rope going to him or her should be laced through the large ring.
5. While in a secure position and facing the brakeman, the practice rescuer takes the main-line rope with a figure 8-

Box 17-1 | Lowering Commands

"ON BELAY?"
(Litter tender to brakeman.)
"BELAY ON."
(Brakeman to litter tender.)
"DOWN SLOW."
  or
"DOWN FAST."
(Litter tender to brakeman.)
"STOP!"
(Generally this command is given by the litter tender to the brakeman, but it may be given by anyone who sees danger or potential problems developing.)
"STOP! STOP! WHY STOP?"
(Litter tender to brakeman. This response is given when, for an unexplained reason and without command from the litter tender, the rope has stopped moving. The brakeman may still be letting out rope, but the rope may be jammed somewhere. This obviously has the potential to create a very serious problem and requires an explanation.)
"OFF BELAY."
(Litter tender to belayer. The litter, rescue subject, and litter tender [or tenders] are on the ground or in a secure position and are in no danger of falling.)

"BELAY OFF."
(Belayer to litter tender.)

The following voice communications also may be used when needed.
"SLACK."
(Litter tender to brakeman or belayer. It means, "The rope is too taut, give us some slack.")
"TENSION."
(Litter tender to brakeman or belayer. It means, "Take up some rope and make it more taut to help us out here.")
When a belay is being used, the tender must specify to which line he or she is referring.
"SLACK ON BELAY LINE."
  or
"SLACK ON MAIN LINE."
When the litter has reached the ground, a voice signal is given.
"OFF ROPE."
(Litter tender to brakeman. It means, "I have unclipped the rope from the litter and no longer need the line.")

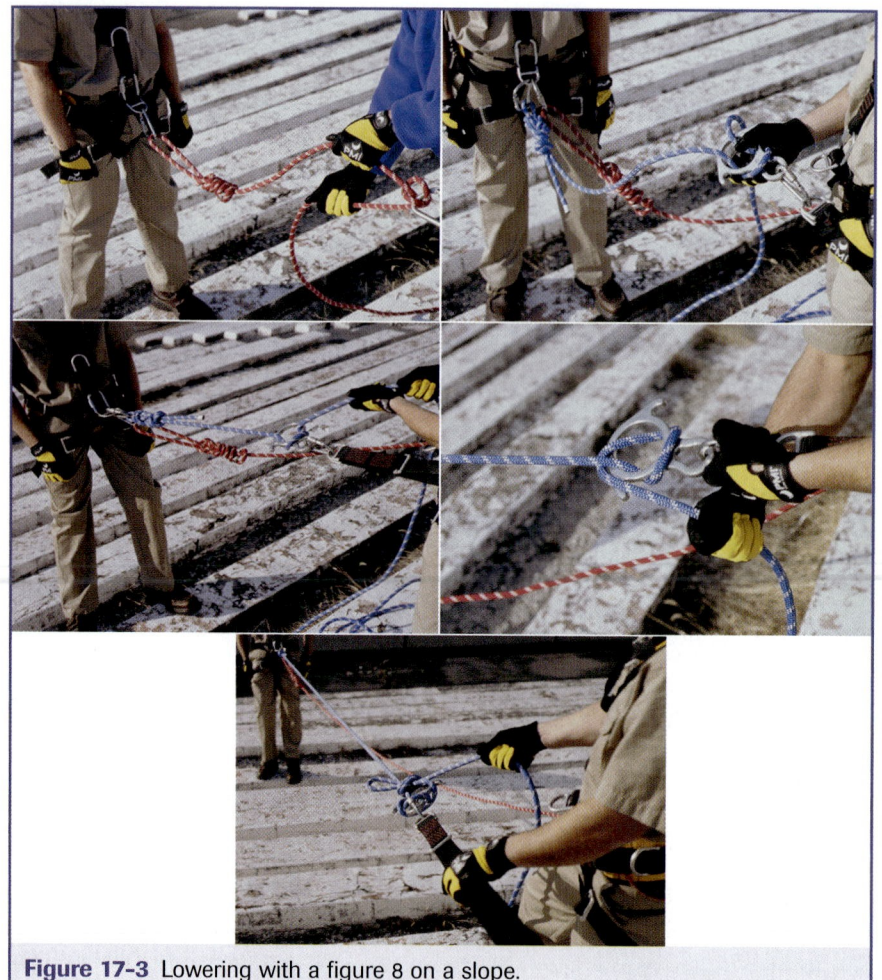

Figure 17-3 Lowering with a figure 8 on a slope.

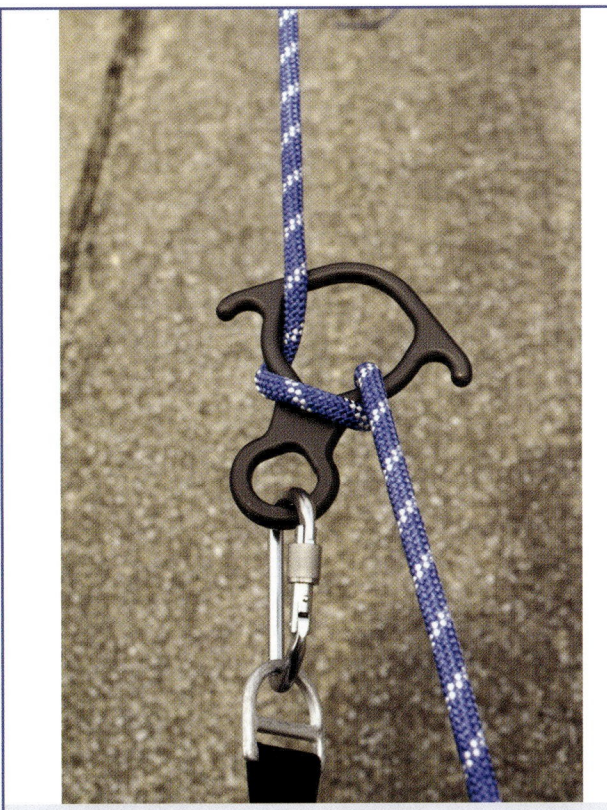

Figure 17-4 Figure 8 laced for lowering.

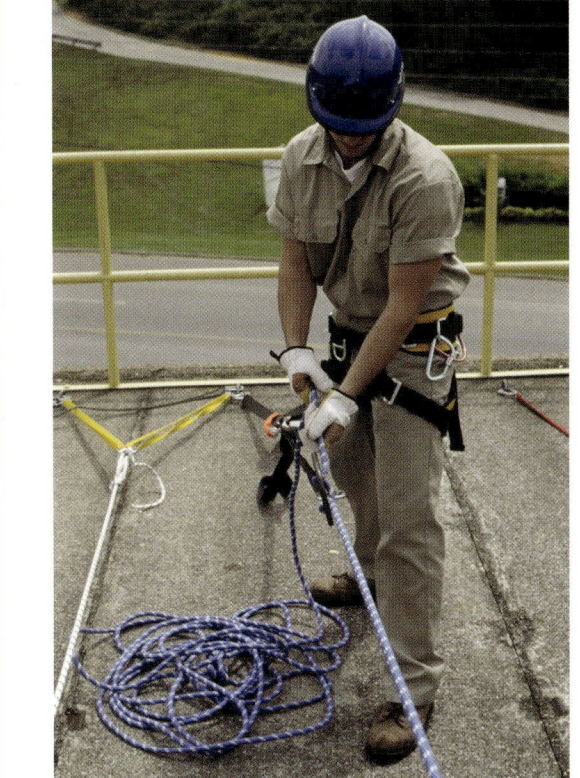

Figure 17-5 Brakeman's stance for lowering.

on-a-bight knot in it and clips it into a seat harness carabiner. He or she secures it by locking the carabiner (Figure 17-3, *B*).

6. The practice rescuer initiates the belay sequence (Practice rescuer: *"On belay."* Belayer: *"Belay on."*)

7. The brakeman pulls out any slack from the section of the main-line rope between the figure 8 descender and the practice rescuer.

8. For the remainder of this procedure, the brakeman should be wearing gloves. The following should all be in a straight line: anchor point, anchor sling, anchor carabiner, figure 8 descender, the rope between the figure 8 descender and the practice rescuer, and the practice rescuer's seat harness tie-in (Figure 17-5).

9. The brakeman's hand is on the rope that is feeding into the braking device. One hand, the *brake hand*, must continue to grip the rope during the lowering operation except when the lowering device is securely locked off. The other hand, the guide hand, can also grip the rope if needed for greater tension on the braking device, or can help manage the rope in back or front of the figure 8.

10. The practice rescuer pretensions the system to make sure all parts of the system have been rigged correctly under load and that no lines will tangle. Pretensioning also removes all slack from the system, which prevents shock loading when the load goes over the edge. To initiate this procedure, the practice rescuer calls, *"Preload."* The brakeman holds tension on the brakes, and the practice rescuer pulls slack out of the system (Figure 17-3, *C*).

11. When the practice rescuer is satisfied that the rigging is correct and when he or she is ready to begin descending, the individual calls to the brakeman, *"Down slow."* The brakeman slowly begins allowing the rope through the figure 8 descender as the practice rescuer walks backward downhill. The brakeman should keep the brake hand approximately 18 inches (45 cm) from the figure 8 descender and should allow the rope to slip slowly through his gloved hand.

    If temporarily there is too much friction for the practice rescuer to pull the rope through the descender, the brakeman's guide hand can help pull rope through the device.

12. The belayer must control the belay rope so that there is enough slack in the belay line and it does not interfere with the movement of the practice rescuer. However, there must not be too much slack in the belay line, so that if the main lowering line fails, the belay line immediately can take the load without severe shock loading.

Locking Off

13. The practice rescuer calls, *"Stop."* The brakeman holds the rope taut, stopping the descent of the practice rescuer. The belayer maintains an *on belay* status.

14. Tying off the figure 8 descender as a braking device is similar to tying it off as a rappel device. *During this procedure, the brakeman maintains a firm grasp on the brake side of the rope and does not allow the rope to slip through the descender.*

With the brake hand, the brakeman swings the brake side of the rope forward toward the load (practice rescuer) until the brake side of the rope is parallel with the rope that goes out of the descender toward the practice rescuer. Still holding the brake side of the rope taut, the brakeman swings it farther around in an arc until it is trapped between the large ring of the figure 8 descender and the rope going to the load (Figure 17-3, *D*).

15. To further secure the rope, the brakeman pulls the brake side of the rope firmly down toward the anchor, across the surface of the figure 8, and around behind one ear of the device. The rope is pulled firmly between the line going to the load and the large ring and above the line first locked off. The brakeman must make sure the rope lies firmly around the device and that there is no slack. The brake side of the rope is brought down and around the figure 8 again, as before, and then behind one ear; however, it is not placed between the line going to the anchor and the large ring. Instead, a large bight of rope is formed from the brake side of the rope. The bight is brought up parallel with the rope going to the load and is used to tie an overhand knot onto the rope going to the anchor (Figure 17-3, *E*). The brakeman must make sure the overhand knot is contoured well and is set firmly against the top of the figure 8 and that there is no slack in the knot (Figure 17-6, *B*).

Unlocking

16. Unlocking the brake device is the reverse of tying it off. The brakeman unties the overhand knot. He or she takes the bight out of the rope and unwraps it from the figure 8 descender *while making sure that the brake side of the rope remains trapped between the large figure 8 ring and the rope going to the load.* Now, *while maintaining firm control of the brake side of the rope with the brake hand,* the brakeman untraps the rope and brings it back to its normal position for lowering.

> ### ⬛ *Caution*
>
> If the practice rescuer is heavy (more than 160 pounds [73 kg]), the brakeman should double wrap the figure 8 descender for the lowering.

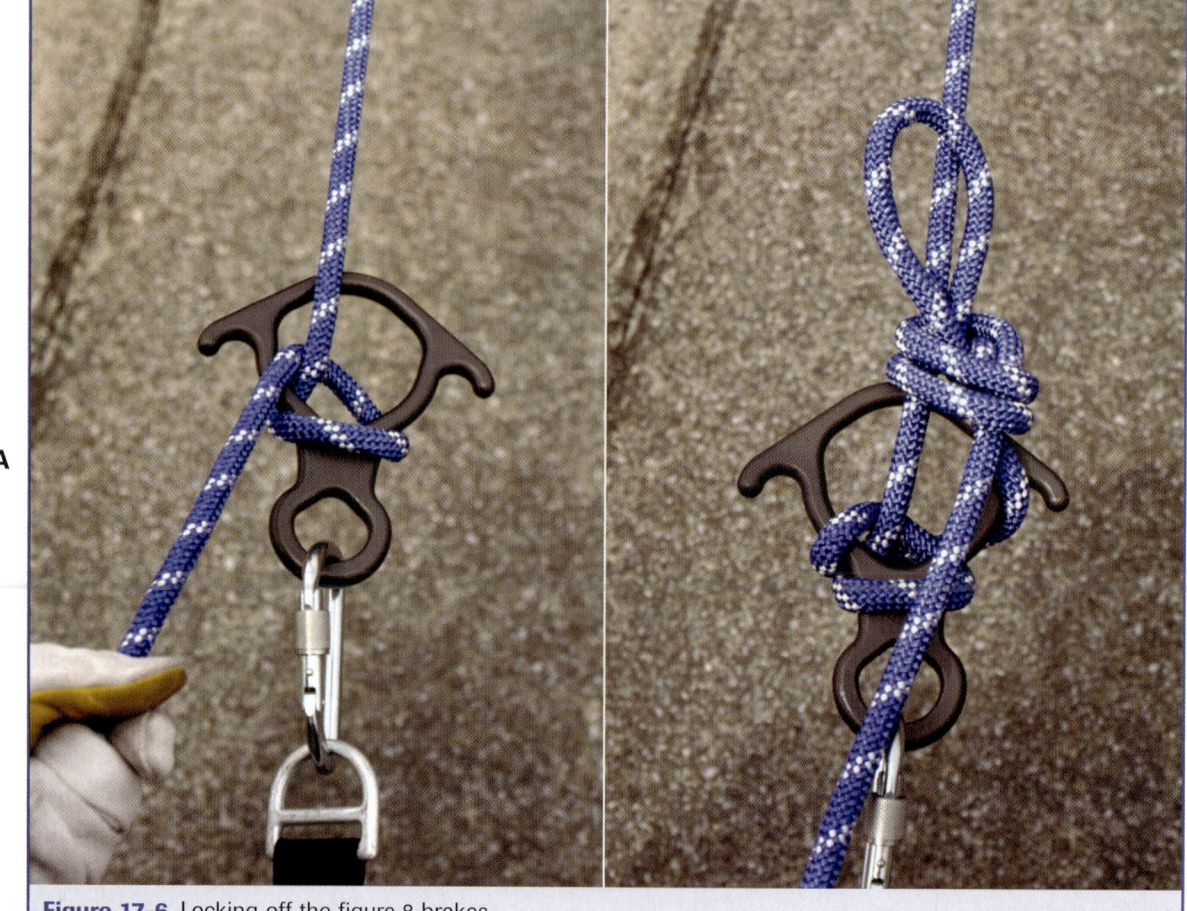

Figure 17-6 Locking off the figure 8 brakes.

17. The practice rescuer gives the voice communication, *"Down slow"* (or *"Down fast"*). The brakeman lowers at the appropriate speed, while the belayer maintains control of the belay rope.

Getting Off Rope

18. When the practice rescuer reaches the ground or other intended secure position, he or she calls, *"Stop."* The brakeman stops rope from passing through the descender. (If the lowering rope is too tight for the practice rescuer to disconnect from it, he or she calls, *"Slack,"* and the brakeman allows slack in the rope.) The belayer maintains the load on belay until the practice rescuer relieves him or her by completing the belay cycle. (Practice rescuer: *"Off belay."* Belayer: *"Belay off."*)

Using a Figure 8 with Ears to Lower a Person down a Vertical Face (Figure 17-7)

1. Choose a short vertical face (approximately 20 feet [6 m]) where the top breaks over gradually into a steep face.

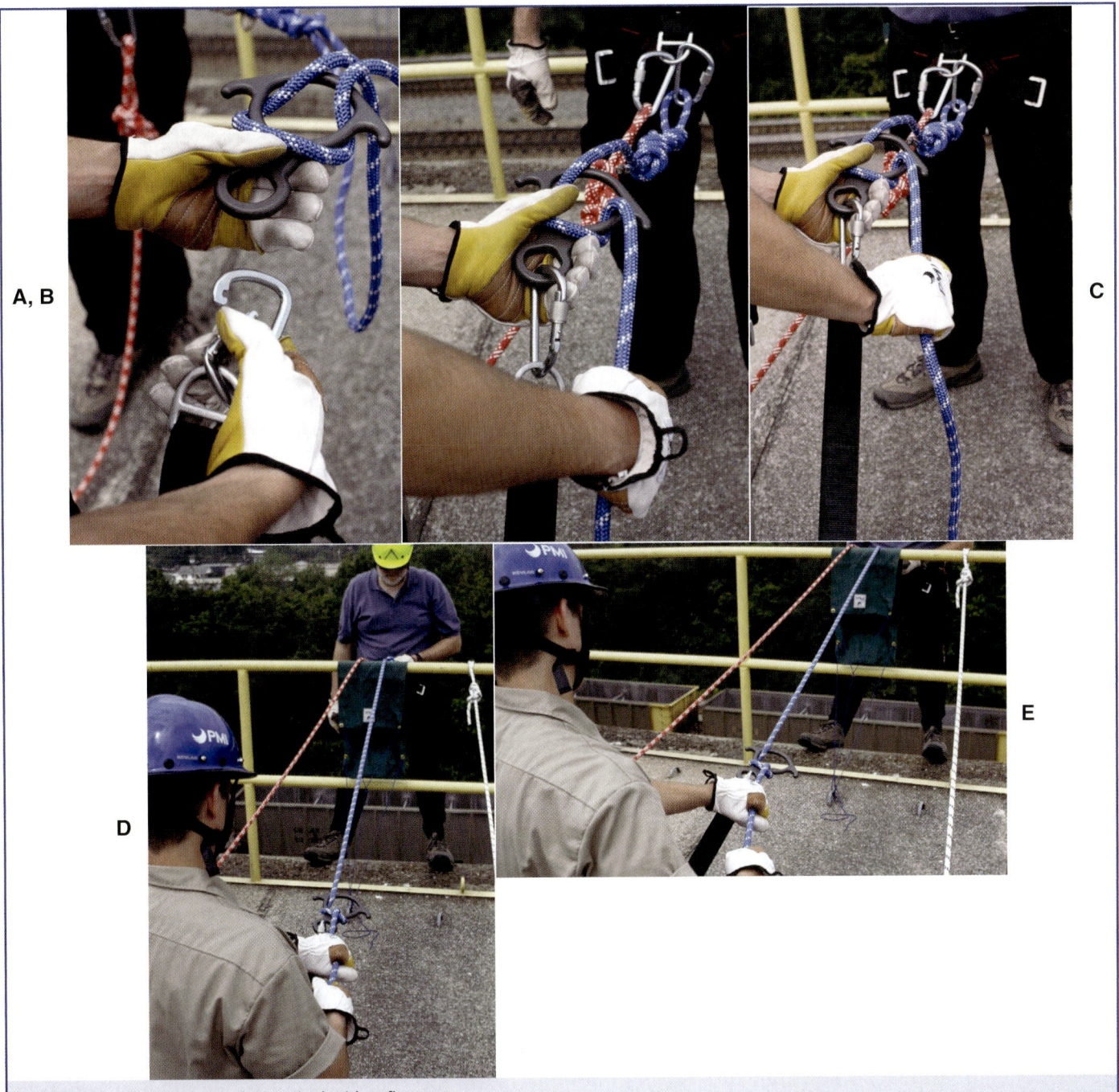

Figure 17-7 Lowering on the vertical with a figure 8.

2. Establish a secure anchor point safely back from the edge. If the brakeman or practice rescuer is too close to the edge, the person should be attached to a safety line connected to a secure anchor point. If possible, have the anchor point high off the ground to assist the practice rescuer in going over the edge. Attach an anchor sling to the anchor point in a way that the practice rescuer can rig into the main line without being too close to the edge. Clip a locking carabiner in the end of the anchor sling.

3. For the belay, attach another anchor sling to a separate anchor point. The belayer should be tied into a safety line that is not part of the belay line. (Ideally, the belayer should be on a separate anchor from the belay. If this is not possible, the belayer may be on the same anchor point but his or her body must not be linked to the belay system.) (See Belaying of One-Person Loads, p. 113.)

4. Place edge protection to protect the rope from abrasion (Figure 17-7, *B*).

5. Now, follow steps 3 through 9 on pp. 253-255 for attaching the practice rescuer into the belay and lowering systems (Figure 17-7, *C* to *E*).

6. The practice rescuer pretensions the system to make sure all parts are rigged correctly under load, that no lines will tangle, and that shock loading will not occur when the load goes over the edge. To initiate this, the practice rescuer calls, *"Preload."* The brakeman holds tension on the brakes, and the practice rescuer pulls slack out of the system.

7. When the practice rescuer is satisfied that the rigging is correct and when he or she is ready to begin descending, the practice rescuer gives the *"Down slow"* voice signal to the brakeman. The brakeman then slowly allows the rope to pass through the figure 8 descender. The practice rescuer leans back against the rope and begins to move backward towards the drop.

Getting Over the Edge

8. Getting over the edge probably will be the most difficult part of the operation for the practice rescuer, therefore the practice rescuer should remain in close communication with the brakeman. The practice rescuer should approach the edge deliberately and slowly. At the edge, the practice rescuer may want to give a *"Stop"* command to the brakeman and examine the situation. The practice rescuer should approach this procedure as he or she would a rappel: feet shoulder width apart, body perpendicular to the slope, and facing the brakeman but looking back over the shoulder at what is about to come.

9. Follow steps 11 through 18, pp. 255-257.

Using a Brake Bar Rack to Lower a Practice Rescuer on a Slope

This practice exercise is designed to give the student the feel of lowering a load using a brake bar rack as the braking device. This lowering sequence again uses a practice rescuer as a load (Figure 17-8).

1. Follow steps 1 through 3, p. 253, except attach the eye of a brake bar rack to the main anchor with a locking carabiner. If possible, align the rack so that the bars are in a horizontal orientation, with the bend of the rack pointing toward the

drop. The hyper-bar (the long bar next to the bend of the rack) should be positioned so that the slot that clips onto the frame faces down.

2. Unclip all the bars except the hyper-bar.

3. Lay the main line rope *on top* of the hyper-bar. *Do not run the rope between the hyper-bar and the rack.* Pull the slack out of the rope between the practice rescuer and the hyper-bar, and with one hand, hold the rack. With the other hand, pull the rope over the hyper-bar and around the bottom, back toward the practice rescuer. This should pull slack out of the rope between the rack and the practice rescuer and out of the anchor sling between the eye of the rack and the anchor point.

4. While continuing to hold the rope taut with one hand, use the other hand to engage the second bar. Slide it up to jam the rope between it and the hyper-bar. As you lace the rope onto the rack, make sure the rope runs on the side of the bar opposite the notch that clips the bar to the frame of the rack. This keeps the bars pressed against the rack frame.

5. While one hand holds the second bar in place against the rope, use the other hand to bring the rope around the second bar, as was done around the hyper-bar, so that the rope holds the second bar in place.

6. Continue this procedure until all the bars needed to lower the practice rescuer down the slope have been laced onto the rack.

7. To lower with the brake bar rack, the brakeman's dominant hand (the right hand on a right-handed person) should be on the portion of the rope feeding into the brake bar rack. This is the brake hand. *The brake hand should never be taken off the rope until the practice rescuer is off rope or the brake bar rack is securely tied off.* The other hand should be on the bars of the rack, cradling them; this is the guide hand. The guide hand can be used to help change the amount of friction by manipulating the bars (Figure 17-8, *A*).

8. After the rope has been laced up in the brake bar rack, take the rope in the brake hand and pull it forward hard in the direction of the load. This should do two things:
   - Take any slack out of the anchor sling
   - Jam the bars together toward the top of the rack

9. After raising the rope and pushing the bars to the top, bring the rope across the end of the hyper-bar and down toward the bottom of the frame to add extra friction. This is known as the *quick stop position;* it prevents rope from going through the rack. Use this position whenever the lowering must be stopped quickly.

   Now, hold the rack in the quick stop position until the practice rescuer is ready to start being lowered.

Lowering the Practice Rescuer

10. When the practice rescuer is ready, he or she initiates the belay cycle. (Practice rescuer: *"On belay."* Belayer: *"Belay on."*)

11. The practice rescuer pretensions the system to make sure all parts have been rigged correctly under load and that no lines will tangle. This also is done to remove all slack from the system to avoid shock loading when the load goes over the edge. To initiate pretensioning, the practice rescuer

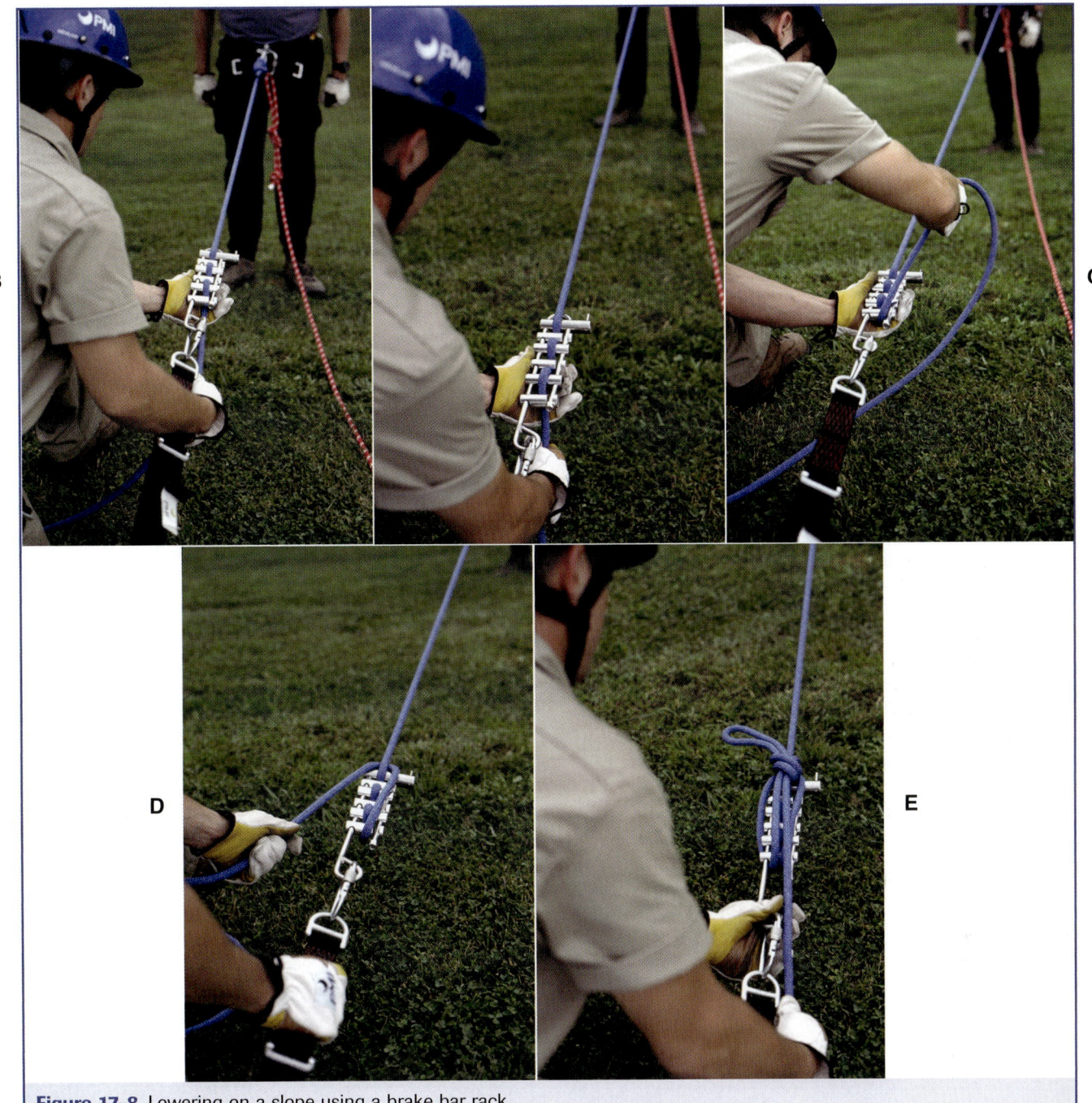

A, B

C

D

E

Figure 17-8 Lowering on a slope using a brake bar rack.

calls, *"Preload."* The brakeman holds tension on the brakes, and the practice rescuer pulls slack out of the system.

12. When the practice rescuer is satisfied that the rigging is correct and when he or she is ready to begin descending, the practice rescuer calls, *"Down slow,"* to the brakeman. The brakeman then begins to allow rope through the brake bar rack. The practice rescuer should lean against the rope to help it move through the brake system. If the rope is not moving through the rack, the brakeman can help it along by reducing rack friction (Figure 17-8, *B*).

Changing Friction when Using the Brake Bar Rack for Lowering

13. As in rappelling with the brake bar rack, it is best to begin a lowering with more bars engaged than are expected to be needed. If friction still must be reduced so that the practice rescuer can descend faster, remove the rope from the end of the hyper-bar and try spreading the bars apart along the length of the rack with the guide hand. The farther apart the bars are, the lower the friction.

If there is still too much friction, disengage the bottom bar. Take the end of the rope in the brake hand and swing in an arc from the quick stop position, first back toward the anchor and then under the rack and toward the load. This maneuver releases the bottom bar from under the rope but leaves the rope pressing the fifth bar against the other bars. Now take the guide hand, squeeze the two legs of the rack together, disengage the last bar, and move it out of the way. Using the guide hand, spread the remaining bars apart to reduce friction.

If still more friction must be reduced, repeat the procedure with the next bar up, the fifth bar. Swing the rope in an arc in a direction opposite from before so that it disengages the fifth bar but holds the remaining four bars in quick stop. Unclip the fifth bar and slide it back on the rack toward the eye and out of the way. *Do not lower a load on fewer than four bars.* If the loaded rope does not move through the remaining four bars, spread the bars with the guide hand to reduce the friction and/or push the rope through the bars with the brake hand.

Locking Off

14. The practice rescuer calls, *"Stop!"* The brakeman stops the rope from going through the brake bar rack. Then, bring the rack into the quick stop position as described on p. 259 (Figure 17-8, *C*).

15. If the practice rescuer is to be stopped for an extended period, the brakeman can tie off the brake bar rack. With the brake hand holding the rope in the quick stop position, pull the rope across the hyper-bar, down between the legs of the rack, and up again behind the section of loaded rope leaving the rack and going to the practice rescuer (Figure 17-8, *D*).

16. Next, bring the rope back toward the eye of the rack, holding the rope firmly to keep all the bars locked together. Then bring the rope through the two legs of the rack and across the bottom bar.

17. Again bring the rope toward the practice rescuer, in the same path as before. Pull it firmly so that all the rope strands are taut and the bars are locked together.

18. The brake bar rack should now be locked in the Stop position. To secure the rope, form a large bight with the strand of rope in the brake hand (the guide hand can be used to help form the bight).

19. Treating the bight as one strand of rope, tie an overhand knot across the strand of the rope going to the practice rescuer. Firmly cinch down the overhand knot against the hyper-bar of the rack. *There must be no slack in the strands of rope running over the rack and no space between the bars.* The brake bar rack now is locked off (Figure 17-8, *E* and Figure 17-9).

Unlocking the Brake Bar Rack

20. When unlocking the brake bar rack, the brakeman must *always keep a firm grip on the brake side of the rope and allow no slack in the brake side of the rope.* To untie the overhand knot, pull slowly on the braking end of the rope, positioning the guide hand at the center of the bight so that the bight comes out slowly.

21. With the brake hand firmly on the rope, pull the brake side of the rope in a 180-degree arc until it is pointing in the direction of the anchor.

22. Still grasping the rope firmly with the brake hand, pull the rope from between the two legs of the rack off the hyper-bar and then back to the normal braking position. *The rope must be kept taut by the brake hand during these steps.* With the guide hand, spread the bars apart and continue lowering the practice rescuer.

Getting Off Rope

23. When the practice rescuer reaches the ground or other intended secure position, he or she calls, *"Stop."* The brakeman stops the rope from passing through the brake bar rack. The belayer maintains the load on belay until the practice rescuer relieves him or her by completing the belay cycle. (Practice rescuer: *"Off belay."* Belayer: *"Belay off."*)

    If the rope is too taut for the practice rescuer to disconnect, he or she calls, "Slack." The brakeman allows some rope through the brake bar rack to create slack in the main line.

    If the practice rescuer has finished with the rope and is ready for it to be used for other purposes, he or she disconnects from it and signals to the brakeman, *"Off rope."*

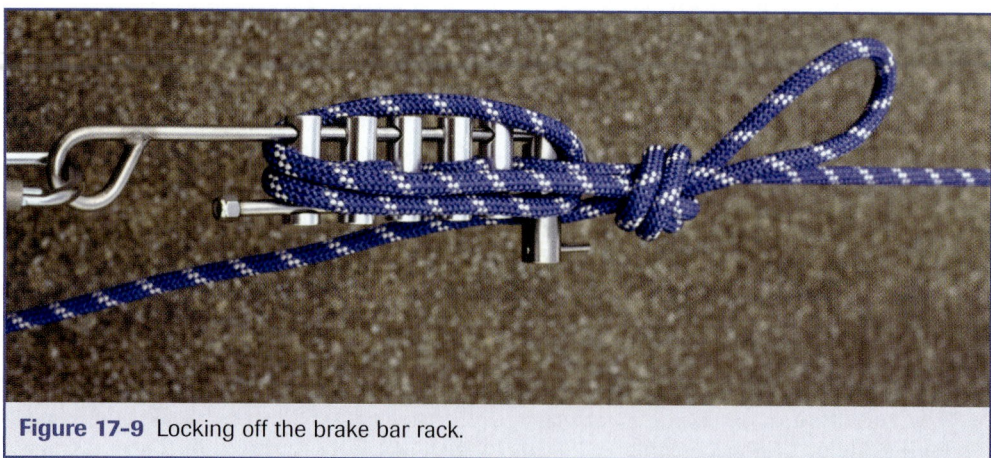

Figure 17-9 Locking off the brake bar rack.

Using a Brake Bar Rack to Lower a Practice Rescuer Down a Vertical Drop (Figure 17-10).

1. Choose a short vertical drop (on the first try, do not choose a face with a sharp edge or one that is undercut).
2. Establish a secure anchor point positioned where the practice rescuer can rig in without danger of falling. To the anchor point, attach an anchor sling with a locking carabiner.
3. To a separate anchor point, connect a belay sling with a locking carabiner. Set a safety line for the belayer and secure him or her to the line (see Chapter 8).
4. Place an edge roller or rope pad to protect the main-line lowering rope.
5. Follow steps 1 through 9, p. 258, for attaching the practice rescuer to the belay and braking systems and for lacing the brake bar rack into the main lowering line (Figure 17-10, *A-D*).
6. The practice rescuer pretensions the system to make sure all parts have been rigged correctly under load and to remove all slack from the system. To initiate pretensioning, the practice rescuer calls, *"Preload."* The brakeman holds tension on the brakes, and the practice rescuer pulls slack out of the system (Figure 17-10, *E*).
7. When the practice rescuer is satisfied that the rigging is correct and when he or she is ready to begin descending, the practice rescuer calls, *"Down slow,"* to the brakeman. As the practice rescuer leans back against the rope and begins to move slowly backward toward the drop, the brakeman allows the rope to pass through the brake bar rack. In order for the practice rescuer to move, the brakeman may need to spread the bars of the rack apart and possibly even remove one or two bars. However, the brakeman must remember: *As the practice rescuer starts over the edge and his or her full weight comes onto the rope and the braking system, more friction will be needed in the brake bar rack* (Figure 17-10, *F, G*).
8. See step 8, p. 258, for guidelines on getting over the edge.
9. On the short vertical drop, continue with steps 10 through 23, pp. 258-260 (Figure 17-10, *H-J*).

Litter Lowering Systems

Litter lowering systems are among the most spectacular of the rope systems. However, they also are among the most complex. They require superior skills in vertical techniques, in rope management, and in teamwork, as well as a complete knowledge of equipment. For these reasons, litter lowering systems must be thoroughly planned, worked out, and practiced before they are needed in a real rescue.

Safety Factors in Litter Lowering Systems

Litter lowering systems bear higher loads than systems involving a load of only one person. In a litter lowering system, the load includes the combined weight of the litter, hardware, and other rescue gear; the rescue subject; and one or two litter tenders (see Chapter 3 for information on calculating safety factors).

This increased load means greater stress on the entire vertical system, including ropes, carabiners, knots, anchors, braking systems, and belay system.

Position of the Litter for Lowering

When possible, a litter is lowered in a horizontal position. This usually is the more comfortable and reassuring position for the rescue subject. It also is less likely to complicate most medical conditions, and it makes it easier for litter attendants to tend to the subject's medical needs.

However, in some cases the litter may have to be lowered in a vertical position, usually in a confined space or when obstructions on the face require a small cross section for the litter.

Single Line versus Double Line Lowering

The many different techniques for lowering litters generally are divided into two categories: single line lowering and double line lowering.

Single line lowering involves one main line for the litter plus a belay line and uses one litter tender. *Double line lowering* involves two main lines for the litter, as well as possibly a belay line, and may use two litter attendants.

Both systems have advantages and disadvantages (Box 17-2).

Litter Rigging for Single Line Lowering

Figure 17-11 shows the litter rigging for a single line lowering.

The Spider

The spider (*bridle* or *harness*) joins the main-line lowering rope to the litter. It consists of a group of lines that first are attached at separate points to the litter rail and then are attached together at the main-line lowering rope. The connection where the spiders and main-line rope come together is the master attachment point (MAP). *For a single line lowering, a spider should have a minimum of four legs.*

A number of manufactured spiders are available that can be adjusted for height and angle and that have tie-in points for litter tenders. Premade spiders should be purchased only from reputable manufacturers who have specifically designed them for rescue purposes.

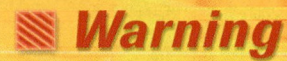

Warning

When using the Sked litter system in a high angle lowering, use the litter's lift slings as a spider; follow the manufacturer's directions for their use.

Constructing Spiders Spiders may be constructed from webbing or rope. Most rescuers who construct their own spiders make them from rope because it is easier to handle and allows for a greater variety of knots.

An improvised litter spider can be created from a bowline on a coil (see Figure 6-14, p. 76) with four loops. Each of the loops can serve as a spider leg.

The lower end of each leg of the spider is attached to the litter rails with a large locking carabiner. The spider should not be tied directly into the litter rail because rope or webbing may abrade

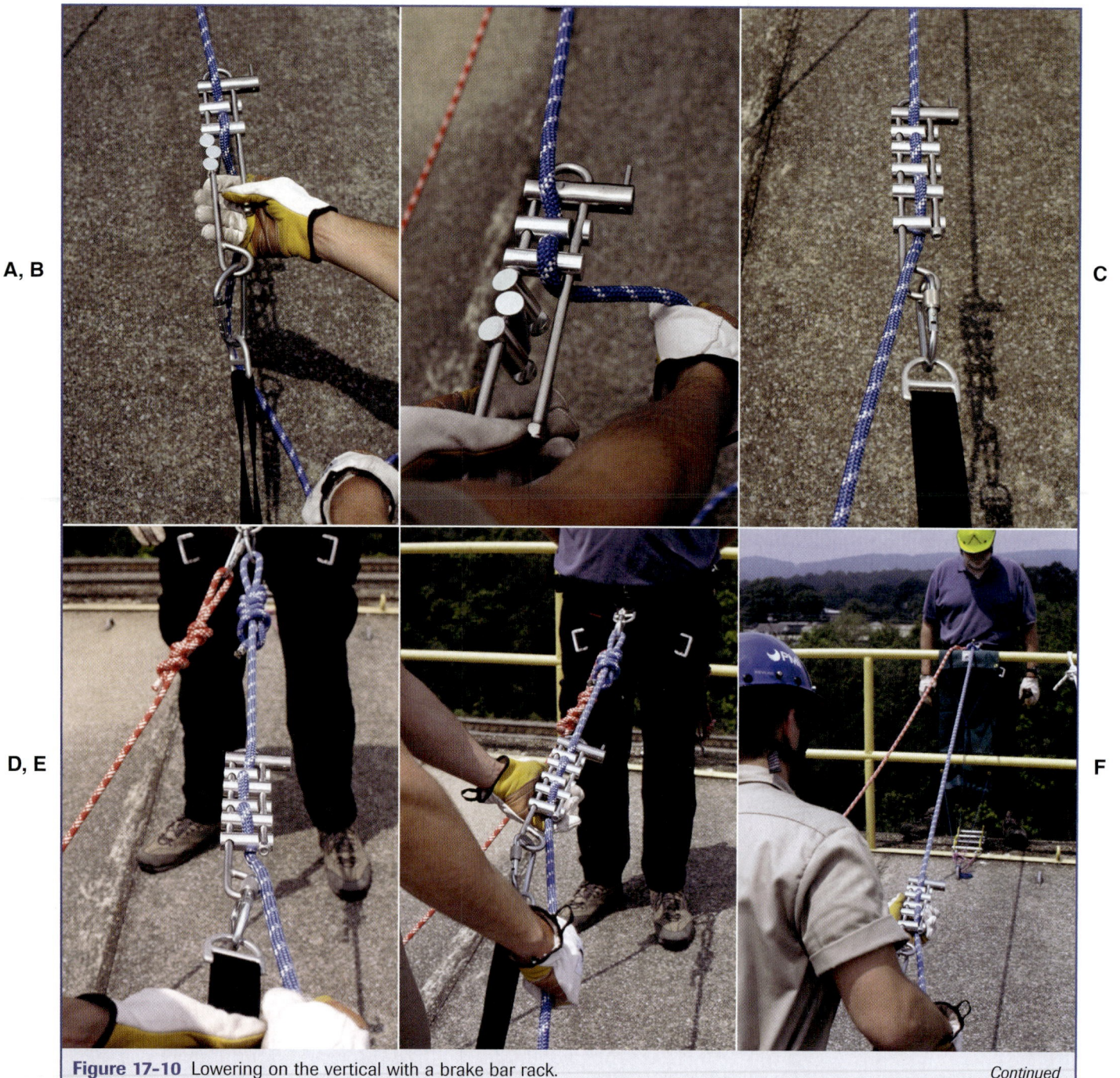

A, B

C

D, E

F

Figure 17-10 Lowering on the vertical with a brake bar rack.

Continued

through when rubbed over the face of a wall or cliff. Also, carabiners give greater flexibility for attaching the spider to or detaching it from the litter rail.

The carabiner gates should be set inward toward the center of the litter. This helps prevent the lock nut on the locking carabiner from being rubbed open on the face of the cliff or wall. The gates also should be oriented so that the locking nuts close with gravity and cannot vibrate to an unlocked position.

The spider should be adjusted so that the subject rides in the litter slightly head up (unless medical reasons dictate head down). Riding head down adds to the subject's anxiety and disorientation.

CREATING A SPIDER FROM ROPE

A simple spider can be constructed from four pieces of rope, each 7 feet (2.1 m) long and at least ⅜ inch (9.5 mm) in diameter (see Figure 17-11). Tie a figure 8-on-a-bight knot in both ends of each piece of rope. Make sure that after the knots have been tied, the spider legs are all exactly the same length.

ALTERNATIVE APPROACH: WEBBING SLING OR ANCHOR STRIP

For an even simpler and quicker approach for creating a non-adjustable spider, a presewn webbing sling or anchor strap can be used for each spider leg (see Chapter 7, p. 85, for information on presewn slings and anchor straps).

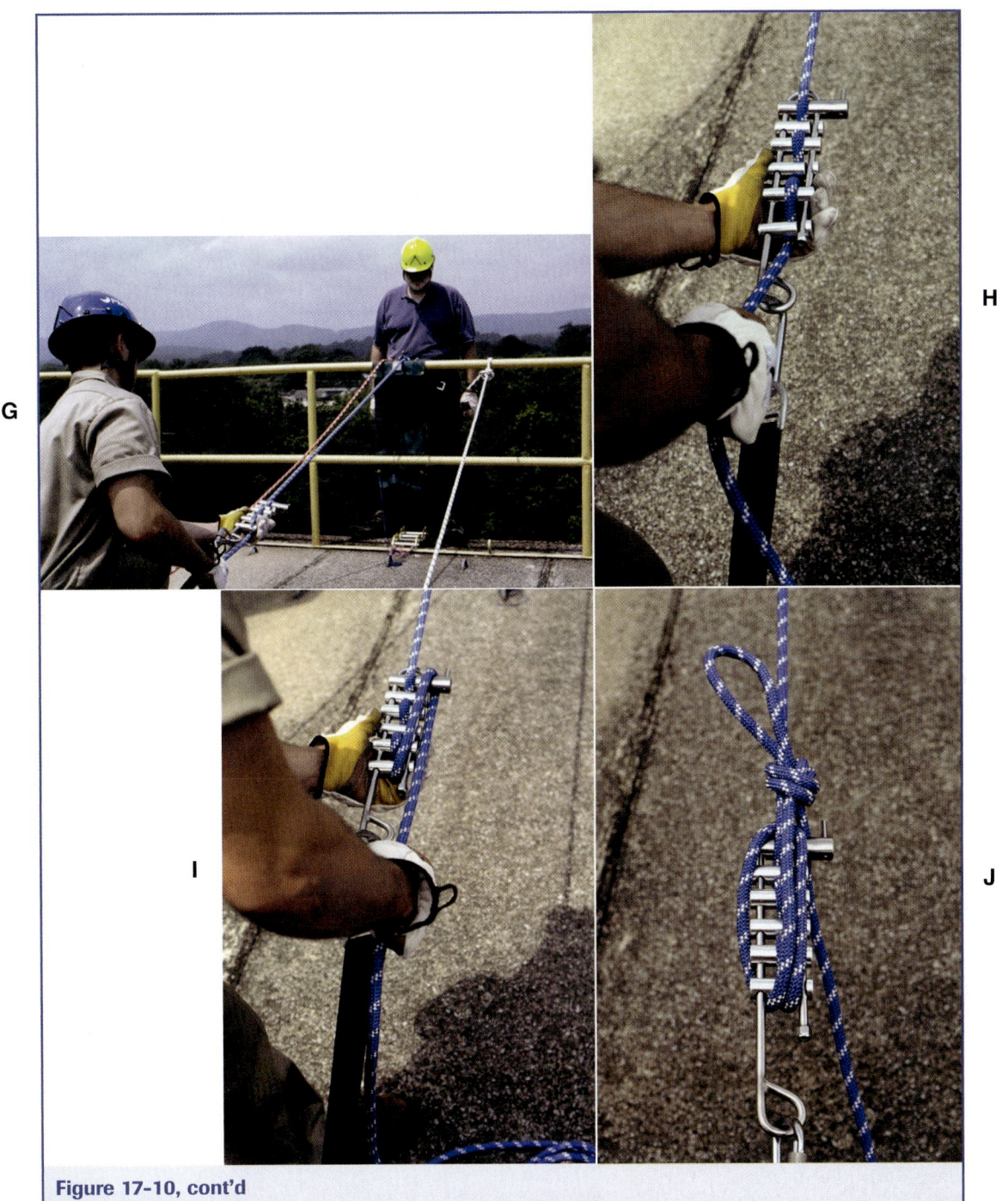

Figure 17-10, cont'd

ATTACHING THE SPIDER TO THE MAIN-LINE LOWERING ROPE (MASTER ATTACHMENT POINT)

1. At the end of the main-line lowering rope, tie a figure 8-on-a-bight knot.
2. Clip a large locking carabiner into this knot (the carabiner must be designed for rescue duty [such as NFPA Class G).
3. Bring all four figure 8-on-a-bight knots in the ends of the spider legs together. Clip the same carabiner across them and lock the gate.

Caution

Not all large locking carabiners fit easily over litter rails. Before purchasing carabiners for this use, measure the diameter of the rail and check the specifications of the carabiner's manufacturer or distributor.

Box 17-2 — Single Line versus Double Line Lowering with Belay

Single Line Lowering

Advantages

- ❏ Rope work and brake management are simpler.

Disadvantages

- ❏ Safety factor may not be adequate for the weight of two litter tenders.
- ❏ Tilting the litter from the horizontal to the vertical position is more difficult (loading of the belay line is required to tilt the litter).

Double Line Lowering

Advantages

- ❏ Technique can be used when two litter tenders are needed, such as for the following:

Complicated medical management of a subject
Vertical face that is too difficult for one tender to manage the litter (e.g., overhangs and gullies)
Shift in the orientation of the litter

Disadvantages

- ❏ Greater stress is exerted on the brake systems and anchors (if both lines run through the same brake).
- ❏ Rope management is more complex.
- ❏ Keeping the litter horizontal may be more difficult if lines come to two different points on the litter.

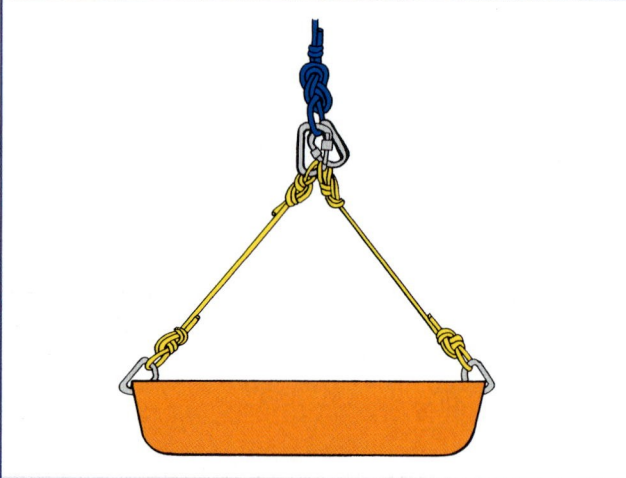

Figure 17-11 Litter rigging view from the end showing two of four fixed legs.

Using a Rigging Plate as the Master Attachment Point

A rigging plate commonly is used as the spider master attachment point, as an alternative to crowding all the bights of rope into one main carabiner (Figure 17-12). The rigging plate provides a strong attachment point and allows for a variety of rigging points.

1. Attach the large hole of the rigging plate to the main-line lowering rope using a general duty rescue carabiner clipped to the loop of a figure 8 on a bight knot.
2. Clip each figure 8-on-a-bight knot at the top of the spider into its own carabiner.
3. Clip each carabiner into a small hole of the brake plate.

Creating an Adjustable Spider from Rope

Figure 17-13 shows an adjustable litter spider made from rope. The adjustable spider can be used in situations in which the litter must be tilted on its axis, as when the wall is not completely

vertical but lies at a steep angle. To compensate for this angle yet keep the litter and rescue subject horizontal, the litter spider can be adjusted.

The materials needed include the following:

- Two lengths of static kernmantle rope, each 12 feet (4 m) long and at least ⅜ inch (9.5 mm) in diameter.
- Four lengths of Prusik material, each 4 feet (1.2 m) long. The Prusik cord must be of appropriate diameter to grip the static kernmantle rope. For example: 7-mm Prusik cord on ⁷⁄₁₆-inch (11.1 mm) rope, or 8 mm Prusik cord on ½-inch (12.7 mm) rope.
- Four locking carabiners with gate openings large enough to fit over a litter rail.

1. At the midpoint of each length of static kernmantle rope, tie a figure 8-on-a-bight knot. Take the figure 8-on-a-bight knots and hold them together with the rope strands hanging down. There should be a total of two figure 8-on-a-bight knots with four rope strands of equal length hanging down from them.
2. Take the center of each piece of Prusik material and tie a Prusik hitch onto each strand of static kernmantle rope about halfway between the figure 8-on-a-bight knot and the end.
3. At each of the four ends of the static kernmantle ropes, attach the two ends of a length of Prusik material. Do this with a figure 8 bend (or a grapevine) knot.
4. There should now be four spider legs. Each should have a loop in its bottom end that can be adjusted by sliding the Prusik knot up or down on the static kernmantle rope.
5. In each loop at the bottom made by the Prusik material, clip a large locking carabiner.
6. Hold the completed spider over the litter.
7. Clip each carabiner into a point on the litter rail that provides equalized loading when the litter is loaded.
8. Clip the two figure 8-on-a-bight knots at the top of the spider into a main-line lowering rope, using a large locking carabiner for the master attachment point, or attach them to a rigging plate as shown in Figure 17-13.

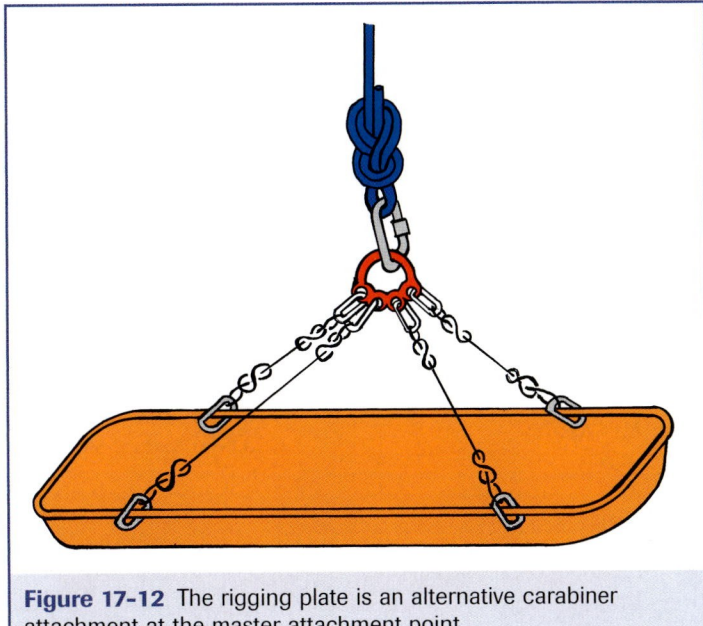

Figure 17-12 The rigging plate is an alternative carabiner attachment at the master attachment point.

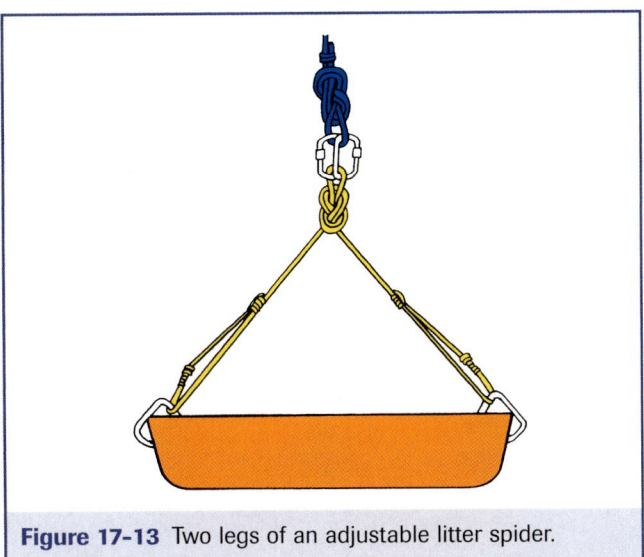

Figure 17-13 Two legs of an adjustable litter spider.

Rescue Subject Tie-Ins

During a high angle rescue, the subject must be attached to a secure safety and belay system. This system must securely connect the subject, his or her packaging, and direct attachments to the spider MAP. If the subject is on a spine board, he or she must be securely packaged onto the board, which, as a unit with the individual, is connected to the safety lines. The subject should also be secured in the litter with lacing across the top to prevent shifting in the litter.

The subject should be wearing a harness, and a safety sling should run from the subject's harness to the carabiners at the top of the spider MAP. This safety sling is designed to catch the subject if the litter fails. Slack must always be left in the safety sling so that the subject is not pulled upward if the litter tilts.

Litter Tender Tie-Ins

A litter tender tie-in serves the following primary purposes:

- Support the weight of the tender so that he or she can have hands free for such tasks as managing the litter and attending to the rescue subject
- Provide safety from falling
- Allow freedom of movement (the tender should be able to move around the litter to clear possible tangles, to clear obstructions under the litter, and to have access to all the subject's anatomy)

Figure 17-14 shows a litter tender tie-in system using two ascenders.

The main attachment to the litter system is known as a ***pigtail***. The pigtail is made of a piece of rope approximately 12 feet (4 m) long. It is attached with a figure 8-on-a-bight knot to the carabiners (or with a carabiner to the rigging plate) at the MAP at the end of the main-line lowering rope.

The litter tender is attached to the pigtail with two ascenders. One ascender is attached with a sling to the tender's seat harness, and the other ascender is attached with a sling to the tender's foot. To prevent the ascenders from accidentally slipping off the end of the pigtail, the lower end of the pigtail is brought back up and clipped into the tender's seat harness.

This rigging of the pigtail gives litter tenders the freedom of movement needed in litter lowering. The tender can use the ascenders to move above the level of the litter to clear possible tangles in the spider rigging, or he or she can move below the level of the litter to remove obstructions, such as loose rock.

Alternative Approach: Prusiks

Many teams do not use ascenders for the litter tender attachment, but instead use Prusiks (to help the litter tender get a leg up, an etrier [i.e., webbing steps] can be added).

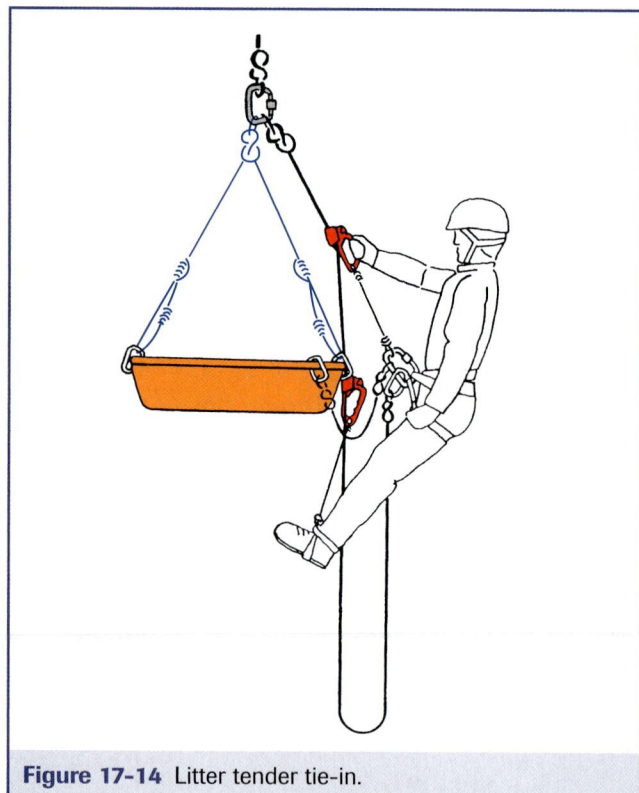

Figure 17-14 Litter tender tie-in.

Alternative Approach: Interlocking Long-Tail Bowlines

An alternative approach for creating a litter belay/tie-in system is the use of interlocking long-tail bowlines. The belay line and main line are tied with interlocked loops. The litter spider main attachment carabiner is clipped through both bowline loops. One long tail becomes the litter tender line, and the second long tail becomes the backup line attached directly to the litter.

Procedure for Lowering a Litter (Single Line with Belay)
Use of a Live Subject for Litter Lowering Practice

Use of a live subject for litter lowering practice can be very dangerous. There is, of course, the danger of practice rescuers dropping the practice subject, and in natural areas there often is an extreme danger from falling rocks. To ensure safety and to simplify the operation, first-time litter lowerings should use a dummy or weights in place of a person.

Many rescue teams, once they have become experienced, do use live practice subjects, because tending a litter with a real person is very different from using a dummy. These teams also feel it is important that all those directly involved in litter lowerings eventually gain experience as the "subject," strapped into a litter that is being lowered, because this is the only way they can fully comprehend the feelings of the rescue subject.

Nevertheless, live practice subjects should be used *only after the rescue team has had the extent and degree of quality practice needed to ensure the safety of the person in the litter.*

Main-Line Lowering System

As noted earlier, both the main line anchor and the belay anchor must have a safety factor appropriate to the load that will be on the system.

In addition, the system must be rigged at the top for safety and convenience. On the main-line anchor system, the lowering device (e.g., brake bar rack) must be attached to the anchor system such that:

1. The brakeman is close enough to the edge to hear voice communication from the litter tender, there is positive radio communication, or an edge tender can relay communications between the brakeman and the litter tender.
2. There is enough room at the top between the brakes and the edge so that the litter can be rigged safely and the tender tied in safely.

Belay Systems for Litter Lowering

Figure 17-15 shows a belay system for litter lowering. It consists of belay attachments at two points:

1. The belay line is first attached to the master attachment point. To do this, move back from the end of the belay rope approximately 12 feet (4 m) and tie a figure 8-on-a-bight

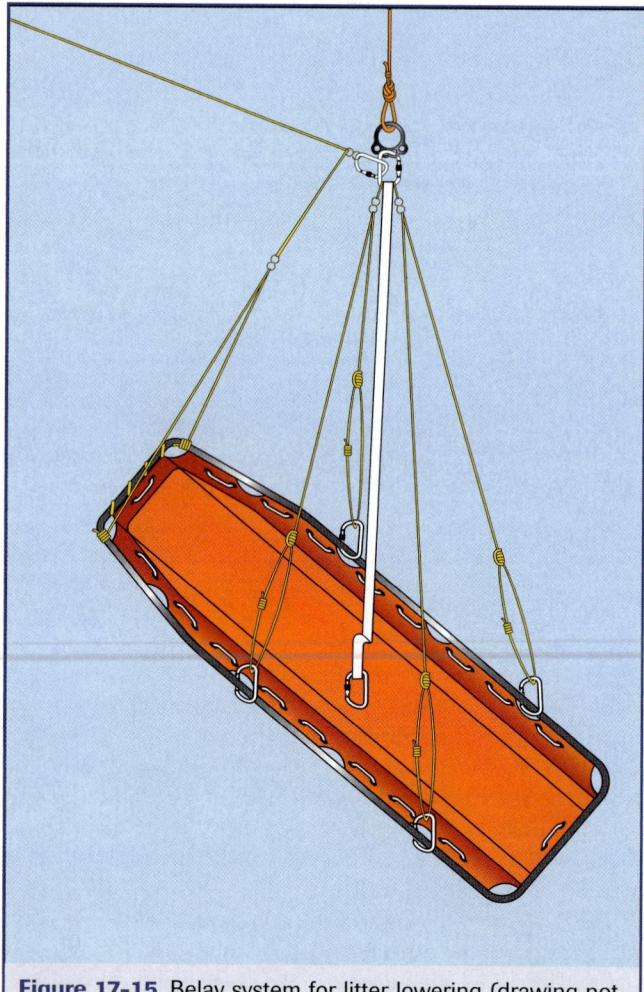

Figure 17-15 Belay system for litter lowering (drawing not to scale).

knot. Clip a large locking carabiner into this knot and then clip the carabiner into the carabiners or the rigging plate at the top of the spider in the MAP. Should anything along the main-line system fail, such as the anchor for the brakes, the belay is rigged to catch at the MAP. In this way, the litter is maintained in its normal horizontal position.

2. The end of the belay line then is attached to the head rail of the litter in the same way as that used for the main-line attachment in slope evacuation (p. 232). This is a backup for possible failure at the top of the spider. Should such a failure occur, the first belay attachment (the figure 8-on-a-bight knot at the spider) would not catch. The second line of safety would be the belay line attachment at the head of the litter. Should this attachment catch, the litter would go into a vertical position with the head up.

NOTE: All those involved in litter lowerings must keep in mind the consequences of the belay catching the head of the litter and arresting a main line failure with the litter ending in a vertical position.

The belay line is *never* tied directly onto the subject in the litter. If the belay line caught the subject directly, it would pull on the person's harness while the subject supported the remainder of the load (litter and tender[s]).

The end of the belay rope should go to the head of the litter. This is to ensure that, should the litter go vertical, the rescue subject remains head up.

The litter tender safety sling that is attached to the litter rail should be attached toward the head end of the litter. If this safety sling is attached at the foot end and the spider fails, the following would occur:

- The tender's pigtail attachment would come loose.
- The litter would go vertical.
- The tender's safety would catch at the foot end of the litter.
- The tender would be dangling helplessly below the foot of the litter.

Rigging the Litter for Single Line Lowering (Figure 17-16)

1. Using a large locking carabiner, anchor a brake bar rack to the main-line anchor sling. The eye of the rack should be toward the anchor, with the bend in the rack and the hyper-bar toward the edge of the drop. Lock the carabiner.
2. Rig a belay system:
    - If the lowering involves only one person (rescue subject only, no tender attached to the litter system) use a system appropriate for belaying one person (see Chapter 8).
    - If the lowering involves more than one person (rescue subject plus one or more tenders), use a rescue belay system (see Chapter 13).
    - Run a belay rope through the belay system with its end where the litter will be rigged.
3. Lace the main-line lowering rope through the brakes (the brake bar rack) with the end of the rope where the litter is to be rigged.

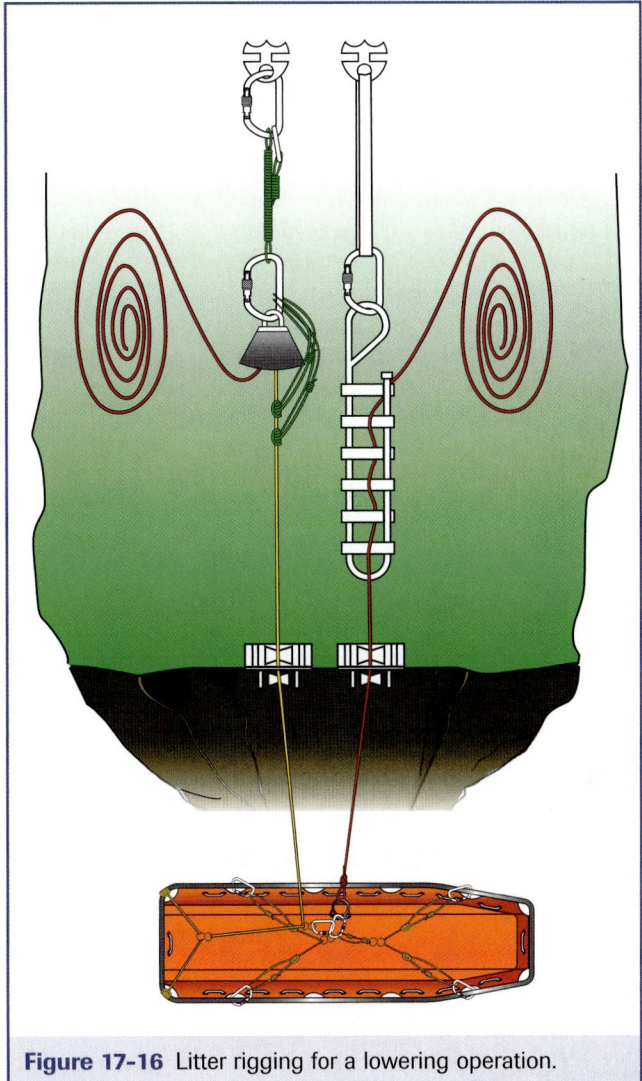

Figure 17-16 Litter rigging for a lowering operation.

4. Rig the litter for a single line lowering as described above. Attach a four-legged spider to the litter. Have ready a pigtail and a separate safety sling for the litter tender.
5. In the end of the main lowering line, tie a figure 8-on-a-bight knot. Make sure to have several inches of tail once the knot has been tied and tightened down. Attach all legs of the litter spider together to the figure 8-on-a-bight knot with a large locking carabiner at the MAP (or attach the spider legs with locking carabiners to a rigging plate at the MAP). Attach the litter tender pigtail, using a figure 8-on-a-bight knot, to the large locking carabiner (or use a locking carabiner to attach it to the rigging plate) in the end of the main-line rope. Lock all carabiners. Attach a separate safety sling for the litter tender to the head end of the litter.
6. Connect the belay line to the litter as described earlier, including attachments both to the top of the spider and to the head rail.
7. Load the litter with a dummy or with weight equivalent to that of a large person and secure the load so that it does not spill out if the litter capsizes.

8. Have the litter tender attach to the pigtail with a seat harness ascender and a foot ascender as described earlier. Have the litter tender attach to the end of the pigtail by tying a figure 8-on-a-bight knot in the end and clipping it into his or her seat harness front tie-in point with a locking carabiner.

9. The litter tender should also attach with a safety sling to a point on the litter rail near the head end.

10. The litter tender initiates the belay cycle. (Litter tender: *"On belay."* Belayer: *"Belay on."*)

11. Before the litter goes over the edge, the litter tender makes a final check of the rigging.

12. The litter tender pretensions the system to make sure that:
    - All parts of the system have been rigged correctly.
    - No lines will tangle.
    - Slack is removed from the system.

    To initiate pretensioning, the litter tender calls, *"Preload."* The brakeman holds tension on the brakes, and the litter tender pulls slack out of the system. If all looks good, the tender prepares for the lower.

13. After checking to make sure all the other lowering team members are ready and alert, the litter tender calls, *"Down slow,"* to the brakeman. The brakeman lets rope through the brake bar rack, and the rope handler feeds rope to the brakeman. The belayer controls the belay so that there is some visible slack in the rope and the belay rope does not interfere with the litter lowering.

NOTE: At the top, before the load goes over the edge, the weight on the brake system may be insufficient to pull the rope through. The litter tender may need to lean back, pulling the litter with him or her, while the brakeman reduces the friction. However, once the tender and litter go over the edge, there will be greater weight on the system, and greater friction will be needed.

Getting Over the Edge

Getting over the edge often is the most difficult step in litter lowering. The best approach is a slow, deliberate one. Whenever the litter tender begins to feel unbalanced, he or she calls, *"Stop!"* to regain equilibrium. The brakeman and belayer must remain very alert to the needs of the tender.

The general strategy is that the litter tender, attached to the litter, backs slowly over the edge, pulling the litter with him or her. The tender leans back on his or her connections to the litter system, and in turn, the lowering system.

To keep the operation as smooth as possible, the tender should avoid shock loading the system. To help with this, the brakeman should lower very slowly as the litter tender moves back over the edge.

As he or she moves back, the litter tender should try to keep all slack out of the main lowering line, the spider legs, and the tender's tie-ins. Leaning back hard against the tie-ins helps with this.

If the top of the drop is flat, the tender may have to lift up the litter by the closest rail, tilting the litter so that the spider legs are evenly taut.

If slack appears in the system faster than the tender can cope with it, he or she should call, *"Stop!"* and remove the slack.

It is important to have the slack out of the litter system before the tender gets completely over the edge. Otherwise, the tender will drop and shock load the system, resulting in:
- Shock loading of anchors, equipment, and rigging
- Fright and perhaps harm to the subject
- Possible injury to the tender

Alternative Approach: Getting Over Undercut Edges and Parapets

Among the most difficult edges to get over with a litter without shock loading are undercut edges and parapets (90-degree edges).

A possible approach is to set the litter on the edge, belayed and with full tension on the brakes, and then have the litter tender climb around the head or foot end of the litter.

1. Make sure the system is on belay and the belayer is alert.

2. Make sure the rope is correctly laced into the brakes and is on tension.

3. Two edge tenders pick up the litter.

4. As the edge tenders move toward the edge, the brakeman (or brakemen) slowly allows enough slack for the edge tenders to maneuver the litter.

5. The edge tenders set the litter on the edge of the wall.

6. The edge tenders make sure the rigging is correct and there is no excess slack.

7. The litter tender checks his or her tie-ins to the litter system.

8. The edge tenders set the litter over the wall with the top rails even with the top of the drop. The brakeman holds the lowering lines tight.

9. The litter tender has the upper ascender line as tight as it will go on the pigtail. With his or her attachment lines tight, the litter tender goes over the wall at the head of the litter. The tender leans back into the tight attachment lines and maneuvers around the litter and into position.

10. The litter tender repositions on his or her tie-ins as necessary.

11. The litter tender places his or her feet against the wall, pulls the litter away from the wall, and gets ready for lowering.

Position of Single Litter Tender

The primary duties of the litter tender are to:
- Attend to the medical needs of the subject in the litter
- Help provide a smooth ride for the subject
- Communicate with and reassure the subject
- Prevent the litter from hanging up
- Shield the subject from environmental factors

These duties are best performed if the tender assumes a natural posture for sitting in a seat harness, with the litter a few inches (or centimeters) above the lap (Figure 17-17). The litter must not rest on the tender's lap or legs, because this restricts the tender's movements and could also trap the tender's legs against the wall.

To help maneuver the litter, the tender uses both hands to grasp the near litter rail. If the tender needs to roll the subject (e.g., to clear the subject's airway), he or she reaches across with one hand, grasps the opposite rail, and pulls it over toward him or her to roll the litter and subject.

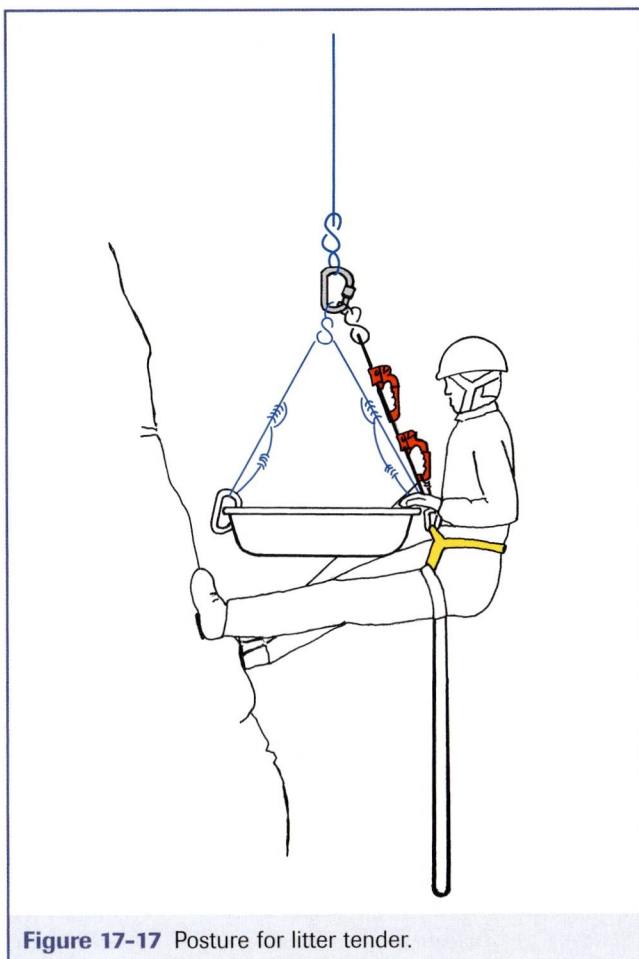

Figure 17-17 Posture for litter tender.

If the litter is against the wall, the tender should have both feet against the wall. By keeping the feet against the wall, the tender can use the leverage to pull the litter away from the wall by grasping the near rail. This helps keep the litter from snagging and bumping against the wall.

At the midpoint on the wall, the litter tender calls, *"Stop!"* The brakeman brings the brake side of the rope forward toward the load, forcing the brake bars together and creating a quick stop on the brake bar rack. If the stop will be a lengthy one, the brakeman can tie off the brake bar rack. However, the brakeman should be ready to respond if the litter tender is not initially in position and needs some additional, very short lowerings to reposition the litter.

When the litter tender is ready to lower again, he or she calls, *"Down slow"* or *"Down fast,"* and the lowering procedure continues.

Once the litter is on the ground, the litter tender calls, *"Stop!"* If the rope is too taut to allow the litter system to be disconnected from the main line, the tender calls, *"Slack,"* and the brakeman allows slack into the main rope.

When the litter tender is in a secure position and in no danger of falling, he or she concludes the belay cycle. (Litter tender: *"Off belay."* Belayer: *"Belay off."*)

When the litter tender (or others on the ground) have unclipped the litter from the rope and no longer need the line, the tender gives the voice signal, *"Off rope."* The brakeman (or others at the top) can then pull the rope back up or, if appropriate, remove it from the anchors.

Positions of Two Litter Tenders

In some situations, such as with a seriously injured subject or rugged terrain, two litter tenders may be required. *With the added weight, it is important to make sure there is an adequate system safety factor, including two lowering lines.* Usually, the medical attendant is positioned at the head end to monitor the subject's condition and provide essential care. On some rescue teams, the medical attendant also is responsible for the rate of lowering and is in direct communication with the lowering personnel at the top. The second tender is at the foot end to manipulate litter around obstructions, push brush aside, and clear loose rock.

NOTE: There are regional variations in how responsibilities are traditionally assigned to litter attendants. The decision on which attendant is to be responsible for movement of the litter must be made before the litter goes over the side.

The medical attendant is positioned at the head of the litter so that he or she can adjust attachments in order to best care for the subject. The second tender is positioned farther down.

Medical Considerations for Rescue Subjects in High Angle Lowering

At this point the student should review the section Medical Considerations for Patients in High Angle Rescue, pp. 185 to 187, in Chapter 12, and the section Medical Considerations: Packaging the Subject in the Litter, pp. 220 to 225, in Chapter 15.

Loading the Subject into the Litter

The procedures for loading the subject into the litter depend both on the individual's medical condition and where the subject is to be loaded.

Topside

Loading of the subject into the litter is easier if it takes place on flat ground, such as at the top of the drop or on a ledge. More personnel may be available to assist, and all members of the rescue team have solid footing. However, the litter loaded with a subject may be more difficult to get over an edge for the litter tender. In this situation, the edge tenders can be of great assistance in getting the litter over the edge smoothly and without causing the subject further apprehension and injury.

Partway Down

If the subject was injured partway down the face of a wall, the person will need to be loaded into the litter at that point. However, this type of litter loading can be very difficult, for the following reasons:

- Often not many rescue personnel will be available (there may only be the litter tender).
- A rescuer hanging from his or her harness will have difficulty getting leverage. If it is a completely free-hanging situation (away from the wall), it will be extremely difficult.

The following are some approaches that can be helpful in this kind of midface loading:

- Stop the litter lowering before you get too low. It is better to start the loading attempt with the litter too high, because the brakeman can always let a bit more rope out to lower. However, if you start out much too low, you may not get another chance. In addition, even low-stretch rope stretches some when the subject is loaded into the litter. Because it is difficult to lift the subject up to clear the litter rails, the optimum level for the litter is equal to the level of the subject.
- Before rigging the litter, have it in line for the subject's position (litter head and foot pointing in same direction as subject's head and feet). If at all possible, have the litter in the correct position before starting over the edge. Otherwise, if the litter has to be turned partway down, the belay and main lowering lines will tangle.
- Clip a safety line onto the subject with a seat harness before he or she is moved for loading into the litter.
- Place the Kendrick Extrication Device (K.E.D.) or Oregon Spine Splint (OSS) on the subject before movement, if possible, because this can help in moving the subject.
- Once the subject is in the litter, run a safety sling run from his or her seat harness to the carabiners at the top of the spider.
- An auxiliary tender is a great help in loading a litter partway down a face.

Use of an Auxiliary Tender

An **auxiliary tender** (sometimes referred to as a *third man*) can be very helpful in litter management and in loading the subject (Figure 17-18). This is particularly true when there is only a single litter tender. The auxiliary tender rappels or ascends on a separate rope system alongside the litter. If local policy or condi-

tions indicate the need, a separate belay may be provided for the auxiliary tender.

The auxiliary tender can be of assistance in several critical ways. He or she can:

- Respond first, before the litter lowering, to assess the subject's medical condition and begin primary treatment
- Assist the litter tender in getting the litter over the edge
- Assist in loading a subject who is partway down a wall
- Help maneuver the litter around obstructions
- Provide medical care unencumbered

Although the auxiliary tender is on a rappel line separate from the litter lowering system, a tether line running between him or her and the litter may help keep this rescuer close to the litter. The tether line should be rigged so that the auxiliary tender can quickly detach from the litter.

Double Line Lowering Systems

In some situations rescuers may choose to use a double line lowering (two lines attached to the litter). The two-line approach can be helpful in the following situations:

- When the position of the litter must be changed from horizontal to vertical and back again (this helps get the litter through obstacles on a vertical space or get through a confined space)
- When use of a two-line system can simplify rigging
- When two tenders need to be attached to the litter; for example, (1) on an uneven, broken up, vertical face, with obstacles such as overhangs and gullies (areas where a single litter tender might have difficulty managing the litter) and (2) when medical considerations or other concerns relating to the rescue subject are too overwhelming for a single litter tender

There are two different systems for double line lowering:

1. Both lines are run through one brake
2. Each line is run through a separate brake, with each acting as a belay on the other

Spiders for Double Line Lowering

Figure 17-19 shows the spider system for a double line lowering. Note that in this case, the spider has six legs: three at the head end coming up to meet one lowering rope and three at the foot end coming up to meet the parallel lowering rope.

The two basic types of spiders that can be used with double line lowering systems are the double line to single point spider and the double line to two points spider.

Double Line to Single Point

With the double line to single point spider, the two lowering lines come together and are attached at a single MAP (see Figure 17-15, in which the two lines would come into the MAP where one line now exists.) In most cases a belay line is not used in a double line lowering.

Double Line to Two Points

With a double line to two points spider, each of the two lowering lines is attached to a separate (usually three-legged) spider

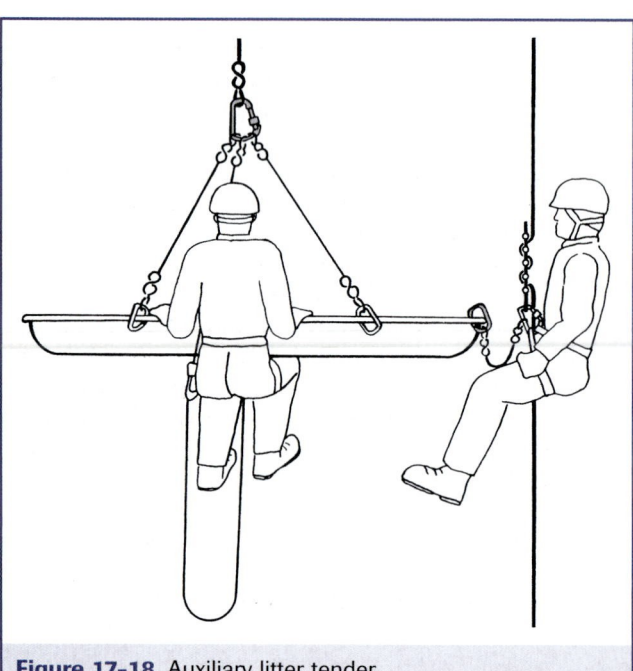

Figure 17-18 Auxiliary litter tender.

component. One is at the head of the litter and one at the foot. A tether connects the two MAPS (see Figure 17-19).

Advantages of a Double Line to Two Points Spider
- A two-point system can provide greater flexibility in maneuvering the litter in some situations, such as getting over the edge.
- The two-point system can provide maneuverability in changing the angle of the litter.

Disadvantages of a Double Line to Two Points Spider
- A two-point system has the potential for high shock loads on dual anchor systems if one anchor fails.
- With a two-point system, it may be difficult to maintain the same speed for both ropes if the ropes run through different braking devices and are attached to the litter with a two-point spider.

Litter Tie-Ins for Double Line Lowering (Two Tenders)

As can be seen in Figure 17-19, each litter tender has his or her own tie-in clipped to a separate lowering rope. As with single line lowering, each litter tender also is clipped in with a separate safety line to a point on the litter rail.

With double line lowering, only one litter tender gives the voice communications to the brakeman. This is the medical attendant, who usually is stationed at the head of the litter so as to best care for the subject.

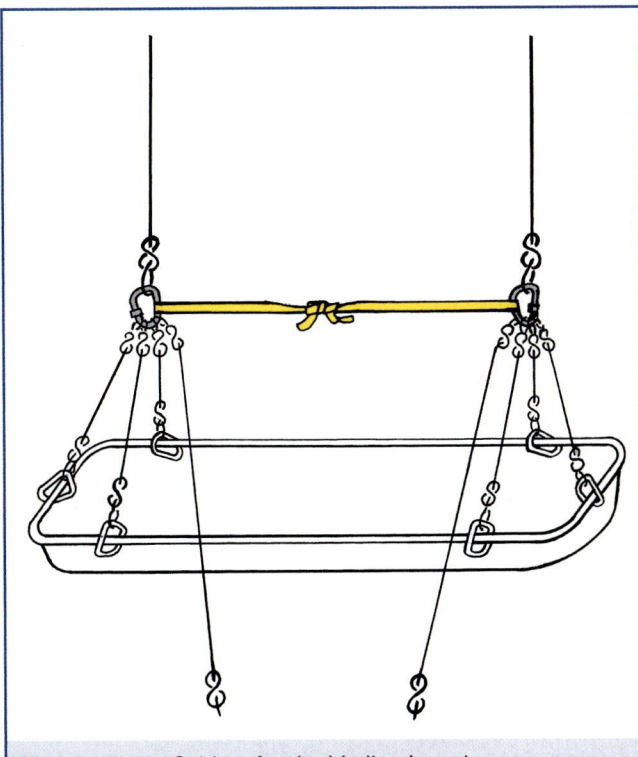

Figure 17-19 Spiders for double line lowering.

Brake Systems for Double Line Lowering (One Brake)

The two main lowering ropes should run through the same brake device and should be controlled by the same brakeman.

Both lowering ropes in a double line lowering should be of the same diameter, design, and wear. If they are not, they may have different rates of friction and elongation, making it difficult to coordinate the lowering. An uneven load on the litter may also cause the ropes to run through the brakes at different speeds. This often is the result of the subject's upper torso being heavier than the lower torso, which means that the head end of the litter often is heavier than the foot end.

To even out the loading in a two line system, the lighter litter tender sometimes can be placed at the head end and the heavier tender at the foot end.

Alternative Approach: Brake Tube

An alternative to the brake bar rack in double line lowering (one brake) is the brake tube (Figure 17-20).

Advantages of a Brake Tube
- Knots can be passed through the device (but double lines should be tied so that their knots do not pass at the same time).
- The device accommodates double line lowering.
- A brake tube affords good control of lowering.

Disadvantage of a Brake Tube
- A brake tube is heavier and bulkier than a brake bar rack.

Changing the Angle of the Litter

The following are typical steps for changing the angle of a litter from horizontal to vertical during a double strand lowering (Figure 17-21).
- The litter has already gone over the edge and is being lowered. It is about to reach an area on the wall through which it cannot fit unless it is tilted at a steep angle (Figure 17-21, *A, B*).
- This sequence assumes that different colored ropes are going to the head and foot of the litter. In this case, the yellow line goes to the head, and the blue line goes to the foot.

1. Litter captain to brakeman: *"Stop!"* (The brakeman stops both ropes from going through the brakes.)
2. Litter captain: *"Down on blue."* (The brakeman allows the rope running to the foot end of the litter to run through the brakes but holds the rope that goes to the head end of the litter. As a result, the foot end of the litter goes down, and the head end remains where it is [Figure 17-21, *C, D*].) NOTE: If the two ropes are the same color, the litter captain calls, *"Down foot."*
3. When the litter reaches the desired angle, the litter captain signals, *"Stop!"* (The brakeman stops the rope going to the foot end of the litter and continues to hold the rope going to the head end. The litter has stopped at a vertical angle with the foot end below the head end. Both litter tenders still hang in the same position, but the litter now is parallel to

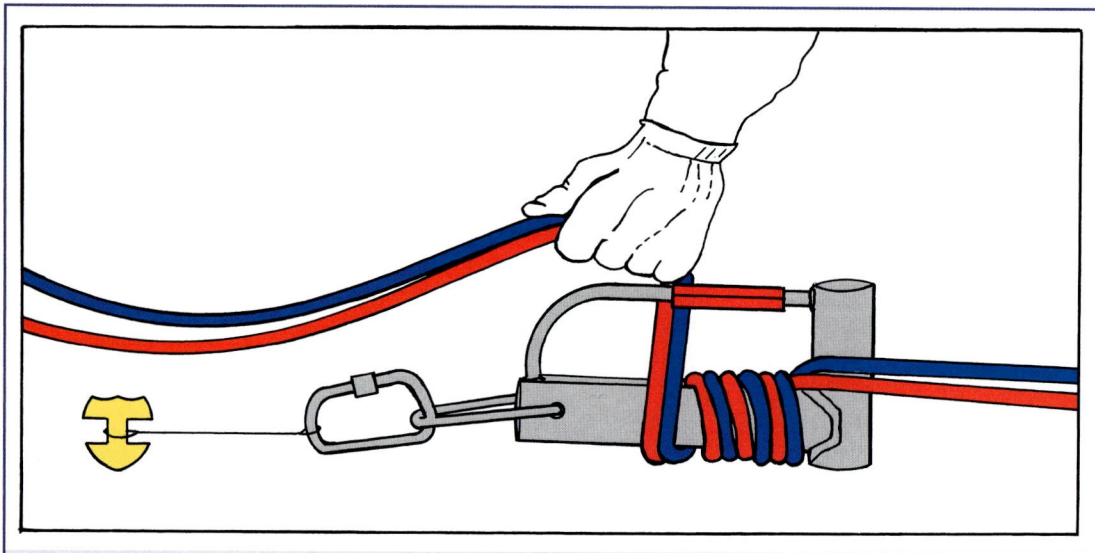

Figure 17-20 The brake tube can be used as an alternative to the brake bar rack in double line lowering.

them. They are still able to reach and tend to the needs of the rescue subject.)

4. Litter captain to brakeman: *"Down slow."* (The brakeman now allows both ropes to run through the brakes at the same speed. The litter maintains the vertical position it has been set at and continues lowering at that angle [Figure 17-21, *E, F*].)

Changing the Angle Back to Horizontal

5. Litter captain to brakeman: *"Stop!"* (The brakeman stops all ropes from going through the brakes. The litter stops completely.)

6. Litter captain: *"Down on yellow."* (The brakeman allows the rope going to the head of the litter to go through the brakes but holds the rope going to the foot. The head of the litter is lowered while the foot end of the litter remains stationary [Figure 17-21, *G, H*].)
   NOTE: If the two ropes are the same color, the litter captain calls, *"Down head."*

7. As the head of the litter becomes even with the foot end, the litter captain calls, *"Stop!"* (The brakeman stops the rope to the head end from going through the brakes and holds the rope going to the foot end. The litter now is horizontal and not moving.)

8. Litter captain: *"Down slow"* (or *"Down fast"*). (The brakeman allows both ropes through the brakes. The litter is lowered in a horizontal position [Figure 17-21, *I*].)

Alternative Approach: Continuous Sequence

A smooth change in the litter angle takes practice, teamwork, and good communication. Once a team has become adept at the procedure, they may be able to skip the "stop/start" steps and keep the litter moving continuously. A continuous sequence might run as follows:

1. Litter tender: *"Down on blue."* (Brakeman stops yellow, continues blue.)

2. Litter tender: *"Down slow."* (Brakeman allows both ropes through the brakes.)

3. Litter tender: *"Down on yellow."* (Brakeman stops blue, continues yellow.)

4. Once the litter is horizontal again, the litter tender calls, *"Down slow"* (or *"Down fast"*). The litter continues lowering in a horizontal position.

Two Brake Lowering System

Some rescue teams prefer to lower a litter using two brakes instead of a brake and a belay device. In this way, should one anchor fail, the second brake system converts to a belay that can more easily be held by the brakeman, and the device can be better used for a controlled lowering than for a belay device.

The advantage of double brake lowering is that the load is shared between two anchors instead of being concentrated on just one. Also, should one anchor fail, loading may be less severe because both ropes are under load rather than one having some slack, as would be the case with a belay.

One disadvantage of double brake lowering is that should one anchor and brake fail, the second anchor and brake will be subjected to shock loading much greater than twice the original load the surviving anchor and brake had before. The remaining anchor must be able to withstand this loading. The remaining brakeman must be using a braking device that can easily and quickly be adjusted to increase the friction as needed. Not all braking devices are capable of quickly giving this extra control. The brakeman must be alert and capable of reacting quickly to this possibility.

When a double brake lowering system is constructed, the two brake stations should be set close enough together to create a small angle between the ropes. In this way, less of a pendulum will result should one side fail. Also, the two brakemen need to be close together to ensure close communication on keeping equal loading on the two braking devices.

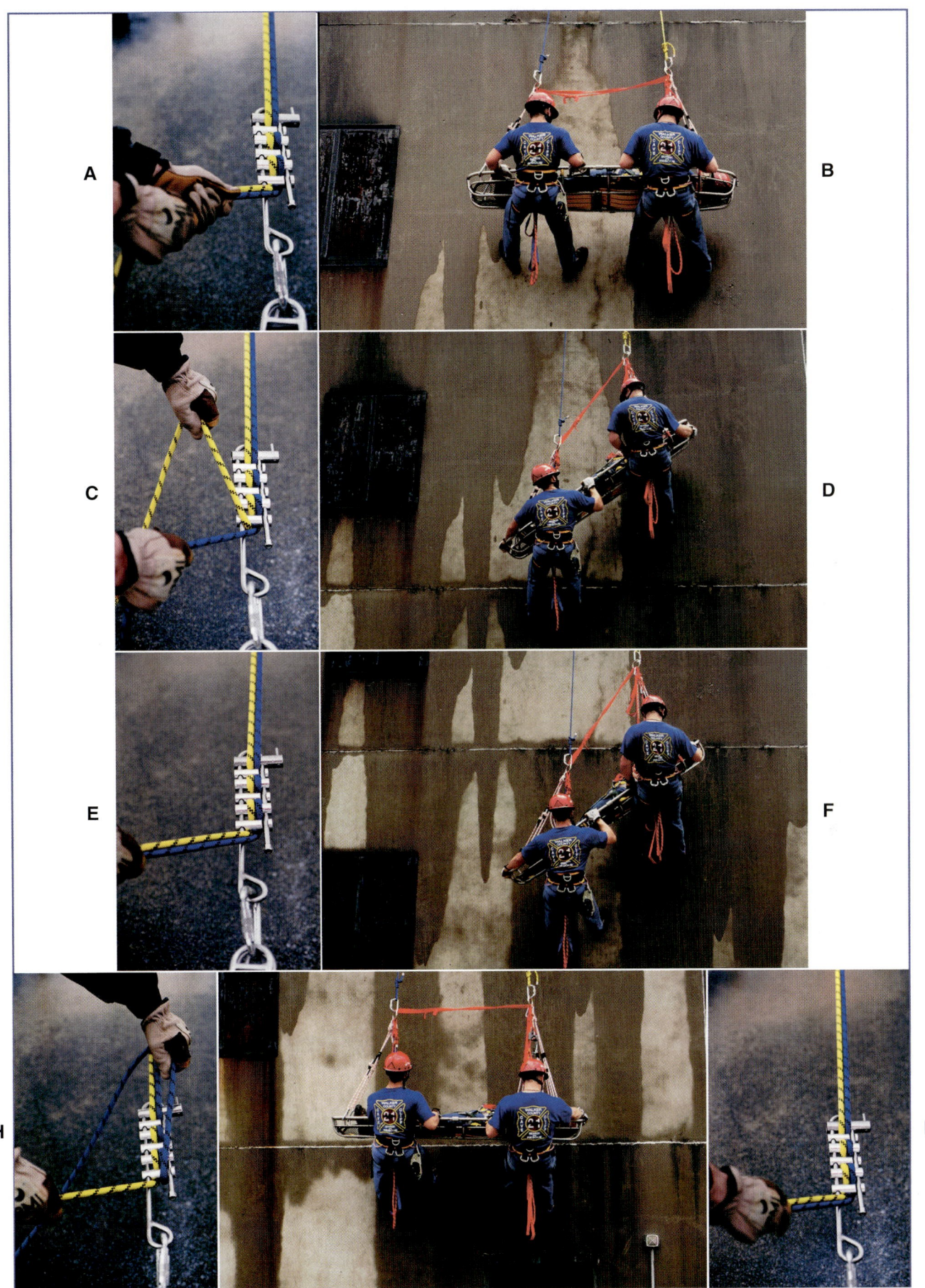

Figure 17-21 Changing the litter angle during a double line litter lowering.

Requirements for Dual Brake Double Line Lowering

- The two spider components must be of equal size.
- The master attachment points must be connected by a sling line. Optimally, this sling should be long enough to allow the litter to be tilted near vertical if necessary but short enough to prevent the two MAPs from spreading too far apart.
- As much as possible, weight must be equalized on each end of the litter. If two tenders are used, they should be of equal size. As an alternative, the heavier tender can be placed at the foot end of the litter. Remember, the upper torso of the subject is heavier than the lower torso. This must be taken into account when balancing the weight of litter tenders.

⬛ *Warning*

When a tether is used to connect both three-legged spiders (see Figure 17-19), the litter cannot be allowed to go completely vertical because this could cause the rigging to press against the subject. In such a situation, team members must be alert and ready to call "*Stop.*"

Sizing of Spiders It is important in a dual line lowering to equalize the lengths of the spiders before starting the lower. The lengths of the spiders depend on the physical conditions of the lowering. The lengths should be a compromise between the following two factors:

1. The spider must be long enough to allow loading and unloading of a subject on the midface if necessary.
2. It must be short enough to allow litter tenders to maneuver the litter in difficult terrain, to enable the tenders to reach the MAP, and to prevent the litter from flopping about while the tenders are trying to maneuver it around obstacles.

Litter Tender Attachments (One Tender) In some situations it is preferable to have two litter tenders. These situations could involve a critical subject requiring full attention by one tender or extremely rugged terrain. One litter tender is preferable because it means less weight on the lowering system, including the brakes and anchors. Also, only a limited number of rescuers may be available.

There are three basic options for a litter tender attachment in a dual line lower with one tender:

1. Have both lowering lines come to a single MAP (see Figure 17-12). This sacrifices some flexibility in adjusting the litter angle.
2. Use two litter attachment points (see Figure 17-19). Attach the litter tender to one MAP as with a single line lower. The disadvantage of this system is that it increases the weight on one end of the litter and therefore on one set of the brakes. This makes it more difficult to keep the litter horizontal. Despite uneven weight distribution, it usually is preferable to place the litter tender on the head end. This gives the tender greater access to the subject, and it is

easier for a litter tender to maneuver the litter while at the heavier end.
3. Attach the litter tender to fixed lines equalized between the two master attachment points. The disadvantage of this system is that it makes it more difficult for the litter tender to move about.

Passing Knots

If the distance of the litter lowering is more than one rope length, it may be necessary to go through a procedure known as *knot pass*. In such a situation, a second length of rope (or more) must be tied to the first rope for the load to reach the bottom. However, some brake systems jam if knots enter them (see the brake tube alternative, p. 271). Therefore a bypass procedure must be used.

Figure 17-22 shows a procedure for passing knots. The system shown uses a single line lower with a belay (which for clarity is not shown).

In addition to a regular lowering system, the following equipment is needed:

- A separate, anchored braking system
- A short length of rope (about 25 feet [8 m]) for interim lowering
- A rope grab for each rope in the main lowering system

1. To avoid delay in the lowering operation, the separate brake system should be rigged and ready before it comes time for the knot pass. The auxiliary braking system is anchored, and the short length of rope is rigged into its own brake system. A figure 8-on-a-bight knot is tied at the end of the short length of rope, and a locking carabiner is clipped into it. The short piece of rope should be adjusted in its brakes so that the cam reaches the main lowering line just below the main brakes.
2. Before less than about 20 feet (6 m) is left on the first rope, the second main rope is tied to it with a figure 8 bend or grapevine knot (Figure 17-22, *A*).
3. Before there is less than 3 feet (1 m) between the knot and the brakes, the lowering is stopped. The knot must not get any closer to the brakes. *If the system slips and the knot enters the brakes, it will jam and will require a difficult hauling procedure to get it unjammed.*
4. The rope grab is placed on the main-line lowering rope just below the main brakes. If a cam is used, the arrow on the cam should point to the load (down the drop) so that the cam grips the main rope. The rope grab is locked on the rope (Figure 17-22, *B*).
5. The auxiliary brakeman holds the auxiliary brakes tight. The main brakeman slowly allows some slack in the main brakes until the load is taken on the auxiliary brake system, and the rope through the main brakes becomes slack (Figure 17-22, *C*).
6. Once the load is fully on the auxiliary brakes, the rope is unlaced from the main brake system (Figure 17-22, *D*).
7. The auxiliary brakeman begins to lower on his or her system until the knot on the main lowering is well past the main brakes.

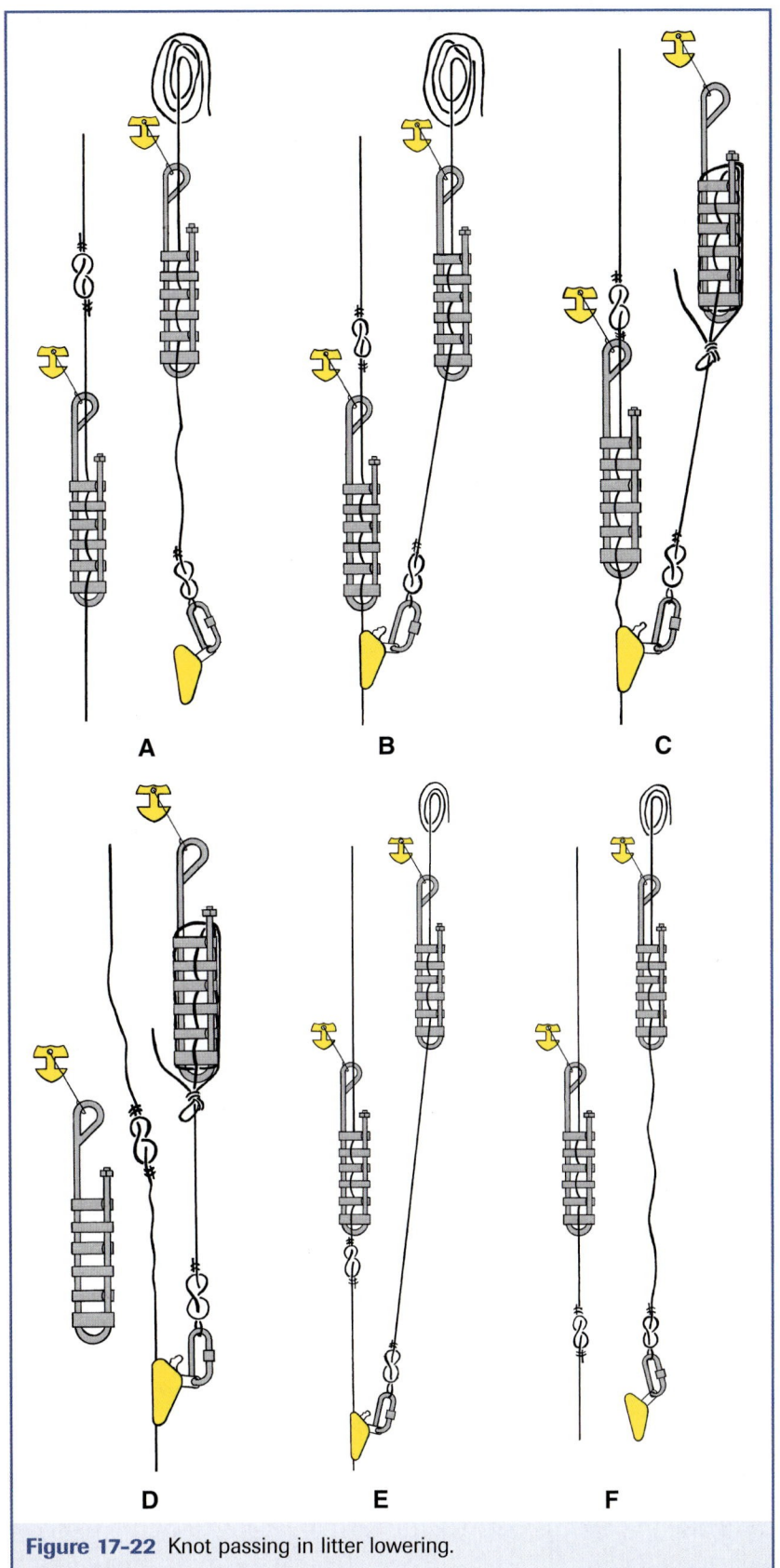

Figure 17-22 Knot passing in litter lowering.

8. The auxiliary brakeman stops the rope from going through the auxiliary brakes. *This must be done before the rope grabs on the main lowering rope get out of reach of the personnel at the top.*

9. Once the knot in the main line is past the main brakes, the main line (now into the second rope) is replaced onto the main brakes (Figure 17-22, *E*).

10. The main brakeman locks off the main brakes. The auxiliary brakeman begins to lower through the auxiliary brakes.

The load is taken onto the main line, and the auxiliary line goes slack.

11. Once the auxiliary line is slack, the auxiliary brakeman stops rope from going through the auxiliary brakes.

12. The now slack auxiliary line, along with the rope grab, is removed from the main line (Figure 17-22, *F*).

13. The main line lowering continues. If an additional knot must be passed, the auxiliary brake system is reset for it.

Evaluation Exercises

Cognitive and Affective Exercises

1. List four environments in which a high angle lowering system might be used in a rescue.

2. A hip belay may serve as a belay in a rescue lowering system.

   A. True
   B. False

3. With a partner, repeat from memory and in sequence the voice signals between litter tender and brakeman and between litter tender and belayer during a high angle lowering.

4. In a high angle lowering, the brakeman's dominant hand should be on the slack rope that is feeding into the brakes. What is the term for this hand?

   A. Belay limb
   B. Dominant hand
   C. Brake hand

5. Describe the position of the hands and the rope for a "quick stop" position of a brake bar rack during a high angle lowering.

6. When the load goes over the edge during a high angle lowering, what significant change occurs that affects the lowering system and the brakeman's ability to control it?

7. Give at least one advantage and one disadvantage for each of the following:

   A. Single line litter lowering
   B. Double line litter lowering

8. In a single line lowering, what is the minimum number of legs for a spider?

   A. Eight
   B. Six
   C. Five
   D. Four

9. From the list below, select the material that would be needed for a spider used in single line lowering of a litter.

   A. Two 12-foot (4 m) lengths of static kernmantle rope
   B. One brake bar rack
   C. Four 4-foot (1.3 m) lengths of Prusik material
   D. Four locking carabiners with gate openings large enough to fit over a litter rail
   E. Two general-use ascenders

10. When a spider is attached to a litter, which direction should the carabiner gate face?

    A. Outward
    B. Toward the cliff face
    C. Toward free air
    D. Toward the subject

11. Describe the attachment system for litter tender tie-ins that includes the use of ascenders to give adjustable height.

12. List five duties of the litter tender during a high angle evacuation of a rescue subject.

13. List four potential duties of the auxiliary tender during high angle lowering of a litter carrying a rescue subject.

14. Name three conditions that might make double line lowering of a litter with a subject preferable to single line lowering.

18

Hauling Systems

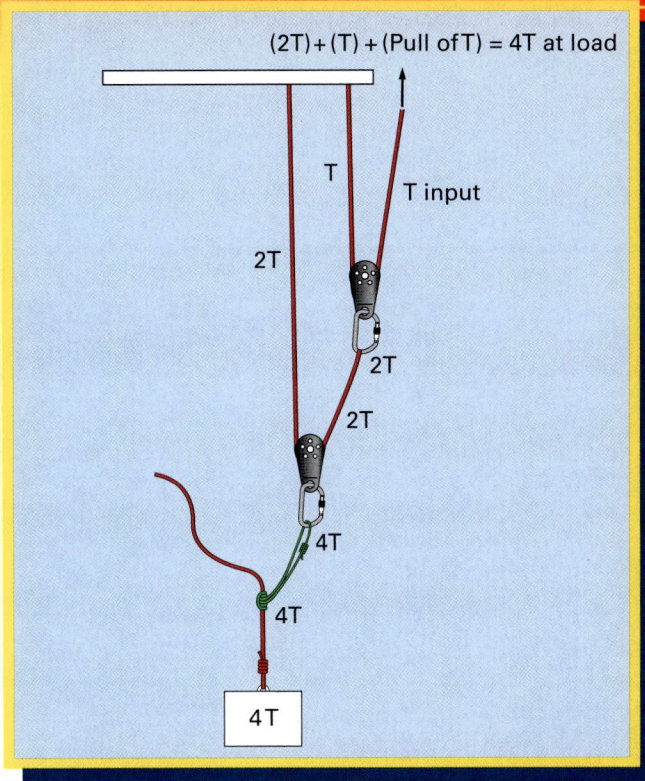

(2T)+(T)+(Pull of T) = 4T at load

T

T input

2T

2T

2T

4T

4T

4T

Prerequisites

Before attempting the activities described in this chapter, you must have demonstrated that you can properly:

1. Use and care for rope.
2. Use and care for other equipment needed in the high angle environment.
3. Tie correctly and without hesitation the knots necessary for safe, effective work in the vertical environment (see Chapter 6).
4. Apply the principles of anchoring and rig a safe and secure anchor.
5. Apply the principles of belaying and safely and confidently belay another person using either a Münter hitch or a personal belay device.
6. Apply the principles of low angle evacuation: correctly set the rigging in any of the elements of slope evacuation and safely and confidently assume the role of litter tender, haul team member, rope handler, brakeman, or belayer.
7. Correctly distinguish between one-person and rescue belays; correctly tie a load-releasing hitch and demonstrate how to release it under load; correctly rig a tandem Prusik belay system and operate it; correctly rig a Prusik minding pulley and operate it.
8. Apply the principles of high angle lowering systems: correctly rig any of the elements of high angle lowering and safely assume the role of litter tender, brakeman, belayer, rope handler, or edge tender.

Objectives

On completion of this chapter, you should be able to:

1. Describe how hauling systems can be used in rescue operations and give some typical examples of situations in which they might be used.
2. Discuss the functions of the following in a rescue haul system: pulleys, haul cam, progress capture device (PCD), tag line, edge protection, haul team, cam tender, and haul captain.
3. Discuss the need for reliable communications in rescue hauling.
4. Describe the principles of a 1:1 haul system, a 2:1 haul system, a 3:1 haul system (Z-rig), and a 4:1 haul system (piggyback rig).
5. Explain how to determine mechanical advantage and define the difference between theoretical and actual mechanical advantage.
6. Discuss the basic criteria for selecting specific haul systems and select the equipment to be used in a hauling system.
7. Repeat from memory the voice communications used in rescue hauling.
8. Describe the primary medical considerations for rescue subjects in hauling operations.
9. Function as a member of a haul team, able to act as a cam tender, haul captain, or belayer for a haul system.
10. Rig a 1:1 hauling system, a 2:1 hauling system, a 3:1 hauling system (Z-rig), and a 4:1 hauling system (piggyback rig).

The material in this chapter conforms to guidelines published by the National Fire Protection Association (NFPA), specifically standard 1006, *Professional Qualifications for Rescue Technicians* (2002), and standard 1670, *Operations and Training for Technical Rescue Incidents* (2004). NFPA standards are revised regularly, and readers are advised to review the latest version of this standard.

Key Terms

Actual Mechanical Advantage (AMA) The useful mechanical advantage of a machine, such as a pulley system. It is calculated by subtracting the effects of friction from the theoretical mechanical advantage (TMA) of the system, or it can be measured by determining the actual input and output forces of the system in use.

Compound Pulley System Any combination of two or more simple pulley systems rigged in such a way that the first acts on the second.

Fixed Pulley A pulley that is anchored and does not move as the load moves. Also known as a *change of direction pulley*. Fixed pulleys do not add mechanical advantage to a system but may make it more convenient to pull.

Haul Cam A rope grabbing device that grips the rope to provide the "bite" in hauling.

Haul System Efficiency The result of dividing the actual mechanical advantage (AMA) of a haul system by the theoretical mechanical advantage (TMA). This value is expressed as a percentage.

Mechanical Advantage (MA) The ratio of the output force produced by a machine to the applied input.

Piggyback System (Pig-Rig) A compound pulley system in which one hauling system pulls (or piggybacks) on another hauling system. The term is often used for a specific type of 4:1 hauling system in which one 2:1 system is attached to (piggybacked onto) another 2:1 system to create a 4:1 system.

Simple Pulley System A simple machine consisting of a pulley and rope that provides a mechanical advantage.

Tag Line A line attached to a load that can be used to maneuver the load and prevent it from snagging and to hold it away from a vertical face.

Theoretical Mechanical Advantage (TMA) Calculated mechanical advantage without allowance for friction and other losses of advantage.

Traveling Pulley A moving pulley that is attached to a load or to a haul cam, which adds to the mechanical advantage.

Z-Rig Common name given to a specific type of 3:1 hauling system. The name is taken from the general shape that the rope makes as it runs through the system.

Rescue Hauling Systems

A knowledge of lowering systems is essential for competent rope rescue personnel; however, not all rescues are performed in high places. In fact, depending on the location, many rescues involve raising a rescue subject out of a lower place, such as the following:

- Silos
- River gorges, canyons, and escarpments
- Grain elevators
- Sewers
- Tank cars
- Basins
- Utility vaults
- Storage bins
- Fuel tanks
- Air vents
- Mine shafts
- Caves
- Tunnels
- Confined spaces

Purposes of Hauling Systems

Rescuers use hauling systems for two basic reasons: (1) to make raising a rescue load easier and more convenient and (2) to make it safer.

Hauling systems, especially those that also provide mechanical advantage, make the job of raising a load easier for the rescue team. The team needs less force to pull the load, though the task probably will take longer and the team will need to pull the rope a greater distance to raise the load. The ability to construct hauling systems in various locations and to use that equipment properly allows rescuers to establish a location for the raising that is most convenient and safest for both the subject and the rescuers.

For example, a hauling system could be established that was:
- Closer to vehicles and roadways
- Away from rockfall and other falling hazards
- Away from potential hostile activity
- Away from bystanders
- At a shorter drop

The most basic hauling system is a direct pull. Note that in Figure 18-1, *A*, a rope has been let down a drop of 10 feet (3 m)

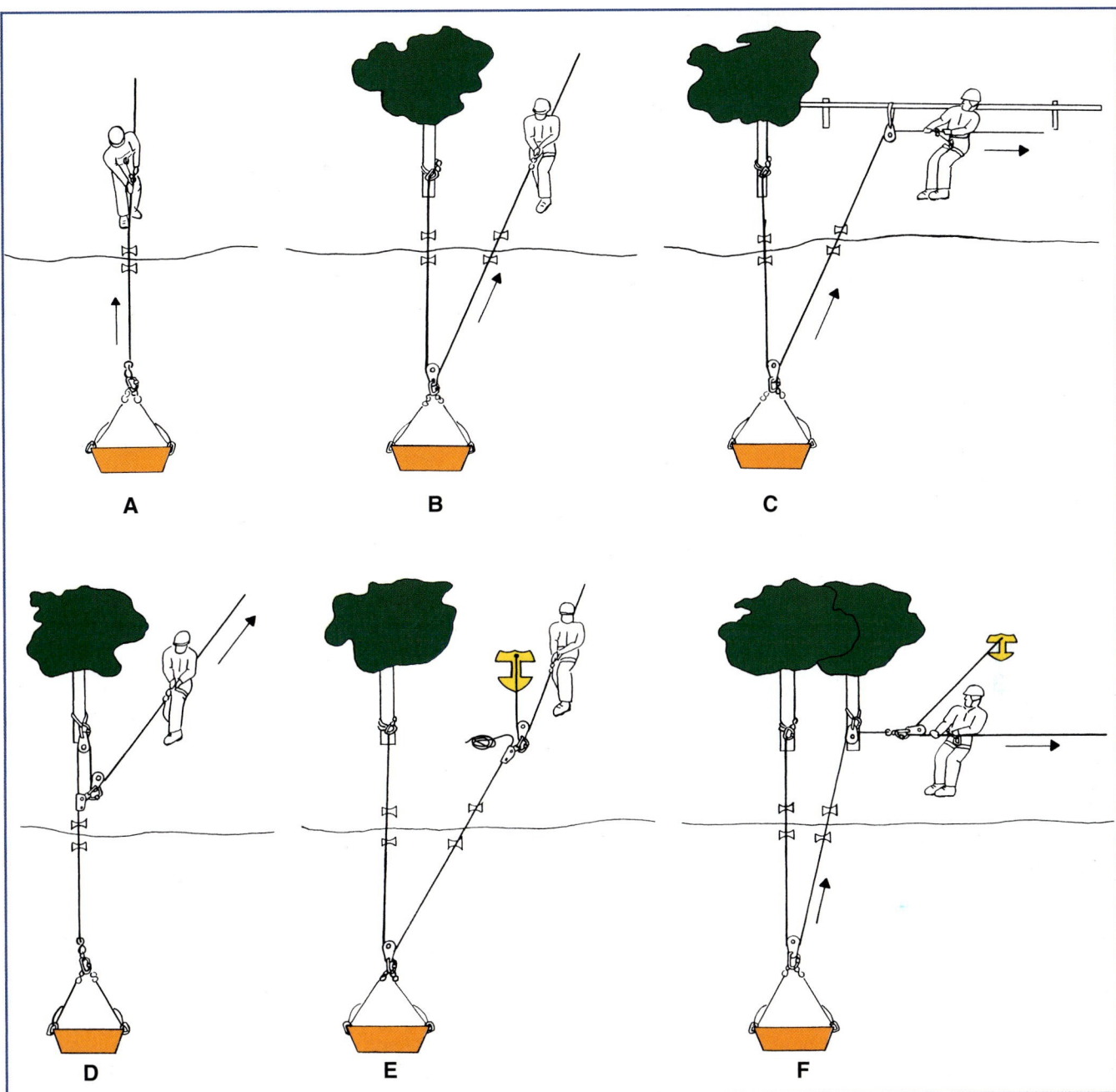

Figure 18-1 Calculating mechanical advantage (MA). **A**, 1:1. **B**, 2:1. **C**, 2:1 with change of direction. **D**, Z-rig 3:1. **E**, Compound 4:1. **F**, Compound 4:1 with change of direction.

and is connected to a load that weighs 100 pounds (444 N). The rope is directly on the load, and it is a straight haul. Therefore, bringing the 100-pound (444 N) load to the top will require 100 pounds (444 N) of force, plus some extra force to overcome the friction of the rope on the edge rollers. It also will require 10 feet (3 m) of rope. (See Box 1-1, p. 5 for a discussion on the distinction between weight and mass.)

Although this is a hauling system, it does not use any less force to move the load than if the rope had not been used. This is so because the force pulling the rope *(input)* must be equal to or greater than the force on the load *(output)* to start the load moving. Adding a mechanical advantage pulley system to a basic

hauling system allows less force on the input side of the system to move a greater load on the output side of the system.

How Hauling Systems Work

Pulleys are essentially wheels on axles with grooves in the wheels to guide the rope. When rigged with rope, a pulley becomes a simple machine, just as a lever or a ramp is a machine. The force required to move a load can be greatly reduced by using pulleys and rope to create mechanical advantage. With a mechanical advantage system, a relatively heavy load can be moved with minimal force. Depending on the configuration of pulleys and rope, varying amounts of mechanical advantage can be produced. The amount of mechanical advantage different systems can produce can be calculated by formulas, which are discussed later in this chapter.

When **mechanical advantage (MA)** is calculated, the result is expressed as a ratio. For example, a system in which a 100-pound (444 N) load could be moved with a calculated 50 pounds (222 N) of force would be a 2:1 mechanical advantage. We refer to this calculated mechanical advantage as a **theoretical mechanical advantage (TMA).**

The calculated mechanical advantage is considered theoretical because rescuers never are able to use the full mechanical advantage of any hauling system. Some of the force exerted in the haul is lost through friction in the pulleys, rubbing or dragging of the rope against an edge, and rope stretch. The mechanical advantage left over from this friction loss is called **the actual mechanical advantage (AMA)**. For discussion purposes in this text, we will discuss hauling systems in terms of the theoretical mechanical advantage and refer to it simply as the *TMA*.

Keep in mind, however, that the actual amount of mechanical advantage derived from a hauling system depends greatly on **haul system efficiency,** which includes how the system is rigged and on the **efficiency** of the components (e.g., pulleys) used to build it. At several points the chapter explains how to avoid loss of MA in hauling.

Calculating Mechanical Advantage

In the simple example in Figure 18-1*, *A,* we can calculate the TMA in simple ratio form as follows:

Load:Force required to move load
100 pounds (444 N):100 pounds (444 N)
Ratio (TMA) = 1:1

Note that in this example, the length of rope pulled by the rescuers (10 feet [3 m]) is the same as the distance the load moves.

In Figure 18-1, *B,* the same load (100 pounds [45 kg]) must be raised, but in this case the rescuers have attached a pulley to the load. A pulley in this position is known as a **traveling pulley** because it travels with the load. To gain a mechanical advantage, rescuers have anchored the rope at the top of the drop and then run it to the load, through the pulley, and back up to the top, where the other end of the rope is held by the rescuers. With the system rigged in this way, the rescuers must pull 20 feet (6.5 m) of rope to move the load 10 feet (3 m). However, because half the load is on the anchor and half on the rope they are hauling, they need to pull only with a force of 50 pounds (222 N).

The TMA in this example would be calculated as follows:

Load:Force required to move load
100 pounds (444 N):50 pounds (222 N)
Ratio (TMA) = 2:1

---

*NOTE: These drawings have been simplified for instruction. For maximum MA efficiency, the ropes through moving pulleys should be as parallel as possible. Wider angles lessen the actual MA. For simplification, the progress capture device (discussed later in the chapter) is not shown.

To see how this haul could be made more convenient, consider Figure 18-1, *C.* Note that the rescuers now have added a second pulley at the top so that they can pull the rope horizontally instead of vertically. This second pulley is stationary and is attached to a sling suspended from a column, a strong tree, or some other, similar anchor. This pulley does not provide any additional mechanical advantage. A pulley that is anchored and that does not change position as the rope moves is called a **fixed** (or change of direction) **pulley**. Fixed pulleys can make work easier by changing the direction of the applied force; however, the same force is needed to move the load. It is important to note that the forces exerted on the anchor of a change of direction pulley can be up to two times the actual load, depending on the interior angle of the ropes running through the pulley. Just as in Figure 18-1, *B,* the rescuers are pulling 20 feet (6.5 m) of rope and the load is moving 10 feet (3 m). In theory, it still requires 50 pounds (222 N) of force to move the 100-pound (444 N) load. Therefore the calculation of mechanical advantage is the same, resulting in a TMA of 2:1.

Although the rescuers have not added any mechanical advantage, they may have made their task more *convenient* and possibly *safer.* They no longer must stand bunched together on the edge of the drop, awkwardly pulling up on the rope and fighting gravity. With the addition of the stationary pulley, which acts as a change of direction, they can walk back in a line away from the drop as they pull the rope and raise the load.

This illustration of the effect of a change of direction on the haul is just one example of how convenience and safety must be considered, in addition to mechanical advantage, when rescue haul systems are rigged.

Multiplying the Mechanical Advantage
Simple Mechanical Advantage Systems

The 2:1 TMA system shown in Figure 18-2, *A,* is known as a **simple pulley system**. In simple systems, all the moving pulleys move toward the anchors at the same rate as each other and the load. A simple 4:1 TMA system is shown in Figure 18-2, *B.* In this system, the two pulleys at the load move at the same speed as the load, and each of the four rope strands moves at the same rate and carries one fourth of the load. A common block and tackle rig (Figure 18-2, *C*) is an example of a simple pulley system. In a simple pulley system, if the end of the rope is attached at the load, the MA will be an odd number (e.g., 3:1). If the end of the rope is attached at the anchor, the MA will be an even number (e.g., 4:1) (Figure 18-2, *D*).

Compound Mechanical Advantage

Another means of increasing the mechanical advantage of a hauling system is to stack a second simple pulley system on the original simple pulley system. This results in an increase in the MA equal to the original system's TMA multiplied by the second system's TMA. Based on the engineering principle that a simple machine acting on a simple machine is a compound machine, a pulley system stacked on another pulley system in this manner is called a **compound pulley system**. The general rule of thumb is this: when two rescue hauling systems are joined at the input of the first, the resulting TMA is obtained by

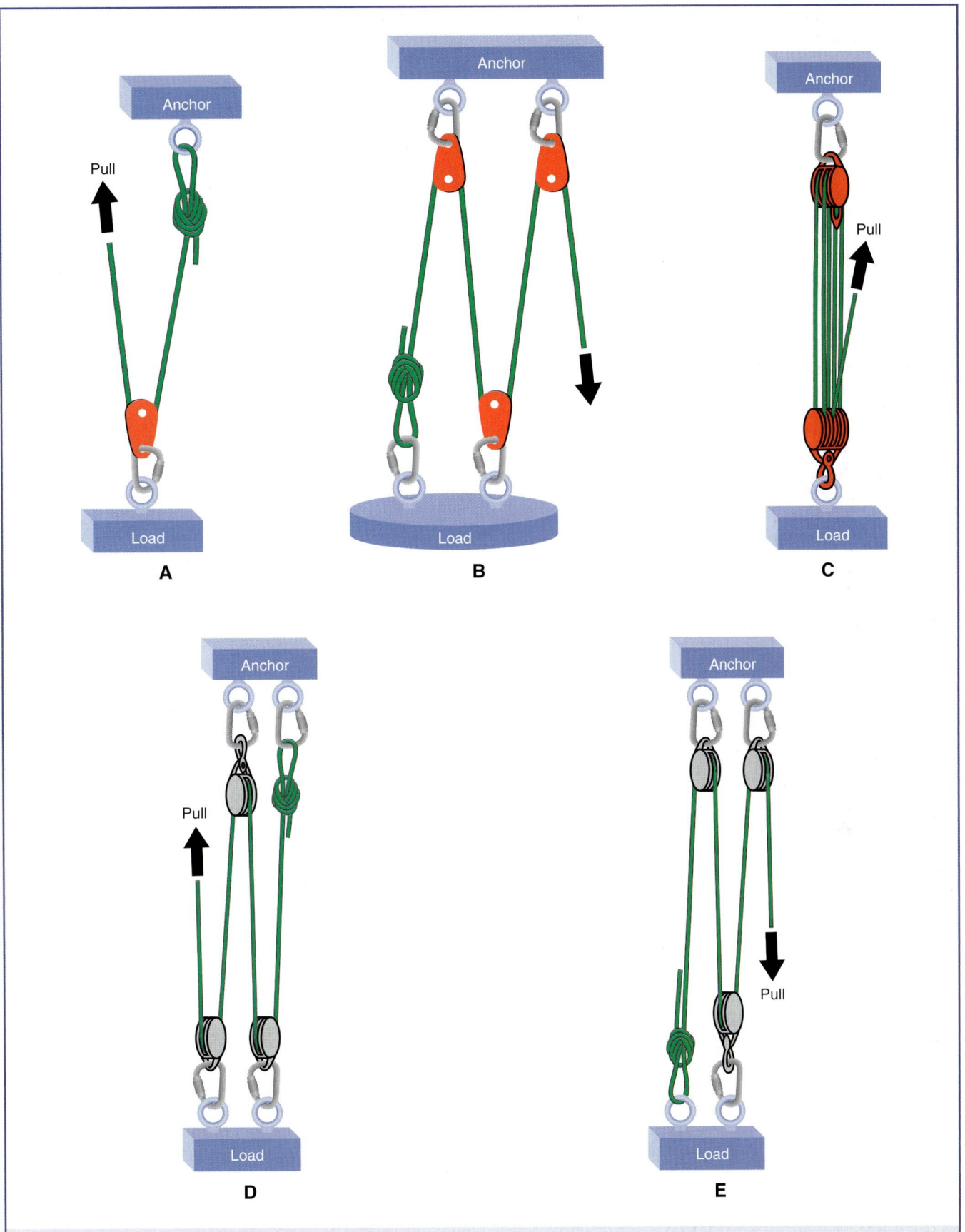

Figure 18-2 Simple mechanical advantage systems. **A,** 2:1. **B,** 4:1. **C,** 6:1 block and tackle. **D,** Even MA–4:1. **E,** Odd MA–3:1.

Box 18-1	Complex Pulley Systems

Although not a true class of machine, a third type of pulley system, known as a complex pulley system, sometimes is discussed. Complex pulley systems do not meet the definition of a simple or a compound system; rather, they involve more variables in rigging. Figure 18-3 is an example of a complex system. Complex systems can have pulleys moving toward the load and the anchor at the same time. They have limited practical use in most rescue applications.

Box 18-2	Exception to the Multiplying Rule

The multiplying rule is a general rule as applied to the basic rescue hauling systems examined in this chapter. There are exceptions to this rule. It may not apply, for example, in certain compound block and tackle systems. The most reliable way to determine a mechanical advantage is to measure actual force required to move a known load or the length of rope pulled against the distance the load moves.

multiplying the two TMAs (Boxes 18-1 and 18-2). For example, if a 2:1 TMA hauling system is added to the input end of a 2:1 system, the result is a 4:1 TMA. If a 2:1 TMA hauling system is added to the input end of a 3:1 system, the result is a 6:1 TMA, and so on. The major advantage of building compound pulley systems as opposed to simple systems is that mechanical advantage can be increased to its maximum potential in a compound system for the number of pulleys used in the system. A simple system takes more pulleys to reach the same TMA as a compound system, and the extra pulleys increase the loss of system efficiency through additional friction. Therefore, compound systems are more efficient than simple systems of the same TMA.

Ways to Add to Mechanical Advantage

Incremental Addition of Mechanical Advantage

Figure 18-1, *D*, shows a means of increasing the TMA from 2:1 to 3:1 simply by rearranging the pulleys used in the 2:1 system with a change of direction (see Figure 18-1, *C*). This particular type of system is commonly called a **Z-rig** because of the general shape made by the rope as it runs through the system.

Note that in the 3:1 system, at point A there is an anchor to which a pulley is attached. This is a stationary pulley, and the main-line hauling rope runs through it. At point *C* there is also a pulley through which the same rope runs. However, this is a traveling pulley, and a rope grab with a carabiner is attached to it. The rope grab is attached to the main strand of the same rope. In this case, though, the pulley and rope grab move as they are pulled by the top end of the rope. The rope grab grips the rope that goes to the load and pulls it up.

In this system, there are three strands of moving rope. For every foot the load moves, the haul team must pull 3 feet (1 m) of rope. The load is supported by three moving ropes, and each

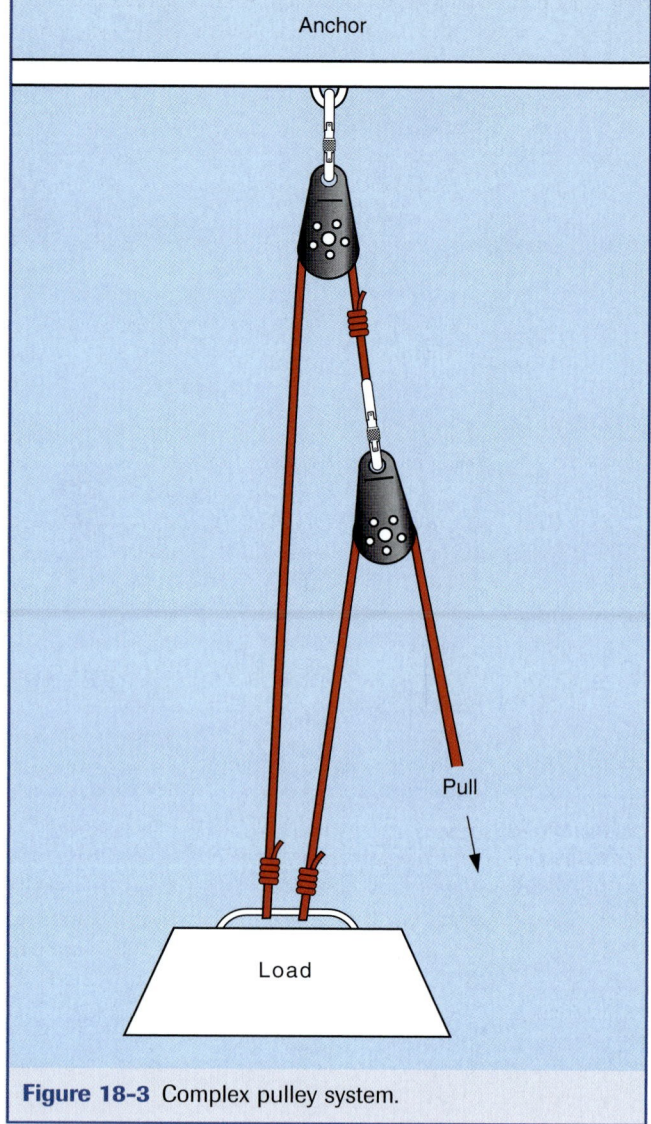

Figure 18-3 Complex pulley system.

rope supports approximately one third of the load. Therefore, to move the 100-pound (444 N) load, the haul team must exert a force of approximately 33.3 pounds (148 N):

Load:Force required to move load
100 pounds (444 N):33.3 pounds (148 N)
Ratio (TMA) = 3:1

Beyond the Z-Rig

As the need for greater mechanical advantage increases, a variety of methods can be considered. Using the 4:1 MA as an example, the following method could be used to achieve the desired result.

To create one type of 4:1 hauling system, take the 2:1 hauling system from Figure 18-1, *B*, and add another 2:1 system. Start by adding a second pulley at the end of the rope where the rescuers had been hauling (see Figure 18-1, *E*). Take a second rope and anchor one end of it at point *A2*. Run the rope through the second pulley at the end of the first rope and bring the second rope back parallel to itself toward anchor *A2*. The haul team now pulls on the second rope at its free end. This is known as a ***piggy back system (pig-rig)***. In this system, the lower pulley makes a 2:1, which is attached to the load via a haul cam, and the upper pulley is a second 2:1, which is piggy backed onto the lower system creating a compound 4:1. As the haul progresses, four strands of rope are moving. To pull the load up 10 feet (3 m), the rescuers must pull 40 feet (12 m) of rope. Moving the 100-pound (444 N) load requires a pulling force of 25 pounds (111 N):

Load:Force required to move load
100 pounds (444 N):25 pounds (111 N)
Ratio (TMA) = 4:1

As with the example in 18-1, *C*, the rescuers could make things more convenient and possibly safer with a change of direction pulley. This time, however, the rescuers still could construct a 4:1 system if they first added a directional at the edge of the drop, as they have in Figure 18-1, *F*. After the directional pulley has been rigged, a second 2:1 TMA system could be rigged (Figure 18-1, *F*).

To accomplish this, they first would set anchor *A2* back from the drop. Next, they would pull the top end of the first rope through the directional (stationary) pulley. Then they would attach the traveling pulley to the end of the first rope (point *TP3*). They would attach a second rope to anchor A2 and run it through the second traveling pulley. They would then haul on the free end of the second rope by walking back away from the directional pulley and edge of the drop.

As mentioned before, the stationary pulley at the top of the drop would serve only as a directional and add no mechanical advantage. However, it would provide greater convenience and safety in the hauling system. The rescuers now would be able to haul by walking back from the drop. The TMA in Figure 18-1, *F*, would be the same as that in Figure 18-1, *E*.

Load:Force required to move load
100 pounds (444 N):25 pounds (111 N)
Ratio (MA) = 4:1

Calculating Mechanical Advantage and System Efficiencies

The T System for Calculating Mechanical Advanatage

The following is a method for calculating the MA of a compound or complex pulley system, the tension in any one part of the system, and the force on each component. If the efficiencies of the various pulleys are known, the AMA of the complete system can be calculated.

Start by drawing a diagram of the pulley system to be analyzed (Figure 18-4). Beginning with the input side of the system, where the haul team will pull, assign the value *T* (for tension) to the loaded rope. The *T* value also is applied to the first pulley in the haul system. Theoretically, the rope tension on one side of the pulley must equal the rope tension on the other side. Assuming that the pulleys are 100 % efficient, the value of the

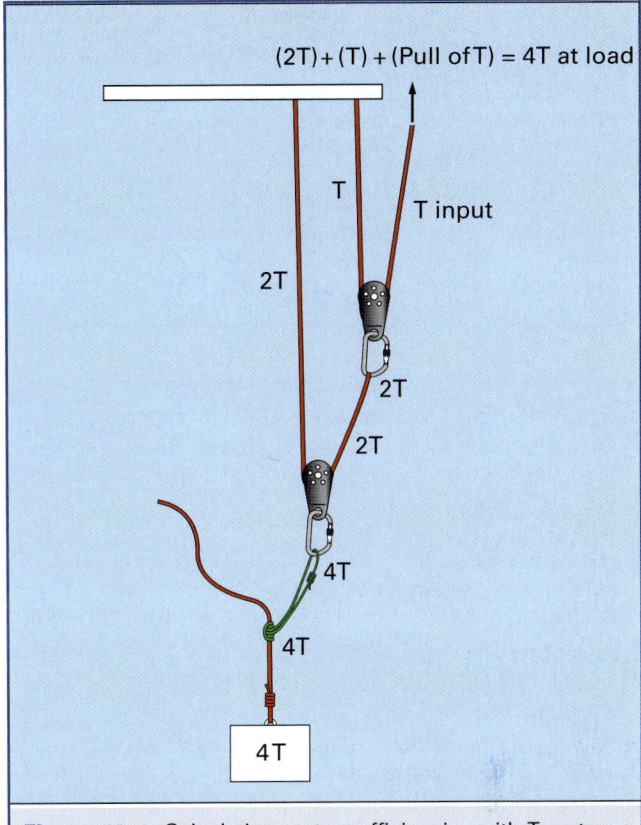

Figure 18-4 Calculating system efficiencies with T system.

rope coming out the other side of the pulley also will be *T*. In the example (Figure 18-4), the tension in the rope from the first pulley to the rope's anchor must be *T* as well.

The output carabiner of the first pulley has a value of *2T*, because if the pulley is to remain in equilibrium, the tension must be equal to the sum of the tensions in the ropes coming out the other side of the pulley. Therefore the input rope tension to the second pulley is *2T*. Likewise, the rope tension out the opposite side of the pulley also is *2T* and is transmitted to the anchor of the rope running in the second pulley. This pulley must also be in equilibrium. The output is the sum of the tensions of the input rope to it *(2T)*, and the anchor side rope tension *(2T)*. This makes a total of *4T* pulling on the rope grab, the same as the load at the end of the rope. The first example (B) in Figure 18-4 is a 4:1 system.

The actual load or input force can easily be inserted into the calculation to determine the expected load on any one component of the system. Figure 18-5 substitutes 125 pounds/ force (lbf) (556 N) for the input of *T* in the previous example.

The same *T* system can be used to calculate the anticipated AMA if the efficiencies of the pulleys are known. Assume that the first pulley on the input side is 95% efficient, and that for the second pulley, a carabiner has been substituted that is only 50% efficient when used as a pulley. Figure 18-6, *A* shows the resulting MA. Now reverse the position of the two pulleys (Figure 18-6, *B*). Note the difference made by the placement of the more efficient pulley. When possible, the more efficient pulley should be placed at the input side of the pulley system.

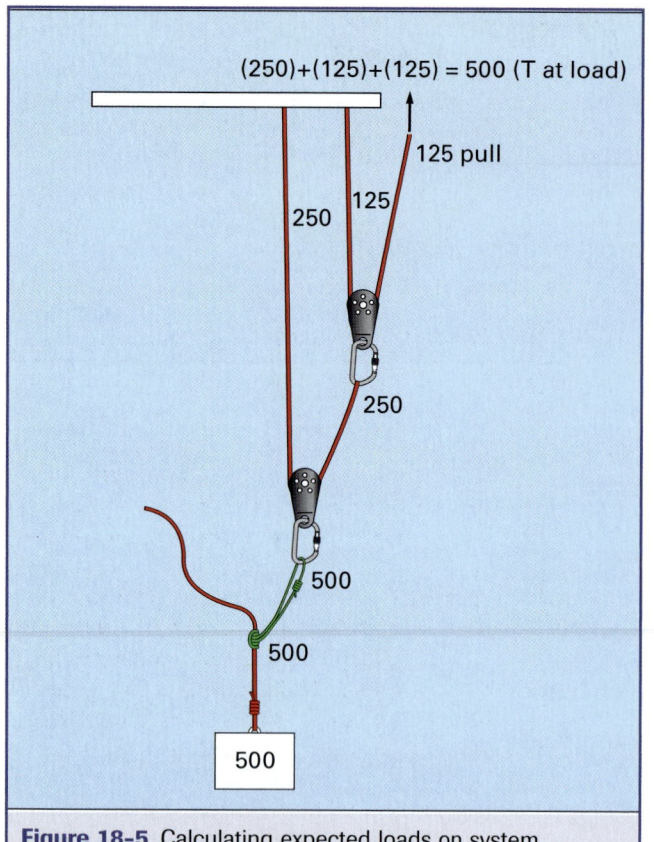

$(250)+(125)+(125) = 500$ (T at load)

125 pull

125

250

125

250

500

500

500

Figure 18-5 Calculating expected loads on system components.

Elements of Hauling Systems
Role of Rope Grabs in Hauling Systems

In hauling systems, devices called *rope grabs* are used to grip the rope. Several types of mechanical rope grabs or soft hitches may be used for this purpose. However, rescuers must consider factors such as the amount of force that will be exerted on the rope grabs, how easy they are to reset, how much friction they provide, whether they meet rescue standards, and the ways they will be used.

Nature of the Rope Grab

Depending on its position in the hauling system, a rope grab serves one of two purposes:
1. It grasps the rope so that it can be pulled by the hauling system; this is known as the **haul cam**. (An example of a haul cam is shown at point *C* in the 3:1 hauling system shown in Figure 18-1, *D*.)
2. It holds the rope while the haul team resets itself to get another bite on the rope; this is known as the *progress capture device (PCD)* or *ratchet cam*.

General-Use Ascenders

General-use ascenders are rope grabs that often are used for loads heavier than those for which light-use (personal) ascenders are designed. In a general-use ascender, a metal cam presses the rope against the metal shell of the ascender. Some well-known

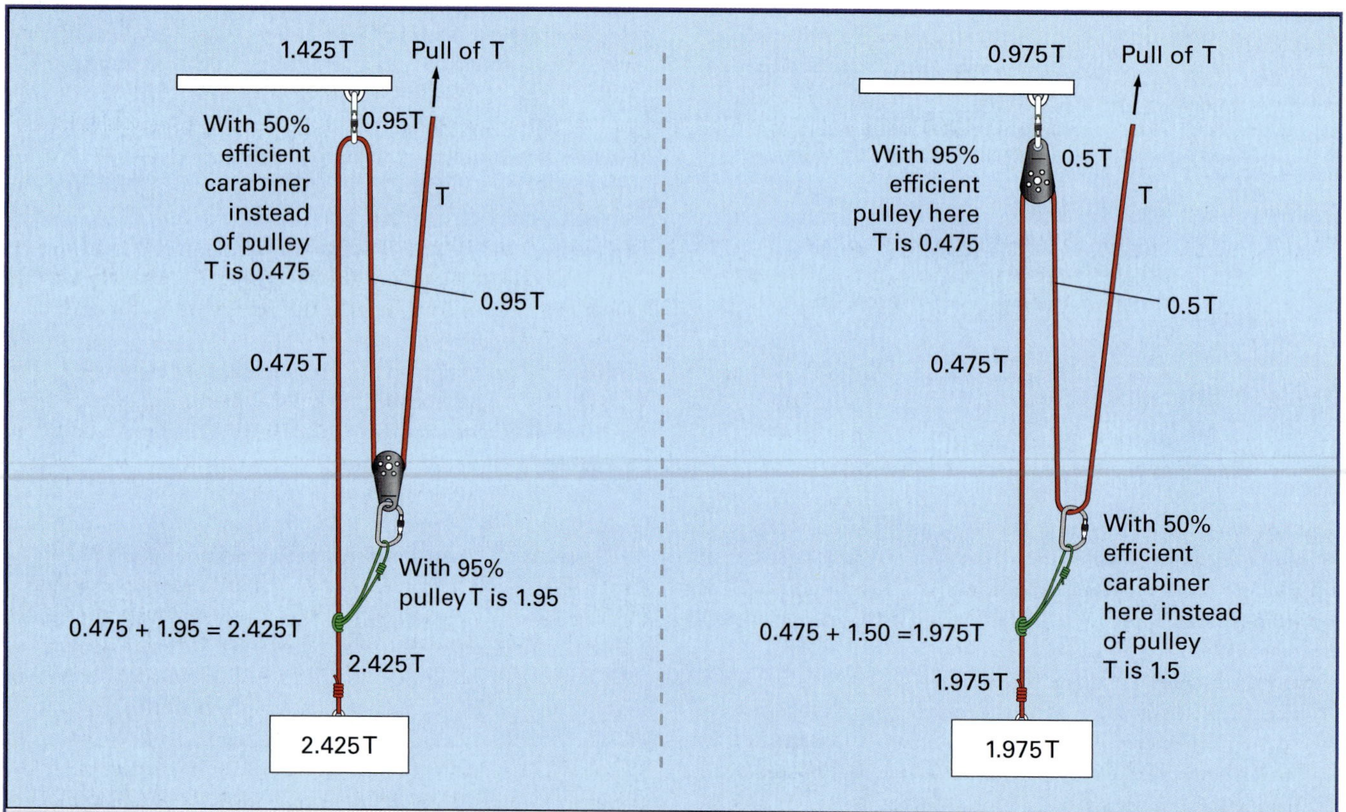

1.425 T   Pull of T

With 50% efficient carabiner instead of pulley T is 0.475

0.95 T

T

0.95 T

0.475 T

With 95% pulley T is 1.95

$0.475 + 1.95 = 2.425T$

2.425 T

2.425 T

0.975 T   Pull of T

With 95% efficient pulley here T is 0.475

0.5 T

T

0.5 T

0.475 T

With 50% efficient carabiner here instead of pulley T is 1.5

$0.475 + 1.50 = 1.975T$

1.975 T

1.975 T

Figure 18-6 Calculating anticipated AMA.

models are the Rescucender (Petzl, France), the Progressor (PMI) and the Ascender (Gibbs).

Advantages

- Easy to use
- Can be rigged to reset automatically
- Can be manipulated quickly, even when used as a PCD

Disadvantages

- Inconsistent design and performance among the various designs (some models are designed to slip when impact loaded and others may cut through the rope)

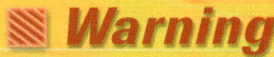

Warning

Light-use (personal) ascenders must not be used in rescue hauling systems. Light-use ascenders are designed only for one person's body weight. They are not designed for the high stresses caused by the multiplication of forces involved in hauling systems. Use of light-use ascenders in hauling systems can result in tearing of the rope or structural failure of the ascender. Either of these circumstances can result in failure of the entire system.

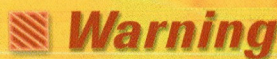

Warning

Never use a single friction hitch or a hard cam for a belay in rescue hauling. Under shock loading, a single friction hitch could fail, and a hard cam could cause the rope to fail (see Chapter 13).

Friction Hitches

Another type of rope grab is the friction hitch. Friction hitches, also known as "soft cams," are created by tying accessory cord in a hitch around the rope to be hauled. The most commonly used friction hitch is the triple-wrapped Prusik hitch. The diameter of the accessory cord used to make the friction hitch should be at least 2.5 mm smaller than the diameter of the rope it grips (e.g., an 8 mm cord would be used for an 11 mm rope) and should have an appropriate safety factor for the intended use.

Advantages

- If correctly sized and used, a three-wrap Prusik will hold until the accessory cord breaks or until it breaks the line it is gripping.

Disadvantages

- May be more difficult to manipulate
- Slippage under load can cause friction heat, which can result in melting and failure
- May not catch in icy or muddy conditions
- Performance varies widely, depending on material used and experience of rescuers

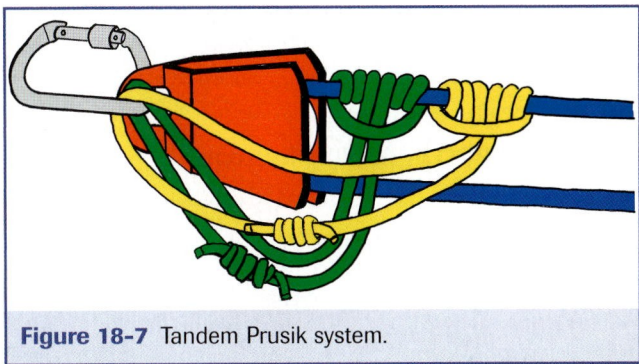

Figure 18-7 Tandem Prusik system.

No single rope grab device or technique is perfect for every rescue situation. Every device has some drawbacks, and any device, whether mechanical rope grab or friction hitch, can be made to fail if used improperly or if stress on the system exceeds its designed capacity.

Because most mechanical rope grabs can be made to fail with high shock loading, some rescue teams prefer to use the tandem Prusik system as an alternative rope grab device for the main haul cam in hauling systems (Figure 18-7). In some tests, the tandem triple-wrap Prusik system was shown to have greater energy absorption capability than a number of other methods used in the belaying of large loads.

A single Prusik (rather than tandem Prusiks) or two-wrap Prusiks (rather than three-wrap Prusiks) may be easier to operate as a main haul cam, but they do not necessarily provide adequate holding power to prevent slippage. Test results are inconclusive, and great care should be taken when these or any other means of static holding are used.

The best system is the one that limits fall potential as much as possible because it was built correctly. *Always test a system before it.*

Positioning the Progress Capture Device

In order to offer the greatest protection against failure in other elements of the hauling system, the PCD should be positioned as far forward of the hauling system (toward the load) as possible while still being safely in reach of the rescuers.

For example, if the rescuers are hauling a load up a vertical drop, the PCD should be close to the edge but not over it and out of reach. Note that where the PCD is set in a slack system is not where it ends up with the system under tension. Locate the PCD where it can be reached and where it is not compromised by the edge *even when under tension.*

It is important to remember that should anything else in the hauling system fail (e.g., anchors, hauling team, haul cam, and pulleys), the PCD is the last hope to grab the main-line rope and prevent the system and the rescue load from falling. For this reason, the PCD cam should be on a very good anchor.

Alternative Approach: Placing the PCD to the Rear in a Z-Rig

In certain cases, it may be impossible to place the PCD forward of a Z-rig hauling system, such as when no anchors are available for attaching the PCD. When a Z-rig (3:1 MA) is used, the PCD can be placed in back of the hauling system (Figure 18-8). This can be done with a rope grab, or if a Prusik minding pulley is used for the rear pulley, Prusiks can be added to make a PCD out of the rear pulley.

Rigging the PCD in Hauling Systems

At this point, the student should review the sections on ascenders in Chapters 5 and 16.

When a PCD is rigged, it should be set so that, as much as possible, its anchor and anchor sling are in line with the rope the PCD is grabbing. If available, the PCD anchor should include a load-releasing (LR) hitch. This should be done without interfering with or jamming the rope (see Figure 18-9, *A*). If the PCD is rigged too far off to the side of the rope it is protecting, too much slack will appear in the PCD anchor sling. This will result in two problems (see Figure 18-9, *B*): (1) dangerous shock loading of the PCD and its sling and anchor may occur; and (2) the hauling team will lose some of the purchase it has gained when it sets the PCD to reposition for another bite.

Setting a PCD Cam

Two primary concerns must be addressed when rigging a PCD:
1. The PCD must clamp the rope when needed.
2. The PCD must not ride up the rope as the rope moves, because this could result in dangerous shock loading.

The specific way in which the PCD is rigged depends partly on the specific type of rope grab used and partly on the specific circumstances of the rigging.

Free Running General-Use Rope Grab Figure 18-10 shows one method of ensuring that the ascender stays in place and clamps the rope when needed. This technique uses a person known as the *cam tender*. As the main-line hauling rope moves

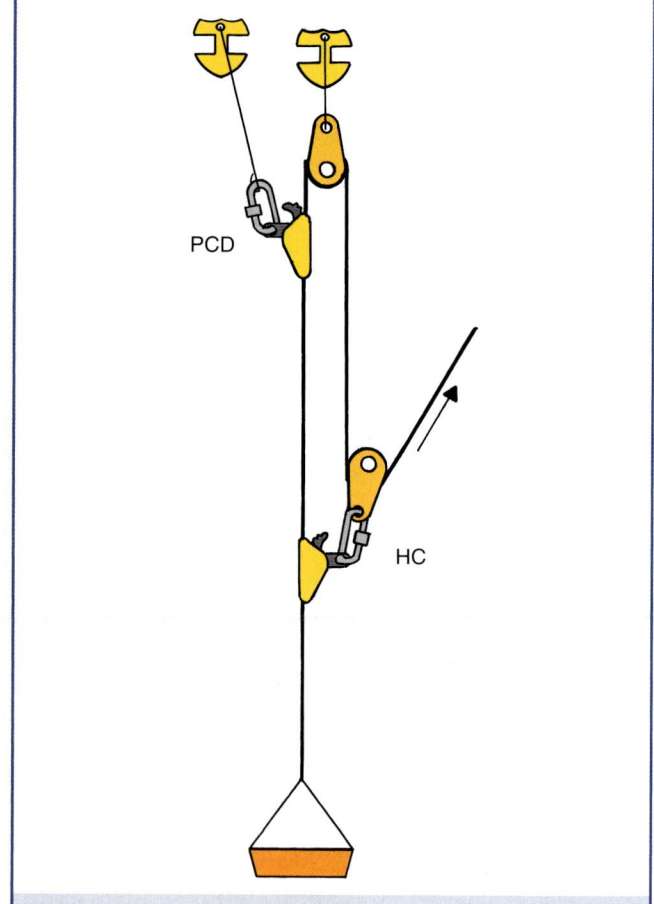

Figure 18-8 Alternative position for a progress capture device.

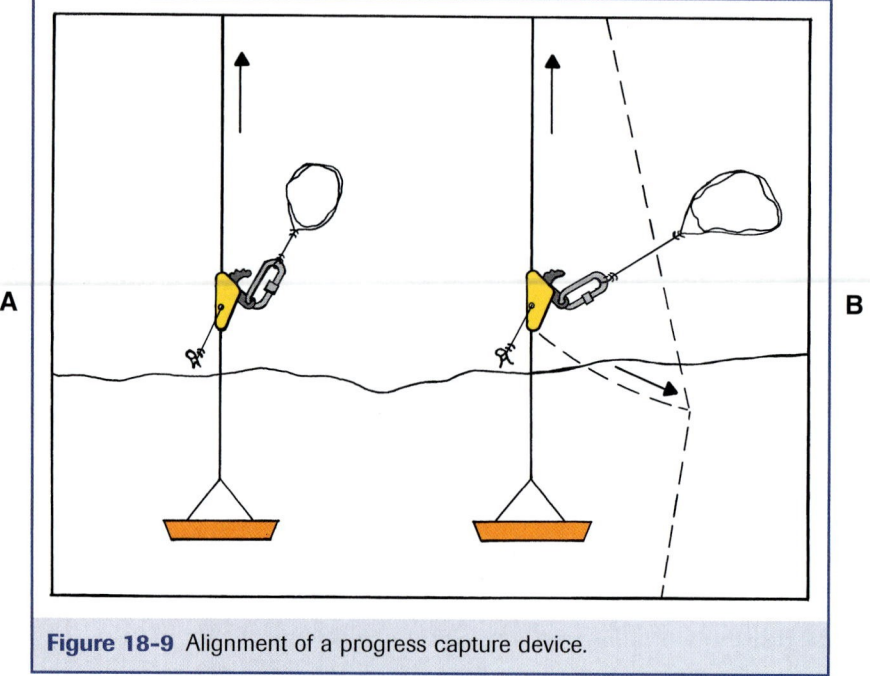

Figure 18-9 Alignment of a progress capture device.

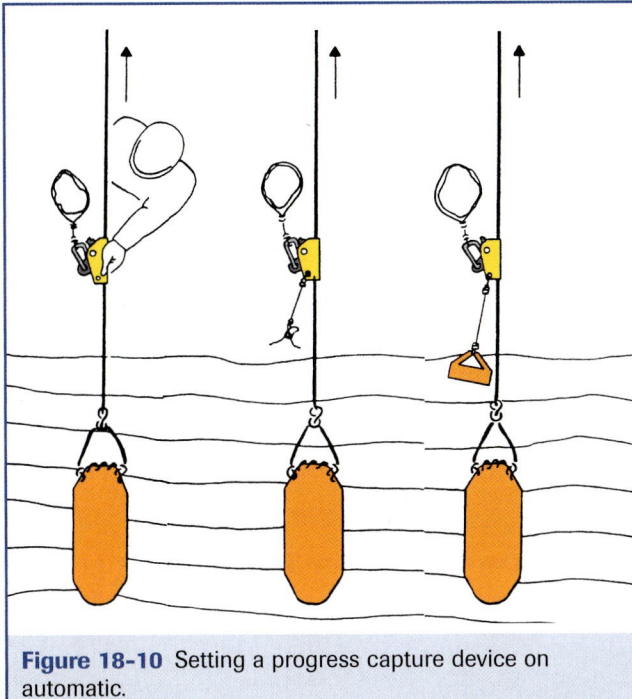

Figure 18-10 Setting a progress capture device on automatic.

up, the cam tender makes sure the ascender does not travel up the rope. To do this, the cam tender holds the backside of the shell with the palm and with the fingers extended out of the way of the cam. The ascender is held in this way so that fingers and gloves do not get caught if the device suddenly shock loads. A finger caught by the cam could be injured, and a glove caught in the cam could prevent it from clamping the rope. Use of a cam tender can be effective, but it requires extra personnel. Also, the potential for human failure or inattention always exists.

A second technique for using a free running cam as a PCD is shown in Figure 18-10. A bungee (elastic) cord is clipped into the empty hole usually found in the point of the arrowhead, and the other end of the bungee cord is anchored securely to a convenient spot toward the load. A great deal of tension is not required on the bungee cord, but there should be enough to prevent the ascender from riding up the rope and to keep the cam clamped on the rope. The bungee cord is tied only to the shell and not to the cam itself. If the bungee is tied to the cam, the cam might not close when it should.

A third alternative for a free running cam is shown in Figure 18-10. A short piece of cord is attached to a weight, and the weight is hung so that it pulls the shell of the cam toward the load.

Preventing Edge Friction in Hauling Systems

A common situation in the rigging of hauling systems often goes unnoticed until it causes problems: this is rope friction over the edge of a drop and elsewhere in the system. Because ropes in hauling systems often are highly loaded, rope friction can cause two significant problems:

1. Friction can increase severely, resulting in a tremendous increase in load for the haul team. Edge friction in hauling often is greater than in lowering over the same edge.
2. Friction can cause severe damage to the rope and other equipment.

Possible solutions to edge friction include edge rollers and directionals, changing the haul rope position, rope padding, and reducing the weight of the load.

Edge Rollers

Edge rollers often may be the most efficient solution to edge friction. However, they must be centered under the rope and securely anchored at each side. Otherwise, they can easily be turned over as the rope moves slightly from side to side.

Directionals

A directional pulley sometimes can be used to hold the rope above the edge and to protect against edge friction. Ways of anchoring a directional pulley include a tripod (Figure 18-11), a strong overhead beam or, in a natural area, a very strong tree.

Changing the Position of the Haul Rope

To change the position of the haul rope, move the haul system to a place where the edge is less sharp or move the rope to a higher angle above the edge so that less friction is generated.

Warning

Make sure directionals are set on a very strong anchor. Some directionals in effect create a 2:1 hauling system on the anchor, exerting higher forces on the anchor than the weight of the load.

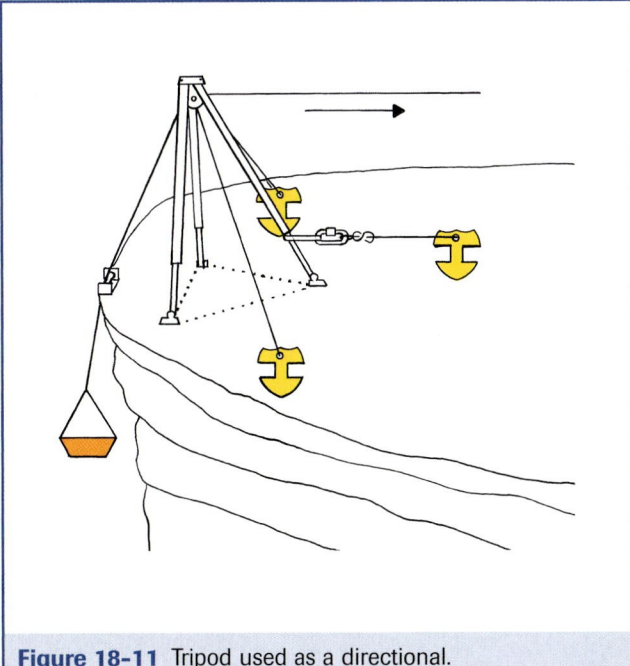

Figure 18-11 Tripod used as a directional.

Rope Padding

Rope padding may only slightly reduce friction, but it may significantly reduce rope damage (see Chapter 4 for tips on padding ropes).

Reducing the Weight of the Load

Keep loads as light as possible. For example, if possible use one tender instead of two on a litter being hauled.

Role of the Haul Team

See p. 241 in Chapter 16 for information on the haul team.

Tag Lines

A *tag line* can be used to better control a load and to prevent it from hanging up during a hauling operation. Tag lines can be used both from the bottom (Figure 18-12) and then from the top to get a load over the edge.

A tag line can be helpful for:

- Positioning a litter when it is hauled through a confined space
- Preventing a litter from getting snagged on an overhanging edge
- Holding a litter away from a wall to ensure a smoother ride for the rescue subject
- Preventing the litter from spinning on free-hanging hauls

Getting Over the Edge

Getting a litter over an edge when hauling can be very difficult. It should be done slowly and carefully, because a hung-up litter can overstress elements of a hauling system and cause failure.

1. Before starting a haul, tie short tag lines onto both the foot and the head of the litter.
2. At the top, station edge attendants *securely tied in*.
3. Make sure the litter attendant is in the best position for getting his or her feet under the litter and against the face (see Figure 17-17, p. 269).

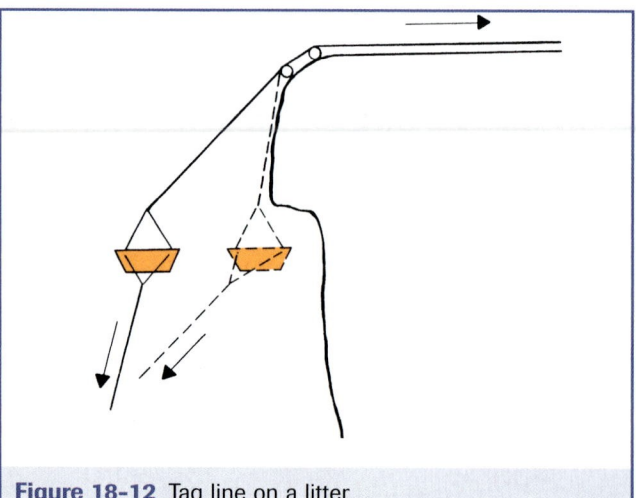

Figure 18-12 Tag line on a litter.

4. Before the litter makes contact under the edge, stop the haul.
5. Have the litter attendant hand a tag line to each of the edge attendants, one at the foot and one at the head of the litter.
6. Restart the haul very slowly and be prepared to stop instantly should the litter hang up. If the litter gets hung up and cannot be freed, you may need to slack off on the system to free it. A load-releasing hitch on the PCD can help resolve a situation in which the litter is hung up and the haul has been pulled tight.
7. As the litter attendant pushes his or her feet against the face and pulls the litter rail away from the face, the two edge attendants help pull the litter up and over the edge.

Communications

See p. 241 in Chapter 16 for information on communications used in hauling systems.

Rigging and Using Hauling Systems in Rescue Operations

> ### ⬛ *Warning*
>
> Hauling systems can create tremendous stress on rope, hardware, and anchors. Hauling team members and other rescuers must keep in mind that forces exerted by the hauling team are multiplied on portions of the system. For example, if a haul team exerts a force of 1,000 pounds (4.45 kN) into a 4:1 system, the resulting force on portions of the system could be around 4,000 pounds (17.8 kN). Higher MA systems could result in even higher forces.
>
> These forces can develop quickly. A mishap, such as a jammed knot or tangled equipment, can quickly lead to system failure. All rescuers must be aware of the forces they are creating and be constantly on guard against problems that may be developing. If a haul suddenly becomes difficult, do not simply pull harder. The system may have become jammed, and pulling harder may cause a failure. Stop the haul and examine the system for problems. As with all rescue operations, one person should act as safety officer, overseeing the safety of rescuers and rescue subjects.

1:1 TMA Hauling System

Figure 18-13 shows a 1:1 hauling system for raising a load up a vertical drop.

Minimum Equipment Requirements

- One main-line rope
- One anchor sling
- Two locking carabiners
- One rope grab (PCD)
- One LR hitch
- Separate belay system appropriate for the load to be hauled

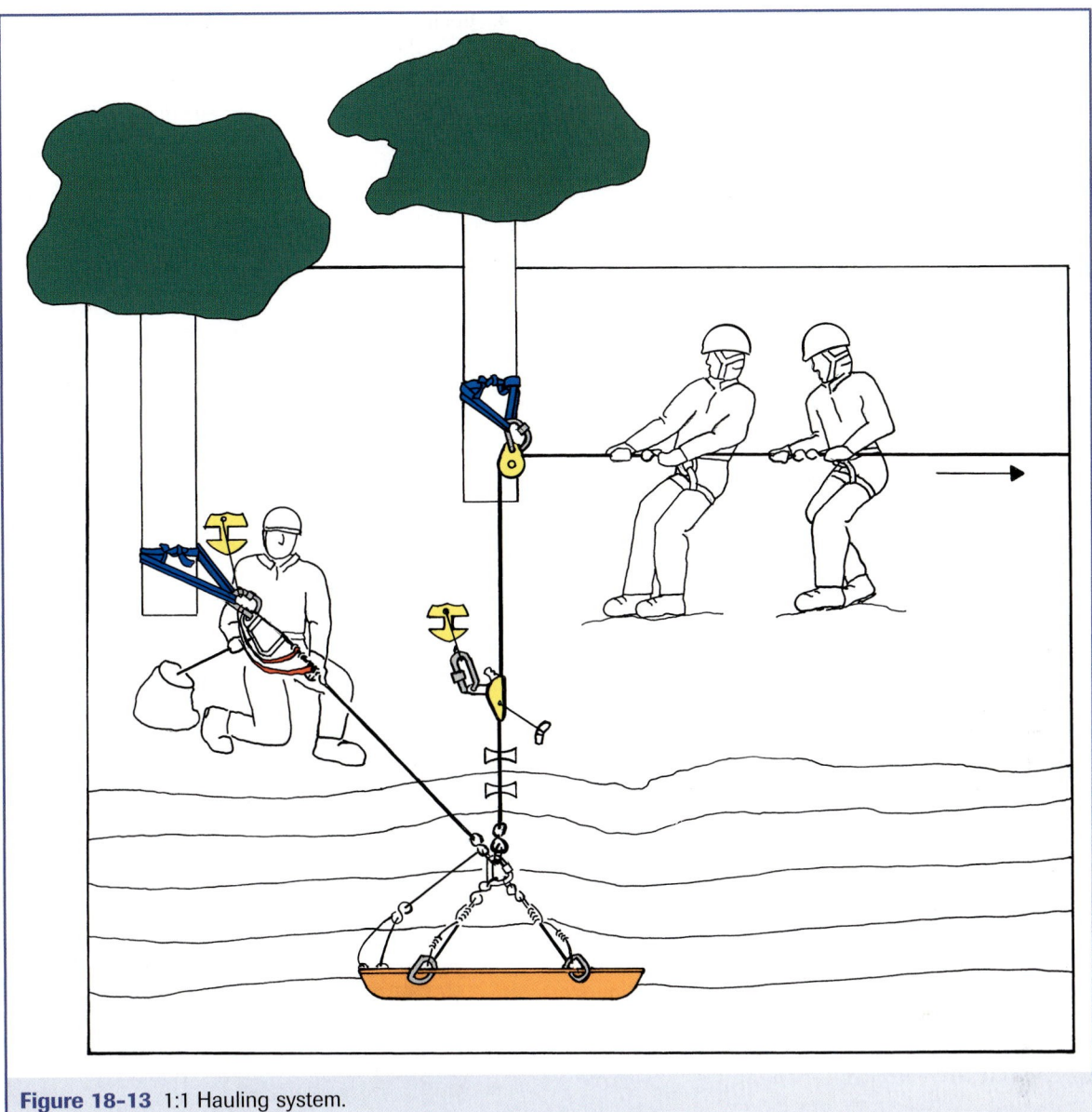

Figure 18-13 1:1 Hauling system.

Rigging the 1:1 System

1. At the top of the drop and back from the edge, establish a secure anchor point. Into the anchor point, securely attach an anchor sling with a locking carabiner. Into the carabiner, clip a pulley for the directional. The directional should be located such that the haul team can move the rope in a convenient direction.
2. Thread the main-line hauling rope into the pulley and tie a stopper knot in the end of the rope or secure the rope by temporarily tying off the upper end.
3. Drop the lower end of the rope over the edge close to where the load is to be hauled.
4. Establish a separate anchor point for the PCD. This anchor should be located close to where the main-line rope will run but slightly off to the side so that the PCD and its anchor sling do not tangle with the rope. To the anchor

point, attach an anchor sling with a locking carabiner in the end of the sling. On the anchor sling, place an LR hitch with the second carabiner. Clip the PCD into that carabiner.
5. Attach the PCD to the rope. If it is a general-use ascender, its arrow should point toward the load. Make sure that after the rope has been loaded, the PCD creates very little bend in the rope. (If the PCD creates considerable bend in the rope, the device is producing a great deal of rope friction, which will increase the load for the haul team.)
6. Check for edge friction and place any devices (e.g., an edge roller) that can reduce it.
7. On a separate anchor point, rig a belay appropriate to the type of load (one-person or rescue load).
8. Attach the lower end of the main-line rope to the load and remove slack between the PCD and the load.

9. Attach the lower end of the belay rope to the load and adjust appropriate slack between the load and the belay device.
10. Position the haul captain such that, if possible, he or she has a field of view of both the load and the haul team. If near the edge, the haul captain should be tied in to a safety line.
11. Position a cam tender to make sure the ascender does not travel up the rope and that it sets on the rope as intended (or set the ascender for "automatic" with a bungee cord or weighted line).
12. Position a belayer with the belay system, ready to establish the load on belay.
13. Position the haul team with the rope in their hands, ready to haul.

Beginning the Haul

14. When all the rescuers are ready, the person on the load (e.g., practice rescuer or litter tender) initiates the belay cycle by calling, *"Haul slow"* (or *"Haul fast."*).
15. The haul captain relays the signal to the haul team: *"Haul slow"* (or *"Haul fast"*).
16. When the haul team has gone as far as it can or as far as the system allows, the haul captain calls, *"Set."* The haul team immediately stops hauling and slowly eases back so that the PCD catches. The cam tender makes sure the PCD is set.
17. The haul captain then calls, *"Slack."* The haul team immediately reverses direction and moves back up the rope to take another bite of rope.
18. The haul captain calls, *"Haul,"* and the cycle continues until the load reaches the top.

Getting the Load over the Edge

One of the most difficult parts of a haul sequence is getting the load over the edge, particularly if the edge is sharp or undercut (or both). As the load nears the top, the main line tends to pull it at a low angle that forces the load against the edge. This also tends to increase friction between the main-line rope and the edge. These factors add to the stresses already present in a haul system.

As in rappelling or lowering, the one factor that affects edge problems in a haul is the angle the rope makes from the anchor to the edge. A horizontal angle usually is the most difficult (i.e., the anchor is on the same level as the load when the load is at the edge), and a vertical angle usually is easier (i.e., the anchor is above the load when the load is at the edge). This angle can be increased in various ways, such as raising the level of the anchor to establish a high directional. However, it must be kept in mind that high directionals tend to multiply forces on anchors and other gear.

Use of a tag line can be very helpful in these situations. As the load reaches the top, those below can hand over the tag line to edge tenders, who can use it to help pull the load over the top.

The following procedures also can be helpful for getting the load over the edge while reducing the potential for equipment failure and personal injury:

■ As the load approaches the edge, the haul captain calls, *"Haul very slowly."* The haul team moves very slowly and is prepared to stop instantly.

■ If necessary, the haul captain can call, *"Stop,"* and size up the situation at the edge.
■ All rescuers should be alert for the development of problems or stresses the edge. Anyone who notices such a situation can call, *"Stop!"*
■ Edge tenders, secured with safety lines, can be very helpful in getting loads such as litters over the edge.

Hauling from a Confined Space

Figure 18-14 shows the use of a 1:1 hauling system that incorporates a large tripod to perform a rescue from a vertical confined space. The chains that come with a tripod should also be used at the base of the legs.

■ The tripod must be securely anchored by a back tie in the direction opposite to the direction of the haul.
■ A pulley (directional) is attached by means of a sling anchored to the apex of the tripod.
■ A PCD is attached to a separate sling that is anchored at the apex of the frame. The PCD should be lower down and closer to the ground. However, it should be high enough that it does not interfere with getting the load out of the hole.
■ A tag line should be attached to the load. Initially this is used by the rescuers below to position the load so that it does not snag on the edge. Once the load is out of the hole, a rescuer at

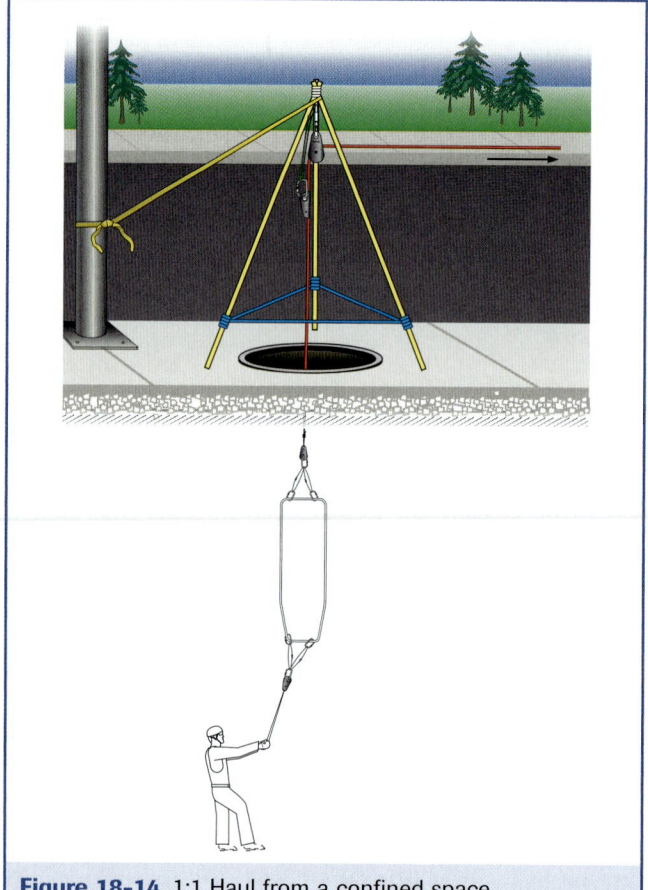

Figure 18-14 1:1 Haul from a confined space.

the top controls the tag line to swing the load from over the hole to an area where it can be safely detached.

- When the load is at the top, the haul team gives slack and the cam tender releases the cam so that the load can be moved from over the hole.

2:1 Hauling System without the Diminishing V

Problems can arise with a conventional hauling system with a traveling pulley on the load (see Figure 18-1, *B*) because it creates a *diminishing* V, which results because the rope runs around the traveling pulley. During the haul, the diminishing V tends to get snagged on brush, rock, building projections, and other objects. Also, there are two strands of rope to create edge friction.

Figure 18-15 shows one way to remove the diminishing V yet keep a 2:1 TMA. Note that only a single haul-line attachment runs to the load, as would be the case in a 1:1 hauling system. However, after the rope has gotten to the top, a short 2:1 hauling system is attached to it with a haul cam. With the diminishing V kept smaller and at the top, the system is less likely to snag, and if it does, rescuers are able to reach it to free it.

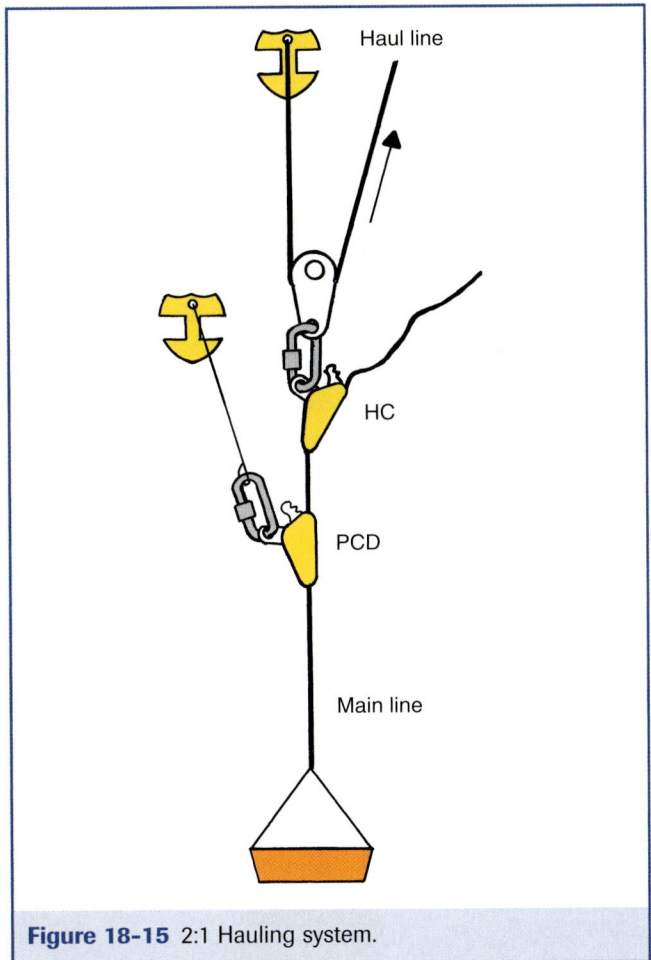

Figure 18-15 2:1 Hauling system.

Setting Up a 2:1 System

1. Follow steps 1 through 9, pp. 289-290, for setting up a simple 1:1 TMA hauling system.
2. At the top, and where rescuers can reach it, attach a haul cam to the main-line rope. This should be placed above the PCD (between the PCD and the anchor). To get the greatest amount of bite possible, the haul cam should be close to the PCD; however, it should be far enough away that the two cams do not jam during hauling operations. Onto the haul cam, clip a locking carabiner. Clip a pulley on to the carabiner.
3. Take a second rope (the haul rope) and fold it in half. Attach one free end of the haul rope to an anchor that is in the direction to be pulled.
4. Thread the haul rope through the pulley attached to the haul cam.
5. Pull the second strand of the haul rope back parallel to the first strand that goes to the anchor. The haul team pulls on the second strand of the haul rope.

Hauling with the 2:1 System Attached to the Main Line

6. If there is a shortage of personnel for this operation, the haul captain may be stationed at the haul cam to manipulate it, but he or she should have a good field of view of the operation. With enough personnel, one person can be assigned specifically to the job of haul cam tender.
7. Follow steps 11 through 16, p. 289.
8. When the haul captain calls, *"Slack,"* the haul team immediately reverses direction and moves back up the rope to take another bite. As they do this, the person attending the haul cam resets the system. He or she also makes sure no slack develops on the main-line rope between the haul cam and the load.
9. When the haul team reaches its original position, the team is ready to begin another haul cycle.

3:1 (Z-Rig) Hauling System

Figure 18-16 shows a 3:1 haul system. This particular 3:1 system is commonly called a Z-*rig* because of the approximate shape the rope makes as it goes through the system.

Minimum Equipment Requirements

- One main-line rope
- Three locking carabiners
- Two pulleys
- Two rope grabs (one for hauling, one PCD)
- Separate belay system appropriate for the load to be hauled

Rigging the 3:1 System

1. Above the load (point *A1* in Figure 18-16), set an anchor point. Attach an anchor sling with a locking carabiner and clip a pulley to the carabiner.
2. Thread the main-line rope onto the pulley and lower an end of the rope to the load.
3. Set a separate anchor point for a PCD with an LR hitch; this anchor should be close to where the main rope will run but

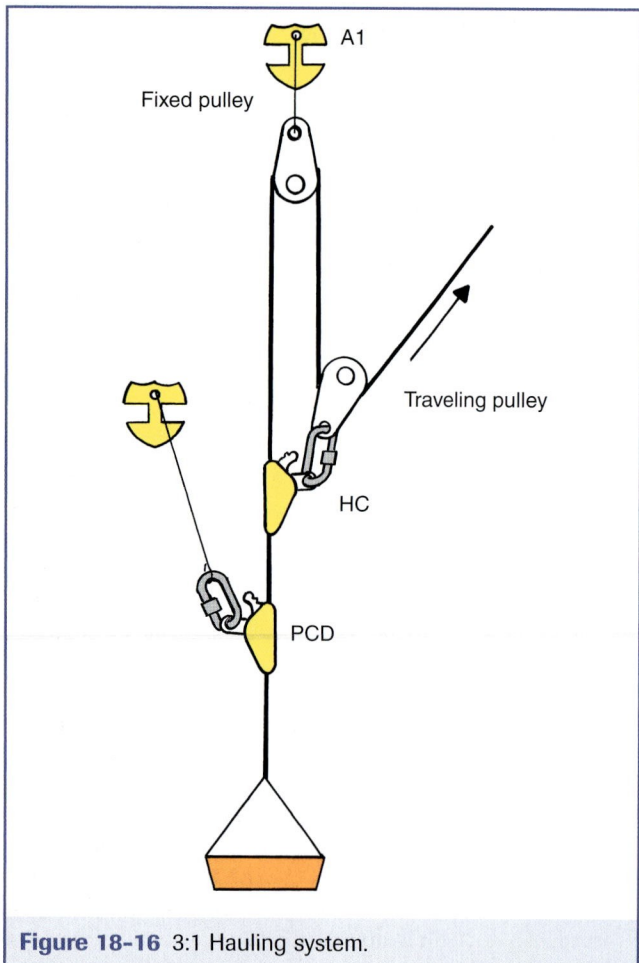

Figure 18-16 3:1 Hauling system.

slightly off to the side so that the PCD and its sling do not tangle with the rope. Attach an anchor sling with a locking carabiner. Into the carabiner, clip a general-use ascender with its arrow pointing toward the load (or attach a Prusik loop to the rope and attach its sling to the carabiner).

4. Thread the PCD (Figure 18-16) onto the rope. After the rope has been loaded, make sure the PCD does not create much of a bend in the main-line rope, which could mean a much higher load for the haul team.

5. At a point just above the PCD, place the haul cam (*HC* in Figure 18-16). (If a general-use ascender is used for this purpose, the arrow should point toward the load.) Clip a locking carabiner into the haul cam and attach a pulley.

6. Bring the upper end of the main rope back in the direction of the load and run it through the pulley on the haul cam.

7. Reverse direction again with the upper end of the rope, bringing it back toward the first anchor and parallel to the other two strands. This is the hauling end of the rope. Remove all rope slack from the hauling system.

8. In this configuration, the haul must be back toward anchor *A1* and parallel to the other strands of the rope. If it is off to the side, some advantage will be lost. If, because of limited space or some other reason, the haul team must go off in another direction, set a directional, using a fixed pulley. In

this way, the only advantage lost is the small amount accounted for by the friction of the directional pulley.

9. Follow steps 11 through 15.

10. Before the pulleys at *A1* and *HC* come together, the haul captain calls, *"Set,"* and the haul team immediately stops hauling and slowly eases back so that the PCD catches. The haul cam tender makes sure the PCD has set.

11. The haul captain calls, *"Slack."* The haul team instantly reverses direction and moves back toward the load with the rope still in their hands. As they do so, the person attending the haul cam resets the system by grasping the carabiner attached to the haul cam and pulling it back down on the rope until it reaches the PCD (or pulls the Prusik knot back down the rope).

12. When the haul team reaches its original position, it is ready to begin another cycle.

4:1 (Piggyback) Hauling System
Minimum Equipment Required

- One main-line rope
- One hauling rope (50 to 100 feet [16.5 to 33 m], depending on the space available for the haul)
- Three locking carabiners
- Two pulleys
- Two rope grabs (one to act as a PCD and one for hauling)
- Separate belay systems appropriate for the load to be hauled

Rigging the 4:1 System (Figure 18-17)

1. Attach the main-line rope to the load. Secure the upper end so that it does not accidentally slip over the edge.

2. Establish a strong anchor point for the PCD, close to where the main rope will run but slightly off to the side so that the PCD and its anchor sling do not tangle with the rope. Attach an LR hitch to the anchor point. Into the end of the LR hitch, attach a locking carabiner and clip a general-use ascender to it (or tie a Prusik to the rope and clip the end of the sling into the carabiner).

3. Establish an anchor point for the hauling system (point *A2* in Figure 18-17). This anchor point should be well back from the edge and in line with the load to allow room for the haul system. Attach a sling to the anchor point and clip a locking carabiner to it.

4. Find the center of the haul rope (the shorter line). At the center, tie a figure 8-on-a-bight knot and clip it into the locking carabiner on the anchor sling.

5. After the figure 8-on-a-bight knot has been tied, the hauling rope will have two strands. Bring one leg of the haul rope back in the direction of the load. About two thirds of the way down this leg of the haul rope, create a bight and clip a pulley into it. Into the pulley, clip a locking carabiner and attach a rope grab to it; the rope grab must be attached on the main-line rope above the PCD (between the PCD and the top end of the main-line rope). If the rope grab is a general-use ascender, the arrow on the shell should point toward the load. This is the point where the hauling system piggybacks onto the main-line rope.

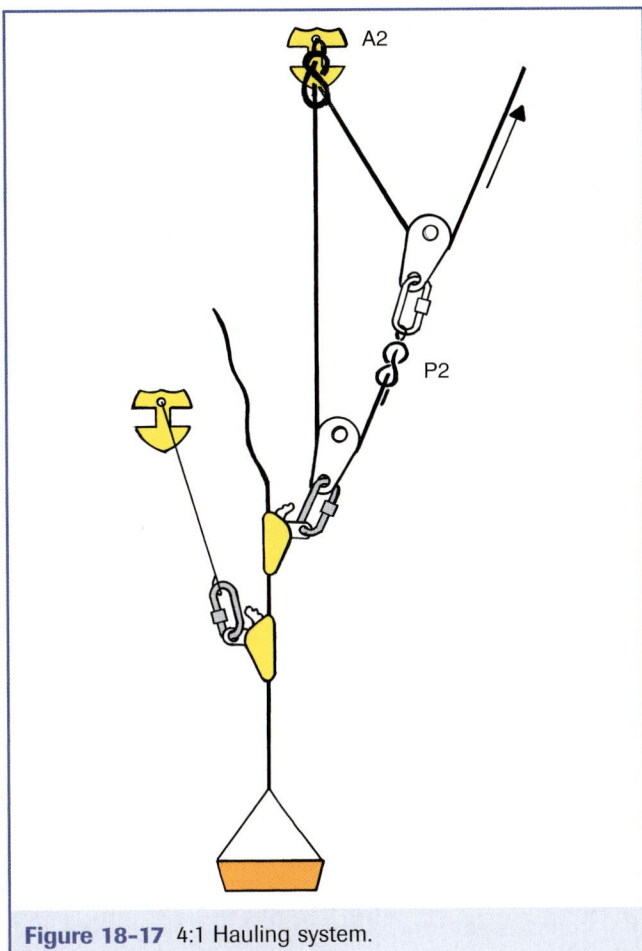

Figure 18-17 4:1 Hauling system.

6. On the same leg of the haul rope to which the rope grab has been attached, find the free end of the rope. In this end, tie a figure 8-on-a-bight knot (point *P2* in Figure 18-17). Clip a locking carabiner into it and attach a pulley to it.

7. Take the second leg of the haul rope and bring it down to the pulley just clipped into the first leg of the haul rope. Thread the second strand through the pulley.

8. Pull the end of the second strand back toward the anchor for the hauling system (point *A2* in Figure 18-17). This is the end the haul team pulls.

9. Follow steps 11 through 15, p. 290.

10. Before the pulleys at *P2* and *A2* come together, the haul captain calls, *"Set."* The haul team immediately stops hauling and slowly eases back so the PCD catches. The PCD tender makes sure the rope grab sets.

11. The haul captain calls, *"Slack."* The haul team instantly reverses direction and moves back toward the load with the rope still in their hands. As they do this, the person attending the haul cam resets the system.

12. When the haul team reaches its original position, it is ready to begin another cycle.

General Considerations for Rescue Hauling Systems

As with all rope rescue techniques, hauling systems must be adapted to the rescue circumstances and environment. A thorough knowledge of equipment and techniques is good, but rescuers should not necessarily rig the most complex system they know. In fact, the simplest system workable under the circumstances often produces an efficient, successful rescue.

The following factors must be considered when a team is deciding on a hauling system:

- If speed is needed, a simple system often means that (1) the system can be set up quickly, and (2) the haul itself can be performed quickly.
- If few personnel are available for a haul team, a higher MA (and therefore a more complex system) may be required.
- If a large number of personnel are available for a haul team, a simpler system can be used. A higher MA system with a large haul team creates the potential for overloading and system failure.
- If only a small amount of gear is available for rigging, a simpler hauling system usually is used.
- If the hauling area is cluttered, the hauling system is more likely to become snagged; a simpler system may not be as easily jammed.
- If the haul team has limited room, a simpler system should be used if possible. Limited space means constant resetting of the system and delay in the rescue.
- If a load is heavy, a higher MA (i.e., a more complex system) may be required.
- If a load is light, a lower MA (i.e., a less complex system) may be sufficient.

Evaluation Exercises

Cognitive and Affective Exercises

1. List five situations in which rescue haul systems might be used.

2. What are the two basic reasons that rescuers use hauling systems?

3. Define mechanical advantage.

4. How does theoretical mechanical advantage differ from actual mechanical advantage?

5. Assuming a load of 400 pounds (1.8 kN), calculate the force that would be needed for a haul team to move the load with the following:

   A. 1:1 hauling system
   B. 2:1 hauling system
   C. 3:1 hauling system
   D. 4:1 hauling system

6. Which type of pulley—fixed pulley or traveling pulley—can be used to create additional mechanical advantage in some hauling systems?

7. In a basic rescue hauling system, if a 2:1 haul system is added to another 2:1 system, what likely is the resulting mechanical advantage? What is the TMA if a 2:1 haul system is added to a 3:1 system?

8. In hauling systems, personal ascenders should not be used for what purpose?

9. What should be the position of the progress capture device in relation to the other elements of the haul system?

10. What might be the possible consequences of rigging a progress capture device so far to the side of a main-line rope that it creates a significant bend in the rope?

11. What are two consequences of edge friction on a rope in hauling systems?

12. Describe two methods of reducing such edge friction.

13. What technique can a rescue team use to help control the movement of a litter that is being hauled and to help prevent it from becoming snagged?

14. List the minimum equipment requirements for rigging the following:

    A. 1:1 hauling system
    B. 2:1 hauling system
    C. 3:1 (Z-rig) hauling system
    D. 4:1 (piggyback) hauling system

15. What significant problem can arise with a 2:1 hauling system that uses a traveling pulley attached to the load?

Psychomotor Exercises

16. Draw a 2:1 hauling system using a traveling pulley on the load. Label the parts and the forces acting on the system.

17. Draw a 3:1 hauling system using a Z-rig. Label the parts and the forces acting on the system.

18. Draw a 4:1 hauling system using a piggyback rig. Label the parts and the forces acting on the system.

19

Tower Rescue

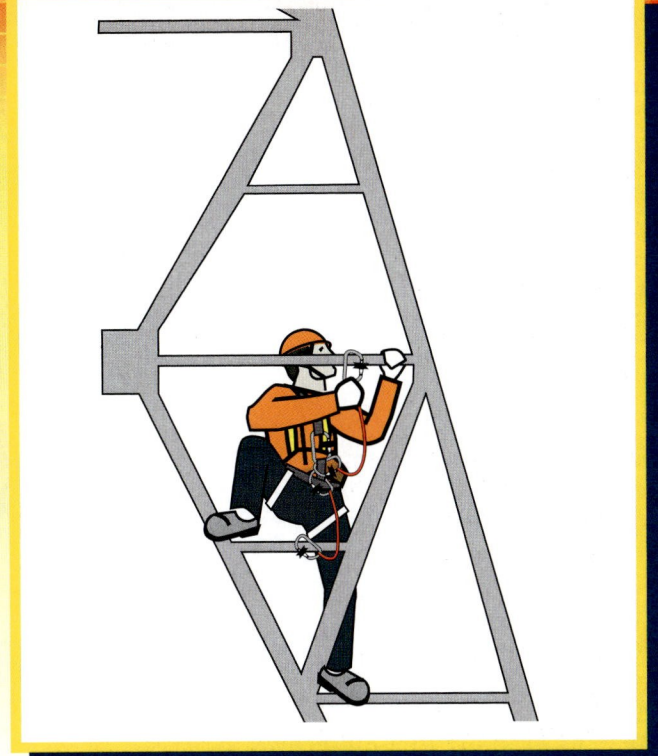

Prerequisites

Before climbing any tower for training or rescue, you should take a tower awareness class that includes information on electromagnetic energy (EME) (nonionizing radiation) and radio frequency (RF) radiation exposure.

Also, before attempting the activities described in this chapter, you must have demonstrated that you can properly:

1. Use and care for rope.
2. Use and care for other equipment needed in the high angle environment.
3. Tie correctly and without hesitation the knots necessary for safe, effective work in the vertical environment (see Chapter 6).
4. Apply the principles of anchoring and rig a safe and secure anchor.
5. Apply the principles of belaying and safely and confidently provide the appropriate belay.
6. Apply the principles of rappelling: rappel safely and under control, tie off the rappel device to operate hands free of the rappel device and rope, and then return to a safe and controlled rappel.
7. Apply the principles of ascending: tie a Prusik hitch correctly and without hesitation and know how to use it; comprehend the uses and limitations of mechanical ascenders; confidently and safely ascend a fixed rope using either friction hitches or mechanical ascenders; confidently and safely change over from rappelling to

ascending and ascending to rappelling; and extricate yourself from a jammed rappel device or similar problem.
8. Apply the principles of high angle lowering: correctly set the rigging in any of the elements of a high angle lower and safely assume the role of litter tender, brakeman, or belayer.
9. Correctly distinguish between one-person and rescue belays; correctly tie a load-releasing hitch and demonstrate how to release it under load; correctly rig a tandem Prusik belay system and operate it; correctly rig a Prusik minding pulley and operate it.

Objectives

On completion of this chapter, you should be able to:

1. Describe the two types of tower rescue.
2. Explain the difference between a lead climb and a lanyard climb.
3. Describe the proper use of a lanyard.
4. Explain the limitations of using lanyards for tower climbing.
5. Explain the limitations of lead climbing on a tower.
6. Describe the hazards associated with a tower rescue.
7. Explain the importance of preplanning in a tower rescue.
8. List the individual skills needed by a tower rescuer.

Key Terms

Drop Zone The area immediately under and around the tower where objects may fall. It could extend out 30 to 50 feet (10 to 16.5 m) or farther from the base of the tower if the object that is dropped bounces off the structure or is blown by the wind.

EME or **RF Exposure** *EME (electromagnetic energy) is* nonionizing radiation. *RF (radio frequency) radiation* is exposure to nonionizing electromagnetic energy at radio frequencies. The major concern with RF energy is tissue heating.

Freestanding Tower A self-supporting structure with three or four legs. It generally is wider at the base and narrower at the top.

Ground-Controlled Rescue A rescue in which the lowering and belay lines are controlled and operated from a ground position and not on the tower.

Guyed Tower A narrow column that sits on a base and is stabilized by a series of guy wires attached to the tower at pre-engineered positions.

Lanyard A piece of rope or webbing that connects a rescuer's harness to a lifeline or anchorage.

Lanyard Climbing The use of one or more lanyards to ascend a structure.

Lead Climbing A two-person climbing method involving protective anchors (protection) placed by the individuals as they climb (see Chapter 1, p. 2).

Monopole A cylindrical, self-supporting column that is larger at the base and narrower at the top. Monopoles usually are associated with PCS (personal communication systems [e.g., cell phones, pagers]) antennas.

Size Up Continuous evaluation of information, resulting in the development of a rescue plan.

Tall Tower As a rule of thumb, some instructors consider anything over 200 feet (66 m) to be a tall tower. This chapter does not address tall tower rescue.

Tower-Based Rescue A rescue in which the lowering and belay lines are controlled and operated from a position on the tower.

Tower Rescues: a Growing Need

Towers serve a number of purposes, including carrying electrical transmission lines and supporting communications networks. The number of towers erected is increasing by thousands each year, and soon these structures will be found in all but the most remote wilderness areas. No one seems to know for certain how many towers currently dot the landscape, but they number in the hundreds of thousands.

Electrical transmission line towers have been built since early in the twentieth century. The construction boom for communications towers began around 1995. On May 25, 1997, the Occupational Safety and Health Administration (OSHA) issued a memorandum stating that, "the industry anticipates that over 180,000 towers will be constructed in the United States in 1997 and another 250,000 in 1998."

Tower rescues can include workers involved with building or maintaining a tower or who have been injured or have suffered a sudden illness. However, other types of people also become rescue subjects. Many are individuals who climb a tower for the thrill of it. Others may be involved with alcohol or drug intoxication or may be having emotional problems.

On January 25, 2002, accounts of two tragedies involving towers appeared in the *Houston Chronicle*. In one case, a teenage girl was seriously burned climbing an electrical tower after an argument with her mother. In the other case, a young man decided to see how close he could get to the energized lines and was killed instantly. His reason for being on the tower was reported to be that he was upset about losing his hometown girlfriend after he'd gone away to college on a football scholarship.

Hazards in Tower Rescues

Tower rescues are dangerous in many ways. Besides the obvious danger of working at height, towers expose rescuers to hazards they may not normally encounter on the ground. The hazards on an electrical transmission line tower involve not just the transmission lines themselves, but also the minimum air distances around those lines. OSHA has published a chart that shows the minimum distance workers, tools, and equipment must be kept clear of for different-voltage lines (Table 19-1).

One of the hazards on an AM radio tower is that the entire tower is energized, and any contact to ground results in a completed circuit through the person's body. The hazards on any tower are the potential for **EME** or **RF exposure**.

This chapter follows the philosophy of this text and focuses on basic and team rope rescue. However, *before attempting any type of tower training or rescue, rescue students should seek competent instruction on the above-mentioned hazards.*

Personal Rescue Equipment

Each rescuer should have the following equipment:
- A rescue helmet with chin strap and three-point suspension (not a fire helmet or construction hard hat)
- A pair of rescue gloves (not fire gloves or cloth utility gloves)
- Sturdy footwear (not fire boots or sneakers)
- A quality harness, one that meets the rescue or fall protection standards of OSHA, the American National Standards Institute (ANSI), the National Fire Protection Association (NFPA), or the European Committee for Standardization

Table 19-1 | Energized Power Lines

The hoist system (gin pole and its base hoists) used to raise and lower employees on the hoist line, shall not be used unless the following clearance distances as recommended by ANSI are maintained at all times during the lift:

Power Line Voltage Phase to Phase (kV)	Minimum Safe Clearance (Feet)
50 or below	10
Above 50 to 200	15
Above 200 to 350	20
Above 350 to 500	25
Above 500 to 750	35
Above 750 to 1000	45

From OSHA CPL 2-1.36 - Interim Inspection Procedures During Communication Tower Construction Activities. http://www.ti0rc.org/biblioteca/se-008.pdf Accessed April 29, 2003.

(CE) (an example would be a full-body harness [for fall protection] with front connection points for the rescuer and side D rings for positioning)

- Appropriate clothing that takes into account both the current and the predicted weather
- Two ways to safety or tie off on the tower
- A descent device
- Self-rescue gear
- An appropriate number of locking carabiners
- A means of safely ascending and descending a tower

Other equipment also may be needed, depending on the time of day or the weather. This equipment may include a helmet light and a secondary source of light, sun glasses or goggles, extra gloves, fluids, high-energy snacks, heat packs, additional foul weather clothing, and possibly a waist pack for carrying the gear.

Rescue Gear

Tower rescue gear consists of the following equipment:

- A radio and radio harness for each rescuer
- Climbing equipment needed to ascend the tower
- Ropes of appropriate length (which depends on the rescue method chosen)
- Anchor material for the lowering and belay systems or for changes of direction if these tasks are to be performed from the ground
- If necessary, a means to secure the rescue subject; this involves a number of factors: the nature of the rescue; whether one or more subjects is involved; whether the subject (or subjects) has been injured and if so, the type of injuries; the current and predicted weather; the number of rescuers available; and whether the subject (or subjects) has a harness, its type and its condition

Tower Climbing

The four common ways to climb a tower in a rescue are free climbing, built-in fall protection, lead climbing, and lanyard systems.

Free Climbing

Free climbing is climbing without the use of any safeties or backup. It is unsafe and is forbidden by OSHA regulations. Free climbing should not be considered or allowed at a rescue.

Built-In Fall Protection

A tower can be safely ascended using the fall protection that is a permanent part of the tower (Figure 19-1). This feature usually is a ⅜-inch (9.5 mm) wire cable fastened to the tower at the top and bottom and at intermediate points in between. The climber must use a mechanical wire rope grab on this cable. Unfortunately, not all towers have built-in fall protection. On those that do, the fall protection cable must be inspected before rescuers trust their lives to it. If for any reason the integrity of the fall protection is questionable, rescuers should use another means of protection.

Lead Climbing

Lead climbing is described in Chapter 1.

Advantages

- The rescuer is securely attached to the rope at all times, and if the individual places his or her protection properly, it will prevent a fall to the ground.
- Once the lead climber has secured the rope at the top, other rescuers may safely climb to that position with the aid of a rope grab.

Disadvantages

- Lead climbing can be difficult and awkward, particularly for those inexperienced in recreational rock climbing.
- The lead climber is exposed while setting protection. He or she may be clinging to the tower with one hand while setting protection and attempting to clip in with the free hand.
- Lead climbing is equipment intensive; it requires slings and carabiners for setting protection, additional pieces of equipment (i.e., weight) that rescuers must transport up the tower.

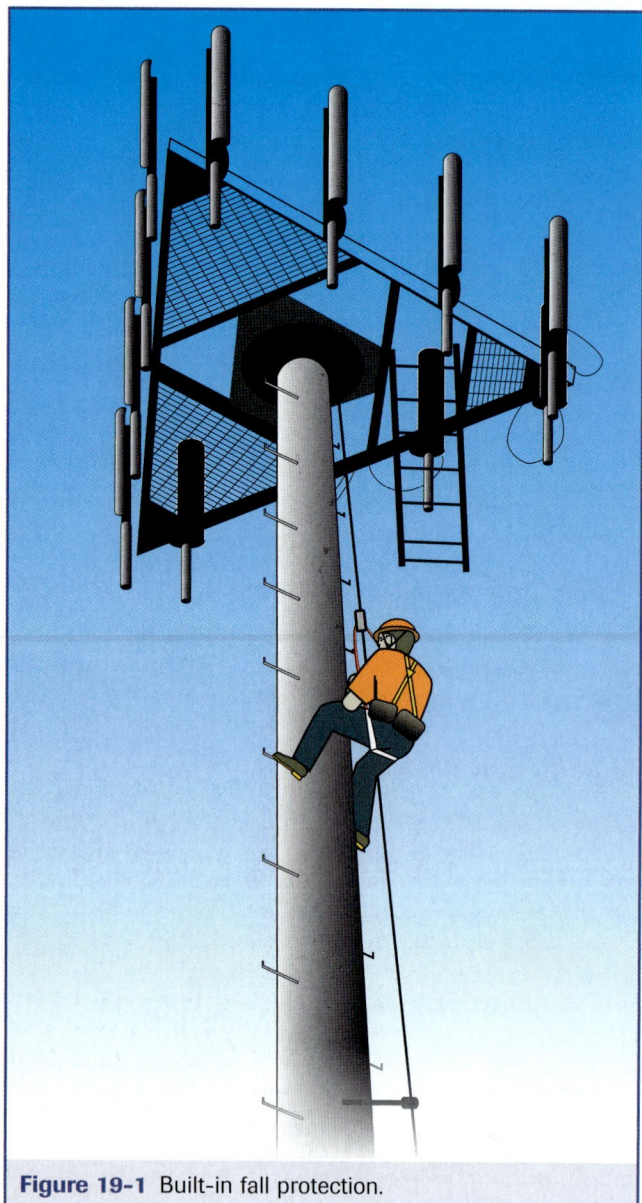

Figure 19-1 Built-in fall protection.

- It requires a team of two, one climber and one belayer, and the team can travel only as fast as the slower member.
- Lead climbing is only as safe as the lead climber and belay make it. The lead climber determines the degree of risk. The higher he or she climbs above the last piece of protection, the longer the fall that could be taken and the more likely he or she is to be injured, which would stop or slow the rescue.
- Lead climbing usually involves high-stretch rope. Many instructors who teach lead climbing on structures use high-stretch rope, the same type of rope used by recreational climbers. However, because of the elongation of high-stretch rope, a rescuer using this rope who falls has a longer fall, with the potential for hitting more objects on the way down.

Lanyard Systems

A *lanyard* system (Figure 19-2) also can be used to climb a tower. If the rescuer is climbing the leg of a tower, the lanyard can be wrapped around the tower leg and moved up as the rescuer climbs the tower. If the rescuer uses two lanyards and climbs a ladder on the tower, the rescuer can clip into the beams of the ladder or onto the rungs if they are suitable. On some towers, and with proper instruction, the lanyard can be used on tower step bolts.

Lanyards of different types and styles can be found in industrial and rescue catalogs. They can be purchased in different fixed lengths or in adjustable lengths. Lanyards can be designed for fall restraint, fall protection, or work positioning. Not all lanyards work in all situations on all towers.

Because of their design and the way they are used, lanyards limit the distance rescuers can fall, as well as their contact with

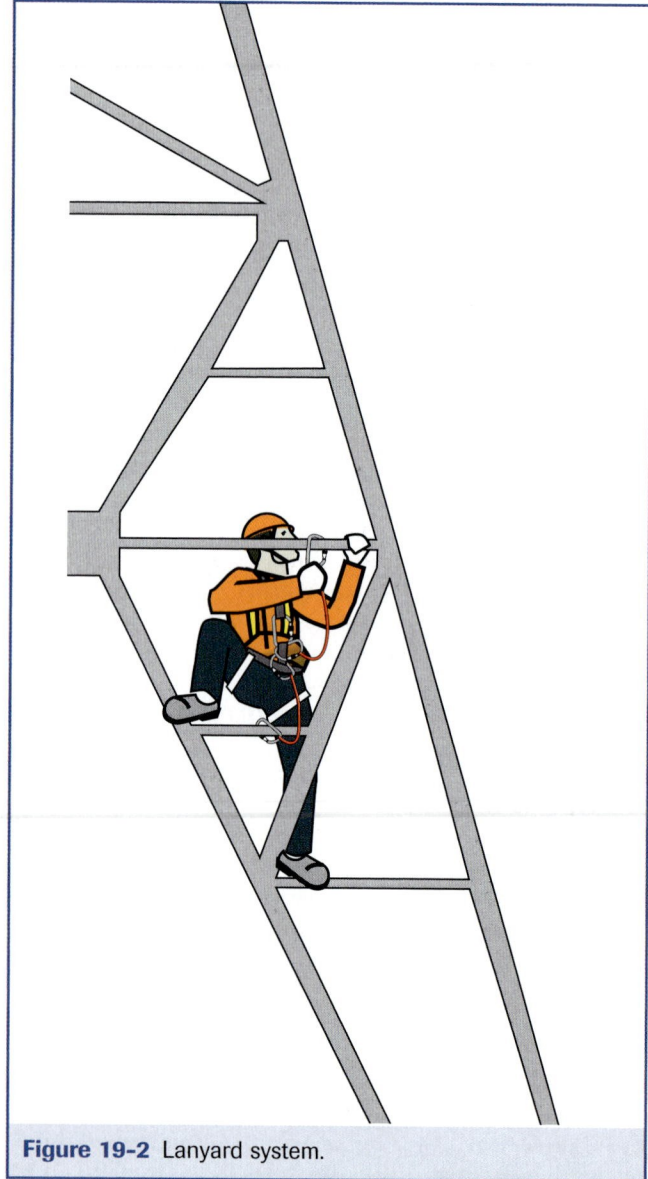

Figure 19-2 Lanyard system.

the structure during the fall. When using a lanyard as a safety for climbing a tower or structure, rescuers should never climb even with or above their connection point. Proper instruction in the use of a lanyard (and observance of those rules) can minimize the potential for injury should a fall occur on a lanyard system. It is important to remember that this book is designed as *a training manual to be used under the guidance of a qualified instructor*.

In a tower rescue, lanyard systems have some advantages over lead climbing:

- **Lanyard climbing** eliminates the need for a dynamic rope, an extra piece of equipment used in lead climbing. High-stretch ropes generally are not used in a rescue operation involving a lowering. High-stretch ropes usually have thinner sheaths, which make them more susceptible to abrasion on the unprotected steel of most towers.

- Use of lanyards eliminates the need for gear to place protection for lead climbing, thus reducing weight and bulk and most likely fatigue on the rescuer.

- Lanyards offer the rescuer more freedom of movement. The rescuer can maneuver within the structure of a guyed tower or traverse across a structural member of a free-standing tower without concern about rope entanglement.

- Lanyards also eliminate concern about rope entanglement caused by the wind, as well as the possibility of ropes contacting electrical equipment or wires.

- A rescuer using a lanyard is not dependent on a second rescuer to act as a belayer. The use of lanyards allows several rescuers to move up or down the tower at the same time, on the same leg or on separate legs of the tower. These rescuers can ascend or descend at their own speed and at a rate within their own comfort zone.

Basic skills for any rescuer working on a tower include the ability to ascend, descend, and traverse. Once rescuers reach their work stations, they must be able to safety themselves off. Lanyards can also be used for this purpose.

Lanyards also have some disadvantages:

- Depending on the design of the lanyard or the design of the tower, the lanyard may not reach around the tower leg (e.g., a **monopole** with a large base).

- A lanyard that is not adjustable could pose a greater fall hazard (the longer the lanyard, the more slack that can result, which could mean a longer fall with more potential objects to strike).

- When lanyards are used with step bolts, the potential for step bolt failure exists.

- Lanyards generally need anchor points above the rescuers' connections on their harnesses.

- Each rescuer needs an independent system, and each rescuer is responsible for his or her own actions (this could be an advantage or a disadvantage, depending on the knowledge and maturity of each rescuer).

Rescuer Safety

As in any rescue operation, the rescuers' safety is a primary concern. However, tower rescue presents some special safety concerns for rescuers.

Climber Exhaustion

Climber exhaustion can be caused by a number of factors, including the following:

- *The height of the climb:* The higher the tower, the longer the ropes needed for lowering and belaying. More rope means more weight. The higher the tower, the farther the increased rope weight and associated gear must be carried.

- *The type of tower construction:* On towers with step bolts, the distance between the bolts makes a difference to each rescuer. Rescuers with short legs must exert more energy when climbing, and the more gear a rescuer carries, the more weight the person must lift with each step.

Freestanding towers (Figure 19-3) are built in sections, which are connected at joints called *flanges*. Generally

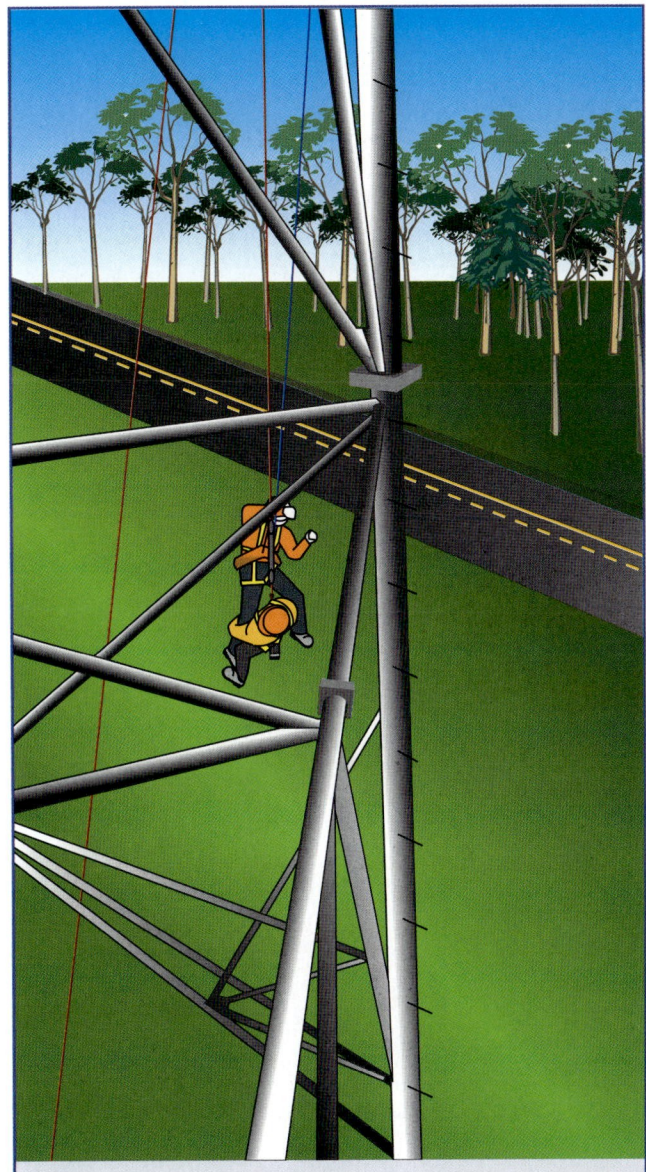

Figure 19-3 Freestanding towers.

speaking, the larger the sections, the larger the flanges. Occasionally the distance between step bolts at flanges varies. The bolts may be farther apart at these points, making it more difficult for shorter rescuers or rescuers with shorter arms or legs to negotiate these flanges.

Guyed towers (Figure 19-4) are stabilized with guy wires, which are connected to the tower at pre-engineered positions. On towers with a narrow face, the rescuer must negotiate around and through these wires and maintain his or her balance while transporting the ropes and rescue gear up the tower.

■ *The physical condition of the rescuer:* Tower climbing is hard work. Climbing with rescue gear is even harder. Cardiovascular conditioning is just as important as upper body and leg strength for tower rescuers. This is particularly true on tall towers.

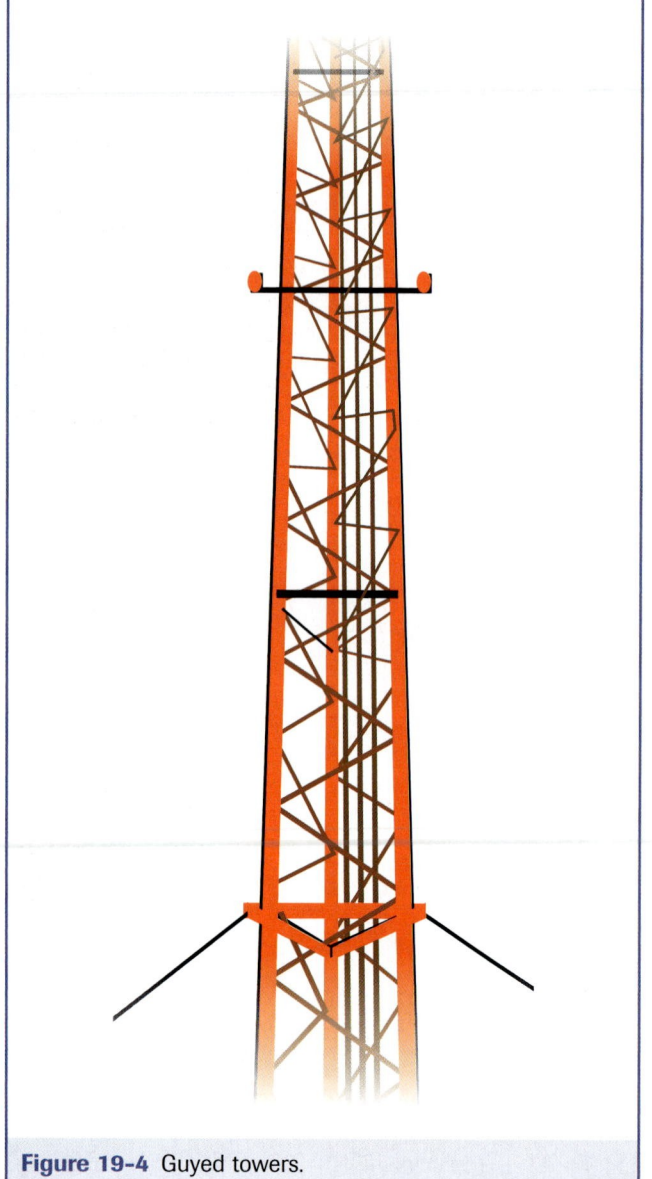

Figure 19-4 Guyed towers.

Other Factors

Other factors that can affect rescuer safety include the weather and the presence of birds, bees, or wasps.

A high air temperature or high humidity (or both) affects all rescuers, and adequate hydration is important. Rescuers should consider carrying fluids for long or difficult climbs, for rescues that may be long and involved, or when weather considerations dictate. Rain, sleet, snow, or ice makes climbing dangerous. Steel is slippery when wet. Low temperatures, a brisk wind, and the cold steel of the tower can numb hands and fingers and make gripping the tower difficult. Ice buildup on towers is especially dangerous. Falling chunks of ice are a danger to all rescuers and equipment. Many if not most tower workers will not climb during periods of high winds, lightning, or heavy ice buildup.

Bee and wasp nests are often found on towers and present a danger to rescuers. Birds have been known to dive bomb workers on towers in the area of the birds' nests.

Caution

Galvanized drippings on towers can cut rescuers or equipment.

Caution

Water from rain or snow makes steel slippery.

Caution

Secure all gear when working on towers (e.g., pagers, knives, cell phones, keys, sunglasses).

Warning

Wear a helmet when working on towers or in the **drop zone** around the tower.

Warning

Never free climb on a tower.

Tower Rescue Size Up

The following steps can help rescuers *size up* a tower rescue situation and respond accordingly.

1. Determine the safety of the tower.

If the structure is a guyed tower, look for loose, damaged, or missing guy wires. Check the tower for any other damage. If a winch or other form of lifting device is on site, gain control of that equipment or perform a lockout/tagout on it.

2. Determine number of rescue subjects.

Allocation of resources depends on the number of rescue subjects.

3. Determine the location of the rescue subject.

The location of the subject on the tower may help in determining the number of rescuers needed on the tower. On a monopole, only a limited number of rescuers will have access to the subject. A small face on a guyed tower doesn't afford the same working room as a freestanding tower might.

4. Determine the medical considerations for the subject.

Is the person breathing? Is he or she conscious or unconscious? Is the individual uninjured, slightly injured but able to help, or injured and unable to help? This information helps determine the number of rescuers needed on the tower.

5. Determine the type of rescue needed.

Is the operation a rescue or a recovery? Does the subject need an attendant? Is this to be a tower-based or ground-based rescue?

6. Determine the number of rescuers needed or available.

How many rescuers can get into position on the tower safely? Are enough trained rescuers available to perform the rescue from the tower?

7. Develop a rescue plan.

Is the operation to be a *ground-controlled rescue* or a *tower-based rescue*? The rescue plan is guided by the previously gathered information. If the rescue is to be tower based, will the lowering be controlled from the tower or by the attendant? If it is to be ground based, are there antennas or dishes around which the rescuers must negotiate? If so, how will that be accomplished?

8. Select the rescuers.

The rescuers must understand and agree to the proposed rescue plan, and they must be able to perform their assigned tasks. They should have previous tower training experience and must be comfortable at the height at which they will be working.

9. Determine the climbing system.

Will the existing fall protection on the tower be used? Will a lead climb or a lanyard climb be done? What are the advantages and disadvantages of the system chosen, and do the rescuers understand them?

10. Consider the current weather and the predicted weather.

As the weather changes so do safety considerations. High winds may necessitate an attendant even if the original plan did not call for one.

11. Consider the time of day.

If the rescue extends into the night, are the rescuers prepared for cooler or colder weather? Do they have two sources of hands-free lighting available to them? Does the rescue plan take into consideration that the rescue may take longer because of darkness? Is an attendant now needed?

12. Develop a backup plan.

Have some alternatives been considered in case the original plan won't work? What is the backup plan if only a limited number of qualified tower rescuers is available and one of them should require help?

Completing the Rescue

After the rescuers have climbed the tower, reached the subject, and secured themselves, they are in a position to complete the rescue. The rescue can be handled in one of two ways: (1) rig lowering and belay systems and perform these operations from the tower, or (2) rig the lowering line and the belay line through anchored changes of direction above the subject and control the lowering and belaying from the ground.

The procedures for lowering and belaying are the same as those outlined in Chapters 8, 13, and 16. The major difference between a tower rescue and other rescues is the environment in which the rescue takes place; the techniques of anchoring, lowering, and belaying remain the same. The only additional skill required of a tower rescuer is the ability to ascend, descend, and traverse the structure safely to reach the subject.

A tower rescue is not a sport or a recreational activity, and the belay technique, the equipment, and the safety factors should take this into account. For a tower rescue, $7/16$-inch (11 mm) or $1/2$-inch (12.5 mm) ropes are used. OSHA considers 310 pounds (140 kg) to be the maximum weight for one worker with equipment. NFPA standards consider 300 pounds (135 kg) to be the maximum weight for one person. This information should be considered when rescuers practice belays, because a tower rescue could involve lowering a subject or a subject plus an attendant. Belaying should be practiced with the same equipment and techniques that will be used at a tower rescue.

Preplanning

Preplanning for tower rescue sites can save valuable time. This is particularly important because climbing the tower to the rescue subject can be very time-consuming.

Contacts and Resources

Obtain the emergency phone number for the site manager or managers. Towers often have more than one *carrier* (i.e., the owner of the equipment on the tower) and therefore more than one site manager. Talk to each carrier and determine the hazards posed by that company's equipment. Determine in advance the quickest way to de-energize and lock out equipment that would be a danger to rescuers and the rescue subject.

Remember, there are no guarantees in preplanning for tower rescue sites. New carriers are added to towers as service increases; up-grades on equipment are performed routinely; and company buyouts and mergers create new companies with new site managers. Site managers should be contacted on a regular basis so that preplans can be updated as much as possible.

Equipment and Personnel

1. Preplan the climbing system.
   - Does the tower have built-in fall protection?
   - Will it be used? (If so, obtain the appropriate rope grabs.)
2. Preplan the rescue operation.
   If it is to be tower based:
   - What lengths of rope will be needed?
   - What size slings will be needed to anchor around structural members?
   - How many rescuers will be needed on the tower?
   If it is to be ground controlled:
   - How long do the ropes need to be?
   - Are anchors available and accessible or must they be improvised?
3. Preplan resources.
   - Is this a rescue the team or department is trained and equipped to handle, or is preplanning required for additional resources?

Training

Tower training must begin with the appropriate hazard awareness training. Whether it is awareness training on the hazards of EME/RF or on the hazards associated with electrical transmission lines, no rescuers or trainees should be permitted on an active tower until they have had this training.

The initial hands-on training should be conducted under the guidance of qualified instructors and should include a top belay for each student until he or she has mastered the different techniques.

Evaluation Exercises

1. List the hazards associated with a tower rescue.

2. List two advantages and two disadvantages of using a lead climb on a tower.

3. List two advantages and two disadvantages of using a lanyard climb on a tower.

4. Describe the basic skills a rescuer should have for working on a tower.

5. Name the three types of towers.

6. When a rescue plan is being developed, what are the two basic forms it can take?

7. Which climbing system recommends that rescuers "never climb even with or above their connection point"?

20
Highlines

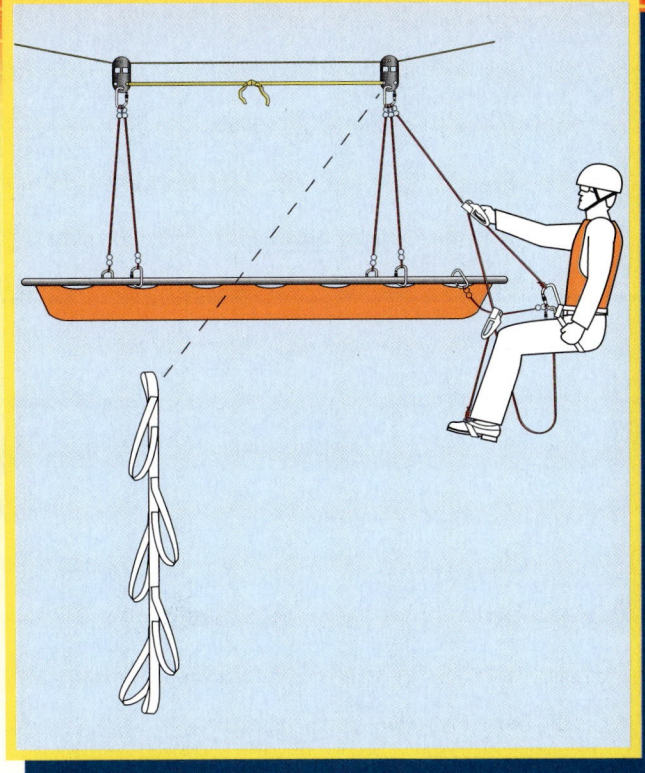

Prerequisites

Before attempting the activities described in this chapter, you must have demonstrated that you can properly:

1. Use and care for rope.
2. Use and care for other equipment needed in the high angle environment.
3. Tie correctly and without hesitation the knots necessary for safe, effective work in the vertical environment (see Chapter 6).
4. Apply the principles of anchoring and rig a safe and secure anchor.
5. Apply the principles of belaying and safely and confidently belay another person using either a Münter hitch or a personal belay device.
6. Correctly distinguish between one-person and rescue belays; correctly tie a load-releasing hitch and demonstrate how to release it under load; correctly rig a tandem Prusik belay system and operate it; and correctly rig a Prusik minding pulley and operate it.
7. Apply the principles of high angle lowering systems: correctly rig any of the elements of a high angle lowering system and safely assume the role of litter tender, brakeman, belayer, rope handler, or edge attendant.
8. Apply the principles of hauling systems: determine the mechanical advantage (MA) required for a hauling system; correctly rig any of the elements of a hauling system; rig for a 1:1 MA hauling system, a 2:1 MA hauling system, a 3:1 MA hauling system (Z-rig), a 4:1

MA hauling system (piggyback rig), and compound versions of MA systems; and safely and confidently assume the role of cam tender, haul captain, haul team member, and belayer.

Objectives

On completion of this chapter, you should be able to:

1. Explain the ways highlines can be used in a rescue operation and give some typical examples of where they might be used.
2. List the basic elements of a rescue highline system.
3. List the major considerations in determining whether a highline is a feasible rescue technique for a specific situation.
4. Explain the possible consequences of overtensioning a highline.
5. Discuss the role of rope sag in highlines and apply the 10% rule to a variety of highline spans and load weights.
6. Explain the functions of the following: main-line rope, load, pulleys, lowering/belay line, and tag line.
7. Select equipment to be used in highline systems.
8. Rig a highline system using a single main line, a lowering/belay line, and a tag line.
9. Describe the circumstances in which a highline constructed of parallel main lines would be preferable to a highline constructed of a single main line.
10. Rig a litter and litter tender attachments for a highline.

The material in this chapter conforms to guidelines published by the National Fire Protection Association (NFPA), specifically standard 1006, *Professional Qualifications for Rescue Technicians* (2002), standard 1670, *Operations and Training for Technical Rescue Incidents* (2004), and standard 1983-01, *Standard for Life Safety Rope and System Components*. NFPA standards are revised regularly, and readers are advised to review the latest version of this standard.

Key Terms

Belay Line A type of tag line set up to prevent an uncontrolled lowering of a load.

English Reeve System One of several rigging systems that can be added to a highline to control the load from either side. Controlling the system's lines from either side, rescuers can raise or lower a load from the carrier at any position along the highline.

Haul Line A type of tag line that the haul team uses for pulling on a load; with highlines, it is used to transport the load across the highline.

Highline (also **Tyrolean** or **Telpher**) A system of using a rope suspended between two points to move people or equipment over an area that is a barrier to a rescue operation. Also known as a *Telpher* or *Tyrolean*.

Horizontal Highline A highline in which the two suspension points are nearly on the same level.

Kootenay Carriage A modified knot-passing pulley that is used on highlines as the main-line pulley for single and double main-line systems or as a high strength tie off.

Lowering/Belay Line The line attached to a load on a highline that is used to control the load from the near-side point.

Main Line The line (or lines) that provide the support of the load.

Steep Angle Highline A highline in which one of the suspension points is considerably higher than the other.

Tag Line A line attached to the load on a highline that is used to maintain contact or control of the load from either side.

Tandem Pulleys Two in-line pulleys on the same rope. Tandem pulleys are used in highlines to stabilize a load and to distribute its weight along the rope.

Highlines in Rescue

A *highline*, also sometimes referred to as a *tyrolean* or a *telpher*, is a rope line suspended between two points on which people, equipment, or other loads can be moved. Highlines can be simple or very complex to rig. Many technical rescue teams regularly practice setting up highlines, not because this rope rescue system is needed so often in real rescue operations, but because rigging a complex highline is a good test of many different rope rescue skills.

A *horizontal highline* is suspended between two points that are nearly on the same level (Figure 20-1, *A*). In a *steep angle highline*, one of the two points is much higher than the other (Figure 20-1, *B*). Highlines also may be suspended from points that produce angles anywhere between a steep one and a horizontal one. Special rigging, such as an English reeve system (discussed later in the chapter), can be added to a basic highline to allow loads to be raised or lowered from the span.

Use of Highlines

Highlines are used to transport rescuers, rescue subjects, and equipment across an area that presents a barrier to customary rescue operations. Some typical uses of highlines include the following:

- To bypass an obstacle (highlines may be used to cross a deep canyon or gorge)
- To avoid hazardous terrain (a highline may be used to bridge a swiftly flowing river; by adding an English reeve system, a rescue subject can be plucked from midstream without any rescuers being placed in the water)
- To avoid difficult terrain (a highline might be suspended over an area clogged with large boulders or thick debris, through which it would be very difficult and time-consuming to move a litter with a rescue subject)
- For emergency evacuation (highlines might be used to evacuate people from a hazard posing the threat of injury or

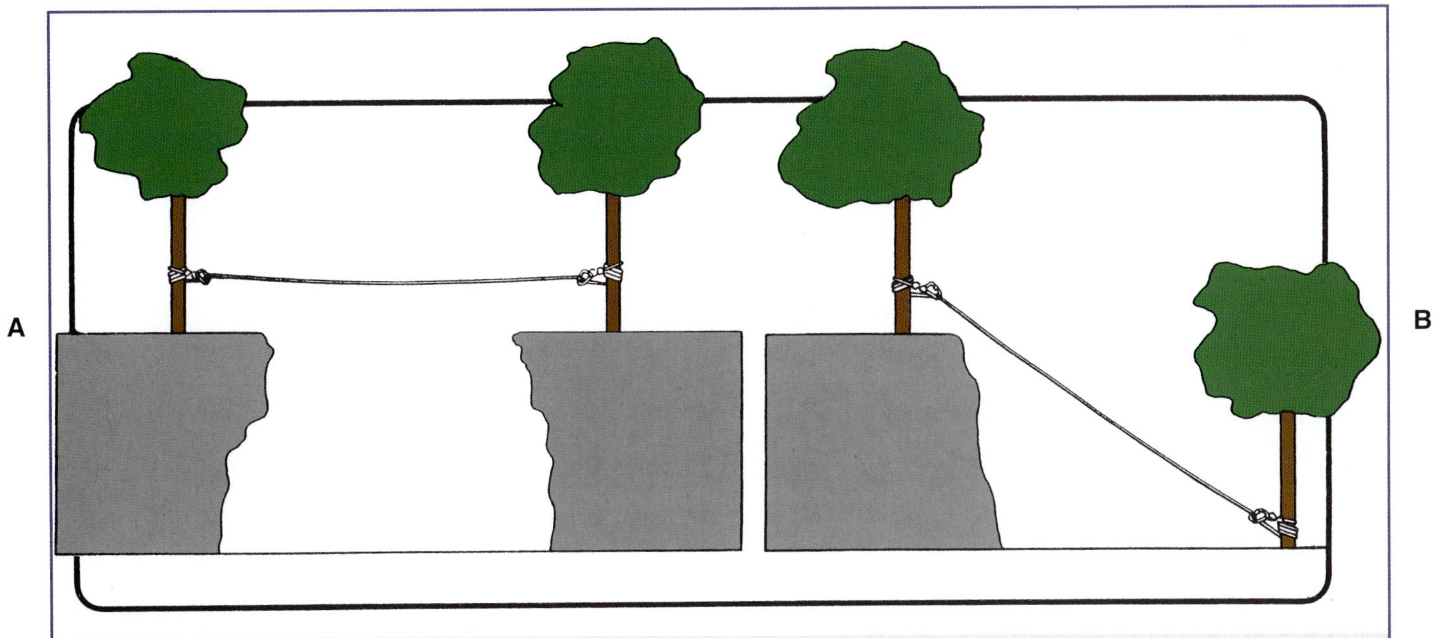

Figure 20-1 **A,** Horizontal highline. **B,** Steep angle highline.

death when no other practical or expeditious means of evacuation is available, such as with a fire in a building)

- In tactical situations (highlines might be used to evacuate civilians and/or bring in tactical personnel in a barricade or hostage situation)

Problems with Highlines

Highlines have several drawbacks:

- *Potential stress on and failure of equipment:* Perhaps more than any other rope rescue system, highlines have the potential to overstress rope, equipment and anchors, resulting in failure of the system. The rigging and use of highlines require a thorough knowledge of the potential forces involved.
- *Lengthy setup:* Highlines require a great deal of teamwork and communications to set up. When they first attempt the task, teams sometimes find rigging a highline to be very time-consuming. When time is crucial, even rescue teams experienced with highlines often find other techniques preferable.
- *Difficulty getting initial personnel and rope across:* One of the most difficult parts of rigging a horizontal highline is getting the initial personnel to the far-side anchorage and getting the rope and equipment across to them.

Elements of a Highline

Figure 20-2 shows the basic elements of a highline system that might be used in a rescue. In this operation, a rescue team is moving a litter with a rescue subject from left to right in a horizontal highline. In many cases it would be desirable to include a litter tender. However, for simplicity, this is not shown in this illustration. (Litter tenders for highlines are discussed later in the chapter.)

Main Line

The ***main line*** is the line that supports the major portion of the weight of the load in the highline. In many cases the main line can be a single line. However, under circumstances of high loading, a double line may be preferable. The rope should be a low-stretch design (e.g., a static kernmantle rope). Otherwise, a great deal of uncontrollable stretch could develop in the system. An appropriate amount of sag must be present in the main-line rope to prevent overstressing of the rope, other equipment, and anchors.

Near-Side Anchor

The *near-side anchor* is the anchor to which the main-line rope initially is attached. It ordinarily is the point from which operation of the highline is initiated and controlled. It also usually is the anchor nearest the arriving rescue personnel. Because of the stresses generated in highlines, the main-line anchors must be extremely reliable. In a horizontal highline, the two main-line anchors are subjected to similar stresses. In a steep angle highline, the upper anchor is subjected to the most stress, much as an upper anchor would be in a lowering system.

Far-Side Anchor

The *far-side anchor* is the anchor to which the main-line rope is attached at the far-side point. This anchor must be at least as strong as the near-side anchor. In a steep angle highline, the far-

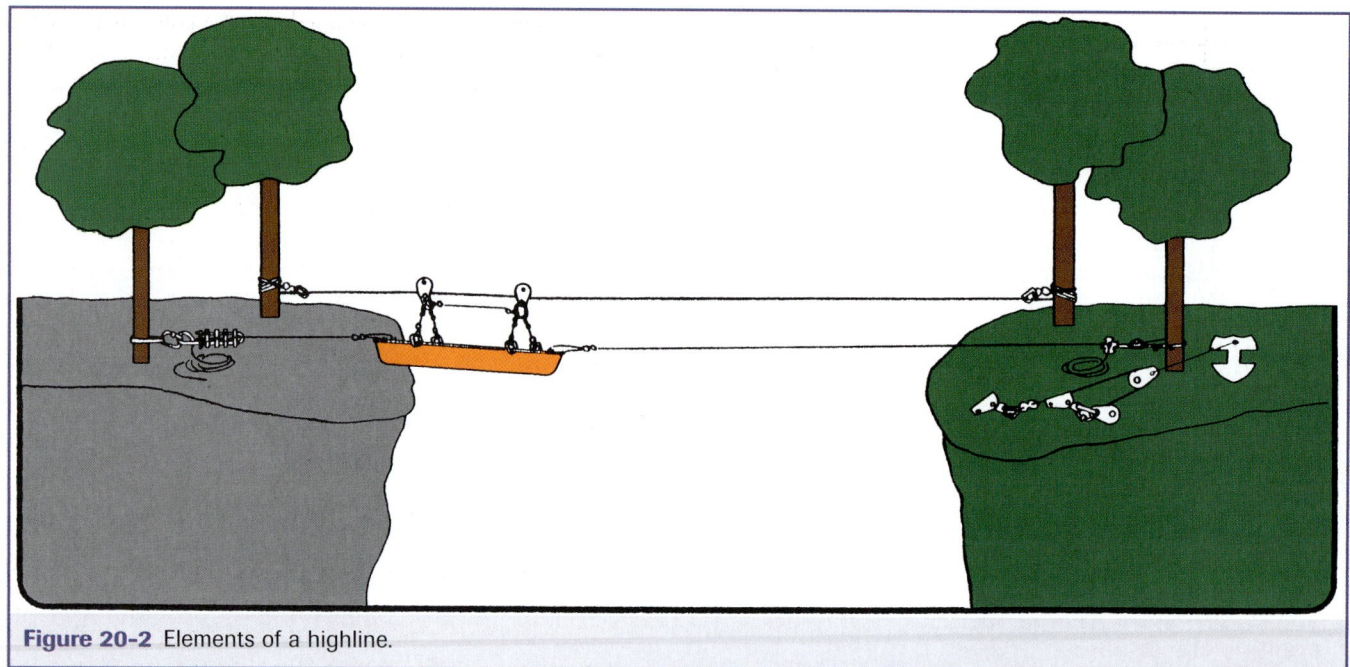

Figure 20-2 Elements of a highline.

side anchor receives less stress while the load remains near the top (Figure 20-3, *A-C*). However, as the load approaches the bottom, the far-side anchor is subjected to greater stress.

Load

The *load* is the mass, including personnel and equipment, that will be riding on the highline at any given time. For example, this may be a litter with the rescue subject and possibly a litter tender. In other cases, the load may be one person, a rescue subject attached to a rescuer, or equipment.

Pulleys

Pulleys are used in various places in a highline. They often are used to create a tensioning system for the highline, and a traveling pulley often is used to attach the load to the main-line rope. A *traveling pulley* allows the load to travel along the rope with minimal friction.

With higher loads, ***tandem pulleys*** are preferable to single pulleys because tandem pulleys create less of a bend in the rope, and they spread the load along the rope. It is important that pulleys be set so that they travel in a straight line along the rope. Otherwise, they may torque and create drag. If a pulley is not available, a large locking carabiner might be used in its place. However, this would mean greater friction and the potential for wear on and damage to the carabiner.

A special large pulley, sometimes called a ***Kootenay carriage***, can be used for the traveling pulley. This pulley can accept double ropes in the same sheave and has additional attachment points for the tag and lower/belay lines.

Tag Line

A ***tag line*** is a non-load-bearing line that connects the load with either side of the highline. A tag line may be used simply for the purpose of maintaining contact with the load, or it may double as a ***belay line*** or haul line.

Haul Line

The ***haul line*** is a tag line that is also used to haul the load. Beyond the center point of a horizontal highline, the load must be pulled upward to overcome the sag in the system. Depending on the situation, this can be quite strenuous and may require the use of a mechanical advantage system. In a steep angle highline, a haul line is needed to bring the load from the low anchor side to the high anchor side.

Lowering/Belay Line

The ***lowering/belay line*** runs from the higher of the two end anchor points and is connected to the load. It is used primarily to control the speed of the load; this is achieved by running the lowering/belay line through a lowering device, such as a large figure 8 descender or a brake bar rack (Figure 20-4, *A*). In a horizontal highline, this lowering effect usually is necessary only until the load reaches the center of the main line (Figure 20-4, *B*). At that point, because of sag and stretch in the rope, the load starts "uphill" toward the far side (Figure 20-4, *C*). After this point, the lowering/belay line performs more in its function of a belay. In a steep angle highline, if the load is traveling from the upper point to the lower one, the lowering/belay line acts primarily as a lowering line until the load nears the bottom. In a steep angle situation, the lowering/belay line requires a lowering device with a great deal of friction and control.

Highline Loads
One-Person Loads

Figure 20-5 shows a highline load consisting of only one person. The essential elements of this load are:

- A support sling that runs up to the rigging plate under the pulley. A large carabiner clips it into the seat harness front tie-in point. At the top end it is clipped into a large locking carabiner.

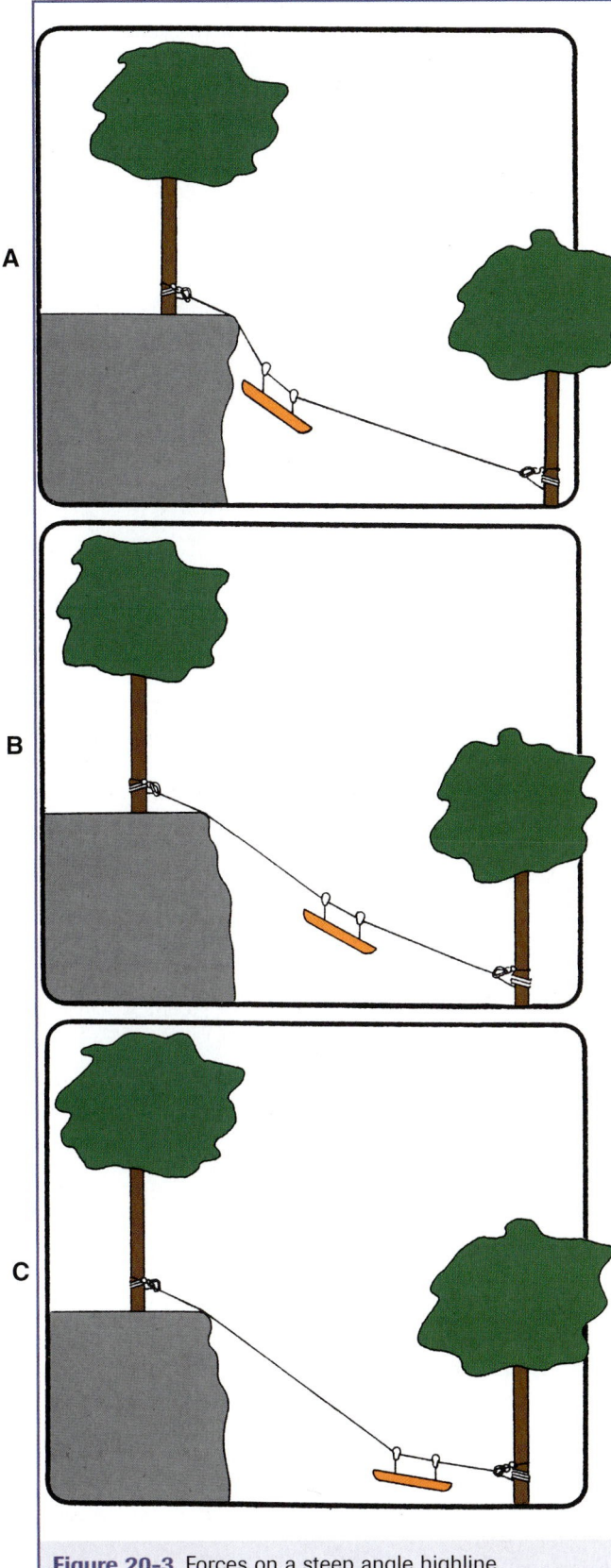

Figure 20-3 Forces on a steep angle highline.

■ A rigging plate that is clipped into the pulley with a large locking carabiner. The rigging plate provides a central tie-in point that can effectively be pulled from either direction without twisting the system. Also clipped into the rigging plate are (1) a lowering/belay line (with a carabiner) and (2) a tag line (with a carabiner).

Note also that the person riding the highline is wearing gloves. This is to prevent rope burns should he need to grab a rope while he is moving, to enable him to grasp the rope and pull hand over hand if necessary, and to prevent injuries to his fingers in the moving pulley. If the person transported on the highline is a rescue subject, it may be wise to make the support sling long enough so that the subject cannot reach the highline and injure his or her hands.

Two-Person Loads

If the person on the highline is rescuing another individual, the rescue subject may be clipped in a variety of ways:

■ The rescue subject may be connected to the rigging plate with his or her own support sling. In this case, an additional short sling should be attached between the rescuer's seat harness and the subject's seat harness. This gives the rescuer some control over the position of the subject.

■ A large rigging plate suspended below two separate pulleys on the main line can be used to connect the rescuer and subject to the main line. The rescuer and the subject are connected with their own support slings clipped into separate places on the bottom of the rigging plate. With this method, also, a sling should connect the seat harnesses of the rescuer and subject. The rigging plate acts as a spreader to keep the pulleys in position with each other. This ensures that the two pulleys have a smoother ride down the rope.

Litter Loads

Figure 20-6 shows the rigging for a litter attached to a highline. Litter rigging has a number of elements.

Spiders

The litter system for a highline uses two spiders, each with at least two legs. One set is clipped into the litter rail at the head end, and the other is clipped in at the foot end. Each set of spider legs comes up to a large locking carabiner, which is clipped into a small rigging plate attached to a pulley on the highline. Litter spiders can be tied from rope or made from webbing. Several commercially made, prerigged spiders are available that can easily be adjusted for various litter designs and terrain requirements.

Litter Tender Attachment

Figure 20-7 shows an attachment system for a litter tender on a highline. It, too, has a number of components.

Pig Tail

The main attachment to the litter system is a *pig tail,* which is made from approximately 12 feet (4 m) of rope. The top end of the pigtail is attached with a figure 8 overhand knot to the pulley carabiner over the head end of the litter. To prevent the tender's ascender attachments from accidentally slipping off the end of

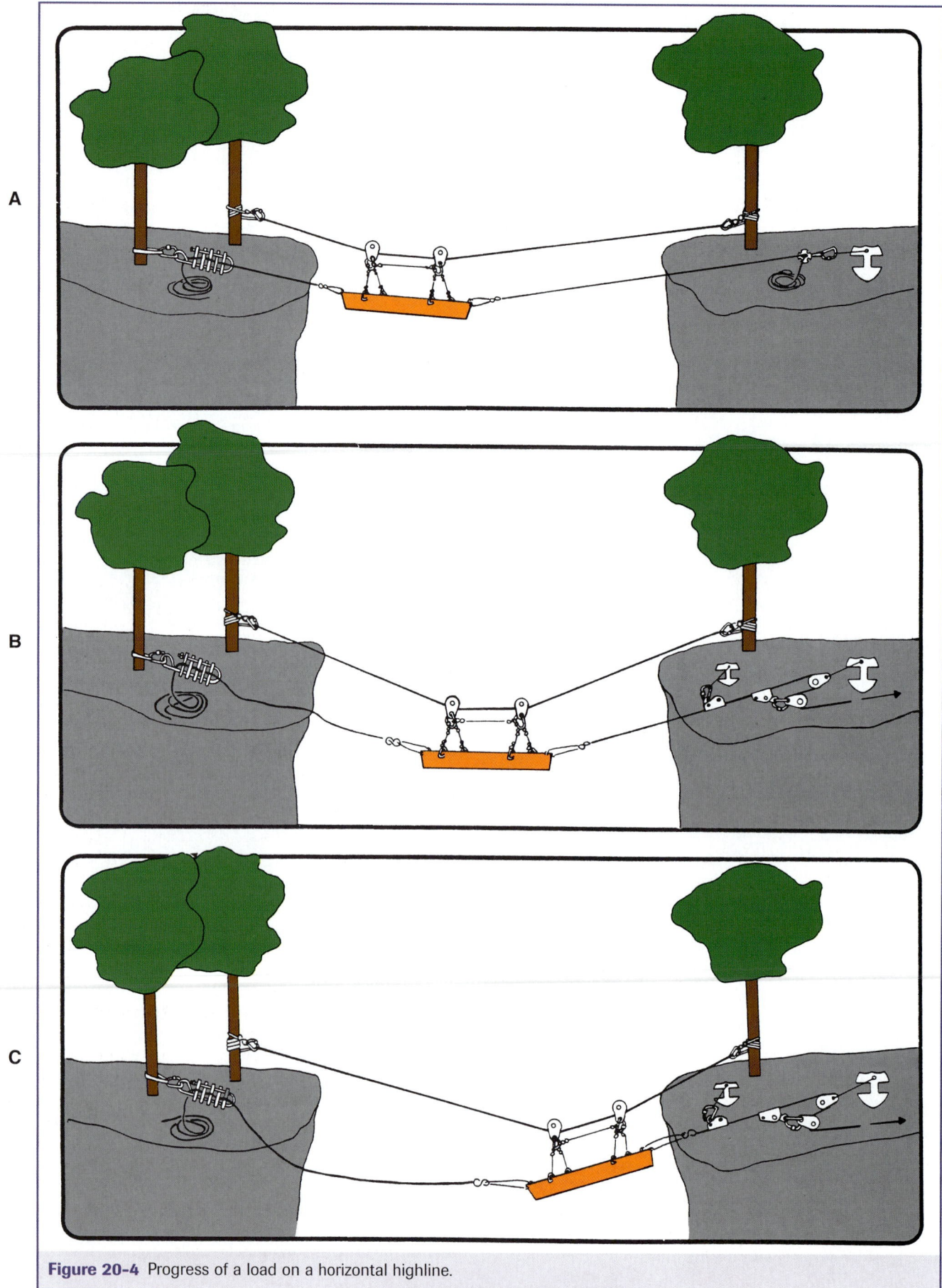

Figure 20-4 Progress of a load on a horizontal highline.

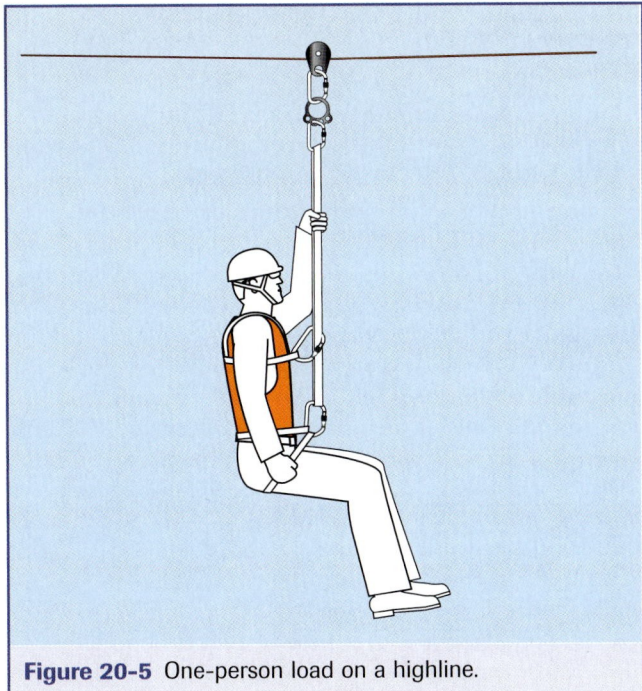

Figure 20-5 One-person load on a highline.

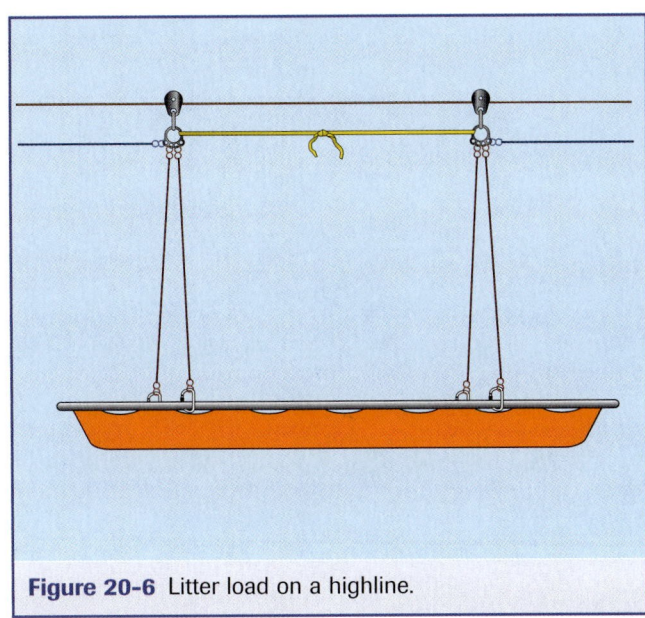

Figure 20-6 Litter load on a highline.

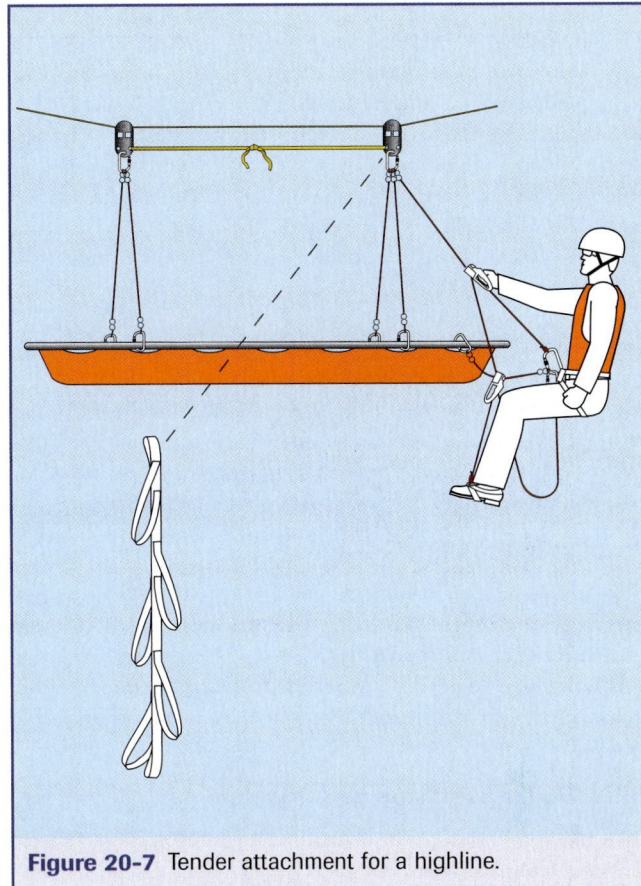

Figure 20-7 Tender attachment for a highline.

the pig tail, the lower end of the pig tail is clipped into the tender's harness carabiner with a figure 8 overhand knot, which also serves as a backup for the ascenders.

Ascender Attachments

The litter tender uses two spring-loaded ascenders that clip into the pigtail to adjust his or her height in relation to the litter. One of the ascenders is attached with a sling to the litter tender's seat harness, the other is attached with a sling to the tender's foot.

Alternative Approach

An alternative litter tender attachment can be created using two Prusik loops, one long and one short. The cord for the longer Prusik loop should be at least 5/16 inch (8 mm) in diameter and at least 3 feet (1 m) long (some trial and error may be required to adapt this loop to individual preferences). This Prusik is attached by a carabiner to the rigging plate and to the harness of the litter tender. The cord for the shorter Prusik should be 7 mm in diameter and 1 foot (0.3 m) long. It is tied around both strands of the longer Prusik loop using three wraps. A second carabiner is used to clip the shorter Prusik into the litter tender's harness. The longer Prusik serves as the tender's primary attachment to the system, and the shorter Prusik allows adjustment in the system.

Some people use a daisy chain as a tender attachment, clipping the end of the daisy chain into the carabiner at the top of the spider and the litter tender into the appropriate pocket on the daisy chain to get the proper position on the litter. This method is not generally recommended, primarily because many daisy chains are not intended to be used as primary life support attachments. Also, use of a daisy chain creates the following drawbacks:

- Once the litter tender is hanging on the daisy chain and the litter is over the side, the tender cannot easily and safely change position on the daisy chain.
- The litter tender lacks the mobility to move below the litter to clear obstructions or perform other tasks.

Etrier (Optional)

The litter tender can also use an etrier as an aid to moving up and down in relation to the litter. An *etrier* is a short ladder made of webbing that may be attached to the rigging plate. It works best in this position if it is extra long. Shorter etriers may be clipped to the outside rail of the litter to facilitate climbing around or onto the litter. In this configuration it can also be used to tip the litter toward the bearer or bearers, for example, to clear a subject's airway or to put the litter bottom against obstacles in order to negotiate edges.

Safety Tie-In (Optional)

A safety sling may be attached to the litter tender's seat harness and clipped into the rail of the litter near the head end. Some organizations do not use this tie-in, because they consider it to add little or no advantage, especially in light of the disadvantages introduced (e.g., reduced mobility, opportunity for tangling).

Position of the Litter Tender

The litter tender's position is similar to that used in a litter lowering (see Chapter 17): sitting comfortably in the seat harness with the litter slightly above his or her lap. The tender may keep both hands on the nearest litter rail to help stabilize the litter or, alternatively, may grasp the litter on the far side underneath skid rail.

Litter/Subject Position on a Highline

When a litter is rigged onto a horizontal highline, it should be set so as to minimize head-down positioning for the rescue subject. Depending on the length of the highline and the intended application, this often means the head should go first. In a steep angle highline, the litter stays at essentially the same angle until it nears the end of its travel at the bottom. In a steep angle highline, therefore, the litter should be rigged with the head up; this can be done by sending the feet first and/or by adjusting the length of the litter spider's legs.

Spreader

A *spreader* may be used to keep the two pulleys on the main line from spreading too far apart and becoming unwieldy during operations. It also may serve as a stabilizer should one of the pulleys fail. The spreader is created from webbing or a short piece of rope. It runs between the two rigging plates under the pulleys.

Attachments for the Lowering/Belay and Tag Lines

A tag line used for lowering or hauling can function most efficiently if it is attached to the rigging plate above the litter. However, it can also be useful to have the line in contact with the litter rail when negotiating edges. A variable system can be created by attaching the tag lines to the rigging plate using a midline knot but leaving enough slack to run down to the head and foot ends of the litter rail.

Determining the Amount of Sag in the Highline

A critical factor in the rigging of a rope for a highline is determining the proper amount of sag in the main-line rope.

⚠ Warning

A highline system must never be stretched very tight and then loaded. This could result in overstressing and failure of the rope, other equipment, or anchors.

Figure 20-8, *A*, shows the forces present in a highline system when a rope has been stretched tight horizontally with no visible sag. This is an unsafe condition.

Figure 20-8, *B*, shows a load of 200 pounds (90 kg) that has been placed in the middle of a 100-foot (33 m) rope stretched taut. Note that although there is a force of 200 pounds (90 kg) in a downward direction on the rope, the resulting forces off to the side at a right angle are multiplied tremendously. This creates enormous stress on the rope, anchors, and hardware and easily could result in complete failure of the system.

Figure 20-8, *C*, shows what happens with the same 200-pound (90 kg) load on the same 100-foot (33 m) rope, which now has been slacked so that a sag of 10 feet (3 m) has been created in the center of the rope. The forces at a right angle have been reduced to tolerable levels. This basic principle of physics must be kept in mind whenever a highline is rigged. The precise amount of sag also is affected by the stretch in the rope used for the main line.

Considerable debate has arisen among some technical experts over exactly how much slack should be allowed in a highline. Complex mathematical equations have been devised for working this out. However, rather than lug a computer with them every time they rig a highline, many teams simply follow the 10% rule.

10% Rule

The *10% rule* is a conservative method of tensioning a highline. According to this rule, the center of the unloaded highline should sag a vertical distance of about 10% of the span for every 200 pounds (90 kg) of expected load and every 100 feet (33 m) of span in the rope.

More experienced riggers may have developed more refined methods of line tensioning, such as the *rule of 12s* (Box 20-1). The 10% rule is very conservative, but other methods may not be

---

Box 20-1	The "Rule of 12s" Guide for Highline Tensioning

For 7/16" (11 mm) rope, the product of the number of people pulling and the MA of any tensioning system used should not exceed 12. Therefore two people pulling on a 6:1, three people on a 4:1, and so on

For a 1/2" (12.5 mm) rope, the product of the number of people pulling and the MA of any tensioning system used should not exceed 18.

Note well that "people pulling" is the per-person hand gripping strength on the rope as the input power to the MA system and not their full weight or with the haul team tied in to the haul system using their weight and legs to pull with.

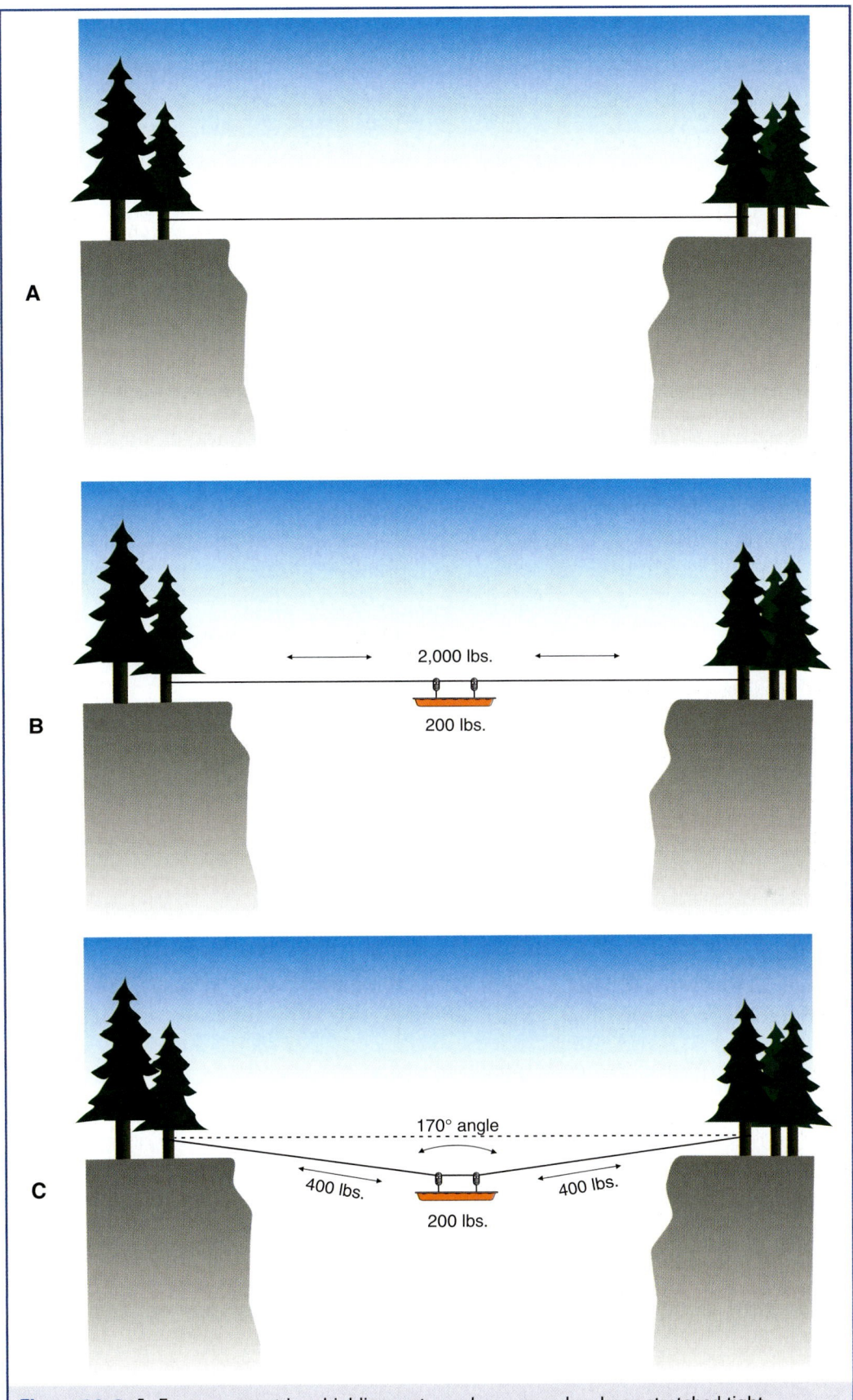

Figure 20-8 A, Forces present in a highline system when a rope has been stretched tight horizontally with no visible sag. **B,** Forces present when a load of 200 pounds (90 kg) has been placed in the middle of a 100-foot (33 m) rope stretched taut. **C,** Result of creating a sag of 10 feet (3 m) with the same 200-pound (90 kg) load on the same 100-foot (33 m) rope.

conservative or produce consistent enough results, especially for riggers using ropes with minimal elongation characteristics. Unless a rescuer is incorporating some sort of force measurement system and is thoroughly experienced in the effects of the rigging system, a conservative approach is recommended.

NOTE: When calculating *rope sag* (the visible amount of sag in the main line before the load is applied) according to the 10% rule, the calculations should be based on the *total weight of the load,* not just the weight of the person or persons on the load. The calculations must also take into consideration the *total length of the span between the two supports,* including the anchors, and not just the width of the gap to be bridged.

The two variables in the 10% rule, therefore, are (1) the weight of the load and (2) the length of the rope span. If either one of these changes, the amount of sag also must change.

Say, for example, that a 200-pound (90 kg) load *(1L)* must be carried on a 100-foot (33 m) span. The formula is:

$$1L \times 100 \text{ feet } [33 \text{ m}] \times 0.1 = 10 \text{ feet } [3 \text{ m}]$$
A 10-foot (3 m) rope sag is required for this load.

In another example, a 200-pound (90 kg) load *(1L)* must be moved on a 200-foot (66 m) span:

$$1L \times 200 \text{ feet } [66 \text{ m}] \times 0.1 = 20 \text{ feet } [6 \text{ m}]$$
A 20-foot (6 m) rope sag is required for this load.

In a third example, a 400-pound (180 kg) load *(2L)* must be transported on a 200-foot (66 m) span:

$$2L \times 200 \text{ feet } [66 \text{ m}] \times 0.1 = 40 \text{ feet } [13 \text{ m}]$$
A 40-foot (13 m) rope sag is required for this load.

Steps in Rigging a Highline

Before the rigging is begun, all equipment must be in order.

Equipment Required

1. 1 Main-line rope. The total length will include:
   - The length of the gap to be bridged plus
   - The length from the edge to the anchor on each side plus
   - The length needed to tie onto anchors on each side
2. 1 Lowering/belay rope. The total length will include:
   - The distance from the lowering device on the near side to the point on the far side where the load will be derigged plus
   - The amount of rope needed to tie to the load plus
   - 20 feet (6.5 m) to spare
3. 1 Tag line/haul rope. The total length will include:
   - The distance from the point where the load is rigged on the near side to the belay device on the far side plus
   - The length needed to attach to the load plus
   - 20 feet (6.5 m) to spare
4. 17 locking carabiners (minimum):
   - 4 (at least) for anchoring (single line system)
   - 2 for attaching the (litter) load to the highline
   - 2 for attaching the pigtail from the lowering/belay and tag lines to pulley carabiners

- 8 for attaching the litter spider to the litter and rigging plate
- 1 for attaching the tender to litter

Anchor Materials

Webbing or anchor ropes (or both) should be used as needed and appropriate for the site. Highlines exert great force on the system. High-strength tie-offs should be used with multipoint anchors or other methods to build bomb-proof anchor systems. Trees used as anchors should be back-tied and pretensioned to provide additional strength (Figure 20-9).

High Directionals

High directionals have come into vogue in rescue rigging and can be quite useful for highline applications. If the highline cannot be rigged well above and clear of the edge using existing natural anchors for high directional pulleys, artificial high directionals may be considered. Examples of commonly used high directionals include prebuilt systems (e.g., the Arizona Vortex, tripods), on-site systems (e.g., a pulley in a conveniently located tree), or site-built systems (e.g., one constructed from three tall poles lashed together). High directionals should be considered a convenience rather than a necessity, and rescuers should learn to rig a highline with or without the aid of such devices.

Rigging a Highline
Litter Rigging

Equipment

The equipment needed to rig the litter includes the following:
- 1 Litter spider (four- to eight-legged set)
- 1 Spreader
- 1 Litter
- 2 Pulleys for the main line
- 2 Small rigging plates (or 1 large one)
- 1 Litter tender pigtail
- 2 Ascenders plus slings for the tender
- 1 Safety sling for the tender (edge protection for both sides)

Procedure

1. Select an appropriate site. It should have:
   - As narrow a span as possible
   - Room on both sides to rig and derig the load and for personnel to get on and off
   - Anchors available that are very strong and secure and high enough so that the load can get over the edge without dragging
2. Get a second team to the far side of the site. All personnel must be thoroughly briefed beforehand on the steps to be followed and on communications. Radios are very helpful in these situations.
3. Get the far-side end of the rope over the span. Depending on the physical circumstances, this may be one of the more difficult parts of the operation.

- If the span is horizontal, one of the following approaches may be necessary:
  - (a) A line gun may need to be used. Usually a smaller diameter line is shot over first, then the end of the main-line rope is attached and pulled over.
  - (b) Rescuers who go across to the far side may have to trail the rope behind them.
- If the setting is an urban one and a line gun is not feasible:
  - (1) Lower the far-side end of the main-line rope to the ground.
  - (2) Have someone pull the end to the base of the structure on the other side.
  - (3) Have the far-side team drop a haul line to the ground. After tying the two ends together, the team pulls up the main-line rope.
- If a steep angle highline is to be used, follow steps (1) and (2) above.
4. Have the far-side team anchor their end of the main-line rope.

5. Have the near-side team pull on the main-line rope until the proper amount of slack is achieved. They then anchor their side of the main-line rope.
6. Get the tag line to the far side. (This may be done at the same time as the main line.) On the near side, secure the end of the tag line so that it does not slip over the edge.
7. Have the far-side team establish an anchor for the tag line belay device.
8. Have the far-side team attach a belay device to the anchor system.
9. Have the far-side team thread the tag line through the belay device.
10. On the near side, establish the anchor for the lowering/belay rope.
11. Attach the lowering system (e.g., brake tube, figure 8 descender, or brake bar rack) to the anchor on the near side.
12. Attach the lowering/belay rope to the load.
13. Thread the lowering/belay rope into the lowering system and lock the rope off.

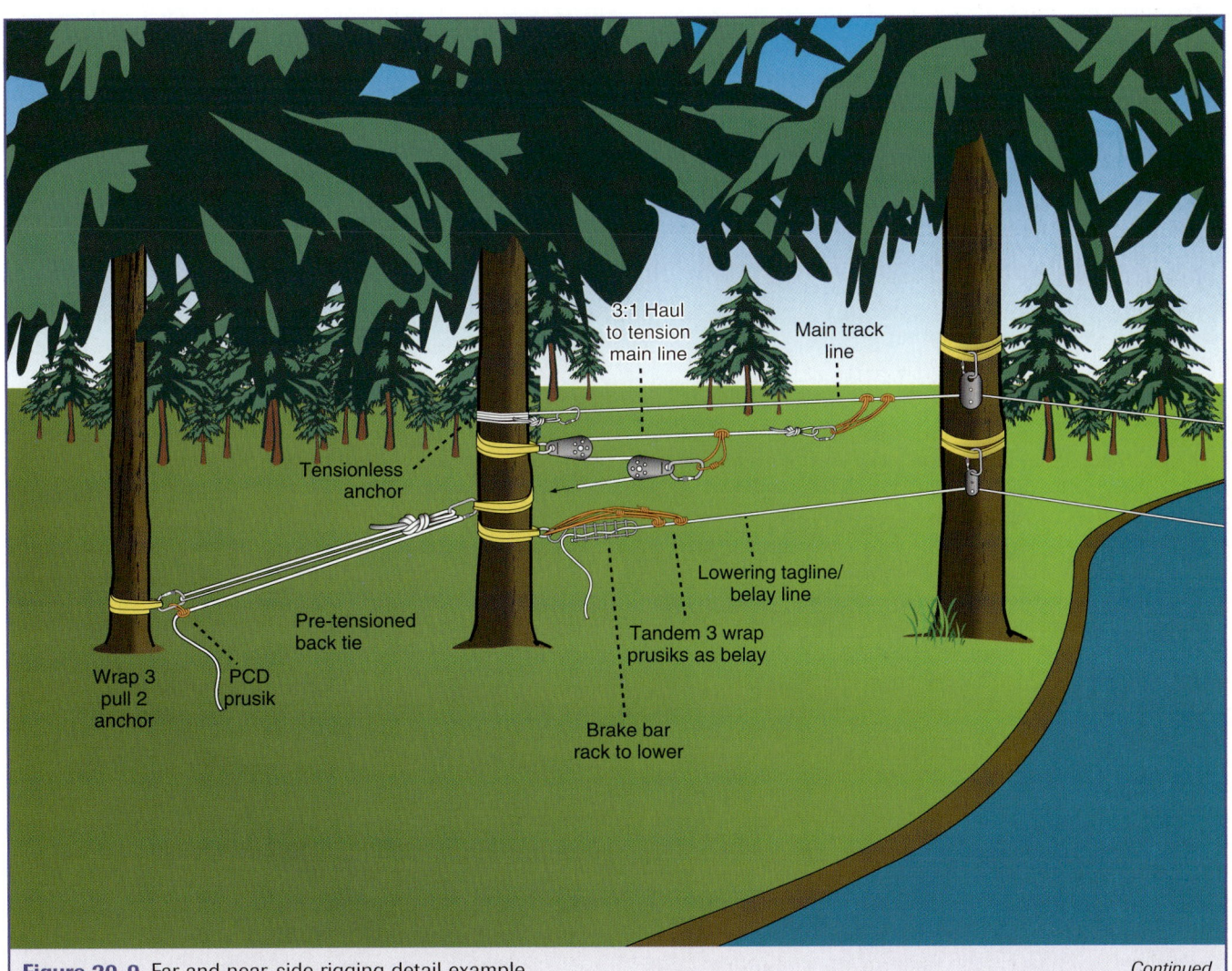

Figure 20-9 Far and near-side rigging detail example.

Continued

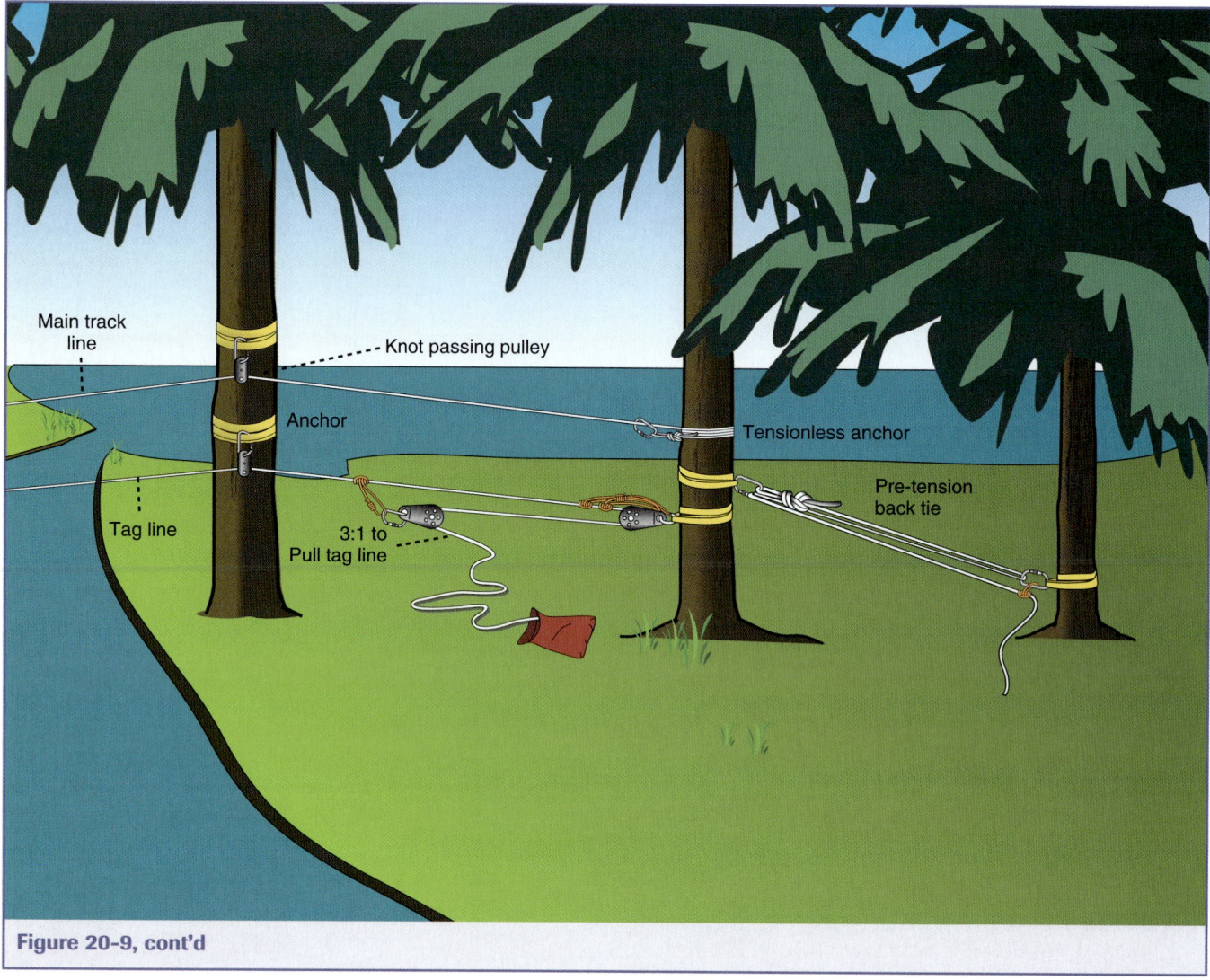

Main track line

Knot passing pulley

Anchor

Tensionless anchor

Tag line

Pre-tension back tie

3:1 to Pull tag line

Figure 20-9, cont'd

14. Rig the litter or the single person who is going to be the load.
15. Set the load on the main line. Make sure the belayer is in control of the lowering/belay line.
16. Attach the tag line to the litter system. Have the tag line belayer on the far side remove slack from the tag line.
17. Have the litter tender attach himself or herself to the litter system.

Beginning Movement of the Load

18. Before beginning movement, recheck the rigging, including the anchors on both sides.
19. Make sure all those involved in the rescue are ready, including:
    - The person attached to the load
    - The brakeman on the lowering/belay line
    - The belayer on the far-side tag line
    - The edge tenders
20. When all personnel are ready, the litter tender or person attached to the load begins the voice signals; he or she calls, *"On belay."*

Lowering/belay line brakeman: *"Belay on."*
Tag line belayer: *"Belay on."*
Litter tender: *"Down slow."*

21. The lowering/belay line brakeman begins allowing rope through the brakes on the near side, while the belayer on the far-side tag line begins taking in slack. It may be prudent to use a line-holding device (e.g., rope grab, Prusiks, or other belay device) at either end. This decision should be based on the potential and consequences of the rope reversing direction and traveling quickly out of control.

Completing Transfer of the Load

22. Once the load has reached the far side and is in a secure position, the litter tender or person attached to the load calls, *"Stop."* The lowering/belay line brakeman stops feeding rope.
23. When the litter tender or person attached to the load is in a secure position on the far side, he or she calls, *"Off belay."*

Lowering/belay line brakeman: *"Off belay."*
Tag line belayer: *"Off belay."*

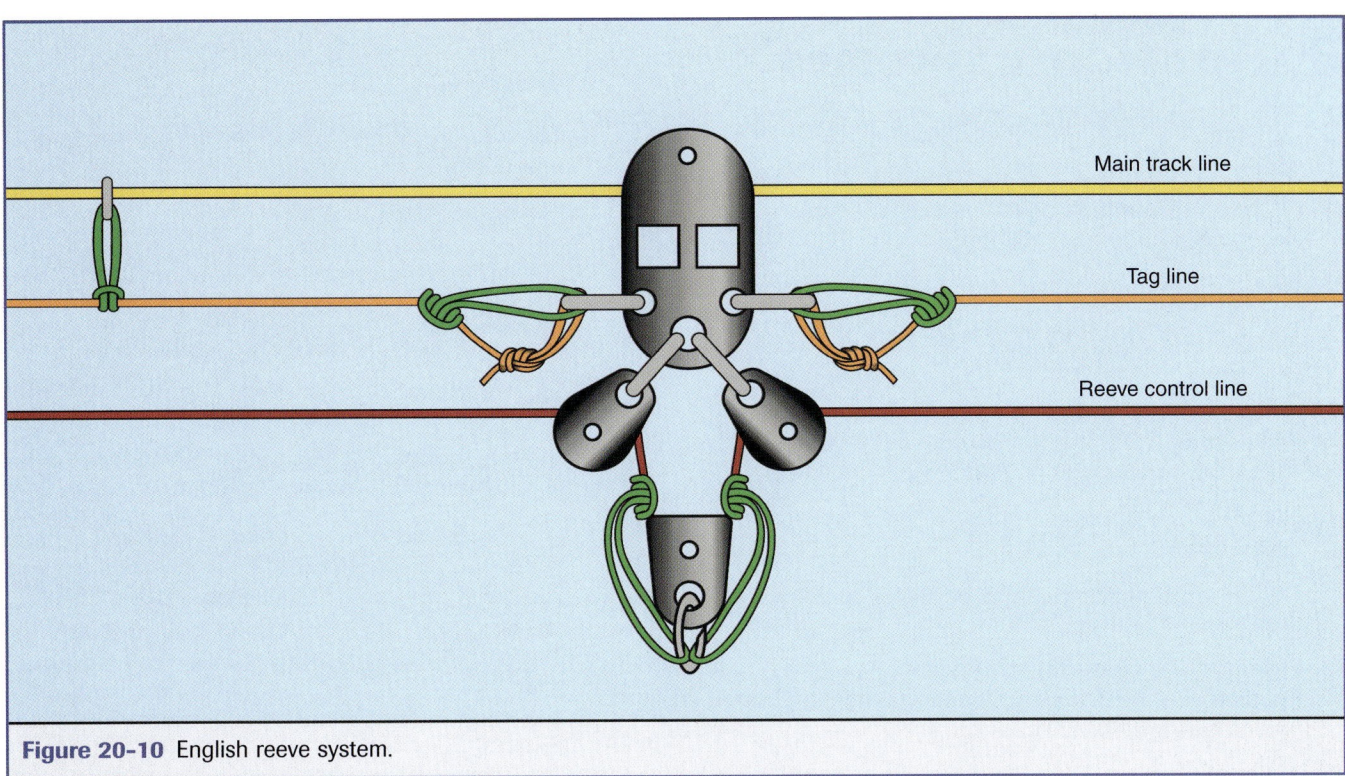

Figure 20-10 English reeve system.

More Complex Systems

Once the rescue team has mastered the basic highline described above, it is a good idea to consider systems that can handle loads greater than one person riding. A litter, subject, and rescuer, with all the extra gear needed to fasten them together, easily can weigh 600 pounds (270 kg) or more. Highlines themselves can create high loads in the main line and all the associated rigging and anchors. Great care should be taken to make sure proper system:load ratios are used and that safety factors are ample for the actual load plus unexpected dynamic loading events.

Helpful Hints

Dual main lines often are a good idea but involve more anchors and good rope management skills. Two parallel 7/16-inch (11 mm) ropes offer more strength than one 1/2-inch (12.5 mm) rope. Special wide sheave pulleys are easier to manage than double sheave pulleys. Dual ropes can flip over each other, and the large sheave pulley can continue on much more easily with less chance of jamming.

As the length of the highline increases, the tag line tends to droop well below the main line and can become a line management problem. Short tag line hangers can be made from Prusik loops about 1 foot (0.3 m) long. Hitch the tag line with the loop and hang the loop from a carabiner clipped to the main line every 33 feet (11 m) or so.

English Reeve System

The ***English reeve system*** is a particular type of arrangement involving ropes and pulleys rigged so as to facilitate movement of the load. This system is useful because it can be used to move a load along either a horizontal or a sloping highline and to raise or lower the load vertically in midspan.

Note that in Figure 20-10 the load is being moved from side to side on the highline using tag lines. The reeve line is tied off. When a load is to be moved vertically, the best control is gained with the tag lines tied off. Applying slack or tension in the reeve line allows the load to be moved up and down. With careful coordination and control of the reeve lines and tag lines, the position of the load can be adjusted simultaneously on both the vertical and horizontal planes.

Evaluation Exercises

1. Describe four situations in which highlines might be useful to rescuers.

2. Name three common problems that rescuers encounter in rigging highlines.

3. Name seven basic elements of a highline system.

4. The litter system for a highline consists of _____ spiders, each with at least _____ legs.

5. Why should two pulleys in tandem be used to support a litter system on a highline?

6. Name two purposes of a spreader for a highline litter system.

7. List the ways in which a litter tender is attached to the litter in a highline system.

8. Assuming the near side of a horizontal highline is the high end, should a litter be moved across head first or feet first? Why?

9. Assuming a steep angle highline, should a litter be moved across head first or feet first? Why?

10. Describe the functions of the following in a highline system:

    (a) Lowering/belay system
    (b) Tag line

11. Describe how the lowering/belay line and tag line should be attached to the litter system in a highline.

12. For a horizontal highline, what kind of device should be used to control the lowering/belay line? The tag line?

13. Explain what happens if a highline is stretched tight and then loaded.

14. The 10% rule states that for every load of about _____ pounds (kg) and for every _____ feet (m) of rope in a highline span, there should be a sag of _____ percent.

15. The 10% rule has two variables, and a change in either of them should mean a change in the amount of sag. What are the two variables?

16. Estimate the amount of visible sag needed in a highline under the following conditions:

    (a) 200-pound (90 kg) load on a 100-foot (33 m) span
    (b) 200-pound (90 kg) load on a 200-foot (66 m) span
    (c) 400-pound (180 kg) load on a 100-foot (33 m) span
    (d) 100-pound (45 kg) load on a 200-foot (66 m) span

17. List the minimum equipment required to rig a highline with a 100-foot horizontal span, having a litter system with tender for a load.

18. List the criteria for an appropriate site for a highline.

19. List three possible techniques for getting the rope across the gap when establishing a highline.

20. Describe the precautions that should be taken before beginning movement on a highline.

21

Helicopter Rescue Operations

Ken Phillips

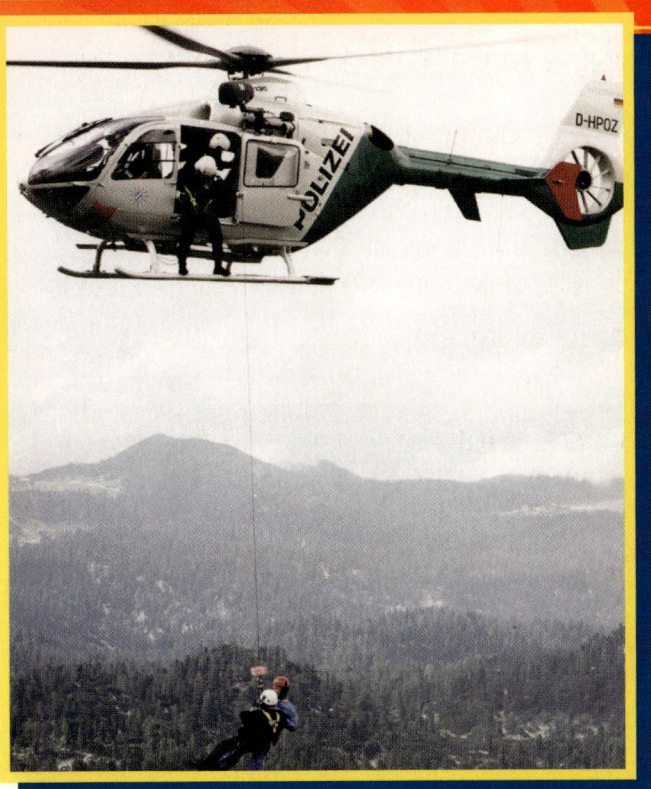

The material in this chapter conforms to guidelines published by the National Fire Protection Association (NFPA), specifically standard 1006, *Professional Qualifications for Rescue Technicians* (2002), and standard 1670, *Operations and Training for Technical Rescue Incidents* (1999). NFPA standards are revised regularly, and readers are advised to review the latest version of this standard.

Objectives

On completion of this chapter, you should be able to:

1. Describe the decision-making and mission planning factors involved in the performance of a safe helicopter rescue.
2. List important considerations in the selection and operation of a functional helispot.
3. Describe safe procedures for operating around a helicopter.
4. List personal protective equipment (PPE) used by a helicopter crew member.
5. Describe rescue subject care considerations that are affected by helicopter operations.
6. Identify the limitations and hazards of helicopter rescue hoists.
7. Identify the limitations and hazards of helicopter short haul operations.
8. Identify "operational red flags" that can occur during helicopter rescues.

Key Terms

Autorotation A rotorcraft flight condition in which the lifting rotor is driven entirely by the action of the air while the rotorcraft is in motion. No engine power is supplied to the main rotor, and lift is developed from the free turning of the rotor blades, which are driven by aerodynamic forces. Rotor inertia is used as the helicopter nears the ground to control the descent.

Center of Gravity (CG) The point in a helicopter where all forces are balanced. In a single-rotor helicopter, this is a range forward or aft beneath the rotor mast. The distribution of the weight of the fuel, the personnel, and the cargo in the helicopter affects this critical balance for safe flight.

Collective Pitch System The flight control mechanisms by which the pitch of all rotor blades is varied equally and simultaneously. The collective pitch control regulates the pitch angle of the main rotor blades. It is used as the primary power control. As the pitch of the blades is increased, lift is induced, causing the helicopter to lift off the ground, hover, or climb, as long as power is available.

Cyclic The flight control mechanism that permits the helicopter to move forward, sideways, and backward by corresponding tilting of the rotor disc.

Density Altitude The actual pressure altitude corrected for temperature and humidity, which provides a measure of the air density.

Flight Following The method and process by which an aircraft is tracked from departure point to destination. Flight following is the knowledge of the aircraft and condition with a reasonable degree of certainty such that, in the event of mishap, those on board may be rescued. It typically is accomplished through a position check on the radio at regular intervals.

Ground Effect When a helicopter is in a low hover, the ground interrupts the airflow under the helicopter, and the velocity of the induced airflow to the rotor system is reduced. The result is less induced drag and a more vertical lift vector. This ground cushion, or ground effect, is beneficial in flight because it increases lift capability for the helicopter, which therefore requires less power to maintain a hover. Ground effect occurs when the helicopter is at a very low altitude, usually one half the rotor diameter. Ground effect is hampered by uneven terrain, vegetation, or water beneath the rotor disc.

Height-Velocity Curve A chart in the helicopter flight manual that indicates the combinations of altitude and forward airspeed required to ensure a safe autorotation.

Helibase Under the incident command system (ICS), a designated facility for conducting helicopter operations that has refueling capability. The U.S. Federal Aviation Administration (FAA) term for a permanent helicopter facility is *heliport*.

Heavy Helicopter A helicopter with a certified gross weight greater than 12,500 pounds (5670 kg). Under the ICS helicopter typing system, a heavy helicopter is a Type 1 helicopter; it must have an allowable payload at 59°F (15°C) at sea level of 5000 pounds (2268 kg) and 15 or more passenger seats.

Helicopter A rotorcraft that depends principally on its engine-driven rotors for horizontal motion.

Helicopter Rappel Insertion of personnel at a site by means of rappelling on a fixed rope from a helicopter in a hover.

Helispot A temporary helicopter landing zone (LZ), which may incorporate a natural or an improved takeoff and landing area.

Hoist Rescue Insertion or extraction of personnel on a lightweight cable using an electric or hydraulic hoist that is anchored to a helicopter.

Hover A condition of flight in which the helicopter remains fairly stationary over a given point, moving neither vertically nor horizontally.

Hover Ceiling The highest altitude at which a helicopter can successfully hover while loaded to its maximum gross weight. In and out of ground effect hover ceilings are computed at maximum gross weight.

Hover in Ground Effect (HIGE) To operate at an altitude (usually equal to one half the rotor diameter above the surface) at which the positive influence of ground effect is attained.

Hover Landing A landing that does not meet the definition of *toe-in, single-skid,* or *step-out* landings. Hover landings are characterized by a need to maintain a substantial amount of hover power while the landing gear is not in contact with the surface. Hover landings normally are required because of the nature of the surface (e.g., swampy ground, tundra or muskeg, snow, or lava rock).

Hover Out of Ground Effect (HOGE) Hovering at a high enough altitude that the added benefit of ground effect is not obtained.

Instrument Flight Rules (IFR) FAA rules governing the operation of aircraft in weather conditions below the minimum for flight under visual flight rules; that is, conditions under which instruments are essential for flight navigation.

Landing Zone (LZ) Any improved or unimproved helicopter landing site that has an adequate touchdown pad and approach and departure paths. Under ICS, a landing zone is referred to as a helispot or helibase.

Light Helicopter A helicopter with a certified gross weight of less than 6,000 pounds (2,721 kg). Under the ICS helicopter typing system, a light helicopter is a type 3 helicopter; it must have an allowable payload at 59° F (15° C) at sea level of 1,200 pounds (544 kg) and four to eight passenger seats.

Load Calculation Calculation of the helicopter's lifting capability for a given altitude and temperature.

Longline A line or set of lines, typically steel cable, used for external sling load operations to deliver supplies to a site where a helicopter could not safely land.

Maximum Gross Weight The certified maximum allowable weight of an aircraft, as determined by the manufacturer and approved by the FAA, at which that particular aircraft can safely fly. This weight is the equipped weight of the aircraft plus that of the useful load (i.e., pilot, passengers, cargo, and fuel).

Key Terms

Maximum Performance Takeoff A steep ascent upon takeoff, done to clear obstacles, that involves limited forward airspeed and that approaches the flight limitations of the helicopter.

Medium Helicopter A helicopter with a certified gross weight between 6,000 pounds (2,721 kg) and 12,500 pounds (5,669 kg). Under the ICS helicopter typing system, a medium helicopter is a type 2 helicopter; it must have an allowable payload at 59° F (15° C) at sea level of 2,500 pounds (1,134 kg) and nine to 14 passenger seats (unless it is in a restricted category).

One-Skid Landing The maneuver of placing one skid of the helicopter on the ground while the other remains above the ground, typically performed in steep terrain. When the skid is in contact with the ground, the center of gravity can shift laterally.

Pilot in Command (PIC) The person who (1) has final authority and responsibility for the operation and safety of the flight; (2) has been designated as pilot in command before or during the flight; and (3) holds the appropriate category, class, and type rating, if appropriate, for the conduct of the flight.

Power-On Landing A landing maneuver in which both skids are in full contact with the ground while full power is maintained; this maneuver is performed to maintain the position of the aircraft on a marginal touchdown pad.

Precautionary Landing A landing conducted by the pilot because of an apparent failure of the helicopter flight systems, which would make continued flight unsafe.

Public Aircraft A government-owned, leased, or hired aircraft that is performing work "exclusively in the service" of any federal, state, or local government agency.

Safety Circle An obstruction-free area on all sides of the helicopter touchdown pad that allows a safe approach to and departure from the touchdown pad.

Short Haul The transport of one or more people externally suspended below a helicopter. Also, the use of a helicopter and an externally attached line to insert or extract personnel in areas that preclude a normal landing.

Situational Awareness The ability of an individual to know what is going on around himself or herself at all times. Situational awareness is maintained by obtaining updated information about the external environment and about all operational conditions in order to form an accurate mental image of a mission.

Sling Load An external load supported by a sling, net, bag, or some combination of these that is attached with a longline to the helicopter by means of a cargo hook.

Step-Out Landing A landing used for dropping off or picking up passengers and cargo (other than the rappel/short haul method) while the helicopter is held in a hover. The helicopter is not in contact with the ground, and the center of gravity can shift laterally and longitudinally.

Supplemental Type Certificate (STC) The airworthiness approval required by the FAA (FAR* – 14 CFR Chapter 1 Part 21.113) when a design modification involves a change in materials, parts, and appliances on the aircraft. Rescue equipment, which is attached to a helicopter, is affected by the scope of this requirement.

Touchdown Pad A designated area, which may have a prepared or improved surface, where the helicopter skids are placed.

Toe-In Landing A landing maneuver in which the helicopter rests on the toes of the skids; toe-in landings are used to drop off or pick up passengers or cargo. To execute the maneuver, a significant amount of hover power (within 15% of hover power) must be held to keep the helicopter from falling backward. When the helicopter is operated in this manner, the potential exists for a significant lateral and longitudinal shift in the center of gravity shift during loading and offloading. In addition, when the helicopter is balanced on the forward one third or less of the skid tube, main rotor blade clearance is another significant concern.

Torque A twisting force that causes a counter-rotating motion. In a helicopter with a main rotor that rotates counterclockwise, the fuselage rotates clockwise. The tail rotor produces anti-torque to counteract this force. The maximum continuous upper torque limit is 100%; however, a transient over-torque may be tolerable to the helicopter power plant.

Translational Lift The additional lift generated as the helicopter transitions from a hover to horizontal flight. Transitional lift is due to the increased efficiency of the rotor system as it generates more lift in forward flight with a higher inflow velocity of air mass comparison with a hover.

Vertical Reference A technique used by the helicopter pilot and flight crew, while operating above the ground, to determine the height of the aircraft and any associated external load through visual clues. Surface landmarks and references are used during approaches, departures, and external-load positioning maneuvers at landing or work areas.

Visual Flight Rules (VFR) The rules for conducting flight operations under visual meteorological conditions (VMC). Aircraft flying under VFR are not required to be in contact with air traffic controllers and are responsible for their own separation from other aircraft. The term also is used in the United States to indicate weather conditions that meet or exceed minimum VFR requirements.

---

*See the section, Applicable U.S. Federal Regulations.

Helicopters in Rescue Operations

As a rescuer, it is necessary that you understand that the consequences of a poorly managed helicopter rescue can be swift and fatal. The **helicopter** truly is an outstanding rescue tool, but it also has specific operating limitations. Rescuer understanding of these limits plus the professional discipline not to exceed them during an emergency is the formula for a safe operation. As accident investigators frequently find, "self-imposed psychological pressure" causes us to make poor decisions when adrenaline clouds our judgment. Poor decision making is preventable, yet, tragically, it is a factor in the vast majority of helicopter rescue accidents.

You cannot disregard the fact that a helicopter is a machine. You might expect it to provide dependable service, but helicopters do break down, disrupting operational plans or leaving rescuers stranded. Always be prepared with backup plans and require field rescuers to be prepared. A helicopter is one more operational tool for rescue, not a panacea to be applied in every rescue situation (Figure 21-1).

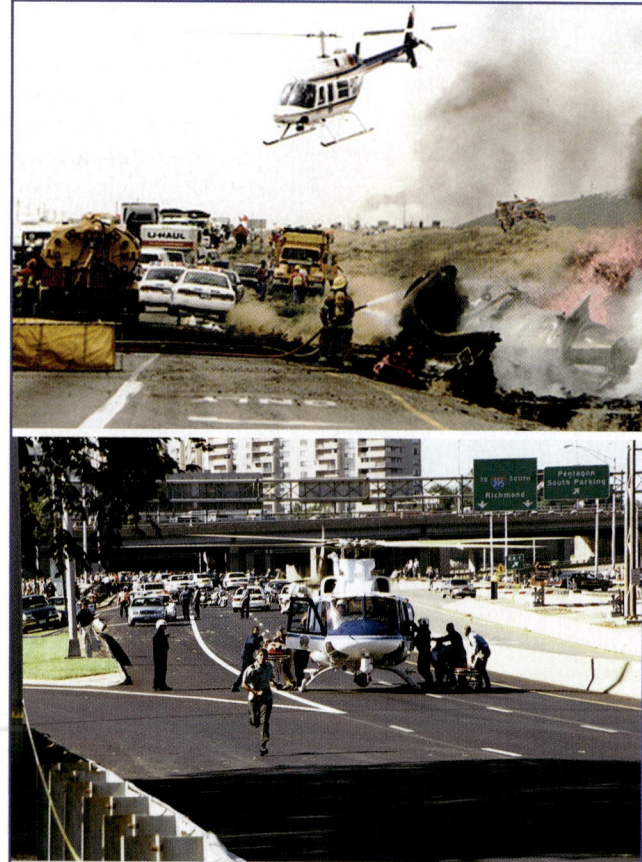

Figure 21-1 A, Arizona Department of Public Safety (DPS) Air Rescue Bell LongRanger III departs from the scene of a motor vehicle accident with a medevac patient. (Courtesy R. Todd Stenhouse, Kingman Daily Miner Newspaper.) B, U.S. Park Police Bell 412 helicopter prepares to take off during a medevac from a helispot on Washington Boulevard, near the Pentagon in Washington, D.C., following the September 11, 2001 terrorist attack. (Courtesy U.S. Army.)

Decision Making and Situational Awareness

Before launching a helicopter for a rescue or requesting the assistance of an outside agency with aviation assets, make sure you are not "wrapped around the axle" by the excitement of the moment. Ask yourself the following three questions:

1. Is this plan in the best interest of the rescue subject (patient) and rescuer safety?
2. Is there a better way to do it?
3. If darkness or poor weather is hampering a helicopter response, will the rescue subject be better served by an evacuation in the morning or in improved conditions?

Rescue crews often show poor judgment by "pressing on" in degraded operating conditions for a non-life-threatening injury that could easily handle a delay. The option of delaying the mission in favor of safer operating conditions is repeatedly overlooked and requires considerable discipline on the part of a rescue team. Remarkably, accidents with the same root cause occur over and over. As rescuers, we must learn from these mistakes and break this dangerous pattern of repetition.

When to Use a Helicopter

Situations that involve remote locations with critical injuries often are appropriate for a helicopter-based rescue. However, when multiple transportation options are available, rescuers should determine which technique offers the least risk and greatest gain both for rescuers and the rescue subject. Evaluate the *totality of the circumstances* surrounding the incident, including the duration and difficulty of a conventional evacuation, rescuer and subject safety, the severity of the subject's injury, current and projected environmental hazards, personnel and aircraft availability, and transport time to a definitive care facility (Box 21-1).

Ask yourself these questions in deciding whether to conduct a helicopter rescue:

- Is a safe landing site available within a reasonable distance of the accident site (Figure 21-2)?

Box 21-1	Mission Decisions

1. **Assess the situation:** Weigh the relative level of urgency, the condition of the rescue subject (or subjects), and stability of the incident.
2. **Determine the alternatives:** Review the various rescue options, including the level of complexity and the risk involved. Greater complexity and risk add significantly to the potential for mission failure.
3. **Select an alternative:** The choice of an appropriate rescue plan should be based on the safety of rescuers rather than the safety of the subject.
4. **Execute the plan:** Initiate the rescue response according to established procedures and reevaluate your ongoing actions. Avoid the "press on regardless" mentality. If the plan is not working, *change* your operational response.

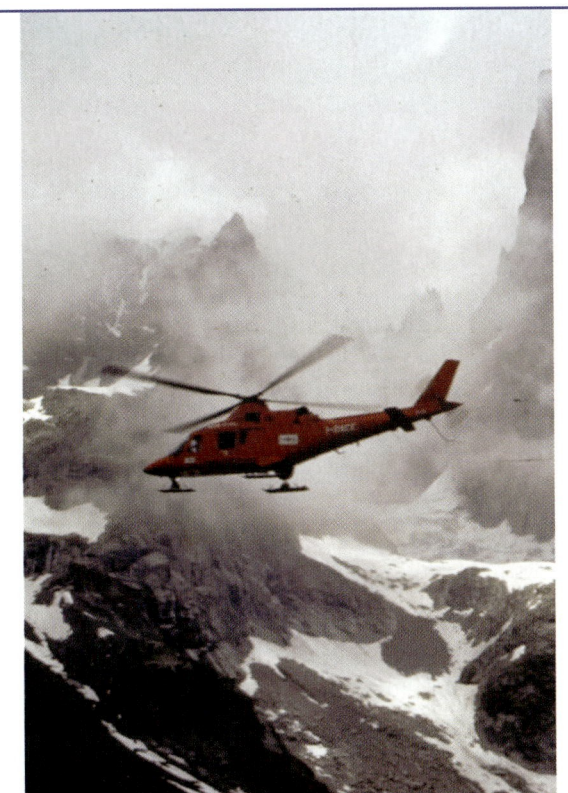

Figure 21-2 Mountain flying operations. An Augusta A109-K2 helicopter operated by REGA (Swiss Air Rescue) flying in the mountainous terrain of the Swiss Alps.

- Does the urgency of the subject's condition require getting someone to the accident site as quickly as possible?
- Would the immediate insertion of advanced life support (ALS) care to the scene convert an urgent medical case to a lower priority ground evacuation?
- Is the risk associated with traversing terrain to the accident scene greater than the risk of using specialized helicopter rappel, short haul, or hoisting techniques?
- Are all the rescuers proficient with the helicopter rescue technique being considered?
- Do extreme environmental factors prevent the use of a helicopter?
- Are conditions adequate for communication with all involved rescue personnel, or do communications barriers exist?

Weather and Nighttime Limitations

Daytime flight operations for aircraft are limited by visual flight rules (VFR) basic weather minimums, which include 1 mile of forward visibility and 500 feet (152 m) of clearance below a cloud ceiling. An exception applies to helicopters in uncontrolled airspace (Class G) *below 1,200 feet (366 meters);* in these areas, helicopters "may be operated clear of clouds if operated at a speed that allows the pilot adequate opportunity to see any air traffic or obstruction in time to avoid a collision" (FAR Part 91.155 b.1).

NOTE: When flying above 1,200 feet (366 m) (i.e., *above ground level [AGL]*) but below 10,000 feet (3,048 m) (i.e., *mean sea level [MSL]*), helicopters need 1 statute mile forward visibility and clearance from clouds that includes 500 feet (152 m) below, 1,000 feet (305 m) above, and 2,000 feet (610 m) horizontal.

U.S. federal land management agencies adhere to the following visibility and wind restrictions for *special use missions* (e.g., mountainous flying, an unimproved **helispot**, or less than 500 feet [152 m] AGL) involving light helicopters: maximum sustained winds of 35 mph (30 knots [56 km]/hour) *or* a wind gust spread (range from minimum to maximum) of 17 mph (15 knots [27 km]/hour) and at least one-half mile (0.8 km) forward visibility.

Night Rescue Operations by Helicopter

Conducting a night rescue by helicopter in a remote setting dramatically multiplies operational risk. Review the option of stabilizing the subject at the scene and initiating the rescue at daybreak. VFR night flight minimum clearances (the visual distance minimums required for nighttime flights) are 3 statute miles (4.8 km) forward visibillity and a minimum of 500 feet (152 m) clearance beneath clouds (FAR Part 91.155).

Night vision goggles (NVG) increase the aircrew's ability to navigate at night. However, they have operational limitations, including difficulty identifying suspended wires, a narrowed field of view, and impaired depth perception. Recurrent training is necessary for aircrews to maintain operational proficiency with night vision goggles. Early vintage night vision equipment used *Generation I* image tube technology. Their relatively large size permitted use only in weapons sight applications.

The first true night vision goggles were produced in the early 1980s using *Generation II* image intensifier tube technology. A drawback of the Generation II tube was that a bright light directed at it caused the tube to shut down as a self-protecting feature. *Generation III* tube technology was a major improvement for all night vision equipment, especially that used in low light conditions. However, earlier Generation III tubes also were adversely affected by bright lights in the field of view, particularly when the user was trying to view a scene in the area of the bright light, the result being a distorted effect known as *halo*.

Newer Generation III night vision goggles, now being delivered to the U.S. military, have an autogating feature for the image tube's internal power supply that provides three times higher resolution in high light levels. In an urban environment, this permits the user to look directly into bright lights (e.g., streetlights) and distinguish a subject.[1]

Mission Planning and Preplanning

For a helicopter rescue operation to succeed, sufficient preplanning must be done well in advance of the initial notification. Rescue teams should develop an in-depth knowledge of and working rapport with outside aviation resources through meetings and advance training. As part of the preplan, consider preparing an aerial hazard map for the local response area, one that identifies wires, power lines, military and operations areas (MOA), in addition to established helisports and staging areas

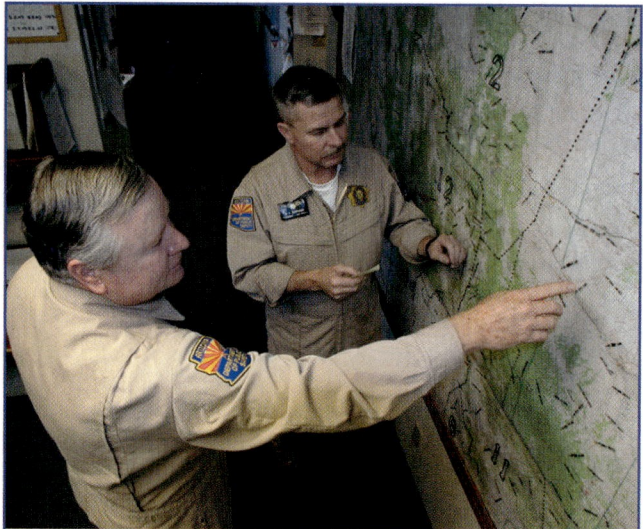

Figure 21-3 Aerial hazard map. Arizona DPS (Department of Public Safety) Air Rescue crew consulting an aerial hazard map before an operational response. (Courtesy Ken Phillips.)

with known coordinates. Such a labeled map (Figure 21-3) is an extremely valuable mission-planning tool.

Outside Helicopter Rescue Assets

Outside helicopter rescue resources can be categorized as follows:

- **Public aircraft** (e.g. police, sheriff, and other public safety agencies): This type of aircraft typically is more readily available and is best configured to support search and rescue (SAR) missions. Develop a working understanding of their capabilities and limitations in advance.
- *Air ambulances:* Commercial air ambulances are a logical air transport choice for a rescue subject suffering from acute trauma because of the aircraft's crew composition, which typically includes a flight nurse and paramedic. The medical configuration of the aircraft, which gives it a higher equipped weight, can hamper its operating efficiency at higher elevations. Be aware that some commercial aeromedical helicopter crews may feel pressured by your request to land at a marginal landing zone in a remote area in order to generate revenue on a mission. Be certain of the appropriateness of your request.
- *Call when needed (CWN) for-hire commercial operators:* For a contracted aircraft, specific provisions are outlined in the procurement document. Considerations include whether the aircraft is capable of handling a litter, whether it is equipped with a wire strike protection system (WSPS), whether a fuel truck is needed to support the aircraft at a remote base, and whether the aircraft is capable of transmitting on public safety very high frequency (VHF). Survey the capabilities and background of local operators (Box 21-2).

- *Military aircraft:* Rescue teams should determine in advance the best contact mechanisms for nearby military units, including after-hours response times, aircraft and crew capabilities, fuel requirements, and radio communication requirements. All requests for federal military helicopter resources are handled through the Air Force Rescue Coordination Center (AFRCC) at Langley Air Force Base.

Helicopter Resource Categories

Helicopters have been classified as follows under the National Interagency Incident Management System[2]:

- **Light helicopter** (type 3 helicopter): A helicopter with a certified gross weight of less than 6,000 pounds (2,721 kg). A light helicopter has an allowable payload at 59° F (15° C) at sea level of 1,200 pounds (544 kg) and four to eight passenger seats (Figure 21-4).
- **Medium helicopter** (type 2 helicopter): A helicopter with a certified gross weight of 6,000 to 12,500 pounds (2,721 to 5,669 kg). A medium helicopter (Figure 21-5) has an allowable payload at 59° F (15° C) at sea level of 2,500 pounds (1,134 kg) and nine to 14 passenger seats.
- **Heavy helicopter** (type 1 helicopter): A helicopter with a certified gross weight over 12,500 pounds (5,669 kg). A

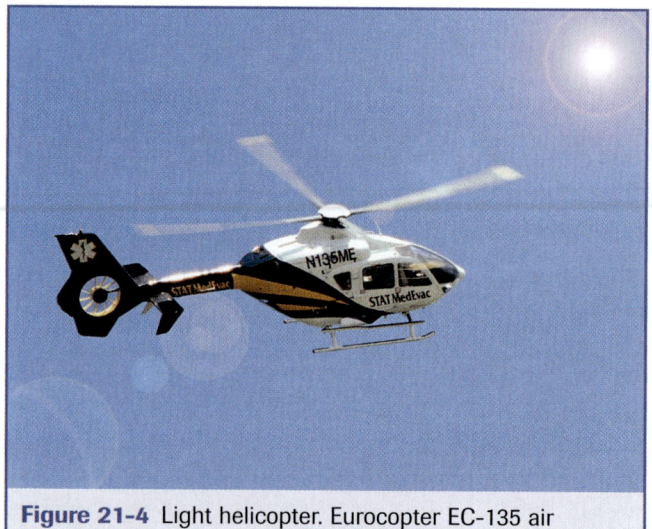

Figure 21-4 Light helicopter. Eurocopter EC-135 air ambulance helicopter operated STAT Medevac of West Mifflin, Pennsylvania. (Courtesy STAT Medevac.)

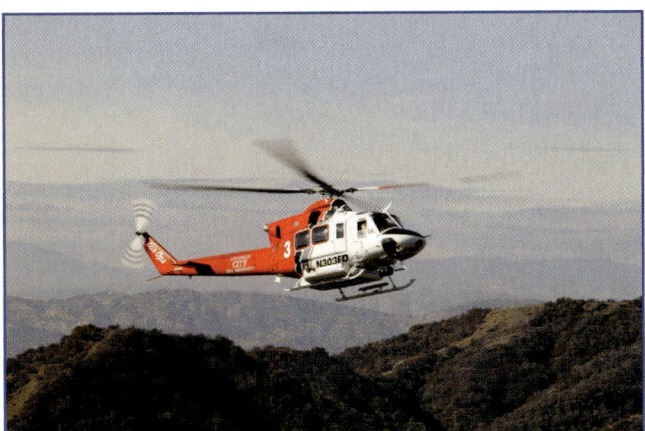

Figure 21-5 Medium helicopter. Los Angeles (California) City Fire Department helicopter during a routine fire patrol flight in the mountains north of Los Angeles. The Bell 412 is equipped with a belly tank for aerial suppression. (Courtesy Glenn Grossman.)

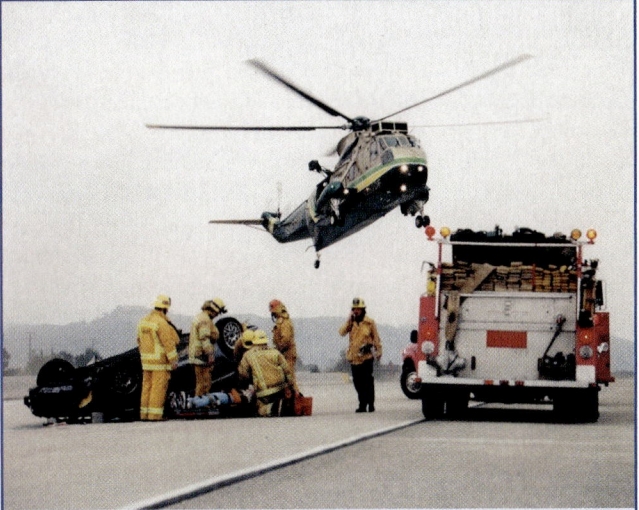

Figure 21-6 Heavy helicopter. The Los Angeles (California) County Sheriff's Department (LASD) Aero Bureau employs "Air 5," for conducting SAR operations and law enforcement support in conjuction with personnel of the Emergency Services Detail (ESD). This hoist-equipped Sikorsky H-3 Sea King is staffed by a crew of five. (Courtesy Los Angeles County Sheriff's Department Aero Bureau.)

heavy helicopter (Figure 21-6) has an allowable payload at 59° F (15° C) at sea level of 5,000 pounds (2,268 kg) and 15 or more passenger seats (unless it is in a restricted category).

Table 21-1 shows the "typing" of helicopter categories used for national incidents involving the incident command system (ICS); this categorization allows rescue organizations to order resources that best meet the needs of the operation.

Mission Management

The success of a mission is directly related to how well it is organized and managed. Establish an adequate incident management structure (ICS or incident management system [IMS]) for the identified response. To achieve this, the role of command must be clearly identified to all personnel; an adequate span of control must be maintained to prevent task overload; and staffing positions must be filled with trained, qualified rescue workers. For large scale responses, activate the positions of air support group supervisor, helibase manager, and helispot manager to coordinate the arrivals and departures of numerous helicopters. This type of positive control of aviation assets prevents the

incident from turning into an unmanaged "air show," in which pilots and air crews are forced to operate without direction.

Flight Following

Flight following is a system of tracking helicopters. It provides an operational safety net in the event a rescue helicopter becomes overdue during a mission. Because the pilot reports the aircraft's radio position at least hourly (every 15 minutes is preferable), a dispatcher or helibase manager has a fixed point from which to start search efforts. This can reduce the response time for reaching personnel who may be injured. Flight following can be maintained through an *instrument flight rules (IFR)* flight plan, a *visual flight rules (VFR) flight plan* with check-in to FAA facilities en route, an agency VFR flight plan with check-ins according to established agency minimums, or even an automated radio or global positioning system (GPS) tracking system.

Table 21-1	Helicopter Type		
	Type I	**Type II**	**Type III**
Passenger seats	15+	9-14	4-8
Allowable payload at 59° F. (15° C) at sea level	5000 pounds (2268 kg)	2500 pounds (1134 kg)	1200 pounds (544 kg)
Example aircraft	Sikorsky S-70 (UH-60) Black Hawk, Sikorsky S-64 Skycrane, Bell 214, Boeing-Vertol BE-234	Bell 212, Bell 412, Eurocopter BK-117, Sikorsky S-58T	Bell Jet Ranger B-3, Bell Long Ranger L-3, Bell 407 Eurocopter AS350 A-Star, Eurocopter EC-135, MD500, MD900 Explorer

Communications

Clear, precise communications eliminate pitfalls that have jeopardized many missions. Radios can be used effectively between the aircraft and rescuers on the ground through incorporation of an interface cable, which connects a handheld radio to a flight helmet. For congested incidents, a designated air-to-ground frequency separates aircraft transmissions from other incident traffic for clear communication; for example, this is standard practice in wildland firefighting aviation operations.

Common hand signals (Figure 21-7) are useful when combined with radio transmissions because they are immediately understood. Hand signals avoid the problems of garbled messages and radio frequency congestion. However, pilots who are not familiar with or confident of the ground personnel using the hand signals may ignore the signals or rely on their own best judgment instead. Working and training in advance builds the necessary trust and familiarity between aircrews and ground rescuers.

Landing Zones

A number of important factors affect the choice of a helicopter **landing zone (LZ):**

- **Touchdown pad:** Room must be available for a designated area, which may have a prepared or improved surface, where the helicopter skids can be in contact with the ground.
- **Safety circle:** An obstruction-free area must be available on all sides of the touchdown pad (Figure 21-8) that allows a safe approach to and departure from the touchdown pad. The safety circle also is a zone free of obstacles and hazards (e.g., wires, tall trees, loose debris) for a helicopter departing at a low angle (Table 21-2).
- *Other considerations:* An exposed ridgeline, outcropping, or clear saddle can provide a landing zone, especially if the approach and departure path are unobstructed (Figure 21-9). However, take into account the fact that winds can be variable. In a deep canyon, a helicopter requires a long forward and unobstructed path to gain altitude. A tight, confined landing area requires a **maximum performance takeoff;** this may approach the operating limits of the aircraft and should be avoided.
- *Slopes:* Avoid slopes of more than 5 degrees or 11% grade. On sloping surfaces, a situation known as *dynamic rollover* can occur. As a helicopter lifts off from a sloping landing zone, if one skid or wheel is still on the ground, the helicopter may pivot around the skid or wheel. When this happens, the pilot can reach the "stop" limit on the cyclic control as he or she runs out of cyclic travel and will be unable to stop the rollover. Dynamic rollover also occurs on level surfaces, for example, when a skid or wheel becomes stuck on a landing zone (e.g., from sinking into mud or warm asphalt) or is restrained by a tie-down or some other obstacle during takeoff.
- *Dust abatement:* For repeated use of a landing zone, especially an unpaved **helibase,** consider dust abatement by using available fire apparatus to wet down the surface. Reducing dusty conditions improves safety, because the pilot can observe the touchdown pad during landing and can receive unobstructed hand signals from ground personnel. Furthermore, dusty and sandy conditions can damage aircraft engines.
- *Wind indicator:* A wind indicator provides the pilot with a visual cue for wind direction and speed. A windsock, flagging, or smoke or dirt thrown into the air as the helicopter initiates a high orbit over the scene can serve as a wind indicator. A helicopter achieves optimum performance when landings and takeoffs are made into the direction of the oncoming wind. Ground rescuers should anticipate this in their selection of a helispot and in the staging of rescue apparatus or personal equipment.
- *Snow landing* Depth perception on snow and glacial ice often is poor. Blowing snow can be reduced by packing down the snow with skis or a snow machine. Equipping a helicopter with snow pads helps reduce uncontrolled settling of the aircraft in snow.

Hot loading or hot off-loading (i.e., with the engine running) of a helicopter sometimes may be required for efficiency, such as for crew shuttles and power-on landings. However, remember that this practice poses greater risk for personnel. Anticipate the situation and secure loose debris and gear in advance. Personnel mentally get in a rush around a running helicopter, and this is when mistakes can easily occur. Shutting down the aircraft to load personnel or a rescue subject dramatically lowers the risk and increases the safety of everyone working near the aircraft.

Load Calculation

Exceeding the operating load limits of a particular helicopter can have devastating consequences. To ensure that a helicopter is not "over gross," a **load calculation** should be prepared before *any* mission. Although it might be viewed as an unnecessary delay during an emergency operation, the load calculation is an essential flight planning tool. Military crews may use a performance planning card to complete the load calculation. The aircrew assumes responsibility for completing the "load calc," using the following mission-specific information:

- *Helicopter equipped weight:* The empty weight of the aircraft, including accessories, without fuel on board.
- *Operating weight:* The weight of the aircraft plus flight crew and fuel load.
- *Allowable payload:* Calculated maximum permitted weight of passengers and cargo.
- *Actual payload:* The true weight of passengers and cargo.

NOTE: Preweighing SAR equipment and marking the weight so that it is clearly visible on the outside of the bags streamlines payload calculations during an operational response.

- *Maximum gross weight:* The certified maximum allowable weight of an aircraft; it is the maximum weight, as determined by the manufacturer and approved by the FAA, at which that particular aircraft can safely fly.

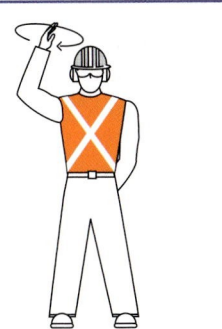

CLEAR TO START ENGINE
make a circular motion above
head with right arm.

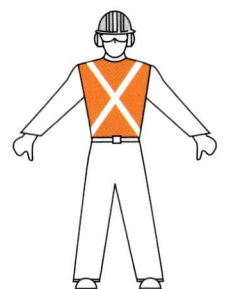

HOLD ON GROUND
stand arms out at 45°,
thumbs pointing down.

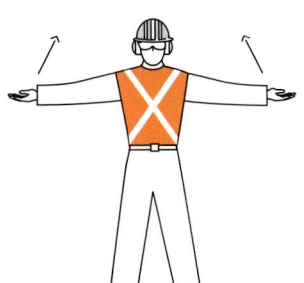

MOVE UPWARD
arms extended sweeping up.

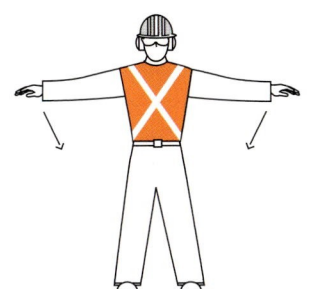

MOVE DOWNWARD
arms extended sweeping down.

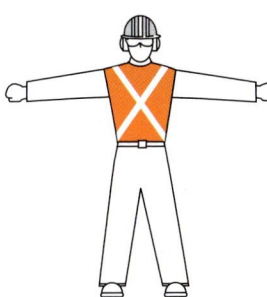

HOLD HOVER
arms extended with
clenched fists.

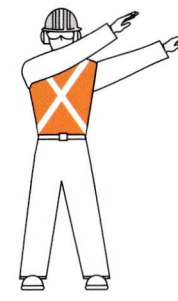

CLEAR TO TAKE-OFF
extend both arms above head

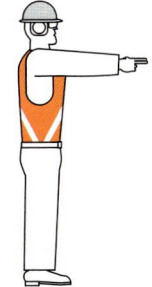

**LAND HERE, MY BACK IS
INTO THE WIND**
extend arms toward landing
area with wind at your back.

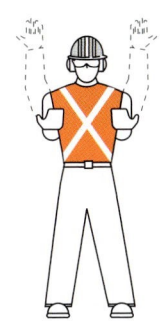

MOVE FORWARD
extend arms forward and wave

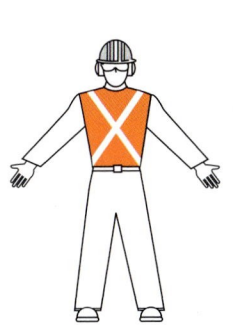

MOVE REARWARD
arms extended downward
using shoving motion.

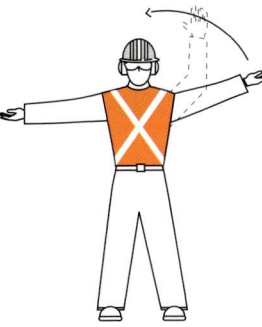

MOVE LEFT
right arm horizontal, left arm
sweeps over head.

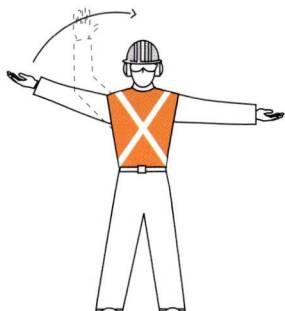

MOVE RIGHT
left arm horizontal, right arm
sweeps over head.

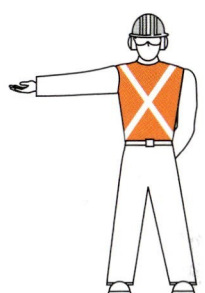

MOVE TAIL ROTOR
rotate body with one arm
extended.

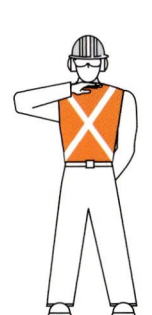

SHUT OFF ENGINE
cross neck with right hand,
palm down.

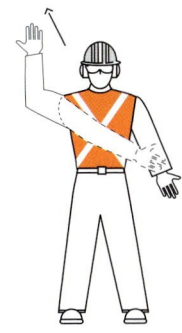

RELEASE SLING LOAD
contact left forearm with
right hand.

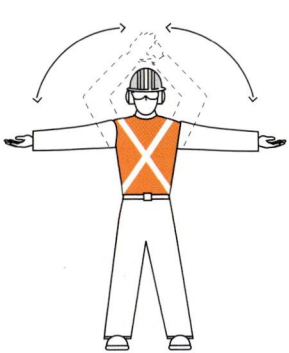

WAVE OFF DO NOT LAND
wave arms from horizontal

Figure 21-7 Hand signals.

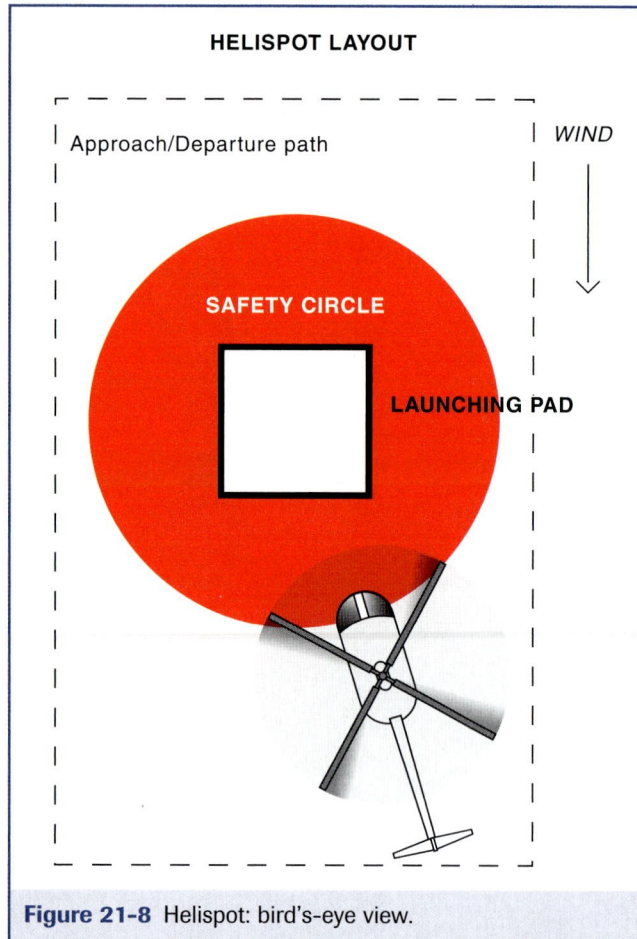

HELISPOT LAYOUT

Approach/Departure path

WIND

SAFETY CIRCLE

LAUNCHING PAD

Figure 21-8 Helispot: bird's-eye view.

- *Fixed weight reduction:* A fixed safety factor amount, used by federal land management agencies, that is assigned to types of aircraft to provide an additional margin of safety. The weight reduction calculation ensures that the maximum gross weight is not exceeded.

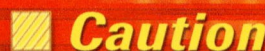

Caution

Perform a new load calculation when environmental conditions change, as with:
- Plus or minus 5° C (41° F) in temperature
- Plus or minus 1,000 feet (305 m) in altitude
- A significant change in the fuel load

NOTE: A pilot responding from a helibase to a remote site can determine the temperature at his or her destination using the *adiabatic rate* (i.e., air temperature decreases 3.5° F for every 1,000-foot [305 m] increase in elevation).

Helicopter Rescue Crews

The key to being a team, rather than just a group of individuals, is a shared mental image among all members. This allows team members to anticipate other members' actions and helps them share knowledge about the incident. Training and working together help foster this heightened level of coordinated teamwork. Mission briefings conducted before a rescue operation (Box 21-3) increase **situational awareness** by developing a shared mental image for all crew members. It is essential to identify who is in charge so that there is no confusion among team members during the emergency response.

Crew Configuration

The exact crew configuration varies based on the agency and aircraft size (Figure 21-10). However, most rescue helicopter crews include the following:

- *Pilot:* The **pilot in command (PIC)** conducts all activities related to flying the helicopter. He or she has final authority over and responsibility for the operation and safety of the flight (14 CFR* Part 1.1).
- *Copilot/helicopter manager:* The copilot/helicopter manager is responsible for performing en route navigation and communication tasks. The copilot serves as second in command of the aircraft during flight operations. This additional front seat crew member also serves as an extra set of eyes for aerial hazards and other aircraft, and they can assist in ground reconnaissance, permitting better flight concentration by the pilot in command.
- Operations chief/crew chief/spotter: This crew member is responsible for all operations in the aft cabin of the helicopter. While operating the helicopter rescue hoist or conducting helicopter rappel or short haul activities, he or she coordinates movement of the aircraft directly with the pilot.
- Rescuer/medic/pararescuer: This crew member performs rescue tasks related to hoist, short haul, or helicopter rappel operations. Once on the ground at the rescue site, this person becomes a link between ground rescuers at the

*See the section, Applicable U.S. Federal Regulations.

Table 21-2	Landing Zones		
Helicopter Type	**Type I**	**Type II**	**Type III**
Touchdown pad dimensions	30 feet × 30 feet (9 meters × 9 meters	20 feet x 20 feet (6 meters × 6 meters)	15 feet × 15 feet (4.6 meters × 4.6 meters)
Safety circle diameter	110 feet (33.528 meters)	90 feet (27.432 meters)	75 feet (22.86 meters)
From Interagency Helicopter Operations Guide (IHOG). NFES # 1885			

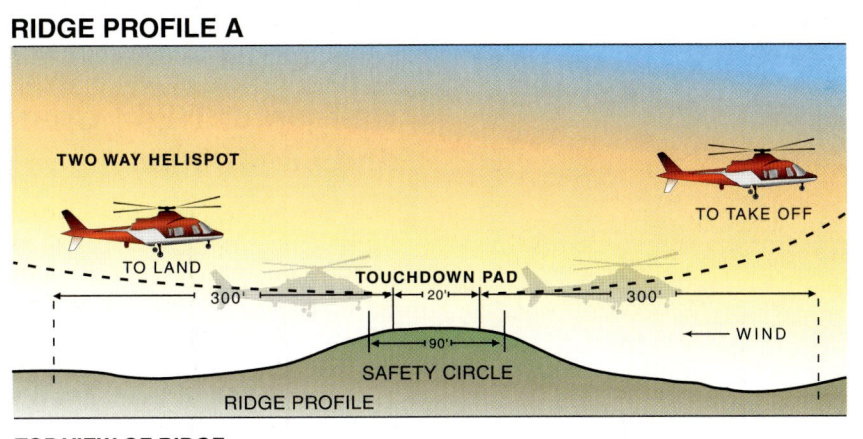

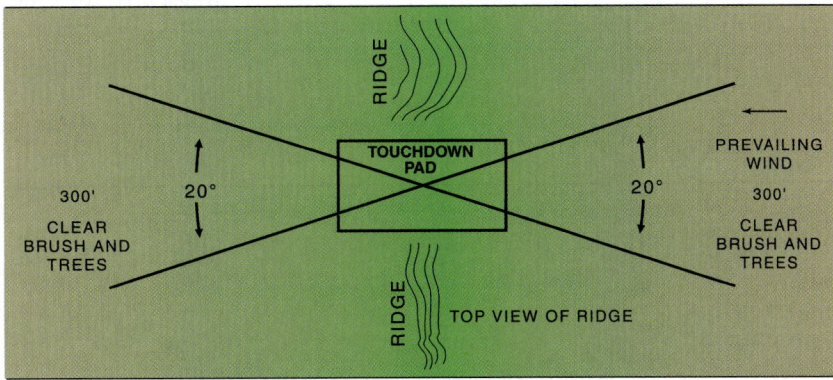

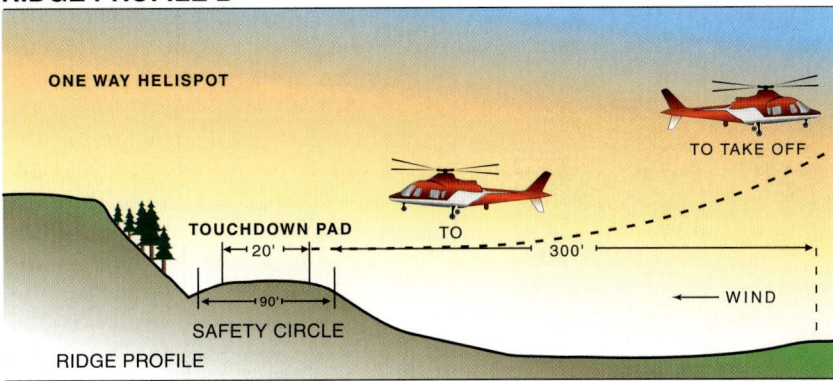

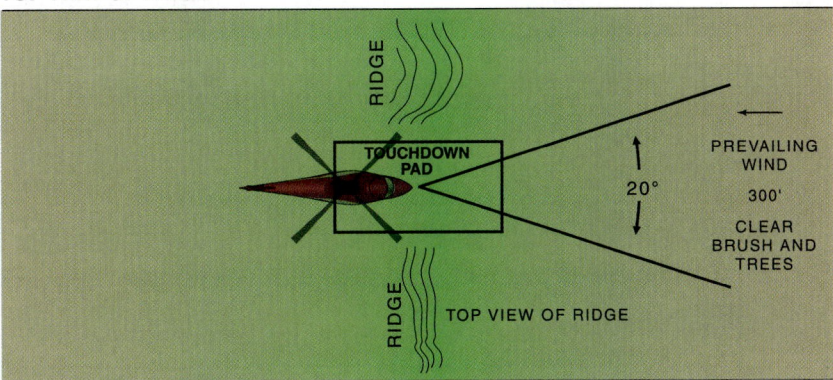

Figure 21-9 Helispot: profile view.

scene and the aircraft. He or she also provides medical care for the rescue subject both on the ground and aboard the helicopter.

Personal Preparedness

Helicopter rescuers quickly can find themselves deployed into an extreme environment in which they are not adequately prepared to function. They are vulnerable to accidents arising from environmental hazards, such as talus, exposed cliff faces, snow or ice, and swift water. The choice of footwear and outerwear, as well as personal survival gear, should be a priority for aircrews that could be exposed to such extremes. Becoming too focused

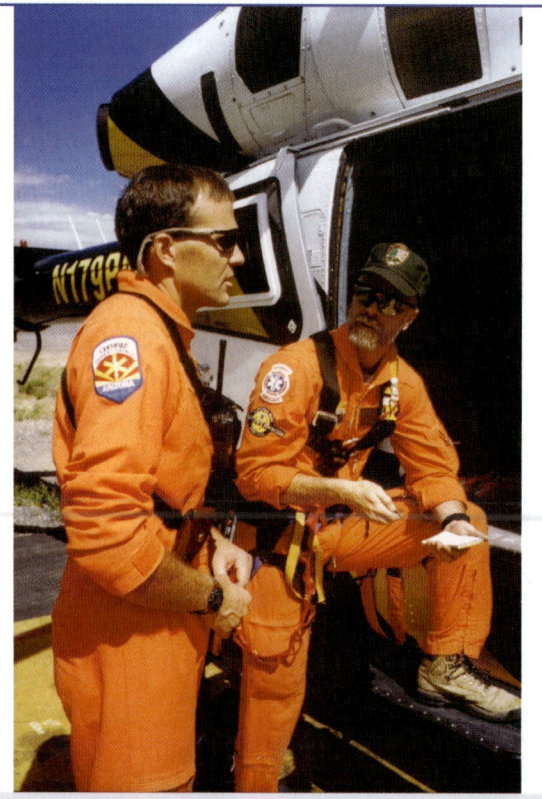

Figure 21-10 Crew briefing. Grand Canyon National Park (Arizona) rangers conducting a mission briefing before initiating a helicopter-based SAR response. (Courtesy NPS.)

on providing a fast emergency medical response for a rescue subject can cause even the most professional aircrews to develop "situational blindness" to their surroundings.

Helicopter Flight Characteristics and Limitations

A basic understanding of the flight characteristics of helicopters allows ground rescuers to make more informed decisions on rescue plans.

Helicopter Aerodynamics

The main rotor blades on a helicopter rotate in a horizontal circular area and act as "wings" or airfoils to create lift for the helicopter. Lift increases as the pitch of the helicopter blades increases. This provides a greater pressure difference between the top and bottom sides of the airfoil. Landing into the wind aids this aerodynamic principle, because with the increased wind velocity over the airfoil, less power is required to achieve the same amount of lift. This is an important concept for ground rescuers to understand, because a pilot will attempt to land and take off into the direction of the oncoming wind.

The circular area defined by the moving tips of the rotor is referred to as the *disc area*. The rotational motion of the rotor blades generates **torque** in the opposite direction. A tail rotor provides *anti-torque* control to compensate and prevent the helicopter from spinning out of control. The use of floor pedals connected to the tail rotor allows the pilot to vary the amount of thrust in the opposite direction.

On helicopters equipped with the NOTAR (NO TAil Rotor) system, the tail rotor is replaced by an adjustable jet thruster. A high-speed, variable pitch fan directs air through the tail boom. Open slots direct air along the exterior of the tail boom, counteracting the torque of the main rotor blades through a force known as the *Coanda effect* (for Romanian scientist Henri Coanda, circa 1910). The tailboom becomes a "wing" flying in the downwash of the main rotor, producing up to 70% of the anti-torque required in a **hover**.[4] The rotating thruster at the end of the tail boom allows the pilot to move the tail boom in either direction.

The pilot can vary the pitch of the main rotor blades to permit the helicopter to climb or descend through the use of the collective pitch control, which is located to the pilot's left (Figure 21-11). At the end of the collective is the throttle, which can be increased manually. The **collective pitch system** also controls power output by demand. As the pitch of the blades is increased, the engine must generate more power to maintain a constant rate of revolutions per minute (rpm).

The **cyclic** control, which is located between the pilot's legs, directs the forward, backward, and sideways movement of the helicopter through corresponding tilting of the rotor disc.

Ground Effect

When a helicopter is in a low hover, the ground interrupts the airflow under the helicopter, and the velocity of the induced airflow to the rotor system is reduced. The result is less induced drag and a more vertical lift vector. This ground cushion, or **ground effect**, is beneficial in flight because it increases the lift

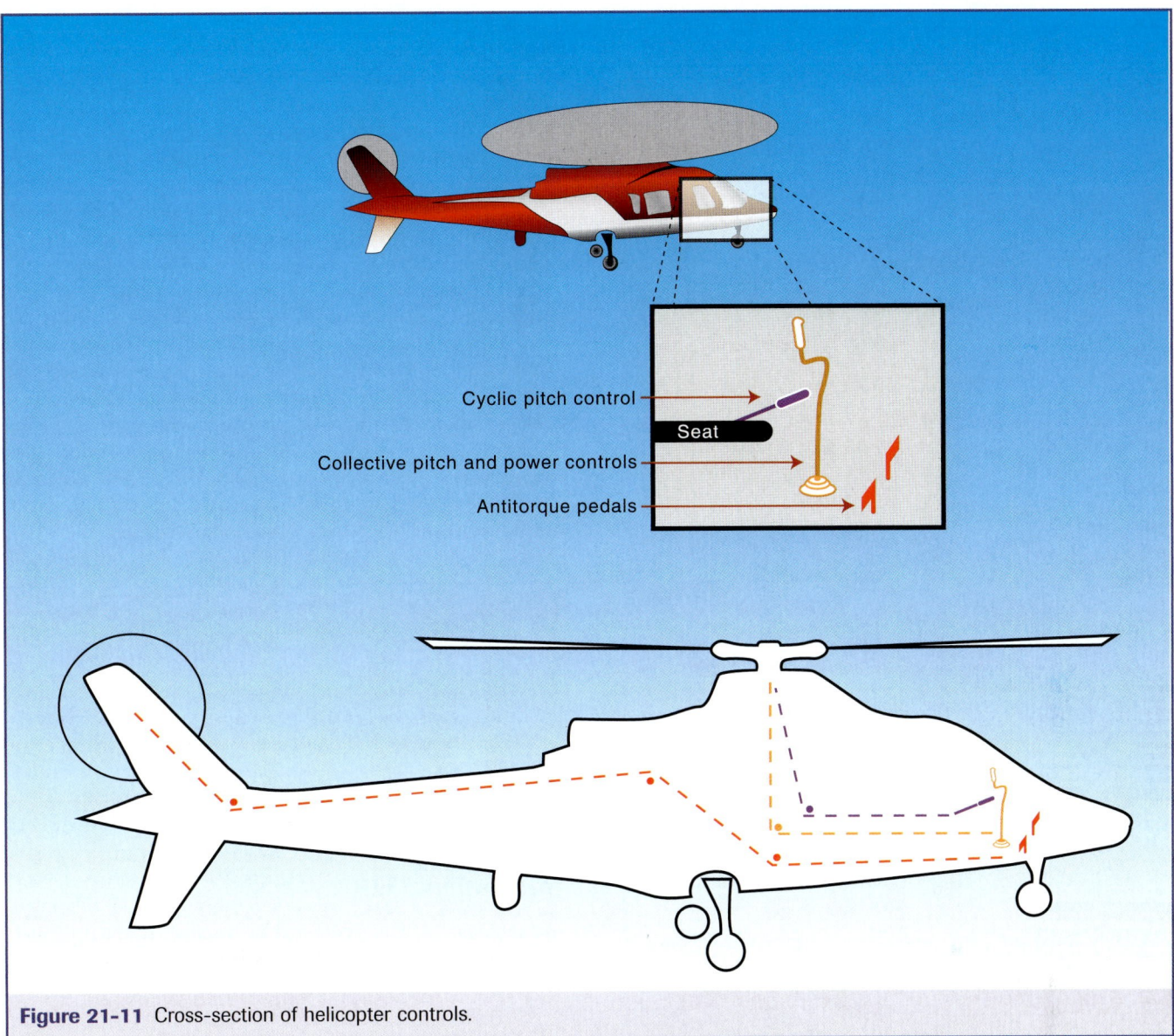

Figure 21-11 Cross-section of helicopter controls.

Labels in figure: Cyclic pitch control · Collective pitch and power controls · Antitorque pedals · Seat

capability of the helicopter, which consequently requires less power to maintain a hover. Ground effect occurs when the helicopter is at a very low altitude, usually one half the rotor diameter. Ground effect is disturbed by uneven terrain, vegetation, or water beneath the rotor disc.

Hover in Ground and Out of Ground Effects

Rescuers should have an understanding of the following helicopter maneuvers:

- *Hover in ground effect (HIGE)* (Figure 21-12): To hover at an altitude (usually one half the rotor diameter above the surface) at which the positive influence of ground effect is attained.
- *Hover out of ground effect (HOGE):* To hover at an altitude high enough that the added benefit of ground effect is not obtained.
NOTE: Tall grass or slopes produce a HOGE hover.

Hovering Over Water

Water dissipates the rotor downwash generated beneath a hovering helicopter, thereby decreasing ground effect hovering capability. Moving water reduces ground effect even more. This decrease in operating efficiency during swift water rescue operations could be significant, because the helicopter actually is hovering out of ground effect. An additional concern during swift water rescue operations is the visual effect of the rushing water, which can lead to pilot disorientation. The pilot can combat this hazard by using a fixed reference point in the water or on the shore.

Autorotation

Autorotation allows a helicopter to land safely, within defined limits, if the engine fails in flight. As the helicopter descends, the airflow is upward through the rotor system, causing a

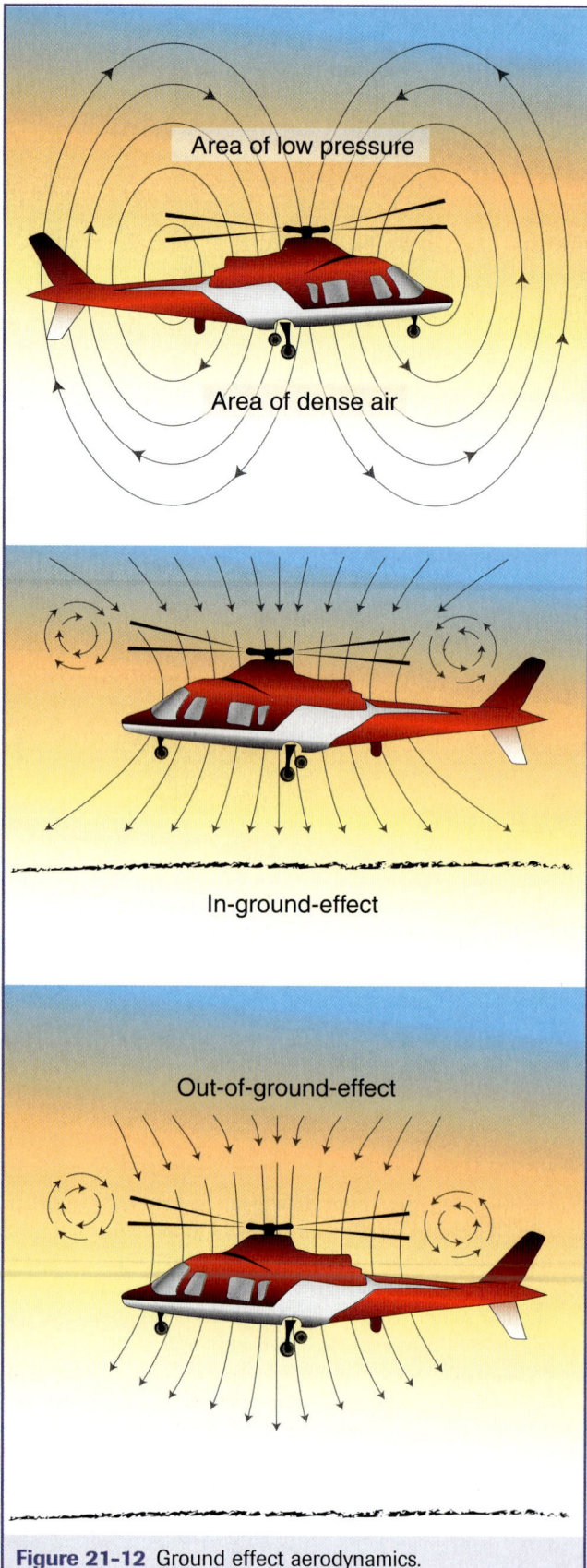

Area of low pressure

Area of dense air

In-ground-effect

Out-of-ground-effect

Figure 21-12 Ground effect aerodynamics.

windmilling of the blades. By changing the pitch of the blades, the pilot can maintain constant rpm. The pilot slows the aircraft using the stored blade inertia and can cushion the helicopter to a landing.

The flight manual for a particular helicopter has a **height-velocity curve,** a chart that shows the airspeed required at given altitudes for a successful autorotation (Figure 21-13). The shaded (cautionary) portions of this chart indicate areas in which it would be unsafe to conduct an autorotation (hence the height-velocity curve also is referred to as the *dead man's curve*).

The minimum altitude for a safe autorotation by most light, single engine helicopters is 350 to 450 feet (107 to 137 m) above ground level with zero forward airspeed, as in a hover.[5] This has serious implications for all helicopter rescue personnel, because the low-altitude hovers used for rappelling, hoisting, and short haul operations all are within the cautionary portions of the height-velocity curve charts. Although multiengine helicopters have quite different height-velocity curves, along with improved capabilities in low hovers, rescuers should be wary and remain alert when working beneath *any* hovering helicopter.

▨ Warning

All rescuers working beneath a low-hovering helicopter must remain aware of the increased risk arising from the pilots' inability to autorotate safely. All ground personnel should have a mental escape plan ready.

Translational Lift

Translational lift is the additional lift generated as the helicopter transitions from a hover to horizontal flight. This additional lift comes from the increased efficiency of the rotor system, which generates more lift in forward flight, which involves a higher inflow velocity of air mass than does a hover.

Types of Helicopter Landings

From a risk management perspective, the preferred helicopter landing is a full touchdown landing at an acceptable landing zone. This method poses less risk to the aircrew and ground rescuers. In some situations the landing zone may be distant from the rescue site; even so, a litter carryout to a removed landing zone may be a better option than other, higher risk extraction techniques such as a helicopter hoist or short haul.

One-Skid Landings

A **one-skid landing** (Figure 21-14) is used in rugged terrain where the topography prevents a normal landing with both skids on the ground. On a steep slope, the pilot may have to put a single skid alongside the slope and allow rescuers to board or exit the aircraft slowly.

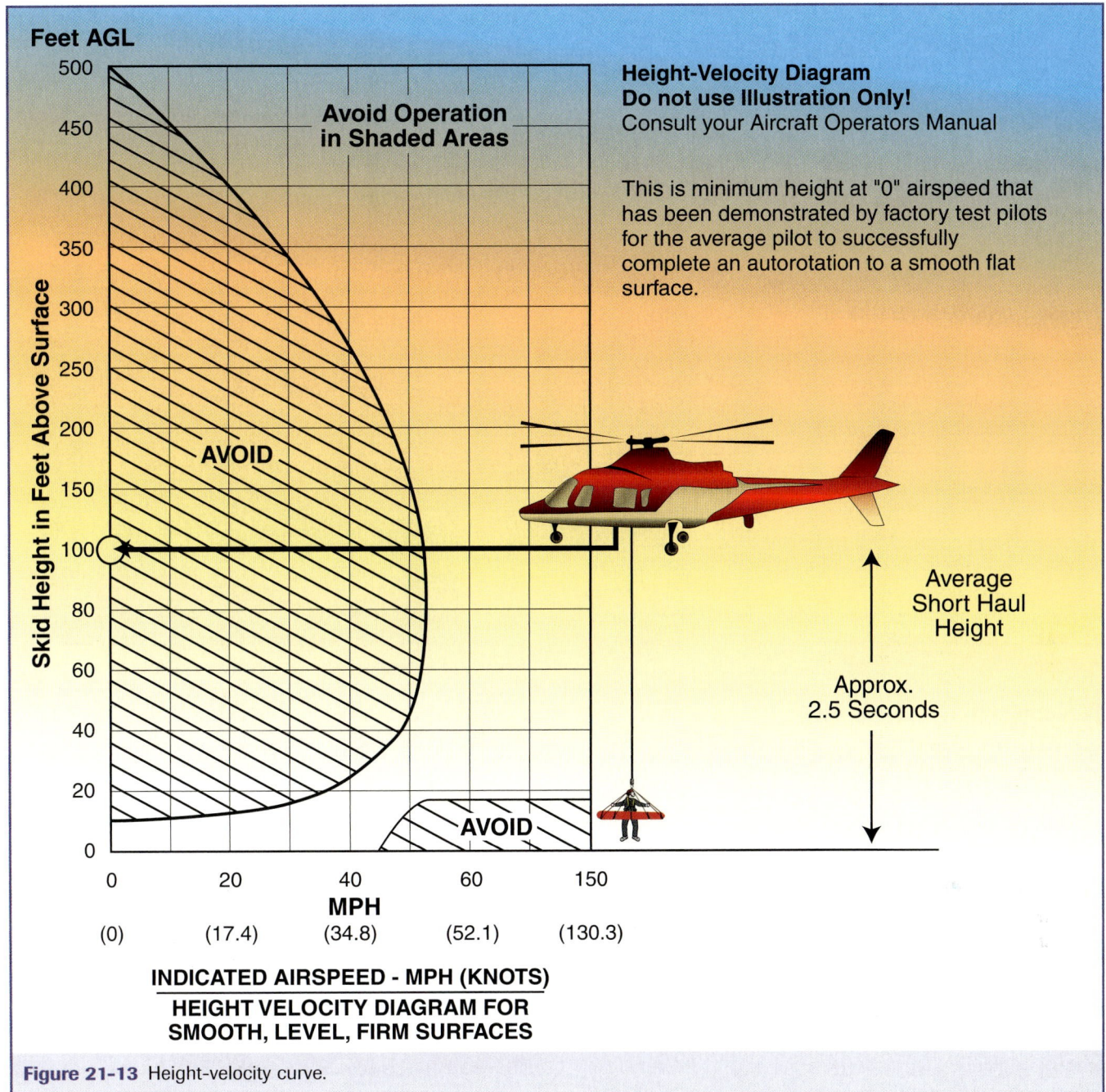

Figure 21-13 Height-velocity curve.

Toe-In Landings

A *toe-in landing* is similar to a one-skid landing in that only the front tips of the skids make contact with the ground. Both of these landing techniques are more risky, because a sudden shift in the internal load of the helicopter may cause the aircraft to become unstable, leading to a crash as a result of contact with the adjacent topography.

One-skid and toe-in landings also put the aircraft close to physical hazards. Although used by many agencies, these techniques require practice and are not a recommended option for most teams, especially those with only intermittent experience with helicopter operations. These landing techniques are not an option to be suddenly improvised during the heat of the moment on a rescue.

Step-out landings and *hover landings* are used to drop off or pick up passengers and cargo while the helicopter is held in a hover. The helicopter is not in contact with the ground, and its center of gravity can shift laterally and longitudinally. This type of landing often is used instead of a toe-in or single-skid landing in terrain where the helicopter cannot land, but it remains a high-risk maneuver that requires considerable practice.

A less risky consideration for a marginal landing zone is a *power-on landing,* in which the pilot places both skids in full

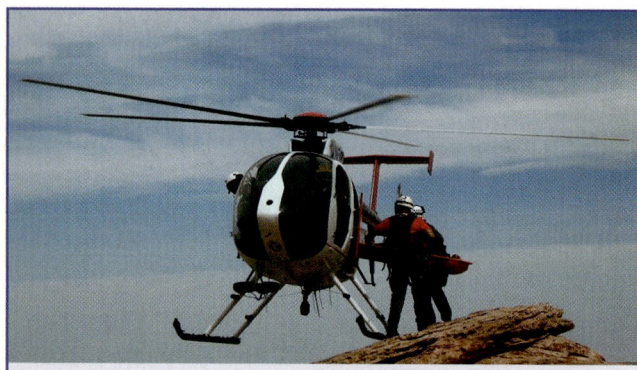

Figure 21-14 One-skid landing. Members of the Las Vegas Metropolitan Police Department SAR Team conduct a one-skid landing. The pilot of the McDonnell Douglas MD530F carefully rests one skid of the aircraft on a rock as SAR personnel load a litter in the aft cabin. (Courtesy Las Vegas Metropolitan Police Department.)

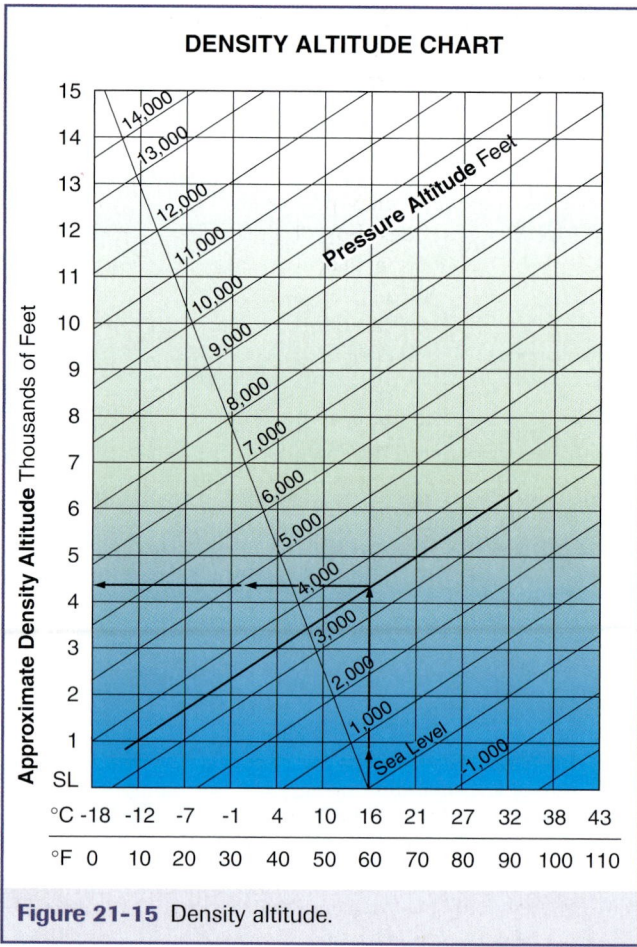

Figure 21-15 Density altitude.

contact with the ground while running full power to maintain the position of the aircraft. This type of landing may be an operational consideration when a minimal touchdown pad is bordered by steep terrain that precludes powering down the helicopter.

Helicopter Performance
Density Altitude

Density altitude provides a measure of the air density (Figure 21-15). The density altitude greatly affects a helicopter's performance. At lower elevations the rotor blade cuts through denser air, which provides a better performance than the air at higher altitudes. At an altitude of 10,000 feet (3,048 m), for example, there are fewer air molecules per cubic foot of air, which results in diminished performance.

Density altitude is defined as the actual pressure altitude corrected for temperature and humidity variations. An easier way of viewing this is that density altitude is the altitude that the aircraft thinks it is at. An increase in humidity has a minor effect on density altitude compared with an increase in the altitude or temperature. Humid air is less dense than dry air, which means that aircraft performance suffers on a humid day. Aircraft performance charts commonly reflect only air temperature and pressure altitude. To understand the dramatic effects of density altitude, consider that on an 80° F (27° C) day at 8,000 feet (2,438 m), the density altitude is 11,100 feet (3,383 m)! High density altitudes may also be present at low elevations on hot days.

Hover Ceiling

The ***hover ceiling*** is the highest altitude at which a helicopter can successfully hover while loaded to its ***maximum gross weight***. In and out of ground effect hover ceilings are computed at maximum gross weight.

Center of Gravity

The ***center of gravity (CG)*** is the point in a helicopter where all forces are balanced. In a single-rotor helicopter, this is a range forward or aft and under the rotor mast. This is a critical balance for safe flight, and it is affected by the distribution of the weight of fuel, personnel, and cargo in the helicopter.

Maximum Gross Weight

The maximum gross weight is the certified maximum allowable weight of the aircraft, as determined by the manufacturer and approved by the FAA, at which that particular aircraft can safely fly. This weight includes the equipped weight of the aircraft plus that of the useful load (i.e., pilot, passengers, cargo, and fuel).

Basic Helicopter Safety
Preboarding

Before boarding a helicopter as a passenger, obtain a preflight briefing from the pilot or aircrew (required by FAA regulations 14 CFR Part 135.117). At a *minimum,* the preflight briefing should include the following information specific to the helicopter:

- Location of the first aid kit and any survival equipment
- Location and operation of the fire extinguisher

- Emergency electrical and fuel shutoff controls
- Operation of doors and seat belts
- Emergency procedures

Safety During Helicopter Operations

Observe the following safety procedures when helicopters are used on rescue operations (Box 21-4):

- Never approach the helicopter until the pilot or crew directs you to do so. Then, approach and depart from the side or front of the aircraft in a crouching position and in full view of the pilot (Figure 21-16). *Never* walk toward the tail rotor.
- To avoid the main rotor, approach and depart on the down slope side of the aircraft.
- Use the door latches as instructed. To avoid damaging fragile aircraft components, be cautious around Plexiglas and moving parts.
- Fasten your seat belt upon boarding the helicopter and leave it secured until the pilot signals for you to disembark. Fasten the seat belt behind you as you leave the aircraft.
- Keep landing areas free of loose debris that rotor wash may pick up.
- Do not throw items from the helicopter, because they could strike the rotor system.
- Provide visual wind indicators for landing and takeoff; stand at the edge of the landing zone with your back to the wind and your arms pointing at the touchdown pad (Figure 21-17).
- When working on the ground around a helicopter, wear eye and hearing protection, along with a helmet secured by a chin strap.

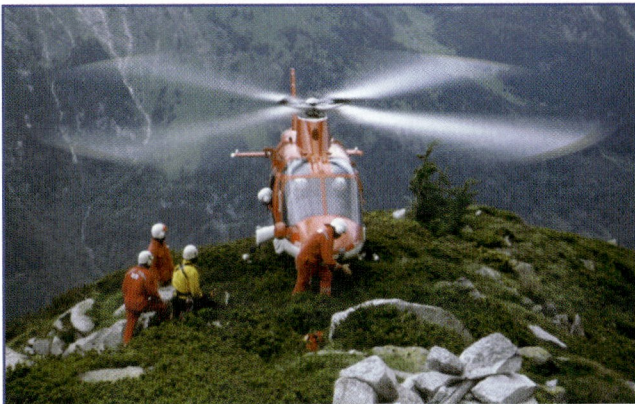

Figure 21-16 Approach and departure around a helicopter. Rescue personnel safely approach a REGA Augusta A109-K2 helicopter at a mountain helispot in Switzerland. (Courtesy Dominik Hunziker.)

- Secure all cargo placed aboard the helicopter; provide the pilot or aircrew with accurate weights.
- Hot loading of passengers or a rescue subject involves greater risk; always be alert when conducting such a maneuver. Consider reducing the risk when practical by shutting down the aircraft.
- Landing zones should have acceptable rotor clearance for the aircraft assigned to the incident, and all incident personnel should be aware of these clearance requirements.
- As a passenger, know the aircraft's location and have a mental plan for what to do in the event of a crash or in-flight emergency.

Personnel Protective Equipment

The military, federal civilian agencies, and most public safety organizations have strict requirements for the personal protective equipment (PPE) that must be worn by the crew and pas-

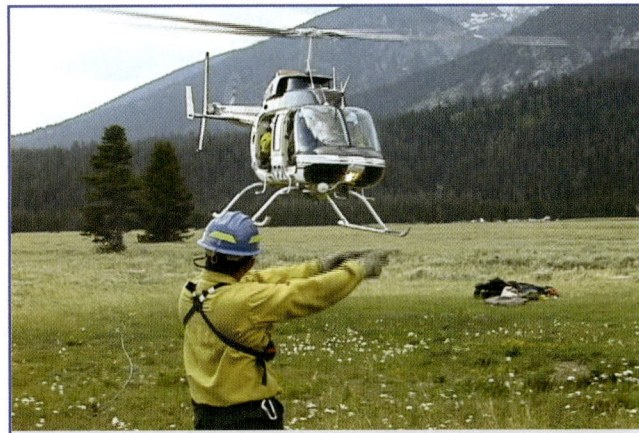

Figure 21-17 Helispot manager. A Yosemite National Park helispot manager, wearing personal protective equipment (PPE), marshals a helicopter using hand signals at a meadow helispot in Yosemite Valley. (Courtesy Yosemite SAR.)

Box 21-4	Twelve Standard Aviation Questions That Could Save Your Life

1. Is this flight necessary?
2. Who is in charge?
3. Have all hazards been identified and have you made them known?
4. Should you stop the operation or flight because of:
   - ❏ Inadequate and unclear communications
   - ❏ Hazardous weather
   - ❏ Turbulence
   - ❏ Insufficient or untrained personnel
   - ❏ Conflicting priorities
   - ❏ Deceased rescue subject
5. Is there a better way to do it?
6. Are you driven by an overwhelming sense of urgency?
7. Can you justify your actions?
8. Are other aircraft in the area?
9. Do you have an escape route?
10. Are any rules being broken?
11. Are communications getting tense?
12. Are you deviating from the assigned operation or flight?

Remember: **WHEN IN DOUBT—DON'T!**

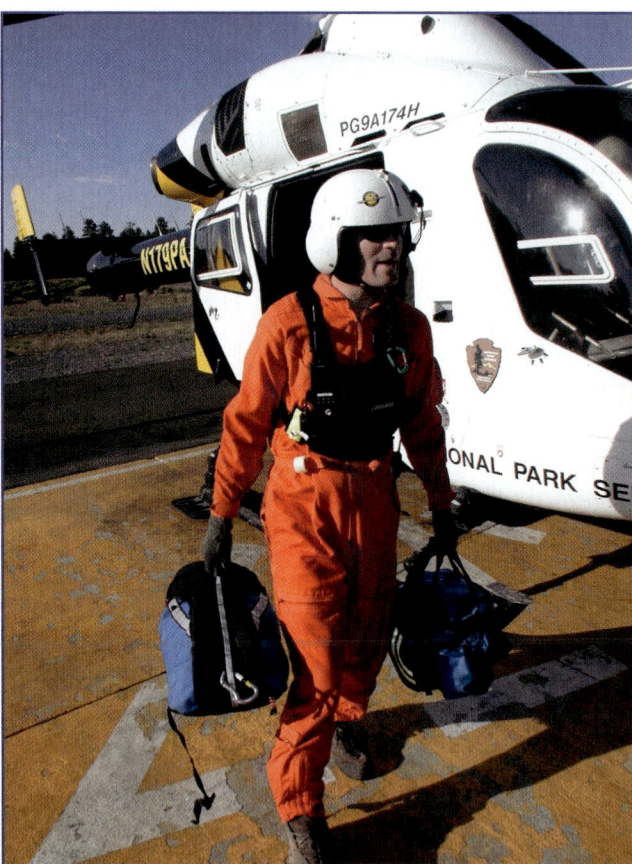

Figure 21-18 Personal protective equipment. Helicopter crew member in personal protective equipment (PPE) including Nomex flightsuit, Nomex gloves, and flight helmet. (Courtesy Ken Phillips.)

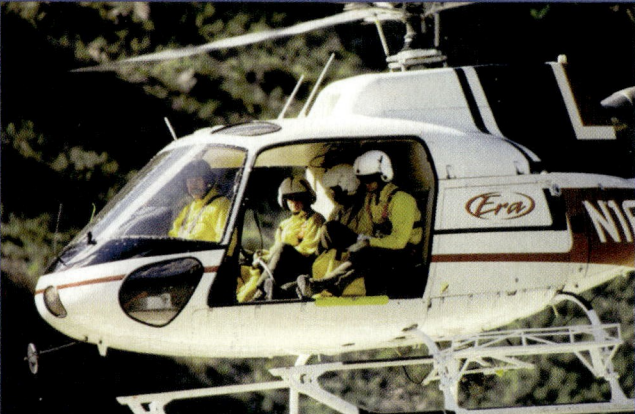

Figure 21-19 Flight helmet. Helicopter rappellers/firefighters with the U.S. Forest Service's Moyer Rappel Crew lift off in a Eurocopter AS350B2 A-Star. Wearing personal protection equipment that includes a flight helmet, these firefighters depart for an initial attack response of a forest fire in central Idaho, west of Salmon. (Courtesy Paul M. Ross, Jr.)

sengers aboard rescue helicopters. Although turbine-powered helicopters are highly reliable, the potential for crash and postcrash injuries still exists. For example, a common risk is a flash fire after the crash, therefore fire-resistant clothing is a necessity (Figure 21-18). Personal protective equipment includes the following:

- *Fire-resistant clothing:* A loose-fitting flight suit or clothing made of Nomex or PBI helps protect against injuries from fire. The loose-fitting style provides an airspace between the fabric and the skin that acts as insulation against heat sources. However, although the fabric reduces the risk or severity of tissue damage, it does not prevent thermal injury to the skin. Nomex is a fire-resistant aramid fiber manufactured by the DuPont Corp. (Wilmington, Delaware). PBI (Polybenzimidazole) is a synthetic fiber produced by Celanese AG. It has no melting point, will not ignite, and retains fiber integrity and suppleness when exposed to flames. The heat transfer through Nomex or PBI could be high enough to melt synthetic undergarments (e.g., polypropylene or Capilene), therefore these fabrics should not be worn next to the skin during flight operations. Flamestop fleece, a fire-resistant, insulating fleece material made from Nomex, is a particularly useful garment material for cold weather helicopter rescue operations.

- *Flight helmet:* Although a costly piece of equipment, a helicopter flight helmet provides the most effective head protection in the event of impact. The Gentex SPH-5 helmet (sound protective helmet), made by the Gentex Corp. (Zeeland, Michigan), is the commercial version of the U.S. Army and U.S. Coast Guard helicopter helmets (Figure 21-19). It provides a maximum peak force deceleration up to 300 Gs (0.4 milliseconds duration) inside the helmet during a sustained impact (single strike using ANSI Z-90.1 test design), which enables the helmet to distribute the impact to a survivable level for the wearer.[6] The flight helmet's design allows communication through a noise-canceling microphone and earphones in the earcups; other features include noise suppression, a protective visor, and an energy-absorbing liner. Even though climbing helmets and firefighter hard hats frequently are worn by ground rescuers aboard helicopters on rescue missions, they are inferior substitutes for a flight helmet, which has been specifically designed for this application.

- *Footwear and hand, eye, and ear protection:* Nomex or leather gloves, as well as leather shoes that are at least ankle height, provide added protection against fire injuries. Nylon components on lightweight hiking boots can melt in a postcrash fire, resulting in burn injuries. The environment of the rescue, such as winter alpine conditions or over-water operations, may dictate footwear (e.g., plastic mountaineering boots) that is more reasonable for outside conditions. Fire-resistant clothing should have sleeves that can be worn over the gauntlet of the gloves and legs long enough to eliminate exposure between the clothing and the tops of the boots. Sunglasses or lightweight, wrap-around skydiving goggles provide excellent eye protection for the blowing prop wash generated by helicopters. Disposable earplugs provide added hearing protection against the high decibel levels of helicopters.

Box 21-5 | Helicopter Rescue Training

1. Review your internal agency aviation guidelines and make sure that written operating procedures are current.
2. Conduct basic helicopter safety training for all personnel who will be involved in aviation activities.
3. Carry out premission training for specific helicopter rescue techniques that will be used.
4. Evolve from ground-based classroom instruction to mock-ups and then actual training flight exercises.
5. Include *typical terrain* training, which is as realistic as possible. This helps highlight deficiencies in equipment or procedures that could become a problem during an actual mission.
6. Maintain skill proficiency on a regular and recurring basis. Without the benefit of repeated exposure to helicopter operations, personnel lose their composure and discipline.

Box 21-6 | European Aviation Regulations

The European Joint Aviation Authorities (JAA), an associated organization of the European Civil Aviation Conference (ECAC), represents the civil aviation regulatory agencies of a number of European countries. Besides working to develop common safety standards, the JAA strives to harmonize its regulations with those of the Federal Aviation Administration (FAA) in the United States. The *Joint Aviation Regulations (JAR)* published by the JAA, make no regulatory distinction between public aircraft and commercial aircraft in Europe.[8]

- *Harnesses:* During hoisting, short haul, and rappelling operations, mission-specific rescue harnesses are worn by crew chiefs/spotters as a tether to the aircraft. Rescuer/medics wear harnesses approved by their flight program. The features of these harnesses can include dorsal attachment points, full-body harness design, and suspension comfort.
- *Personal flotation device:* When over-water flights lack sufficient glide distance to shore, the aircrew should don an aviation life vest for personal safety. An inflatable, FAA-approved personal flotation device (PFD) is preferable to the bulky, U.S. Coast Guard–approved, foam-filled PFD, which would actually restrict a user's ability to safely exit an aircraft that becomes immersed in water.

Applicable U.S. Federal Regulations

Unlike with other high angle rescue techniques, personnel using helicopter rescue methods are affected by statutory regulations. These regulations include the U.S. Federal Aviation Regulations (FAR) in Title 14 of the Code of Federal Regulations (CFR). The European equivalent of the FAR is the Joint Aviation Regulations (JAR) (Box 21-6). Of interest to most rescue agencies is FAR Part 133, Rotorcraft External Load Operations, specifically section 133.1, which exempts "a federal, state, or local government conducting operations with *public aircraft*" from the rotorcraft regulations.

The FAA designates rotorcraft-load combinations as Class A through Class D. "Class D" refers to rescue operations in which the human external load is suspended below the helicopter.

If a private operator (non–public aircraft) were to consider trying a short haul operation, another obstacle exists in the form of Part 133.45(e), 1-4, which requires the use of a twin-engine aircraft with "hover capability with one engine inoperative at that operating weight and altitude." In addition, aircraft-to-rescuer communications are required, along with an FAA-approved "personnel lifting device" that has an emergency release that

requires two distinct actions. "FAA approved" means that a piece of equipment, such as an anchor point, has received a **supplemental type certificate (STC)** verifying that it does not affect the airworthiness of the aircraft.

FAR Part 133.31, Emergency Operations (a), states, "In an emergency involving the safety of persons or property, the certificate holder may deviate from the rules of this part to the extent required to meet that emergency."

This regulation *does not* give rescue organizations, when confronted with a life-threatening emergency on the ground, clearance to violate FAA rules in order to accomplish a mission.

It is important to understand that Part 133.31(a) refers to in-flight emergencies and the helicopter pilot's deviation from rules to handle such an emergency. Rescue organizations unfortunately have sometimes interpreted this regulation as a loophole that allows them to improvise a rescue operation. However, the fact is, such a practice removes the critical need for advance training, and crews may end up carrying out a mission without the requisite proficiency.[7]

In-Flight Emergency: Survival Plan Checklist

The following measures are important in the event of an in-flight emergency:
- Follow the instructions of the pilot and aircrew.
- Secure your seat belt and harness.
- Keep clear of the controls, secure loose gear, and note emergency exits.
- Make sure in advance to wear appropriate head protection.
- Forward-facing passengers with a shoulder harness should sit in the full upright position with the head and back against the seat and the arms folded across the chest.
- Forward-facing passengers without a shoulder harness (lap belt only) should bend forward until their chests rest on their thighs. Arms should be clasped together under their thighs to hold this position.
- Passengers with lap belts and shoulder harnesses should sit with their backs straight and against the seat back as much as possible. If a manual inertia reel lock is available, and time and conditions permit, the reel should be manually locked.

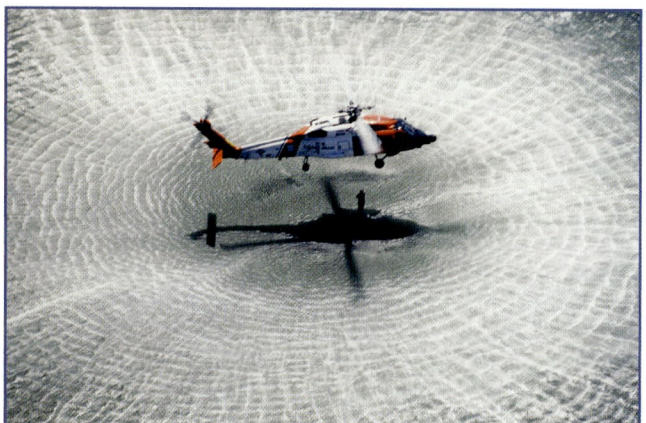

Figure 21-20 Over water operations. An aviation survival technician (AST) and a rescue swimmer are hoisted by an HH-60J helicopter from Air Station Elizabeth City during a search and rescue demonstration for Coast Guard Missions Day at Reserve Training Center Yorktown. (Courtesy United States Coast Guard.)

- Side-facing passengers should bend forward at the waist, grasp the arms under legs, and place the head between the knees.
- Assist any injured individuals who cannot leave the aircraft.
- Exit the helicopter only after the rotor blades have stopped or when instructed to do so by the aircrew.
- Assess the situation and render aid as needed.

Water Ditching Survival Training

Aircrews involved in over-water operations must be thoroughly trained in water ditching procedures (Figure 21-20 and Box 21-7). This very realistic training involves the use of a "dunker" device, which can be brought to a swimming pool, to simulate a water ditching emergency. This training helps participants develop the confidence to survive a water ditching incident without panicking.

Rescue Subject Care and Transport Considerations

Providing effective medical care to a packaged rescue subject while using an external helicopter technique (e.g., hoist or short haul) is significantly more difficult than in conventional rope-based rescue (Figure 21-21). Helicopter operations require the litter attendant simultaneously to contend with rotor wash, flying debris, preventing litter spin, the forward motion of the aircraft, *and* the subject's medical needs (see Chapter 15 for further medical considerations related to attended litter operations).

During hoisting and short haul operations, a litter attendant is not in a practical position to perform extensive medical care in-flight. However, the litter attendant is very important in these types of operations. A subject who vomits and aspirates in-flight is a very real potential problem. Why would an apparently stable subject vomit and aspirate? Aeromedical researchers have found that eight *classic stressors* of flight can lead to profound effects on human physiology[9] (Box 21-8).

A rescue subject is affected by the noise, vibration, and thermal changes that occur during helicopter rescue operations. Low-frequency vibration can induce motion sickness, which stimulates the "vomiting center" of the medulla. In addition, vibration can cause fatigue, shortness of breath, and abdominal and chest pain. Vibration against a subject causes mechanical energy to be transformed into heat energy as body tissues provide dampening, resulting in increased metabolic and respiratory rates. Temperature changes, both hot and cold, in conjunction with exposure to vibration, can inhibit the body's compensation mechanisms.[9,10]

Visual stimuli and anxiety, compounded by motion, precipitate an attack of motion sickness, leading to nausea and vomiting.

Box 21-7 | Water Ditching Checklist

Remind yourself that you can survive a water ditching incident. Most important, **DON'T PANIC!** Panic can be avoided by remaining calm and thinking clearly.

1. Secure loose items. Put your flight helmet visor down and sweep the boom microphone to the side.
2. Unplug your flight helmet.
3. Establish a reference point with your hand (e.g., a door handle). Do not let go of your reference point.
4. Just before contact with the water, crack open the aircraft door.
5. As the aircraft settles in the water, count slowly to five to allow rotor movement to cease.
6. Release your seat belt with your free hand.
7. Exit the aircraft, following your reference point hand.
8. Hand up, look up, and come up toward the surface, following the air bubbles.
9. Survey the surface for hazards and survivors.
10. Inflate your flotation device (don't inflate it inside the aircraft).

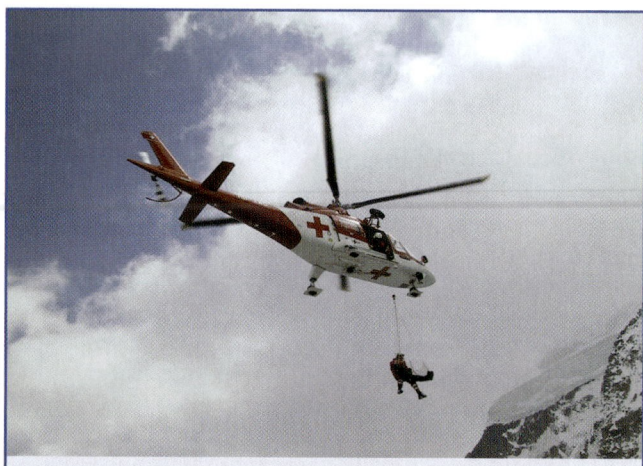

Figure 21-21 Litter attendant. A rescuer suspended beneath an Augusta A109-K2 attends to a patient during a hoist rescue by REGA (Swiss Air Rescue). (Courtesy Dominik Hunziker.)

Box 21-8 | Classic Stressors of Flight

- Noise
- Vibration
- Thermal changes
- Fatigue
- Barometric pressure
- Decreased humidity
- Decreased partial pressure of oxygen
- Gravity (G) forces

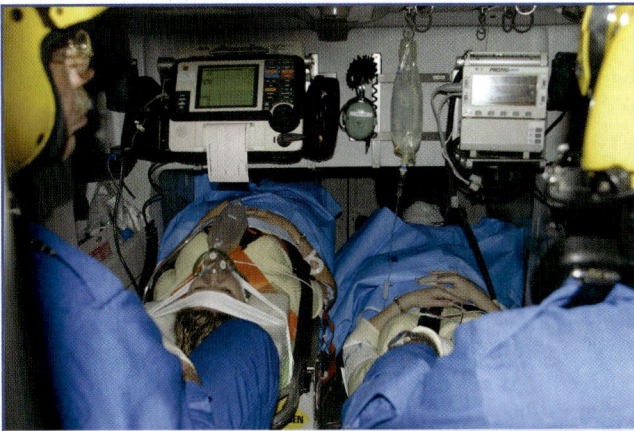

Figure 21-22 Medevac transport. An aeromedical flight crew with Austin/Travis County EMS treats two subjects in flight. (Courtesy Austin/Travis County EMS.)

Visual fixation on other moving objects may also precipitate an attack. This is distinctly different from another malady that affects helicopter transport of subjects with a head injury, a disorder known as *flicker seizures,* which occur when a recumbent individual is affected by the visual strobing effect of rotor blades overhead.

If an adequate power margin exists with the helicopter, a litter attendant is beneficial for an injured subject during hoisting and short haul operations. Simply riding along to share the flight and scenery with the subject is wrong! However, just the presence of an attendant has a considerable positive influence in reducing the rescue subject's anxiety level.

Practice and ensure proper attendant positioning in relation to the subject. Using an inclined, head-up position for the litter and providing an accompanying attendant to clear the subject's airway manually could make a critical difference. The litter attendant should have a manual suction device (e.g., V-Vac or Res-q-vac) readily available on a tether. Unlike other forms of vomiting, vestibular emesis is not relieved by throwing up, therefore continual suctioning and being prepared to clear the airway several times are absolutely vital.

Performing effective cardiopulmonary resuscitation (CPR) in-flight is simply not practical. A subject who is already in cardiac arrest at a rescue scene is best served by good resuscitation efforts there, rather than by attempts at wild heroics in the air.

Additional Rescue Subject Care Considerations

Antiemetics (Antinausea Drugs)

When antiemetics are administered before a helicopter hoisting or short haul extraction, allow for the time of onset required for the drug to take effect. Although aeromedical crews routinely use antiemetics in the prehospital setting, it may be more practical to forgo such delays at the site before a hoisting or short haul extraction and to monitor the subject's airway closely in-flight. In addition, many antiemetics have side effects, such as hypotension or lowering a subject's seizure threshold, which make them less suitable for certain helicopter evacuations.

Oxygen

When on-board oxygen is delivered to a rescue subject, FAA regulations require that, for safety, the oxygen tanks be "appropriately secured" (14 CFR, Part 135.91).

Other Considerations

The unpressurized helicopter cabin affects care of the subject during changes in elevation because of the principles of common gas laws (Figure 21-22). Boyle's law states that under conditions of constant temperature and quantity, there is an inverse relationship between the volume and pressure of a gas. As a helicopter climbs to higher altitude, a volume of gas is forced to expand. This can lead to changes in the subject's respiratory rate and depth and in the performance of intravenous lines and also can affect the rigidity of equipment such as the balloon cuffs of endotracheal tubes, vacuum mattresses, and air splints. Elevation changes also can lead to impairment of already injured subjects, including worsening of a pneumothorax or embolism, as well as onset of hypoxia. The best course of action is to maintain an index of suspicion for a possible change in the subject's status and to be prepared for such a change. A subject with a head injury or one who is combative must be physically and possibly pharmacologically restrained so that there is no chance the person could make contact with the flight controls or personnel.

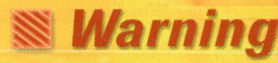

Warning

Be aware that some constrictive hoisting appliances (e.g., horse collar, lifting ring, or rescue strap style), depending on the specific configuration, can impair a rescue subject's circulation and cause him or her to black out.

Helicopter Rescue Techniques

The scope of this text is limited to coverage of hoist rescue, helicopter rappel, short haul, rescuer lowering, and cargo letdown. Other specialized tactical techniques used in military and law-enforcement deployments (e.g., "fast roping" and "helocasting") have their own added risks and require specialized training. Each of the following techniques is fraught with danger in the hands of improperly trained rescuers. This text is designed to provide an overview and to identify the drawbacks and hazards so that ground rescuers understand the limitations of these techniques. Many hours of continual training are necessary to maintain proficiency in these techniques. Understandably, the expense and availability of properly equipped aircraft puts such training out of the reach of most rescuers.

Helicopter Hoist Rescue

Because it works efficiently both for insertions and extractions, the helicopter **hoist rescue** certainly is the most efficient helicopter rescue procedure at a rescue site. The first helicopter hoist rescue was performed on November 29, 1945, to save two men stranded on an oil barge who were in danger of being washed overboard (Figure 21-23). An early Sikorsky production model R-5 helicopter pulled off the rescue in Long Island Sound, a short flight from the Sikorsky factory.[11]

Preconfiguring the rescue hoist on the aircraft for the mission increases operational efficiency, even though the weight of the rescue hoist adds to the overall equipped weight of the helicopter, thus reducing the available payload. Other helicopter rescue techniques require delays for reconfiguring the aircraft for the mission. Unfortunately, the high cost of helicopter rescue hoists means that they usually are available only through the

military and through public safety agencies in larger metropolitan areas.

The most common helicopter rescue hoists are electrically powered units, which provide the best alternative for smaller helicopters (Figure 21-24). A hydraulic hoist requires an onboard hydraulic pump system, frequently found on larger helicopters. The design for the attachment of rescue hoists includes both internal and external mounting styles, and although an internal hoist can be changed over quickly to other serviceable aircraft, it does take up useful internal cabin space.

The hoist operator (Figure 21-25) works in the open aft doorway, secured by a safety tether strap, or *gunner's belt,* that runs form the operator's harness to a fixed hard point in the aircraft. Handheld (pendant) hoist controls can provide a visual display of the amount of cable in use. Older electric hoists may have *cycle limits* imposed by the manufacturer as low as two hoist uses because of overheating of the motor. Newer hoist technology has produced more efficient motor designs with unlimited duty cycles.

The steel cable used on rescue hoists is constructed with a spin-resistant feature. The seven strands of the core are wrapped clockwise, and the 12 outer strands are wrapped counterclockwise.[12] This arrangement prevents the cable from unwinding while a load is suspended during use. A free-spinning hook at

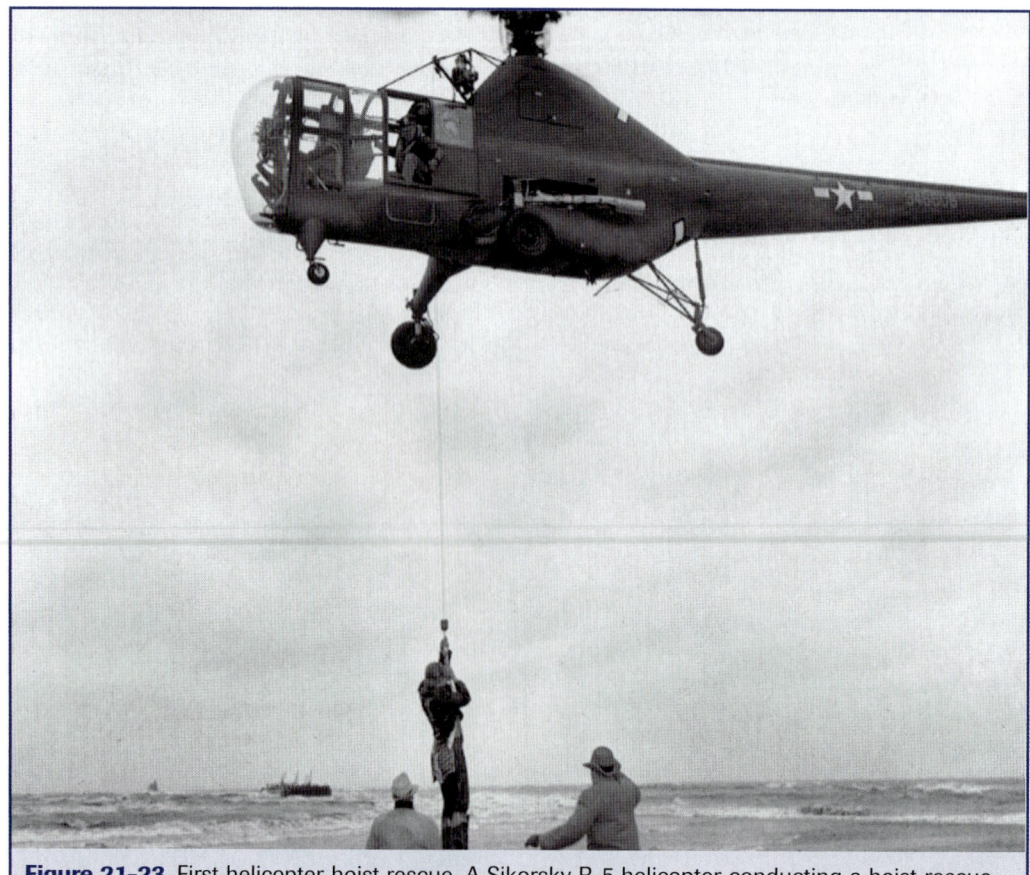

Figure 21-23 First helicopter hoist rescue. A Sikorsky R-5 helicopter conducting a hoist rescue in Long Island Sound on November 29, 1945. (Courtesy Sikorsky Aircraft Corporation.).

the end of the cable also serves as a swivel between the load and the hoist cable, eliminating twisting of the cable.

If the cable becomes entangled, the hoist operator can activate an *emergency cable cutter,* which is an electrically activated squib charge that propels a chisel-end cutter, severing the cable at the bellmouth where the cable exits the hoist.

The lateral CG limits on the helicopter limit the maximum load rating for the hoist. As excessive loads are placed out away from an imaginary line drawn down through the rotor mast, the helicopter becomes out of balance.

Hoist cable lengths vary considerably, but 245 feet (75 m) of usable cable is a common working length for many rescue helicopters. The diameter of hoist cables varies as well, ranging from 1/8 inch (3 cm), rated at a 300-pound (136 kg) capacity, to 3/16 inch (5 cm), rated at a 600-pound (272 kg) capacity.

The hoist cable is truly a lifeline and as such must be treated with respect. Although it is a rare occurrence, a hoist cable can fail. The factors leading to cable failure include environmental exposure, mistreatment or poor maintenance, operator inexperience, and cable malfunction. Some agencies use a separate belay line with the rescue hoist for operational redundancy. Higher end hoist models have a *slip clutch,* which serves much like the drag on a fishing reel, to prevent a shock force on the hoist cable.

A major hazard in helicopter hoist rescue operations is entanglement of the hoist cable, which becomes a concern as the cable reaches the ground or structures. In addition, when rescue work must be done close to active power lines, the potential exists for electricity to energize the hoist cable and injure personnel on the ground. A poorly maintained rescue hoist is a serious concern that threatens operational safety.

The rescue litter on the end of a hoist cable can quickly develop an uncontrollable spin in certain configurations. A

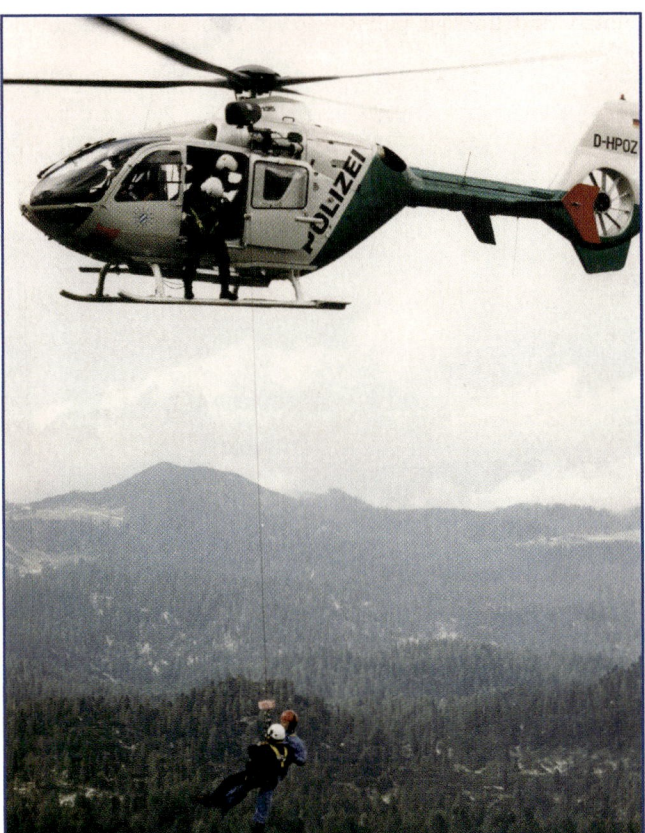

Figure 21-24 Helicopter rescue hoist. A German Police Eurocopter EC-135 helicopter conducts a hoist rescue in the mountains of Bavaria. (Courtesy HRC Heli-Rescue Consult Gmbh.)

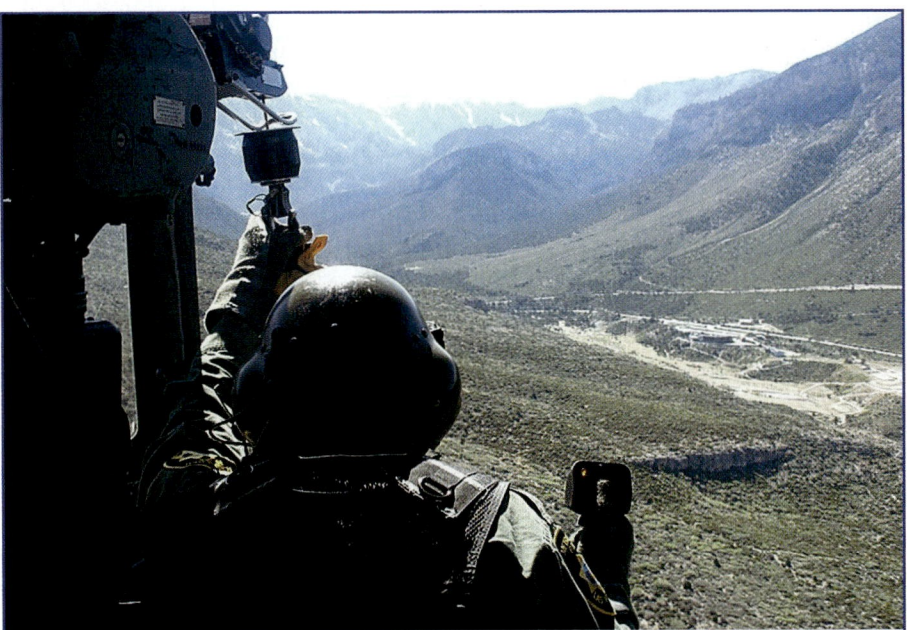

Figure 21-25 Hoist operator. While holding the pendant controls, a Las Vegas Metropolitan Police Department SAR officer prepares for a helicopter hoist evolution. (Courtesy Las Vegas Metropolitan Police Department.)

▓ *Warning*

Beware of static discharge! Helicopters generate static electricity because of the interaction between air particles and the surface of the fuselage as the air moves over the fuselage. A larger helicopter in drier air generates significantly more static electricity because a greater surface area is interacting with air particles and an increased air mass is moving over the fuselage. Composite fuselages, other than graphite, increase the potential for static charge buildup. Blowing snow or dust also increases the interaction with the aircraft and the risk of static discharge. Forward flight causes some of the static to bleed off the tail of the aircraft. However, in a hover, the static does not bleed off. The practice of keying the radio microphone on board the aircraft to discharge the static has only a limited effect, because it relives only the static in the immediate vicinity of the antennas.

If static is present, the hoist cable becomes grounded when touched by ground personnel, who may receive a harmful jolt as the static electricity is discharged. Rescuers can prevent this by allowing the hoist cable to contact the ground before they touch it. However, it is important to remember that a static charge rebuilds quickly (in a matter of seconds) after the helicopter is no longer grounded.[12]

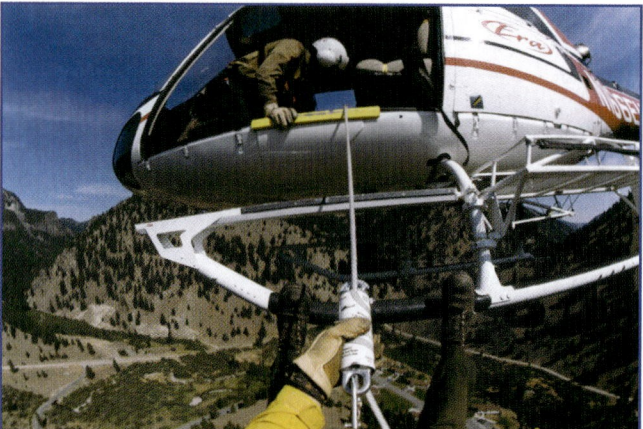

Figure 21-26 Heli-rappel. Moyer Helitack member prepares to exit the skid of a Eurocopter AS350B2 A-Star, during a proficiency rappel at the Moyer Helibase on the Salmon-Challis National Forest. This unique point-of-view shows the Sky Genie device being employed and coordinated by the rappellers with the spotter aboard the helicopter. (Courtesy Ben Croft, USDA Forest Service.)

tended tag line between the litter and an attendant on the ground can eliminate rotational spinning. Open mesh–style litters, depending on the packaging configuration, may also reduce the likelihood of spinning.

Be alert when working beneath heavy-lift helicopters during hoist rescue operations, because the increased rotor wash can easily cause debris from slopes or the forest canopy to strike ground rescuers.

Helicopter Rappel

Early use of the **helicopter rappel** included military operations in combat. The earliest combat use of helicopter rappelling in combination with troop ladders was introduced by the 11th Air Assault Division in 1964-1965. This was initiated into combat in December, 1965, near An Khe in Vietnam by the 1st Airborne Brigade of the 1st Cavalry Division (Airmobile).[14] Helicopter rappelling, also known as *heli-rappelling,* has also been used in law enforcement tactical operations and wildland fire suppression. It was first tested for wildland fire suppression in 1964 at Shasta Lake in Northern California.[15]

Rescuer insertion can easily be accomplished with helicopter rappelling (Figure 21-26), which reduces the exposure time of the rescuer beneath the aircraft compared with a helicopter short haul. Helicopter rappelling mishaps have involved loss of descent control, with subjects striking the ground; a jammed descender caused by entanglement with clothing or hair; a rappel rope that does not reach the ground; and rappeller injury caused by striking the door threshold or skid when exiting the helicopter.

Other factors that must be kept in mind with heli-rappelling include the following:

- From the vantage point of the spotter and pilot above, it is difficult to determine the height of the load. Depending on the ambient lighting, the shadow of the load provides a good reference for estimating height as the rappeller descends.
- An overhead anchor point, which must be FAA approved, provides the easiest departure for the rappeller from the aircraft.
- Most agencies use the figure 8 descender for heli-rappel procedures. The U.S. Forest Service and the Department of the Interior restrict their wildland fire helicopter rappelling programs to use of the Sky Genie (Descent Control, Inc.) for standardization; they also specify use of a *Wildland Fire Helicopter Rappel Harness,* which is a proprietary design.
- The length of a helicopter rappel varies by agency preference and by environmental considerations, which may include insertion into tall forest canopy. Rappels of 75 to 150 feet (23 to 46 m) are most common. Although longer rappels are possible, increased distance extends the required hover time of the helicopter.

A helicopter rappel mission commonly involves a mission briefing, preflight inspection of equipment, and a rappeller safety "buddy check" of personal equipment. Upon arrival at a rescue site, a reconnaissance flight is completed. The pilot establishes hover above the insertion site, and the rappel rope is deployed. The spotter signals the rescuer to move from his or her seat to the exit position with the descender connected to the rappel line.

Procedures for exiting the aircraft vary based on the make of the aircraft and its configuration; descents are made either inside or outside the helicopter skid. The size and allowable payload of the helicopter may allow rappellers to depart from both sides of the aircraft simultaneously. Egress from the aircraft should be coordinated to be as smooth as possible.

As a rappeller initiates the descent on the outside of a helicopter skid, his or her weight is transferred laterally away from the aircraft's center of gravity. This has the potential to exceed the safe operating requirements of the helicopter. With the assistance of the pilot, determine the lateral CG limits in advance to prevent a catastrophic situation. A notable characteristic of wildland fire helicopter rappel programs is that the rappel rope is disconnected and dropped to the ground after rappeller deployment; this eliminates the need to retrieve an unweighted line, which can become entangled in the rotor system.

Helicopter Short Haul Operations

A helicopter *short haul* rescue allows the insertion of personnel, suspended beneath a hovering helicopter on a fixed line, as well as the extraction of a subject or rescuers from a site where a helicopter cannot land. As early as November 1952, the so-called "helicopter lift" technique was utilized by Swiss Air Rescue (later REGA). Swiss Air-Rescue REGA, founded in 1952, is a non-profit foundation, which is a corporate member of the Swiss Red Cross. REGA is derived from the German word *Rettungsflugwacht,* and its French name, *Garde Aérienne,* which involved a large hot-air balloon basket suspended directly beneath an early model Hiller helicopter, carrying a rescuer. Although military extraction techniques (Box 21-9) were being developed simultaneously, Swiss Air Rescue introduced the knotted rope technique (Figure 21-27) in 1966 for use in mountain rescue. This predecessor to helicopter short haul involved a line knotted at intervals that a rescuer would climb down and then sit on a disc seat at the end of the line beneath the helicopter.

The following points must be kept in mind with helicopter short haul operations:

- The short haul cannot be improvised during a rescue operation. *Accidents and near-misses both have occurred*

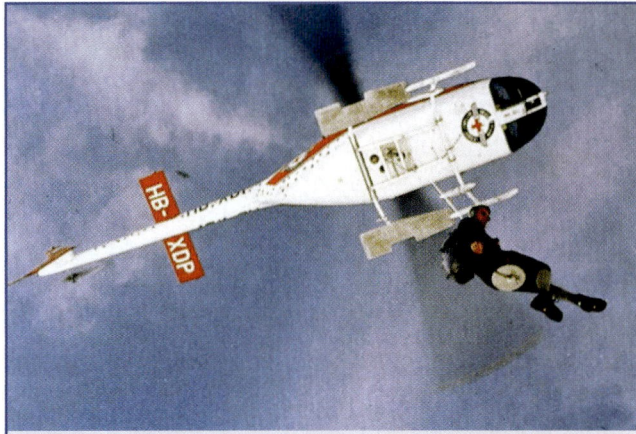

Figure 21-27 REGA knotted rope technique. A reenactment of the original "knotted rope technique" developed by Swiss Air Rescue in 1966. (Courtesy REGA.)

when agencies decided to cobble together a short haul during an incident.

- Helicopter short haul requires pilot proficiency in **vertical reference** flight operations.
- The exposure time of the rescuer during forward flight is greater than during a helicopter rappel. To minimize this exposure time, short haul flights should be limited to the shortest possible flight distance practical. The name "short haul" is derived from this distance factor, rather than from the length of line used (Figure 21-28).
- An advantage of helicopter short haul is that hover time is shorter than with heli-rappelling or hoist rescue.
- The shadow of the load provides a reference for the pilot and spotter in determining the height of the short haul load above the ground.
- Rescuer proficiency is easier to maintain with the short haul technique than with helicopter rappelling because the former requires fewer rescuer manipulations. However, pilot proficiency is significantly more critical.
- A single-strand configuration for a short haul line is common with most rescue organizations. Multiple-strand configurations have been used for redundancy but tend to be cumbersome because of the risk that the strands will become entangled when they become slack. A prerigged short haul line with a solid metal ring at the terminus provides rescue personnel with a point for easy attachment during a hook-up sequence.
- The use of spring-loaded, autolocking carabiners for all connection points, both at the aircraft and on the end of the line, prevents in-flight vibration from accidentally unlocking a carabiner.
- Rescue harness selection for short haul operations should evaluate how the rescuer will fly when encumbered with a loaded pack. The best option is a configuration that does not require the rescuer to grasp the line to maintain an upright orientation. This can be accomplished by using a full-body harness or a seat and chest harness with

Box 21-9	Military Extraction Techniques

Military helicopter extraction techniques, such as McGuire and STABO rigs, were developed during the Vietnam War. These techniques, as well as the Palmer rig or the jungle operations extraction system (JOES), which served U.S. Special Forces troops during the 1960s, have been refined and now are known as the fast rope insertion/extraction system (FRIES).[16]

Originally, an insertion or extraction system was referred to as a special procedure insertion and extraction system (SPIES), but the U.S. Army has combined the two methods into one term. FRIES now includes insertion of troops by means of *fast roping* (sliding down a large braided rope to the ground) and then extraction on a single, fixed rope lowered from the helicopter. Several soldiers, wearing special harnesses, attach themselves by means of rings woven into the rope at 5-foot intervals on the line. The soldiers are lifted en mass away from the extraction site by helicopter (Figure 21-30).

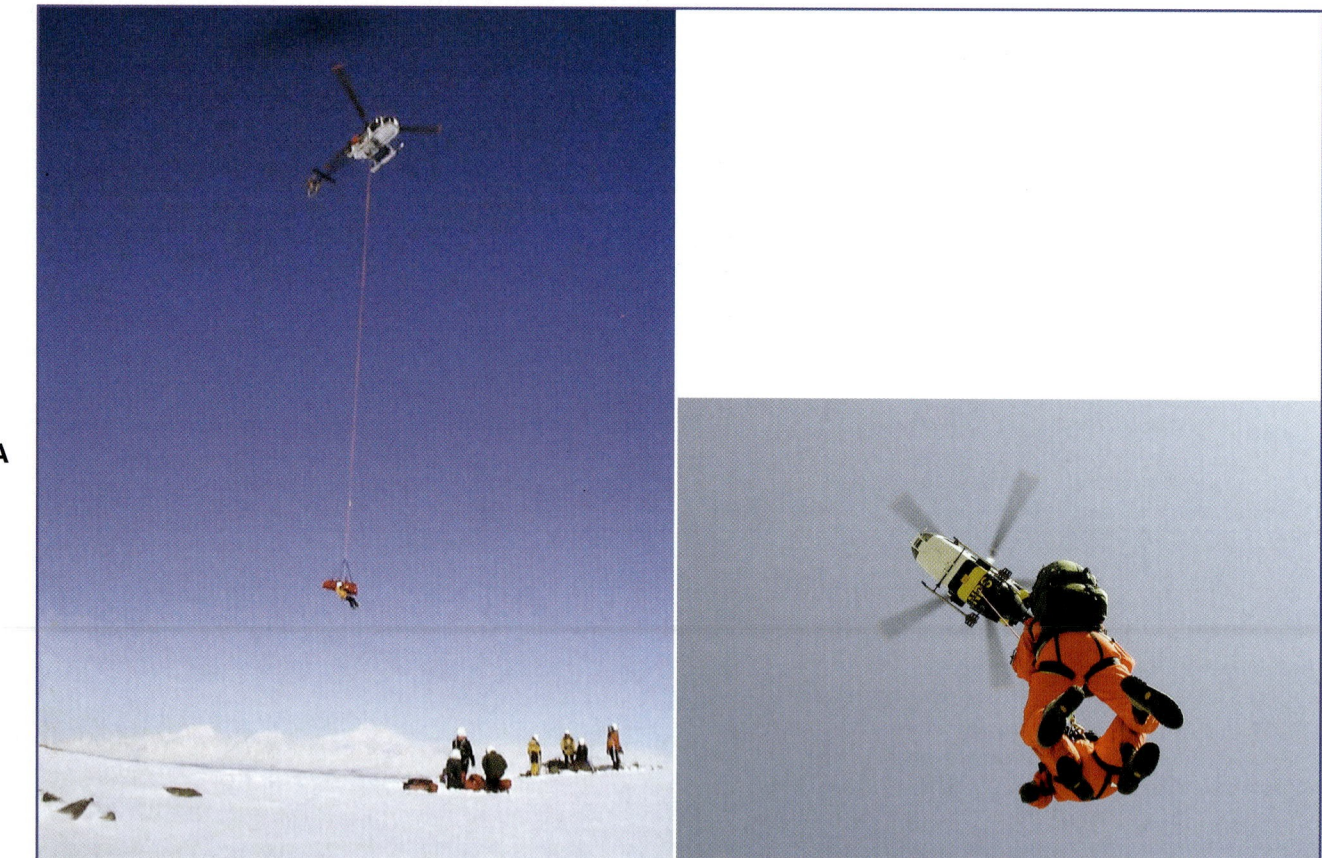

Figure 21-28 Helicopter short haul. **A,** Denali National Park Rangers using an Aerospatiale AS315 Lama helicopter to conduct helicopter short haul training at the start of the mountaineering season. (Courtesy NPS.) **B,** Grand Canyon National Park Rangers are flown in tandem beneath a McDonnell Douglas MD-900 during a short haul training evolution. (Courtesy NPS.)

preconfigured straps (e.g., daisy chains) that can quickly be attached to the short haul line.

NOTE: When not in use, these attachment straps create a possible entanglement hazard if left dangling from the harness. Secure the loose ends immediately when the attachment straps are not in use.

Hazards of Short Haul Operations

The danger of entanglement exists, because the short haul line can easily become snarled in vegetation or ground obstructions. The short haul anchor point should be releasable in the event of line entanglement. During extraction operations, all rescuers must be clear of potential for entanglement. Use mental projection to ask, "What could go wrong, and how can we avoid it?" Also, remember that a low-hovering helicopter is operating within the "dead man's curve," which hinders the pilot's ability to execute an autorotation safely.

A very serious problem is the rotational spinning of a loaded litter during a short haul evolution. Several factors can affect in-flight litter spinning, including the manner in which the litter is rigged (off center rigging worsens spin), an attendant off balance when lifted off the ground, rotor wash, and forward airspeed.

Although many rescue organizations use a Stokes-style litter for short haul rescue operations, a Bauman bag (Figure 21-29)

provides a more aerodynamic subject transport device. The Bauman bag is a hammocklike stretcher constructed of Cordura that has suspension straps, which join to a single connection point overhead.

Known generically as a *helirescue bag* in Europe, the Bauman bag is a Parks Canada evolution of the European Jenny bag, which originated from the hammocklike "lifesaving rescue net" developed by Fritz Buhler of Swiss Air Rescue in 1966. A rescue subject is protected from rotor wash when packaged in the Bauman bag, but some sort of spinal immobilization device (e.g., backboard) is required to give the bag rigidity. A Europeean helirescue bag design by Tyromont also incorporates a built-in vacuum mattress for rigidity. The stability of the Bauman bag in flight makes it a superior choice for rescue subject transport during helicopter short haul rescues.

According to FAA regulations, under no circumstances may a person be carried as part of the external load under IFR conditions (14 CFR-Part 133.33[f]).

Helicopter Short Haul Emergency Procedures

In the event of an in-flight emergency, jettisoning a human load from beneath a helicopter *is not a reasonable strategy*. A crash event is incredibly quick, and the reaction time of the spotter probably will be inadequate. The greatest chance for survival is

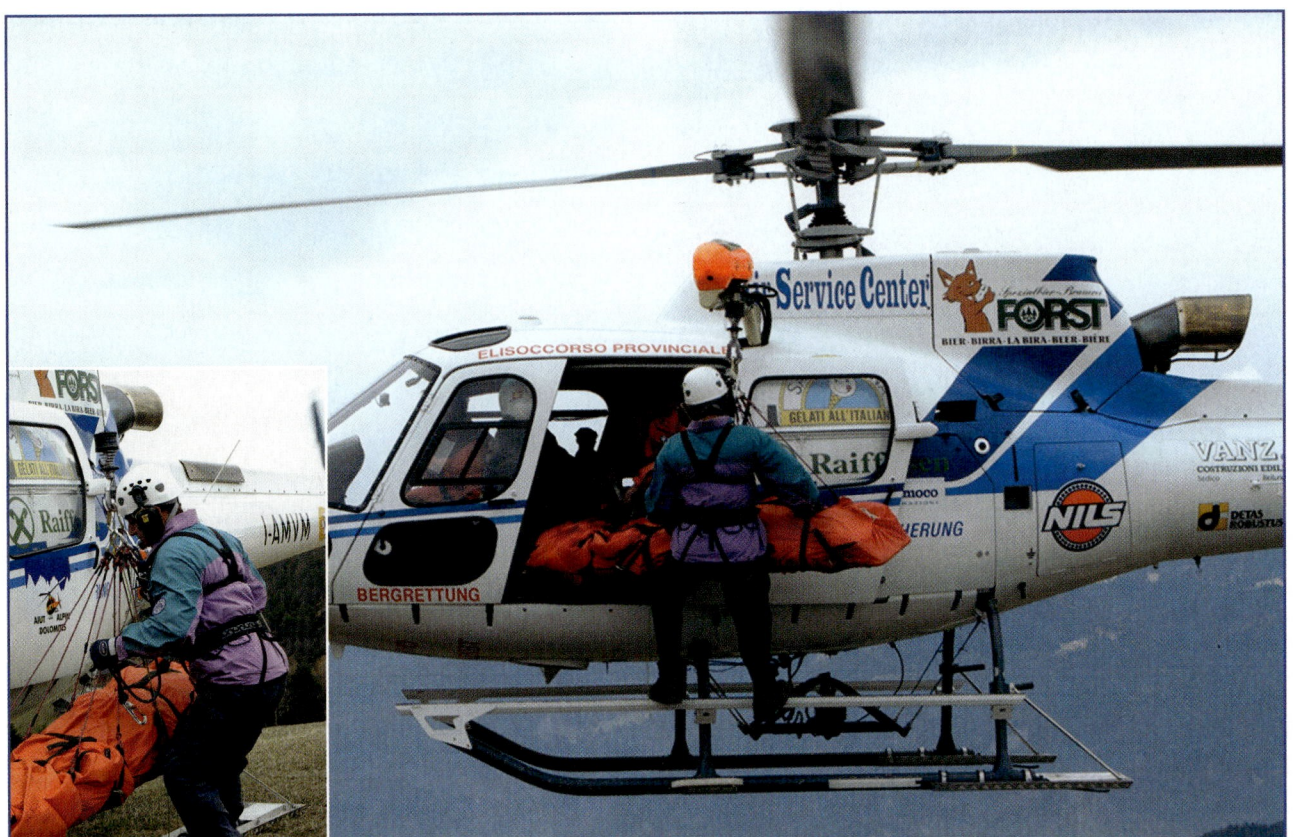

Figure 21-29 Bauman bag. **A,** Italian mountain rescue personnel conduct a hoist rescue. Rescuer attends a patient in a "heli-rescue" bag, otherwise known in North America as a Bauman Bag. **B,** (inset.) (Courtesy HRC Heli-Rescue Consult Gmbh.)

to have the load go with the helicopter to the ground. Rescuers should train in advance using the parachute landing fall (PLF) technique as a means of dissipating the energy of a hard impact. During a mission briefing, it is important that this danger be discussed openly, as well as the planned actions of all team members.

Rescuer Let-Down/Lowering (Dynamic Short Haul)

The let-down/lowering rescue technique involves lowering an aircrew member from a hovering helicopter using a descender/lowering device anchored in the helicopter. This method is used by the California Department of Forestry and Fire Protection, which refers to it as *dynamic short haul.*[17] This procedure has a couple of distinct advantages over helicopter rappelling; for example, the rescuer has the hands free during the descent, and no rope is hanging beneath the rescuer that could become entangled. The rescuer uses a full-body harness. An anchor system inside the helicopter is designed with two points of attachment and is releasable in the event of entanglement. An obvious drawback of this technique is the risk of uncontrolled descent if the aircrew member handling the lowering fails to adequately control the rope through

the descender. After the lowering deployment, the rope, which has a weight attached, is pulled back into the aircraft (Figure 21-31).

Cargo Let-Down

Cargo let-down involves lowering cargo from a hovering helicopter using a let-down line or rope controlled through a descent device. This technique has evolved in conjunction with wildland fire helicopter rappel programs for the delivery of firefighting equipment. Cargo let-down can provide for delivery of rescue equipment to a rescue site by lowering of a cargo package on a descender anchored at the aircraft. An advantage of this technique is that it does not require ground personnel to receive the load.

Typically, land management programs use tubular ¾-inch (19 mm) webbing for cargo let-down operations in conjunction with a figure 8 descender. Limitations for cargo let-down include the weight and bulk of the load to be delivered. Pilot proficiency in vertical reference flying is essential for reliable cargo let-down operations while hovering over a site. Cargo let-down is not meant to replace external **sling load (longline)** operations but simply to provide an alternative for helicopter equipment delivery in special situations (Figure 21-32).

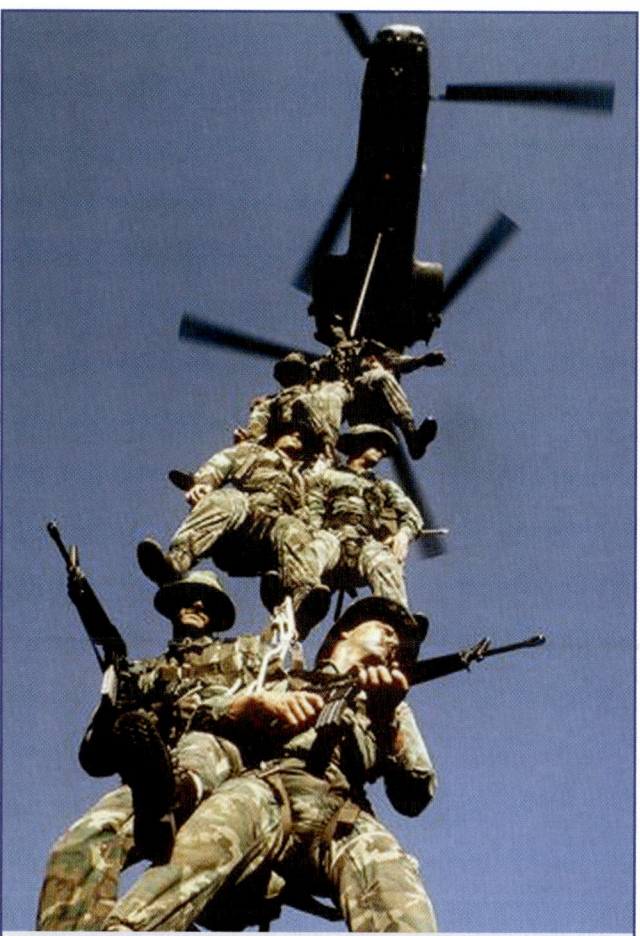

Figure 21-30 SPIE Extraction. A team of Marines is lifted off the ground by a Boeing CH-46 Sea Knight helicopter during special patrol insertion/extraction (SPIE) rig training. (Courtesy Department of Defense.)

Box 21-10 | Operational Red Flags

- ❑ Using media aircraft
- ❑ Conducting a rescue with an unknown crew or aircraft
- ❑ Exceeding the operating capabilities of the aircraft or crew
- ❑ Improvising with an unpracticed or unrecognized technique
- ❑ Radio incompatibility (e.g., VHF versus UHF)
- ❑ Becoming preoccupied with minor details (i.e., not maintaining the "big picture")
- ❑ Inadequate leadership and failure to designate command
- ❑ "Pressing" (i.e., "mission-itis" dictates operational decision making)
- ❑ Failure to delegate tasks and assign responsibilities
- ❑ Failure to communicate intent and plans (i.e., lack of a briefing)

Conclusion

This overview alone cannot provide all the insight and knowledge required to train personnel adequately in helicopter rescue techniques. It is essential that interested rescue personnel contact other agencies currently using these techniques to learn from experienced personnel. Aggressively seek out information, cross-train with other rescue units, and share ideas. *Progress slowly and cautiously in developing a helicopter rescue program. Improvisation in the middle of a rescue is a recipe for an accident.*

Be disciplined with the use of a helicopter and don't violate safety practices in the heat of battle. Trust your instincts, and remember the words of human factors authority Sheryl L. Chappell, "If something doesn't look or feel right, it probably isn't."

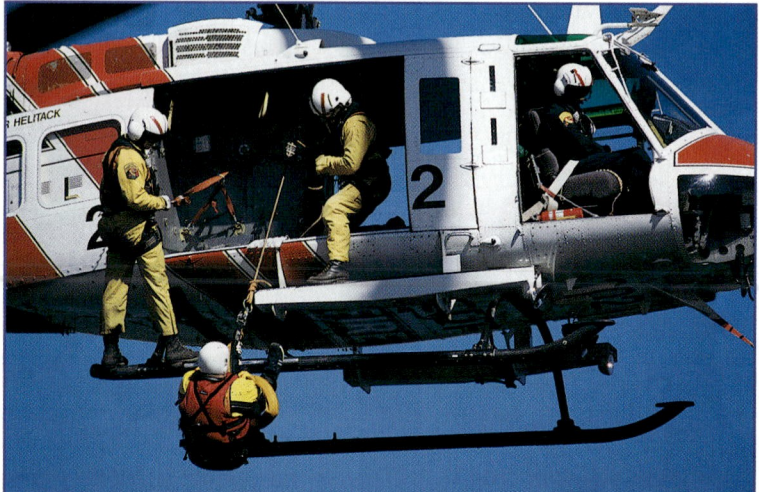

Figure 21-31 CDF "dynamic short haul." Members of California Department of Forestry and Fire Protection (CDF) Vina Helitack practice dynamic short haul during a water rescue drill. Operating from the medium sized UH-1H Super Huey helicopter, a crew chief stands on the skid and directs the lowering of a firefighter with a rappel rack. (Courtesy Barry D. Smith.)

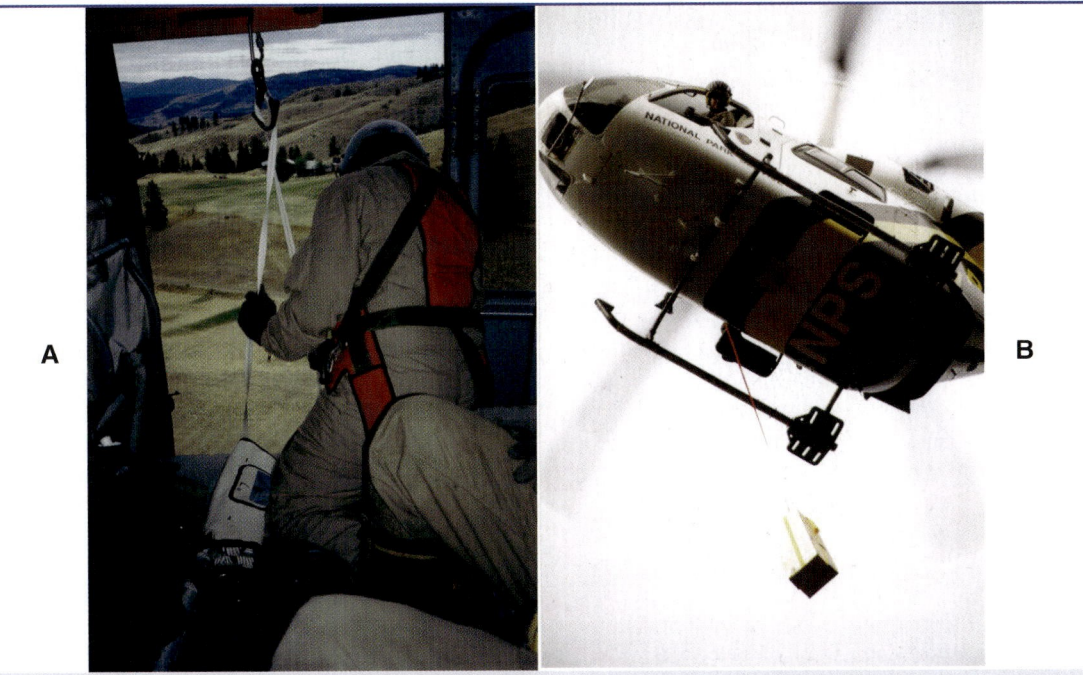

Figure 21-32 Cargo let-down. **A,** Cabin view showing cargo letdown operation. Figure 8 with ears is attached to the ceiling as a friction device, with the 250-foot webbing/letdown strap running through. The cargo is attached with a carabiner to the end of the letdown line. The spotter moves the cargo out the door and lowers inside the skid. The webbing packet is detached from the floor anchor and dropped once the operation is completed. (Courtesy Paul M. Ross Jr.) **B,** Cargo letdown operations are a good option for delivery of needed rescue equipment. Here, equipment in a preconfigured letdown box is lowered on a 250-foot webbing/letdown strap from a McDonnell-Douglas MD 900 Explorer helicopter. (Courtesy Paul M. Ross, Jr.)

Evaluation Exercises

Cognitive and Affective Exercises

1. What three questions should you ask yourself before requesting a helicopter for a rescue or requesting the assistance of an outside agency with aviation assets?

2. Give the dimensions of the touchdown pad and safety circle for type 1, type 2, and type 3 helicopters.

3. List seven safety procedures for working around a helicopter.

4. List the personal protective equipment (PPE) a helicopter crew member should use.

5. List seven potential stresses on a rescue subject during helicopter operations.

6. List four hazards of helicopter rescue hoists.

7. List three potential hazards of helicopter short haul operations.

8. Identify seven operational red flags that can occur during helicopter rescues.

References

1. Isbell W, Manager, Night Vision System Engineering, Litton, Electro-Optical Systems (subsidiary of Northrop Grumman): Personal interview, Garland, Texas, March 14, 2003.

2. US Department of the Interior, Bureau of Land Management: Interagency helicopter operations guide (IHOG), National Interagency Fire Center (NIFC), NFES item #1885, USDA Forest Service Boise, Idaho, January 2002.

3. Weick K: South Canyon Revisited: Lessons from High Reliability Organizations, Published in workshop proceedings; Findings from the Wildland Firefighters

Human Factors Workshop- Improving Wildland Firefighter Performance Under Stressful, Risky Conditions: Toward Better Decisions on the Fireline and More Resilient Organizations, Pages 40-51, Workshop sponsored by USDA Forest Service, Missoula, Montana, June 12-16, 1995. Published by MTDC (Missoula Technology Development Center) USDA Forest Service, Missoula, Montana, July 1996.

4. MD Helicopters (web site): http://www.mdhelicopters.com/Rotorcraft/MDExplorer/MDExplorer_Technical_Description_Contents.htm.
5. US Department of the Interior, Office of Aircraft Services: Basic Aviation Safety, National Interagency Fire Center (NIFC), NFES (National Fire Equipment System) item #2097, DOI, Boise, Idaho, September 1991.
6. Montenegro J, Lead Quality Engineer, Gentex Corp: Interview, Carbondale, Pennsylvania, June 13, 2002.
7. Harrington N, Aviation Safety Inspector, Federal Aviation Administration, Las Vegas Flight Standards District Office (FSDO): Personal interview, Las Vegas, June 14 2002.
8. Joint Aviation Authorities, Hoofddorp, the Netherlands (web site): http://www.jaa.nl, June 2002.
9. Holleran R: Flight nursing: principles and practice, ed 2, St Louis, 1996, Mosby.
10. Samaritan Air Evac and ASHBEAMS (American Society of Hospital Based EMS Air Medical Services), Air-Medical Crew National Standard Curriculum: Instructor Manual, Pasadena, Calif., 1988, U.S. Department of Transportation.
11. Sikorsky Aircraft Corp., Archives (web site): First helicopter civilian rescue, November 29, 1945, http://www.sikorskyarchives.com/first.html.
12. Donaldson P: Down the wire, Helicopter World, Buckinghamshire, UK. 21(3): 23-24, April 2002, Shephard Press Limited.
13. Martin A, Aeronautical Engineer, Advanced Design Division, Sikorsky Aircraft Corp: Personal interview, June 7, 2002.
14. Mertel K: Airmobile-style rappel and troop ladder, US Army Aviation Digest, U.S. Army, Fort Rucker, Alabama, (15(2), 10-13, February 1969.
15. US Forest Service and US Department of the Interior: Interagency helicopter rappel guide, USDA Forest Service, Boise, Idaho, 1990.
16. Pushies F: US Army Special Forces: the power series, St Paul, Minnesota, 2001, Motorbooks International (MBI).
17. California Department of Forestry and Fire Protection, Office of the State Fire Marshall (CDF-SFM) Helicopter Air Rescue Training Program: Instructor Manual, State of California, Sacramento, June 24, 1998.

Bibliography

Chartres J: Helicopter rescue, Surrey, London, Great Britain, 1980, Ian Allan Ltd.
US Department of the Interior, Office of Aircraft Services: Aviation policy: 350 through 354 DM (Departmental Manual), Operations procedures memoranda, Office of the Secretary of the Interior, Washington, DC., December 26, 1996. http://www.oas.gov/library/dm/350dm2.pdf
Haagensen RE et al: Lung function during hoist rescue operatons, Journal of Prehospital and disaster medicine-complete paper, Medical Journal of the World Association for Disaster and Emergency Medicine and the Nordic Society for Disaster Medicine 13(1), March 25, 1997 http://pdm.medicine.wisc.edu/haagensen.htm
Department of Medicine of the University of Wisconsin-Madison.
Phillips K: Short haul helicopter rescue, Rescue Magazine 6(3): 30-41, May/June 1993, Jems Communication, Carlsbad, California.
Phillips K: Helicopter safety, Rescue Magazine 10(1): 38-44, January/February 1997, Jems Communication, Carlsbad, California.
Shimanski C: Helicopters in search and rescue operations: basic and intermediate levels, Evergreen, Colorado, October 1998, Mountain Rescue Association. www.mra.org/HeliInt/HeliInt.html

Web Site Resources

National Interagency Fire Center: http://www.nifc.gov/
US Department of the Interior, Bureau of Land Management: Interagency helicopter operations guide (IHOG): http://www.nifc.gov/ihog/
US Department of Interior, Office of Aircraft Services: http://www.oas.gov
US Department of Transportation, Federal Aviation Administration: Federal aviation regulations (FAR), electronic code of federal regulations: title 14—Aeronautics and space: http://www.access.gpo.gov/nara/cfr/cfrhtml_00/Title_14/14tab_00.html
USDA Forest Service-Aviation: http://www.fs.fed.us/fire/fire_new/aviation/

22

Testing of Systems and Equipment

Loui McCurley

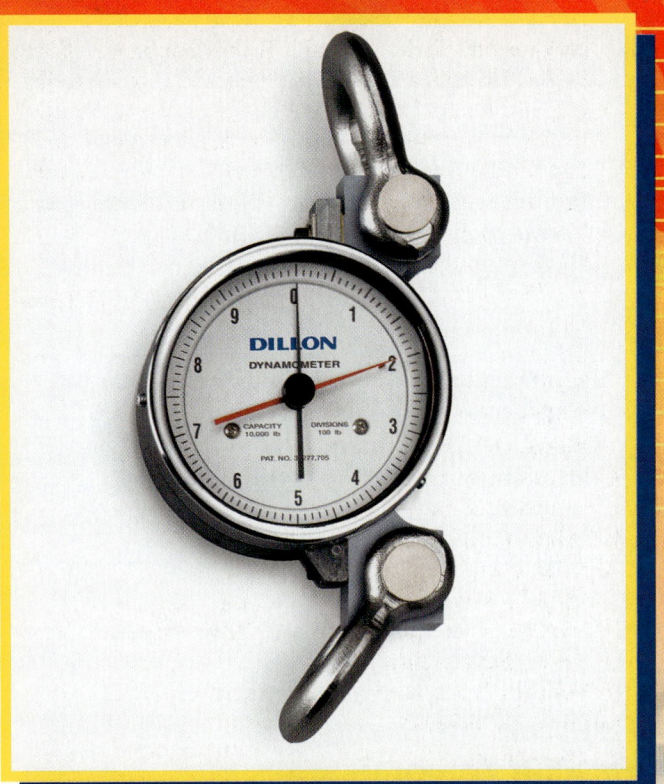

Objectives

On completion of this chapter, you should be able to:

1. Discuss the limitations of product specifications (such as strengths) provided by a manufacturer or third-party test house.
2. Explain why rescuers must have a basic understanding of system forces before they enter the high angle environment.
3. Explain the difference between component testing and system testing.
4. List several factors that can affect the performance of a *component* when it is used in a *system*.
5. Define and explain a *null hypothesis*.
6. Discuss the advantages and disadvantages of mechanical dynamometers and the advantages and disadvantages of electronic load cells.
7. Provide examples of test methods or programs that might be appropriately applied using each of the following: mechanical dynamometers, electronic load cells, and no-force measurement.

Key Terms

Backyard Testing Testing performed by field-type personnel in a less than ideal or an uncontrolled environment.

Component Testing Measurement of how a single piece of equipment performs under a certain set of criteria.

Dynamic Relating to a moving force.

Dynamometer A type of spring scale with mechanical action.

Electronic Load Cell A force measurement device with electronic measurement capabilities.

Hypothesis A tentative explanation for an observation, phenomenon, or scientific problem that can be tested by further investigation.

Null Hypothesis A statistical hypothesis formed to determine whether obtained results are significant.

Static Testing For the purposes of this chapter, the term refers to testing performed with the subject at rest and without motion or momentum created in the system; the opposite of *dynamic testing.*

Systems Testing Assembly of all the components of a rescue system in the manner in which they are to be used and then testing the system to see if actual performance meets expectations.

Reasons for Testing Rescue Equipment

Some rescuers may feel that the performance and verification testing done by equipment manufacturers is sufficient for field use. However, conscientious rescuers devote themselves to a study of the equipment they plan to use as they actually intend to use it in rescue systems. This usually leads to some form of equipment testing. Sometimes such testing is supported by highly refined analysis equipment and technology. Other times, testing consists of using bricks to weight a system and tossing it off a cliff to see what happens. Both kinds of testing can be extremely valuable. The key is to balance any conclusions the testers might be tempted to make with the capabilities and limitations of the testing procedure.

Rescue systems testing is a fine balance between practical application and technical analysis. Few rescue professionals hold second jobs as physicists, but it is important that every rope rescuer thoroughly understand and be capable of estimating forces in a rope rescue system.

Much information might seem intuitive or can be gleaned by estimating forces using simple drawings and general rules of thumb; however, it has been proven many times over that a rescuer's assumptions about system forces are not always accurate. The reasons for this include any number of the forces of reality, such as friction, elasticity in rope and other system elements, working conditions, and interrelationships among gear. The rescuer who wants to become adept at calculating system forces and safety in rope rescue will study the test methods used, as well as the test results, for a given product. In addition, he or she will endeavor to understand the relationships and differences between laboratory test results and real-world use.

The two general categories of testing that are appropriate to rescue systems are component testing and systems testing.

Component Testing

Component testing is the measurement of how an individual piece of equipment performs under a certain set of criteria. Most manufacturers do some type of this testing. In fact, many individual products are tested according to nationally or internationally accepted test methods. To take this concept a step further, many manufacturers submit their equipment to third-party engineering laboratories, which test and certify the equipment as meeting a national or international standard, such as those set by the National Fire Protection Association (NFPA), European Committee for Standardization (CEN), or the American National Standards Institute (ANSI). The most reputable manufacturers adhere to a carefully documented quality assurance program, of which component testing generally is a part.

Component testing most often is performed in laboratories under highly controlled and repeatable conditions. Clearly this has many advantages, especially the ability to verify and confirm test results. A well-made product generally performs consistently in a relatively narrow window when tested repeatedly under the same parameters. However, this advantage must be carefully weighed against the value of the component test results in field applications. After all, most rescues are not performed in highly controlled and repeatable laboratory conditions. Rescuers must consider, therefore, if and how component testing performed in a laboratory relates to use of the equipment in the field.

Carabiners: an Example of Component Testing

Carabiner testing is an excellent example with which to illustrate the comparison of laboratory results to field performance. The long-axis test is a case in point. Current test procedures for carabiner certification vary, but in general, the long-axis test requires that a carabiner be placed in a test fixture in a precisely defined way. Force is applied to the carabiner by means of two narrow pins, called *test pins,* for which the diameter and friction characteristics are closely defined by a standard test method. The loading pins are placed opposite each another per the specification, and force is applied to the pins at a specified rate, pulling them apart until the carabiner fails (Figure 22-1). (Of course, a poorly written test method results in a poorly controlled test environment and perhaps significant differences between the same standard test performed by different laboratories.)

It can be concluded from the description of the long-axis laboratory test that the test is quite repeatable and the test results usually are closely related. However, with a little field experience, a rescuer also can conclude that the likelihood of loading the carabiner at the precisely specified rate and at a point consistent with the test pins is slim to none. Laboratory tests, therefore, can provide guidance, but they cannot provide a precise performance measurement under any conditions other than those used in the test method.

Carabiners are tested and often certified to specific standards by third-party testing agencies, a practice that helps provide users with some consistency and predictability. Most rescue carabiners in the United States are tested to standards set by

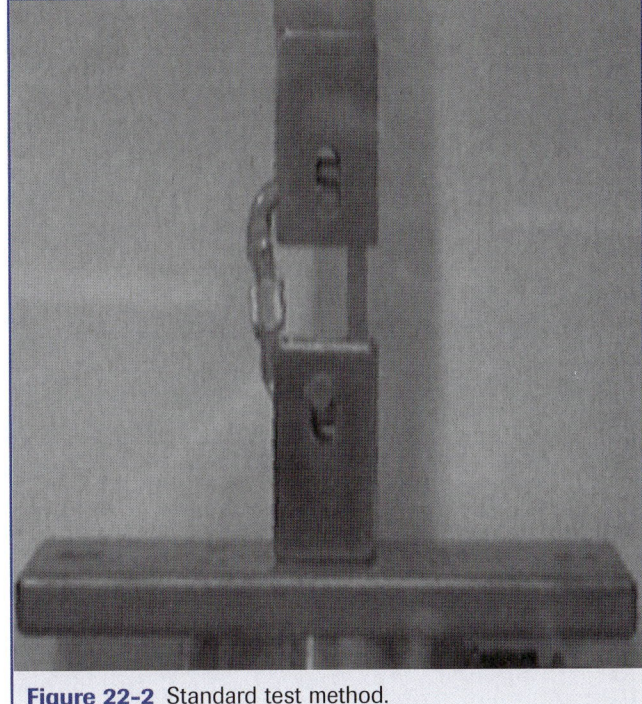

Figure 22-2 Standard test method.

ASTM or to National Fire Protection Association (NFPA) standards, which specify, among other things, that for testing, a carabiner be pulled end-to-end by two steel pins, each having a radius of 6.4 mm (Figure 22-2).

Rescue professionals have expressed concern that the methods used for such laboratory testing and certification do not adequately represent or replicate actual field use, in which carabiners often are overloaded, occasionally to extremes (Figure 22-3).

In response to customer inquiries and concerns about this issue, Seattle Manufacturing Co. (SMC) of Seattle, Washington, a leading U.S. maker of carabiners, launched a research project

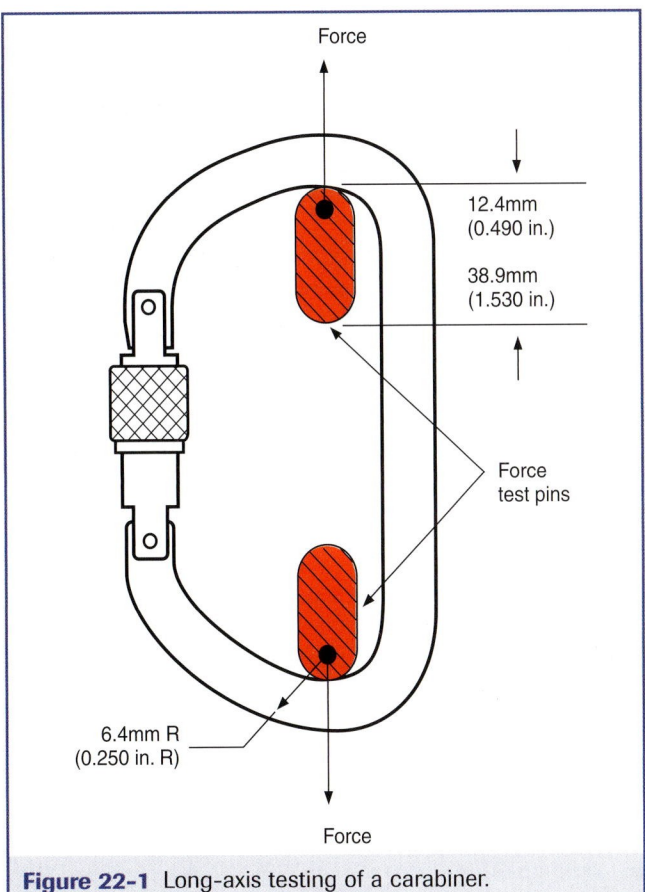

Figure 22-1 Long-axis testing of a carabiner.

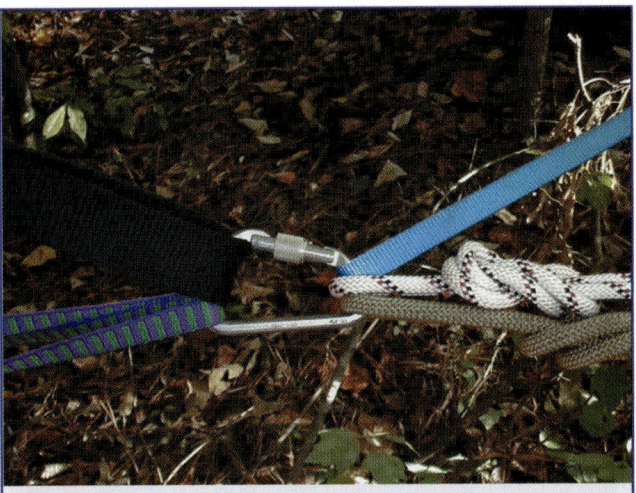

Figure 22-3 Extreme example of real-world carabiner overloading.

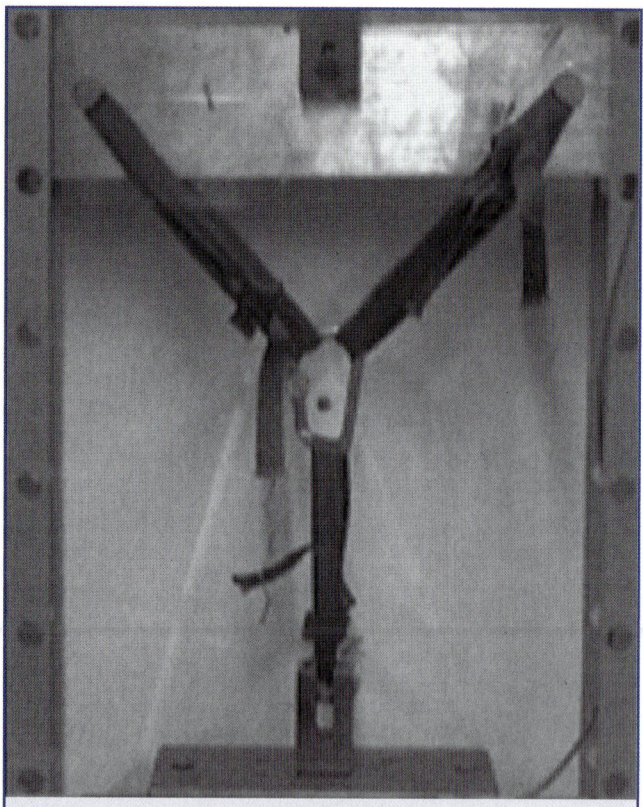

Figure 22-4 Testing for real-world abuse and overloading.

Most reputable manufacturers are willing to share test results from their own laboratories, as well as certifications and test results they have paid for from third-party test laboratories. Before you start any testing on your own, request this information from any manufacturer whose equipment you will be testing.

Recognize that test results are only test results as they relate to the test method used. Familiarity with the test method used, therefore, is as important as the resulting measurements and figures. This may sound somewhat elementary, but overlooking the differences between test methods (and interpretation of results) can result in a great deal of confusion and controversy in backyard testing.

Systems Testing

Perhaps of most interest to field personnel is the category of systems testing. **Systems testing** is the piecing together of all the components of a rescue system in the manner in which they are to be used and then testing the system to see if actual performance meets expectations. Manufacturers seldom prepare information on systems testing, because appropriate systems testing must be specific to the precise rescue system used. Rescuers tend to customize rescue systems for their own environments, resulting in systems that can be very different from one another, even when they look quite similar. For this reason, even when data on rescue systems testing are available, you should carefully analyze the test methods used and the results.

Systems testing most often is performed by curious rescuers in an actual or simulated rescue environment. This can be done either in the field or in a laboratory setting. By nature, this type of testing is less controlled and less repeatable than laboratory testing.

Backyard Testing

The rescue industry commonly refers to any testing performed by field-type personnel in a less than ideal or an uncontrolled environment as **backyard testing**. This term is not meant to be derogatory. Rather, it is used only to differentiate between laboratory testing and the less technically controlled testing more commonly done by those who use rescue equipment.

Planning the Test Project

To be most effective, a testing project must be well thought out in advance. This helps ensure that the necessary equipment and personnel can be scheduled and that adequate time is planned into the project. A sample test project planning sheet is shown in Figure 22-6.

It is useful to give every project a title, particularly if you plan to do much testing. This helps distinguish the projects from each other. Also, one individual, known as the *research coordinator*, should be put in charge of each project. The research coordinator is responsible for knowing how things are progressing at all times and for ensuring that all aspects of the project are assigned. The research coordinator may be the entire project staff or may have additional volunteers under his or her supervision.

to see how well standard carabiner test methods correlated with real-world applications (Figure 22-4). Their findings were disturbing to say the least.

Using a wide variety of carabiners from several manufacturers, SMC performed standardized ASTM/NFPA tests as a baseline. The tests then were repeated using means to replicate real-world field concerns that users had expressed, such as three-way loading, cross loading, and gate open configurations. According to SMC's data, the field-use replication tests showed a reduction in breaking strength of as much as 40% compared with standardized pin testing (Figure 22-5).

Performing Your Own Tests

Many manufacturers already test most components, sometimes even to an established industry standard. The best way to start a testing program is to request information from the manufacturer, specifically the test results and the details of the testing methods used. In some cases, especially if appropriate test methods have not yet been developed, manufacturers write a test method by which to test their equipment.

Rescuers also can write test methods by which to do testing, although it usually is not necessary for component testing. However, developing your own test method has a downside. Because many factors must be considered in equipment testing, a test method written from a single perspective can easily miss important criteria. On the other hand, in some cases it may be more specific than is necessary or appropriate.

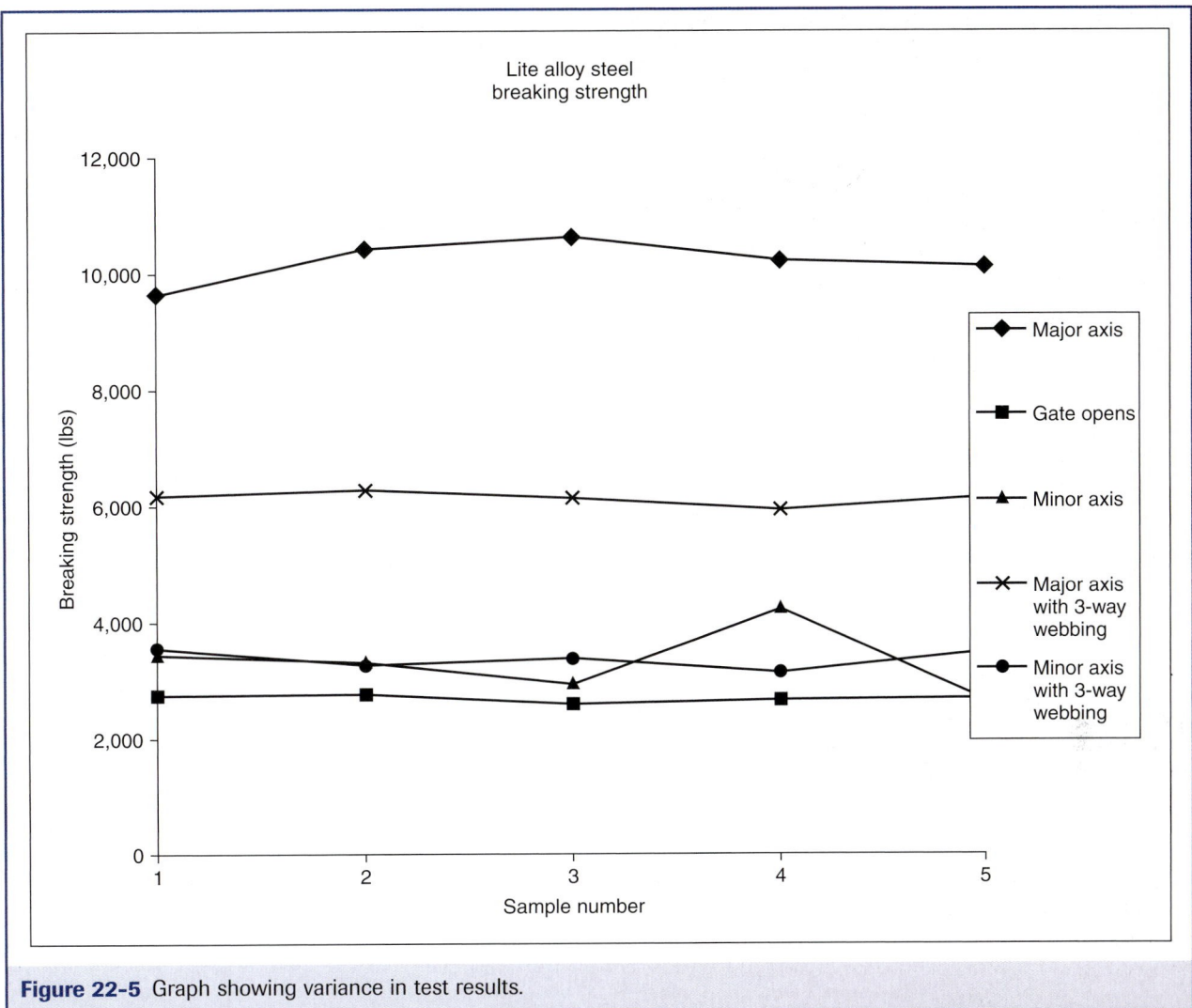

Figure 22-5 Graph showing variance in test results.

The research coordinator can enlist other agencies, personnel, and resources to participate in the project. It is helpful to write down each task or step, the person who will handle it, and when it should be done. Some common tasks that need co-ordination at this stage are (1) conducting a literature search to determine if similar tests have been done; (2) establishing appropriate laboratory and field testing procedures; (3) securing test equipment and samples to be tested; (4) devising a means of collecting the information; and (5) determining how and where the data will be used.

The first step in developing a project plan is to establish a *study objective*. The study objective can be as simple as one question that you hope to answer during the course of your project. This can be more difficult than it sounds. For example, if you begin with a study objective that is too broadly stated, such as "What are the forces in a rescue system?" you will soon find the project becoming unwieldy and cumbersome in the subsequent steps of development. If the study objective is more narrowly stated, however, such as "What are the forces at the anchor in a scree evacuation system with four litter bearers?" the project more quickly comes to a focus and to fruition.

Forming a Null Hypothesis

At this stage, you can form a null hypothesis regarding any single closely defined aspect of your experimentation. A *null hypothesis* is a statistical *hypothesis* that is formed to determine whether obtained results are significant. The end result is really that you will try to *dis*prove this null hypothesis. Alternatively, the null hypothesis can wait until statistical analysis of the test results has been completed. However, forming the null hypothesis early on may help focus the study.

Hypothesis testing begins with the formation of the null hypothesis. Data then are collected, and the viability of the null hypothesis is weighed in light of the data. Based on how closely the data correlate with what might reasonably be expected if the null hypothesis is true, the null hypothesis is either rejected or not.

It is important to remember that failure to reject the null hypothesis is not necessarily the same thing as accepting the null hypothesis. If you do not reject the null hypothesis, you must decide just how convincing the results are (this is discussed further at the end of the chapter).

Test Project Proposal

Project
title:_____

Research
coordinator:_____ Tel:_____

Contact
Address:_____

Study objective: *(State one question that you hope to answer)*

Null hypothesis: *(Rephrase the objective as a statement that you will try to <u>disprove</u>)*

List additional factors that may affect results:

1.

2.

3.

4.

List any other agencies, entities, or personnel who will be assisting in the project, and who will
need to be contacted for updates, permission, etc.

NAME   ADDRESS   PHONE

TYPES OF RESEARCH   Responsible person

[ ] Literature search   _____

[ ] Test procedure   _____

[ ] Laboratory testing   _____

[ ] Field testing   _____

[ ] Data collection   _____

[ ] Test report   _____

[ ] Publication/presentation   _____

Figure 22-6 Sample test project planning sheet.

Continued

Note: the "Responsible Person" need not necessarily be the person who will perform the work. This is simply the person who is responsible for ensuring that the objective is accomplished in a timely and efficient manner.

TEST PROCEDURE - LABORATORY

Briefly describe the nature of the testing to be performed.

What equipment will be needed for this testing?

Location: Time required:

TEST PROCEDURE - FIELD

Briefly describe the nature of the testing to be performed.

What equipment will be needed for this testing?

Location: Time required:

ESTIMATED DATES	BEGIN	END
Literature search	_____/_____/_____	_____/_____/_____
Test procedure	_____/_____/_____	_____/_____/_____
Laboratory testing	_____/_____/_____	_____/_____/_____
Field testing	_____/_____/_____	_____/_____/_____

Figure 22-6, cont'd   *Continued*

Data collection   _____/_____/_____   _____/_____/_____

Test report   _____/_____/_____   _____/_____/_____

Publication/presentation _____/_____/_____   _____/_____/_____

DIAGRAMS:
Please attach a page(s) with drawings or diagrams of test methods or procedures, including anchors, loads, load cells, secondary systems, mechanical devices, etc.

PROPOSED: (date) _____/_____/_____

BY:_____   _____
           (Print)   (Sign)

Figure 22-6, cont'd

Although this may seem a bit negative, there is a reason for it. As any parent can attest, human beings are incredibly adept at creating justifications for things we wish to be so. To avoid the inherent tendency to see everything as "proof," those conducting the test must always ask themselves what is wrong with what they are seeing. For example, if the hypothesis is posed that "Scree evacuation forces with four litter bearers generally are lower than 600 lbf," a test quickly can be devised to prove that this is true. If testers take a statement that they believe is true and then prove it to be true, their job is finished. However, if they take a statement that they believe is not true and then prove it to be true, they must keep searching for ways to prove it is *not* true. In doing so, they are in effect removing all possible contradictions to their hypothesis.

Next comes a brainstorming session. List all the possible factors that you think may affect your results. Stop at nothing. This list becomes invaluable as you develop your test methods.

Test Method

As the first step in creating a test procedure, determine whether the testing to be done falls into the category of component testing or systems testing.

Next, enlist the assistance of experienced testing technicians, manufacturers, or others in the field to establish an appropriate test method for your project. Whether you are considering laboratory testing or field testing, a good piece of information with which to begin is a collection of whatever applicable test methods might be available or have been used or published in

the past. For some types of gear or systems, you may need to wade through a flood of information. For example, in the case of belay testing, you may need to read reams of testing specifications for such things as belay devices, personal belay testing, heavy systems belay testing, manned belay testing, unmanned belay testing, testing on towers, testing in laboratories, testing in field conditions, and testing with a variety of acceptable parameters. For other types of testing, you may be unable to find any test methods at all (see Appendix A for a list of resources for test methods).

If you are unable to find specific test methods for the equipment, a good rule of thumb is to test it *in the manner of use*. This means that if the device operates by having a rope wrapped through it in some way, it should be tested with the rope wrapped through it in that way. In this case especially, engage the assistance of experienced test technicians and consider all the variables at play.

Diagrams are especially useful at this stage. Drawings or diagrams of test methods or procedures and of the elements of the system (e.g., anchors, loads, load cells, secondary systems, mechanical devices) help ensure that nothing is forgotten, and they serve as a good reference on test day.

In your test method proposal, briefly describe the nature of the testing and the equipment needed. You may estimate how many times you might need to repeat the tests to achieve appropriate confidence in your results, but bear in mind that this estimate may need to be revised as you see how far apart (or how close together) your actual test results fall. You can use this information to help determine the amount of equipment and the number of personnel needed for the test, how much time it might take, and where it can most appropriately be done.

Armed with what you have collected thus far, you should be able to analyze your project and set a timeline for completion. Don't forget to include all aspects of the project, such as the literature search, procurement of equipment, arranging of a location, date and personnel needed, completion of the testing procedure, and a summary of the results.

Test Results

Results are a critical part of testing. After all, they are the whole reason for doing the project in the first place. Keep this in mind, because it is where most testing projects fall apart. For best results, create a form on which the results of each and every sample test can be recorded. Leave plenty of room to record unusual events or important notes. Make sure to tabulate the results in such a way that they can be compared against the null hypothesis.

Numeric measurements of forces are not critical for a test series to be valuable. Some tests can give useful data on the "what if" principle. An example of null hypothesis for a "what if" series of tests might be, "If a helmet is dropped, will it exhibit signs of cracking?"

Static Versus Dynamic Measurement

If force measurement is used, note whether the test is *static* or *dynamic* in nature. Although a mechanical *dynamometer* may be appropriate for static forces, an *electronic load cell* is the preferred mechanism for measuring where dynamic loading (or unloading) is a factor.

Dynamometers

Because mechanical dynamometers are so widely used, it is worth taking a moment to discuss their application. The mechanical dynamometers commonly owned by rescue organizations were designed for tensioning lines and are inadequate for measuring dynamic forces (Figure 22-7). These dynamometers can be compared with other spring scales, such as produce scales or bathroom scales, which have several inherent problems.

Drawbacks of Dynamometers Consider a bathroom scale, a type of spring scale gauge. Let's say that your cat runs through the room and bounces on the scale as it goes by. Because the scale is mechanical and because the cat is moving fast, by the time the needle gets halfway to the actual force being created by the cat, the cat is gone and there is no more force to measure. The needle returns to zero.

The technical term for this is *frequency response,* which is the speed at which the pressure mechanism communicates with the readout mechanism. If the frequency response is not fast enough, the peak force is missed.

Another, almost contrary issue can also be demonstrated with the bathroom scale. Consider that this time you want to weigh yourself. When you first step onto the scale, the needle bounces. So what do you do? You hold your breath and stand *very still* while it settles at a more readable number. Where does this needle bounce come from?

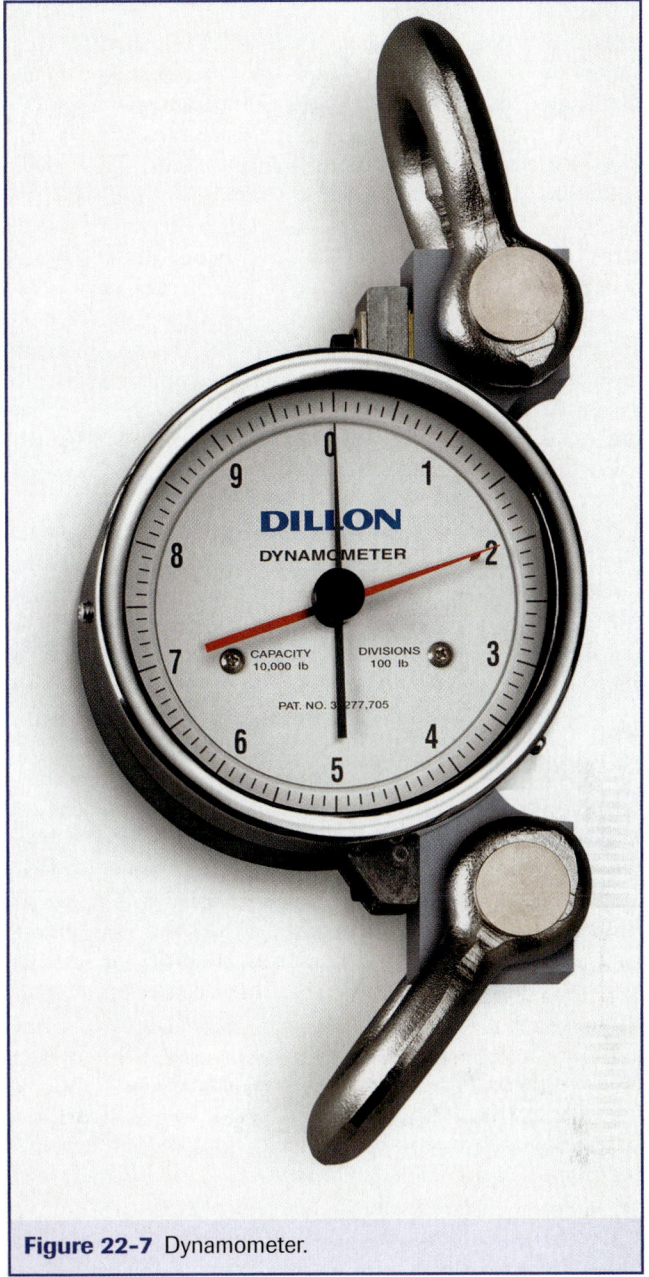

Figure 22-7 Dynamometer.

For starters, it comes from the fact that when a person steps onto a scale, the individual creates more force than his or her actual weight. That's just a simple fact of physics. However, in addition there is a certain amount of momentum that can cause the needle to go higher still. How much higher the momentum can carry the needle depends on several factors, such as the amount of friction in the needle mechanism, how close the person is to the maximum range of the scale, how fast the person hopped on the scale, and the angle at which the scale is resting. The bottom line is, if you were measuring your weight with a *peak force indicator*—such as the little movable needle that stops at the highest force measured on a dynamometer—the result would be affected by this momentum.

The crux of the problem is that these two errors conflict. Furthermore, with a mechanical device such as a dynamometer, a tester can't know which of these is occurring at any given time. During one test a low reading may result because the frequency response wasn't fast enough; during the next (identical) test, a high reading may result because momentum carried the needle farther than it should have gone.

Uses of Dynamometers The drawbacks of mechanical dynamometers do not mean that they shouldn't be used. They do mean that the figures obtained with a static pull are more accurate than those obtained during a dynamic event. Therefore the figures obtained with dynamic testing should not be taken as absolutes. Trends certainly can be measured with a dynamometer, and the more tests the better (as, hopefully, you start to narrow in on a common result). However, the actual figures are not to be trusted.

Furthermore, testers should do their best to design the above-described potentials *out* of the test methods; for example, they should try to minimize "bounce" in the test method. Remember also that peak forces in dynamic loading might be higher than assumed. Try to keep the dynamometer from bouncing off anything after a dynamic unloading event (e.g., rope failure) because this action may jiggle the peak force needle.

Electronic Load Cells

Simply resorting to an electronic force measurement system (i.e., an ***electronic load cell***) does *not* necessarily resolve the problem described in the previous section. The up side of electronic force measurement systems is that they are designed with a specific frequency response in mind which, therefore, the tester usually knows. For field-type rescue systems testing, a frequency response of at least 4 times/second catches most events, although 8 times/second is better.

Be aware that it also is possible to have *too fast* a frequency response, one that picks up every vibration or electrical impulse. In this case, the reading can be very erratic and overly high. If forces in the tests are to be measured with load cells, whether electronic or mechanical, it is best to obtain the services of a person experienced with this equipment.

In either case, verify calibration periodically during the test cycle by hanging a known weight or a recently calibrated instrument on the measuring device. Also, have the instrument recalibrated at recommended intervals by a certified laboratory.

Crunching the Test Results

The results of any test series should be tabulated appropriately and can be analyzed in any number of ways. Be careful at this stage not to deviate too far from the intended goal; it is all too easy to see new projects as the results are tabulated. However, it is most useful to complete the current task before engaging in another.

One appropriate way to analyze the results is to compare them with a null hypothesis. If one has not already been created, now is the time to do it. The question then becomes: What did your actual testing show in relation to your hypothesis/null hypothesis?

Using statistical analysis, the viability of the previously stated null hypothesis can be tested in the light of the experimental data. Depending on the data, the null hypothesis is or is not rejected as a viable possibility.

How much "proof" is needed to make test results statistically significant? The more the actual results deviate from the anticipated results, the greater their significance. Determining an acceptable level of consistency is a rather arbitrary procedure that is left completely to the discretion of the project manager.

Most of the scientific community accepts deviations between 1% and 5%. If, for example, 100 tests were performed, then at the "generous" end of variation, if the results of more than five tests varied from the null hypothesis, the null hypothesis would be rejected.

Few organizations have the resources to perform 100 identical tests. Ten tests are more within the scope of most groups, and if the results of even *one* of these should vary, the testers would be outside the 5% acceptable limit. Clearly, this points out the importance of not drawing definitive conclusions from inconclusive testing. It is human nature to have a tendency to look at a group of tests and, if more than half of them are similar, to begin to see patterns and draw conclusions. Scientifically this is unacceptable, and it is particularly intolerable when dealing with life safety equipment and scenarios. The more samples that can be obtained using precisely defined parameters, equipment, and test methods and the more the results are the same, the more reliable the results are considered.

On the other hand, there is nothing wrong with having inconclusive results. They, too, can be enlightening, and the current project may be a great stepping-off point for someone else's project.

Data from the tests should be presented clearly and in a manner that is easy to comprehend, whether this is done in writing or as a presentation. Completely describe the test methods, the processes, the equipment, the limitations, and the results. Be very specific. Giving examples of results and tabulated data usually is more useful than simply giving conclusions. If the data are presented to a group of your peers, enlightening comments and questions often are forthcoming.

It cannot be stressed enough: be wary of drawing definitive conclusions from testing. It often is useful to have a person who is not affiliated with the project look over the results. This individual can help identify points that need clarification, as well as any potential holes in the process.

With careful forethought and by keeping yourself open to the experience of others, you quickly can learn to correlate test data with field applications in a practical, meaningful way.

Evaluation Exercises

1. One reason for not totally relying on the product specifications provided by a manufacturer or third-party test house would be:

   A. No manufacturer can know your exact field problems.
   B. The manufacturer's laboratory tests may not completely reproduce your field conditions.
   C. The manufacturer's tests may have covered only individual components and not systems.
   D. All of the above.

2. Some of the factors that influence the performance of a component when it is used in a system are:

   A. Friction
   B. Elasticity in the rope
   C. Interrelationships among gear
   D. All of the above.

3. The first step in developing a project plan is to:

   A. Find a place to do the testing.
   B. Obtain grant money.
   C. Obtain the equipment to be tested.
   D. Establish a study objective.

4. A hypothesis is:

   A. A problem that occurs during a rescue.
   B. An initial idea for testing that nobody else has done.
   C. A tentative explanation for an observation, phenomenon, or scientific problem that can be tested by further investigation.
   D. A statistical hypothesis formed to determine whether obtained results are significant.

5. A *null hypothesis* is:

   A. An argument that shows that an idea is invalid.
   B. A hypothesis formed to determine whether obtained results are significant.
   C. An idea that later proves to be null and void.

6. The first step in creating a test procedure is to:

   A. Enlist the assistance of experienced testing technicians, manufacturers, or other qualified personnel.
   B. Determine whether the testing to be done falls into the category of component testing or systems testing.
   C. Apply for grant money.
   D. Order equipment.

7. The disadvantages of a dynamometer include:

   A. They usually measure only peak force.
   B. They are very expensive.
   C. They use only metric measurements.
   D. Poor at measuring dynamic loading.

Appendix A
Standards Setting Organizations and Further Reading

Standards Setting Organizations

American National Standards Institute (ANSI)

American National Standards Institute, Inc.
25 West 43rd Street, 4th Floor
New York, NY 10036
Telephone: 212-642-4900
Web site: www.ansi.org

ANSI sets standards for safety belts, harnesses, lanyards, lifelines, and drop lines for industries such as construction, manufacturing, window cleaning, and arboriculture.

ASTM

100 Barr Harbor Drive
West Conshohocken, PA 19428-2859
Telephone: 610-832-9585
Web site: www.astm.org

ASTM is the facilitator for standards created through the full consensus method. Standards for equipment and techniques used in search and rescue currently are developed through the ASTM process.

European Committee for Standardization (CEN)

Web site: http://www.cenorm.be

CE sets standards for a wide variety of products traded in the European Union, including personal protective equipment. Rescue equipment falls into this category. European standards are available from *national standards bodies,* which are responsible for selling European Standards.

National Fire Protection Association (NFPA)

National Fire Protection Association
1 Batterymarch Park
P.O. Box 9101
Quincy, MA 02269-9101
Telephone: 617-770-3000
Web site: www.nfpa.org

NFPA sets standards specific to fire service applications, including rope and related equipment, along with performance standards for rescuers in the fire service.

Union of International Alpine Associations (UIAA)

Postfach
CH-3000 Bern 23
Switzerland
Web site: www.uiaa.ch
The U.S. representative of the UIAA is:
American Alpine Club
710 10th Street, Suite 100
Golden, CO 80401
Telephone: 303-384-0110
Web site: www.americanalpineclub.org

UIAA represents mountaineers and climbers worldwide on international issues. The UIAA safety commission sets standards for rope, helmets, hardware, and other equipment used in recreational climbing.

Occupational Safety and Health Administration (OSHA)

U.S. Occupational Health and Safety Administration, Department of Labor
200 Constitution Avenue
Washington, DC 20210
Telephone: 800-321-6742
Web site: www.osha.gov

OSHA sets safety standards for the workplace in the United States.

The Cordage Institute

994 Old Eagle School Road, Suite 1019
Wayne, PA 19087
Telephone: 610-971-4854
Web site: www.ropecord.com

The Cordage Institute is a trade association that sets standards for rope and cordage in the United States.

Further Reading

Brown, M: *Engineering Practical Rope Rescue Systems,* Stamford, CT, 2000, Delmar.

Cox M, Fulsaas K, editors: *Mountaineering: the freedom of the hills,* ed 7, Seattle, 2003, The Mountaineers.

MacInnes H: *International mountain rescue handbook,* ed 3, 1999, Constable & Co.

Marbach G: *Alpine caving techniques: a complete guide to safe and efficient caving,* 2002, Speleo Projects, Caving Publications International.

Ray S: *Swift water rescue: a manual for the rescue professional,* Ashville, North Carolina, 1997, CPS Press.

Roop M, Vines T, Wright R: *Confined space and structural rope rescue,* St Louis, 1998, Mosby.

Setnicka TJ: *Wilderness search and rescue,* Boston, 1980, Appalachian Mountain Club.

Smith B, Padgett A: *On rope: North American vertical rope techniques,* Huntsville, Alabama, 1996, National Speleological Society.

Wheelock W: *Ropes, knots, and slings for climbers,* Glendale, California, 1967, La Siesta Press.

Appendix B
Checklists for Rescuer Skills

Skills Checklist
Chapter 6: Knots

Instructions

As each student completes a skill check, the evaluator notes the date in the Evaluator column. If the student demonstrates the prescribed level of competence in the skill, the evaluator signs his or her initials, and the student signs his or her initials in the adjacent column to the right. If the student fails, the evaluator writes "U" (unsatisfactory) in the Evaluator column.

Student _____

Evaluator(s) _____

_____

_____

	First try		Second try	
	EVALUATOR	STUDENT	EVALUATOR	STUDENT
Tie a simple overhand knot.				
Tie a simple figure 8 knot.				
Tie a figure 8-on-a-bight knot.				
Tie a figure 8 follow-through knot.				
Tie a figure 8 bend.				
Tie a ring bend (water) knot in webbing.				
Tie a double overhand (barrel) knot.				
Tie a double fisherman's (grapevine) knot.				
Optional: Tie a bowline on a coil.				
Optional: Tie an Interlocking long-tail bowline.				

Skills Checklist
Chapter 7: Anchoring

Instructions

As each student completes a skill check, the evaluator notes the date in the Evaluator column. If the student demonstrates the prescribed level of competence in the skill, the evaluator signs his or her initials, and the student signs his or her initials in the adjacent column to the right. If the student fails, the evaluator writes "U" (unsatisfactory) in the Evaluator column.

Student _____

Evaluator(s) _____

_____

_____

	First try		Second try	
	EVALUATOR	STUDENT	EVALUATOR	STUDENT
Tie and rig a tensionless hitch on an anchor point.				
Tie and rig a figure 8 on a bight on an anchor point.				
Tie and rig a figure 8 follow-through on an anchor point.				
Tie and rig a ring bend (water) knot in webbing on an anchor point.				
Using rope, tie a pretensioned back-tie between two anchor points.				
Tie and rig a load-sharing anchor on two anchor points.				
Rig a load-distributing anchor on two anchor points.				
Rig a load-distributing anchor on three or more anchor points.				

Skills Checklist
Chapter 8: Belaying of
One-Person Loads

Instructions

As each student completes a skill check, the evaluator notes the date in the Evaluator column. If the student demonstrates the prescribed level of competence in the skill, the evaluator signs his or her initials, and the student signs his or her initials in the adjacent column to the right. If the student fails, the evaluator writes "U" (unsatisfactory) in the Evaluator column.

Student _____

Evaluator(s) _____

_____

_____

	First try		Second try	
	EVALUATOR	STUDENT	EVALUATOR	STUDENT
Repeat from memory and in correct sequence the belay voice communications.				
On level ground, use a Münter hitch to belay a person moving away from the belayer.				
Using a belay practice system, use a Münter hitch to catch a dropped weight that is being lowered.				
On level ground, use a one-person belay device to belay a person moving away from the belayer.				
On level ground, use a one-person belay device to belay a person moving toward the belayer.				
Using a belay practice system, use a one-person belay device to catch a dropped weight that is being raised.				
Using a belay practice system, use a one-person belay device to catch a dropped weight that is being lowered.				

Skills Checklist
Chapter 9: Rappelling

Instructions

As each student completes a skill check, the evaluator notes the date in the Evaluator column. If the student demonstrates the prescribed level of competence in the skill, the evaluator signs his or her initials, and the student signs his or her initials in the adjacent column to the right. If the student fails, the evaluator writes "U" (unsatisfactory) in the Evaluator column.

Student _____

Evaluator(s) _____

_____

_____

	First try		Second try	
	EVALUATOR	STUDENT	EVALUATOR	STUDENT
Rappel using a figure 8 with ears and:				
1. Attach it to the harness and rope correctly.				
2. Maintain control during the entire rappel.				
3. Part way down, come to a complete stop.				
4. Lock off the figure 8 descender securely.				
5. Unlock the descender and complete the rappel.				
Rappel using a brake bar rack and:				
1. Attach it to the harness and rope correctly.				
2. Maintain control during the entire rappel.				
3. Part way down, come to a complete stop.				
4. Lock off the brake bar rack securely.				
5. Unlock the descender and complete the rappel.				

Skills Checklist
Chapter 10: Basic Ascending Techniques

Instructions

As each student completes a skill check, the evaluator notes the date in the Evaluator column. If the student demonstrates the prescribed level of competence in the skill, the evaluator signs his or her initials, and the student signs his or her initials in the adjacent column to the right. If the student fails, the evaluator writes "U" (unsatisfactory) in the Evaluator column.

Student   _____

Evaluator(s)   _____

_____

_____

	First try		Second try	
	EVALUATOR	STUDENT	EVALUATOR	STUDENT
Correctly tie a Prusik hitch onto a fixed rope.				
Ascend a rope safely and efficiently with an ascending system using three ascenders.				
Tie off short while ascending a fixed rope.				
Safely and efficiently change over from ascending to rappelling.				
Safely and efficiently change over from rappelling to ascending.				
Extricate yourself from a simulated jammed rappel device using ascenders.				

Skills Checklist
Chapter 13: Rescue Belaying

Instructions

As each student completes a skill check, the evaluator notes the date in the Evaluator column. If the student demonstrates the prescribed level of competence in the skill, the evaluator signs his or her initials, and the student signs his or her initials in the adjacent column to the right. If the student fails, the evaluator writes "U" (unsatisfactory) in the Evaluator column.

Student   _____

Evaluator(s)   _____

_____

_____

	First try		Second try	
	EVALUATOR	STUDENT	EVALUATOR	STUDENT
Correctly tie a load-releasing hitch.				
Correctly release a load-releasing hitch with a simulated load.				
Correctly rig a tandem Prusik belay system.				
Correctly rig a Prusik minding pulley.				
Correctly operate a Prusik minding pulley.				
Correctly operate a 540° Belay Device.				

Skills Checklist
Chapter 14: Pickoff Rescue Techniques

Instructions

As each student completes a skill check, the evaluator notes the date in the Evaluator column. If the student demonstrates the prescribed level of competence in the skill, the evaluator signs his or her initials, and the student signs his or her initials in the adjacent column to the right. If the student fails, the evaluator writes "U" (unsatisfactory) in the Evaluator column.

Student _____

Evaluator(s) _____

_____

_____

	First try		Second try	
	EVALUATOR	STUDENT	EVALUATOR	STUDENT
Safely and efficiently perform a pickoff rescue of a person wearing a seat harness.				
Tie onto a subject either a hasty seat harness, a hasty seat harness with a chest harness, or a hasty body harness.				
Safely and efficiently perform a pickoff rescue of a person not wearing a seat harness.				

Skills Checklist
Chapter 15: Use of Litters in High Angle Rescue

Instructions

As each student completes a skill check, the evaluator notes the date in the Evaluator column. If the student demonstrates the prescribed level of competence in the skill, the evaluator signs his or her initials, and the student signs his or her initials in the adjacent column to the right. If the student fails, the evaluator writes "U" (unsatisfactory) in the Evaluator column.

Student   _____

Evaluator(s) _____

_____

_____

	First try		Second try	
	EVALUATOR	STUDENT	EVALUATOR	STUDENT
Package a rescue subject in a litter so as to protect the individual from major environmental hazards.				
Using webbing, secure a rescue subject in a litter, taking into consideration the subject's comfort and concerns about adequate breathing and circulation.				

Skills Checklist
Chapter 16: Low Angle Evacuation

Instructions

As each student completes a skill check, the evaluator notes the date in the Evaluator column. If the student demonstrates the prescribed level of competence in the skill, the evaluator signs his or her initials, and the student signs his or her initials in the adjacent column to the right. If the student fails, the evaluator writes "U" (unsatisfactory) in the Evaluator column.

Student _____

Evaluator(s) _____

_____

_____

	First try		Second try	
	EVALUATOR	STUDENT	EVALUATOR	STUDENT
Repeat from memory and in correct sequence the voice communications used in slope evacuation.				
Correctly rig a litter for slope evacuation.				
Package a rescue subject for slope evacuation.				
Correctly rig and anchor a brake system for slope evacuation using a figure 8 with ears.				
Correctly rig and anchor a brake system for slope evacuation using a brake bar rack.				
Correctly rig and anchor a belay system for slope evacuation.				
Correctly rig and anchor a 1:1 (counterbalance) hauling system for slope evacuation.				
Optional: Correctly rig a tree wrap brake system.				

Skills Checklist
Chapter 17: High Angle Lowering

Instructions

As each student completes a skill check, the evaluator notes the date in the Evaluator column. If the student demonstrates the prescribed level of competence in the skill, the evaluator signs his or her initials, and the student signs his or her initials in the adjacent column to the right. If the student fails, the evaluator writes "U" (unsatisfactory) in the Evaluator column.

Student _____

Evaluator(s) _____

_____

_____

	First try		Second try	
	EVALUATOR	STUDENT	EVALUATOR	STUDENT
Repeat from memory and in correct sequence the voice communications used in high angle lowering.				
Correctly rig a litter for high angle lowering.				
Package a rescue subject for high angle lowering.				
Using a litter that has been rigged and with a simulated rescue load:				
1. Correctly anchor a brake bar rack for lowering.				
2. Correctly attach the litter to the lowering rope.				
3. Correctly rig and anchor a belay for the litter.				
4. Correctly lace the lowering rope to the brake bar rack.				
5. Correctly lower the litter with the simulated load, stop the lowering, bring rack to a full stop, tie off the brake bar rack, and then unlock the brake bar rack to continue lowering.				
6. Correctly belay a simulated rescue load during a lowering.				
7. Perform a knot pass during a simulated lowering.				

Skills Checklist
Chapter 18: Hauling Systems

Instructions

As each student completes a skill check, the evaluator notes the date in the Evaluator column. If the student demonstrates the prescribed level of competence in the skill, the evaluator signs his or her initials, and the student signs his or her initials in the adjacent column to the right. If the student fails, the evaluator writes "U" (unsatisfactory) in the Evaluator column.

Student _____

Evaluator(s) _____

_____

_____

	First try		Second try	
	EVALUATOR	STUDENT	EVALUATOR	STUDENT
Repeat from memory and in correct sequence the voice communications used in rescue hauling.				
Using a simulated rescue load, rig the following with appropriate anchors, pulley placement, haul cams, and progress capture device:				
1:1 haul system				
2:1 haul system				
3:1 haul system (Z-rig)				
4:1 haul system (piggyback)				
Optional: Compound 3:1 and 2:1 systems				

Skills Checklist
Chapter 20: Highlines

Instructions

As each student completes a skill check, the evaluator notes the date in the Evaluator column. If the student demonstrates the prescribed level of competence in the skill, the evaluator signs his or her initials, and the student signs his or her initials in the adjacent column to the right. If the student fails, the evaluator writes "U" (unsatisfactory) in the Evaluator column.

Student _____

Evaluator(s) _____

_____

_____

	First try		Second try	
	EVALUATOR	STUDENT	EVALUATOR	STUDENT
Rig a horizontal highline system using a single main line, a lowering/belay line, and a tag line between two anchor points at approximately the same elevation.				
Rig a litter and litter tender attachments for a highline.				
Move a litter across the horizontal highline and return, reversing the lowering and tag line functions as the litter moves back and forth.				
Rig a steep angle highline system using a single main line, a lowering/belay line on the high side, and a tag line on the low side.				
Optional: Rig a highline system using dual main lines (twin track lines), a lowering/belay line, and a tag line on each end.				
Optional: Rig an English reeve to the horizontal highline system.				

Answer Key

Chapter 1: The High Angle Environment

1. Any five of the following:
   - Mountaineering—uses outdoor skills, usually to reach a summit
   - Climbing—uses specialized vertical skills to climb a face
   - Vertical caving—uses the rope as a means of travel
   - Rope rescue—uses rope and associated gear to remove a subject from hazard
   - Fire service rescue—fire service personnel use of rope skills and equipment in a rescue
   - Tactical operations—law enforcement personnel use of rope and associated equipment in law enforcement operations
   - Industrial rescue—use of rope and associated skills for rescue in the industrial environment
   - Rope access—uses rope and associated equipment to access work sites
2. A
3. B
4. D
5. C
6. A
7. A

Chapter 2: Personal Equipment and Protection

1. C
2. D
3. B
4. D
5. C
6. E
7. A
8. C
9. B
10. A
11. C
12. A
13. D

Chapter 3: Rope and Related Equipment

1. A
2. A
3. C
4. C
5. C
6. C
7. B
8. A
9. C
10. A
11. B
12. C
13. B
14. D
15. B

Chapter 4: Care and Use of Rescue Rope and Related Equipment

1. D
2. D
3. A
4. D
5. B
6. C
7. A
8. A
9. D
10. B

Chapter 5: Basic High Angle Hardware

1. C
2. B
3. A
4. D
5. B
6. D
7. A
8. C
9. C
10. B
11. A
12. D
13. A
14. B
15. C
16. D

Chapter 6: Knots

1. A
2. C
3. (a) Either of the following: as a foundation knot for beginning other knots, such as the ring bend (water) knot; as a backup to secure other knots.
   (b) Either of the following: as a stopper knot for certain types of security; as a foundation knot for beginning the figure 8 follow-through or the figure 8 bend.
   (c) As a secure loop in a rope for clipping into.
   (d) To create a loop at the end of a rope when a figure 8 on a bight cannot be tied.
   (e) To join two rope ends.
   (f) To join two webbing ends.
   (g) To back up other knots.
   (h) To join two rope ends.
   (i) For an improvised litter spider.
   (j) In litter lowering and raising

operations, to bring the main line and the belay line to a single point.

Chapter 7: Anchoring

1. (1) Condition of the anchor; (2) structural nature of the anchor point; and (3) location of force on the anchor point.
2. (1) Where rocks or other dangerous objects might fall on the rescue subject or the rescuers; (2) when conditions between the anchor point and the rescue subject could endanger rescuers or damage equipment, such as rope; (3) where no suitable anchors can be found directly above.
3. A technique for bringing a rope into a more favorable position or angle.
4. It reduces flexibility of use and limits the ability to modify the anchor system.
5. (1) It is simple; (2) it reduces stress on rope and equipment; (3) it provides flexibility for dealing with changing conditions.
6. Root system
7. (1) The rescuer may not know who tied the knot and what kind of knot it is; (2) knots in webbing may eventually work their way out; (3) in webbing that has been shock loaded, the knots may have been spot-welded.
8. Tie an interior loop in the webbing using a wrap 2, pull 1 or a wrap 3, pull 2 technique.
9. Any of the following: corroded metal; weathered stonework; deteriorated mortar in brickwork; vents constructed of sheet metal; flashing, gutters, downspouts; and brickwork without bulk (e.g., small chimneys or fire hydrants).
10. Any of the following: structural columns; projections of structural beams; supports for large machinery; stairwell support beams; brickwork with large bulk (e.g., corner walls).
11. (a) Bumpers and tow hooks; (b) axles and cross members.
12. (1) When one anchor point is insufficient to withstand the anticipated forces; (2) when one anchor point is inconveniently placed.
13. 90 degrees; 120 degrees.
14. Two of the following: (1) Try to keep anchor points close to one another; (2) keep the outside angle to less than 90 degrees; even better, limit angles to 60 degrees; (3) Rig load-distributing anchors with a minimum of slack in the system.

Chapter 8: Belaying of One-Person Loads

1. (1) A person at risk of falling; (2) the rope attached to the person; (3) a harness worn by the person and attached to the rope; (4) a belay device; (5) the belayer; (6) an anchor to which the belay device is attached.
2. Any six of the following: (1) When a person is rock climbing or mountaineering; (2) in a rescue situation in which there is a danger of falling; (3) when a person is crossing an area not generally dangerous but that has a small area that could result in a fall; (4) when individuals are unsure of themselves in attempting a new skill, such as rappelling for the first time; (5) when a person's physical or mental capabilities are diminished; (6) when environmental factors, such as potential rock falls or areas slick with ice, increase the danger of falling; (7) when one or more individuals are being lowered by rope, such as in a rescue; (8) when one or more people are being raised by rope, such as in a rescue.
3. (a) A belay is a safety to catch a person should he or she fall. A lowering is the controlled lowering of people and equipment using rope through a lowering device and hardware.
   (b) A belay rope can be run either way (up or down) and does not have weight on it unless there is a fall on it. A lowering rope goes one way, down, and has weight on it throughout the lowering operation.
   (c) A one-person belay uses specialized equipment such as a personal belay device or special knots such as the Münter hitch. A lowering uses a friction device such as the large ring of a figure 8 descender or a brake bar rack.
4. (1) Climber: *"On belay?"*
   (2) Belayer: *"Belay on."*
   (3) Climber: *"Climbing"* (or *"Rappelling"*).
   (4) Belayer: *"Climb"* (or *"Rappel"*).
   When the climber is in a secure place and no longer needs the belay, he or she initiates the exchange to end the belay:
   (5) Climber: *"Off belay."*
   (6) Belayer: *"Belay off."*
5. (1) The slot in the figure 8 may not be the correct size for the rope used; (2) on some figure 8s, the slots are not well designed for use as a belay plate; (3) a figure 8 is not as well balanced as some belay devices and may not be as easy to use.
6. When a top belay is not available.

Chapter 9: Rappelling

1. Any five of the following: (1) The ability to control the descent with minimum physical effort; (2) the rope is not damaged by heat buildup in the rappel device; (3) anchors are not damaged by shock loading; (4) the ability to stop the rappel at any time; (5) the ability to tie off securely and operate hands free of the rope and rappel

device; (6) the ability to operate in any body position, including upside down.

2. They both use friction of the rope on the body to slow the descent.

3. Brake

4. Guide

5. Short, low angle slopes

6. (1) The rope could become unwrapped from the leg, possibly resulting in a free fall to the ground; (2) rope abrasion and pressure can injure body parts, particularly the crotch and shoulder.

7. Any two of the following: (1) The smaller version cannot be used with larger diameter rope; (2) it may be difficult to use the smaller figure 8 descender double wrapped; (3) the rope wraps can slip up and around the larger ring to form a girth hitch.

8. Set an ascender or Prusik loop on the rope above the figure 8 and step into an attached sling.

9. Use a figure 8 with ears.

10. Keep the rope on the side of the descender away from the edge.

11. To prevent tangling and to prevent damage to the rope from heat fusion as a result of rope cross.

12. If the main-line rappel anchor failed but the belay caught, there would be a possibility of a pendulum fall.

13. (1) Keep your body generally perpendicular to the slope; (2) keep your feet apart, about the width of your shoulders; (3) keep your knees relaxed and slightly flexed; (4) take slow, deliberate steps backward; (5) keep your body slightly turned in the direction of your brake hand, looking down slope to select a path of travel; (6) use your guide hand for balance (do not support your weight with the guide hand); (7) never take your brake hand off the rope unless the belay device is securely locked off.

14. Double wrapping the device.

15. The rope may run across seat harness webbing and damage it.

16. The preferred stance is on both feet (or alternatively, on both knees).

17. Generally, the most difficult angle is a horizontal angle (the anchor on the same level as or lower than the rappeller); the easiest is a vertical angle (the anchor above the rappeller).

18. The descender may become jammed, and the rappeller will be stranded in a precarious position.

19. *Advantages:* (1) It offers greater friction and therefore greater control than most descenders; (2) it allows the rappeller to change friction once he or she has begun to rappel; (3) its variable friction allows the rappeller to rappel longer drops more comfortably than with most descenders. *Disadvantages:* (1) It is somewhat more complex than descenders such as the figure 8; (2) it takes a bit longer to put on the rope; (3) it is somewhat bulkier and heavier.

20. Should not.

21. Instead of being on the rope above the device, as with other descenders, the guide hand should be resting on the bars of the rack.

22. Never less than four bars.

23. (1) If the rope wraps are not put onto the carabiner correctly, they can spiral out of the carabiner gate, resulting in a free fall; (2) the wraps can bear on the carabiner gate and break it.

24. The device could lock itself out of reach, possibly leaving the person stranded on the rope.

25. In the bottom end of the rappel line, tie a stopper knot, such as a figure 8 knot.

Chapter 10: Basic Ascending Techniques

1. Friction hitches and mechanical ascenders.

2. General-use ascenders grip the rope primarily by squeezing it against the inside of the ascender shell. Personal ascenders grip the rope with teeth on a cam and also press the rope inside the shell of the device.

3. Slings; webbing, rope.

4. At least two.

5. Friction hitches.

6. Smaller.

7. (1) Frame breakage; (2) rope damage; (3) rope slipping out of an ascender.

8. Safety lever.

9. Any three of the following: (1) The system should allow the person to use the legs and feet more than the arms and hands; (2) the system should hold the person upright on the rope with the body weight over the legs; (3) the system should allow the person to sit and rest while on rope; (4) the system should have attachments to the seat harness, not only to the feet.

10. Tying off short.

11. Chicken loop.

12. The legs.

13. Go over an edge.

14. Change over to ascending.

Chapter 11: Rescue Preplanning and Response: Rescuer Safety and Situational Awareness

1. Any seven of the following: (1) Notification procedures for team leaders and members; (2) contacts for backup resources and outside agencies; (3) procedure for handling requests for emergency assistance; (4) who initiates an operational response for rescue incidents; (5) how a rescue team fits in and to whom they report; (6) the command structure on scene; (7) communications setup, including radio frequencies; (8) medical control contacts and protocols; (9) standardized operating procedures and

techniques to be used by the team during rescue incidents; (10) established landing zones and known aerial hazards; (11) how the rescue team conforms to regulations and standards; (12) established protocols and guidelines for recovery operations.

2. (1) Local rescue needs; (2) locations that generate incidents or have existing hazards; (3) who has jurisdictional and operational responsibility for rescue in a local area.

3. Incident command system (ICS).

4. Five.

5. Incident commander (IC).

6. Any three of the following: hazards; personal safety equipment; safe work practices for specialized equipment; rescue rigging; personal rigging; fatigue; hydration levels; environmental exposure.

7. Standard 1561 *(Standard on Emergency Services Incident Management System)*.

8. One

9. (1) Here's what I think we face; (2) Here's what I think we should do; (3) Here's why; (4) Here's what we should keep our eye on; (5) Now, talk to me.

10. The ability to maintain an accurate perception of the external environment, as well as to detect and act on any problems encountered.

11. (1) Actively question and evaluate the mission's progress; (2) analyze your situation; (3) update and revise your image of the mission; (4) use assertive behavior when necessary.

Chapter 12: Medical Considerations in High Angle Rescue

1. (a) Type 2; (b) type 1; (c) type 2; (d) type 2; (e) type 2.

2. (1) Medical personnel; (2) medical skill; (3); medical control; (4) financial resources.

3. Any three of the following: (1) Immediate assistance with the care of difficult subjects; (2) constructive feedback on past rescues; (3) help with evaluating and adapting new medical protocols or devices; (4) having a visible medical backstop to support field medical operations.

4. Benefit, weight, durability, training, adaptability.

5. (1) Light; (2) portable; (3) easily accessible; (4) provides resources for a short period; (5) designed to be replenished in the field from the team medical kit.

Chapter 13: Rescue Belaying

1. (1) The operators must be extremely alert and prepared for failure; (2) it is very difficult to change the direction of rope travel.

2. Any two of the following: (1) it does not require special equipment solely for the belay; (2) the skills of the brakeman and belayer are the same and are easily interchangeable; (3) a brake belay usually does not accidentally engage and hang up; (4) it does not require load-releasing hitches; (5) it provides a soft catch; (6) it is predictable in the way it will perform.

3. Two triple-wrapped Prusiks anchored securely and placed in-line on the belay rope.

4. Any three of the following: icy rope; muddy rope; high impact; inappropriate Prusik material.

5. To shift the load off the Prusiks should they jam.

6. (1) The Prusiks are tied correctly; (2) they are neat and dressed; (3) they are the appropriate distance apart; (4) they grip the rope with the appropriate tightness.

Chapter 14: Pickoff Rescue

1. The subject is uninjured or only slightly injured.

2. Evaluate and stabilize the subject in terms of injury.

3. Any three of the following: (1) It is appropriate for only one person to perform the rescue; (2) there is a shortage of personnel and/or resources; (3) the urgency of the situation leaves no time to await additional personnel; (4) the benefits of a pickoff rescue outweigh the risks involved.

4. (1) The rope could hit the subject and knock him or her off; (2) if the rope is dropped close to a panicky subject, the person might grab the rope, stopping your rappel or causing injury or death to himself or herself and you.

5. Have the rope in a bag that is attached to you.

6. Assessment

7. (1) One main-line rope with an adequate safety factor for a two-person load; (2) one sewn, manufactured seat harness with thigh/leg supports for the rescuer, (3) one rappel device with enough friction to handle the weight of two people and, preferably, with variable friction; (4) two large locking carabiners (in addition to a locking carabiner already in the rescuer's seat harness tie-in point); (5) one short sling (approximately 2 feet [0.6 m]) with a loop in both ends or an adjustable rescue pickoff strap that will support one person's weight with an adequate safety factor.

8. Directly into the rappel device tie-in point, not into the seat harness.

9. Safety check.

10. Always above.

11. (1) Continued attention to keeping the airway clear; (2) spinal precautions if the injury has resulted in unconsciousness.

12. Any three of the following: (1) It must hold the subject upright; (2) it must prevent the subject from sliding out; (3) it must be simple to put on; (4) it must be usable in adverse conditions (e.g., cold, darkness, wind).

Chapter 15: Use of Litters in High Angle Rescue

1. Any three of the following: (1) It was designed and constructed for rescue; (2) it has the strength to be rigged for rescue and to support the weight of the subject and litter attendant; (3) it has strong, convenient tie-in points where rescuers can attach rigging; (4) it is durable enough to resist damage and protect the subject; (5) it has at least three handholds on each side and two at each end.

2. *Advantages:* (1) They slide easily along rough surfaces and snow; (2) they offer more protection for the subject. *Disadvantages:* (1) The plastic material may degrade with time; (2) they may retain water and snow if not properly drained

3. Any one of the following advantages and disadvantages: *Advantages:* (1) They can be taken to the rescue site more easily; (2) they can be transported in a vehicle space smaller than that required for one-piece litters. *Disadvantages:* (1) They are slightly heavier than the one-piece designs; (2) they are more expensive than one-piece litters.

4. Any three of the following advantages and disadvantages: *Advantages:* (1) They are lightweight; (2) they can be stored or carried in a compact backpack; (3) they are adaptable; (4) they drag easily over rough surfaces even when pulled only from one end; (5) the cost is reasonable. *Disadvantages:* (1) They require additional spine immobilization; (2) they are not rigid enough to be carried by two people at either end; (3) they are not as convenient as basket litters for litter teams to carry when loaded with a subject; (4) they catch wind and rotor wash; (5) they cannot be used with most litter wheels.

5. Any three of the following: (1) Protection of the subject from physical and environmental hazards; (2) subject comfort; (3) physical stabilization of the subject to prevent harmful movement; (4) protection of medical equipment (e.g., IV access sites, bandages).

6. Any three of the following: It must: (1) be accurately shaped and narrow enough to allow placement inside the litter; (2) be rigid, to prevent movement of the spine; (3) be made of strong material that is easy to clean; (4) have attachment points to allow attachment to the litter; (5) have handles for lifting; (6) allow insulation of the subject.

Chapter 16: Low Angle Evacuation

1. *Low angle evacuation:* (1) Most of the litter tenders' weight is on the ground; (2) the weight of the litter is supported both by tenders and by rope; (3) three or more litter tenders may be used; (4) rope is attached to one end of the litter. *High angle evacuation:* (1) Litter tenders' weight is supported by the litter and rope; (2) the weight of the litter is supported by rope; (3) at most, two litter attendants are used; (4) the litter hangs from vertical ropes.

2. Breakage of a butt weld and failure of the litter rail.

3. D

4. B

5. B

6. D

7. (1) The length of the main-line lowering rope; (2) the availability of anchor points.

8. The rope handler assists by feeding the brakeman the rope and removing kinks and tangles before they reach the brakes.

9. Any three of the following: (1) How steep is the slope? (2) Is the footing particularly loose and treacherous? (3) Is the slope icy or muddy? (4) What would be the consequences of a fall by the litter team? (5) Are the main-line brake anchors questionable? (6) Are there plenty of anchors? (7) Is thick underbrush or large boulders a factor?

10. (1) Litter captain to belayer: *"On belay."*
    (2) Belayer to litter captain: *"Belay on."*
    (3) Litter captain to brakeman: *"Down slow"* or *"Down fast."* (The brakeman should repeat this signal to the litter captain so that the captain knows the brakeman understands.)
    (4) *"Stop!"* (Usually the litter captain to the brakeman, but this signal may be given by anyone who sees danger or a potential problem developing.)
    (5) Litter captain to brakeman: *"Stop! Stop! Why stop?"* (This signal is given when, for an unexpected reason and without command from the litter captain, the rope has stopped moving.)
    (6) Brakeman to litter captain: "Two-oh." (This signal means there is only about 20 feet [6.5 m] of rope left.)
    (7) Litter captain to belayer: *"Off belay."*
    (8) Belayer to litter captain: *"Belay off."*

11. Such use of a personal ascender can result in failure in two potential ways: (1) the frame or some other portion of the ascender may fail; (2) the sharp teeth on the cam can tear the rope sheath.

12. D

13. Any three of the following: (1) Knots on moving rope could jam in cracks; (2) broken gear could cause system failure; (3) systems can reach their limit; (4) arms and legs can become pinned.

14. D

Chapter 17: High Angle Lowering

1. Any four of the following: (1) Cliffs; (2) buildings; (3) industrial sites; (4) construction sites, such as tower cranes; (5) other structures, such as stacks, silos, or towers; (6) vertical caves.
2. B
3. (1) Litter tender to belayer: *"On belay."*
   (2) Belayer to litter tender: *"Belay on."*
   (3) Litter tender to brakeman: *"Down slow"* or *"Down fast."*
   (4) *"Stop!"* (Generally the litter tender to the brakeman, but this signal may be given by anyone who sees danger or potential problems developing.)
   (5) Litter tender to brakeman: *"Stop! Stop!"* (This signal is given when, for an unexplained reason and without command from the litter tender, the rope has stopped moving.)
   (6) Litter tender to belayer: *"Off belay."* (The litter, rescue subject, and litter tender or tenders are on the ground or in a secure position and in no danger of falling.)
   (7) Belayer to litter tender: *"Belay off."*
4. C
5. Take the rope in the brake hand and pull it forward hard in the direction of the load.
6. There will be greater weight on the system, and greater friction will be needed.
7. (a) Single line lowering with belay:
   Advantages: (1) Simpler rope work; (2) less complicated brake management.
   Disadvantages: (1) safety factor may not be adequate for the weight of two litter tenders; (2) More difficult to tilt the litter from the horizontal position to the vertical position (i.e., requires loading of the belay line to tilt the litter).
   (b) Double line lowering:
   Advantages: (1) Can be used when two litter tenders are needed, such as for complicated medical management of a subject or for a vertical face that is too difficult for one tender to manage litter; (2) useful when orientation of the litter must be shifted.
   Disadvantages: (1) Puts greater stress on brake systems and anchors (if both lines run through the same brake); (2) requires more complex rope management; (3) may be more difficult to keep the litter horizontal if the lines come to two different points on the litter.
8. D
9. A, C, D
10. D
11. (1) The main attachment to the litter system is a pigtail. It is attached with a figure 8-on-a-bight knot to the carabiners at a master attachment point at the end of the main-line lowering rope. (2) The litter tender is attached to the pigtail with two ascenders. To prevent the ascenders from accidentally slipping off the end of the pigtail, the lower end is brought back up and clipped into the tender's seat harness.
12. (1) Attend to the medical needs of the subject in the litter; (2) help provide a smooth ride for the subject; (3) communicate with and reassure the subject; (4) prevent the litter from hanging up; (5) shield the subject from environmental hazards.
13. (1) Respond first, before the litter lowering, to assess the medical condition of the subject and begin primary treatment; (2) assist the litter tender in getting the litter over the edge; (3) assist in loading the subject part way down the wall; (4) help maneuver the litter around obstructions.
14. (1) When the position of the litter must be changed from horizontal to vertical and back again to get the litter through obstacles on a vertical space or to get through a confined space; (2) on an uneven, broken up, vertical face, where two tenders need to work the litter. (3) when medical considerations or other concerns relating to the rescue subject are too overwhelming for a single litter tender.

Chapter 18: Hauling Systems

1. Any five of the following: (1) Silos; (2) river gorges; (3) canyons; (4) escarpments; (5) grain elevators; (6) sewers; (7) tank cars; (8) basins; (9) utility vaults; (10) industrial storage bins; (11) fuel tanks; (12) air vents; (13) mine shafts; (14) caves; (15) tunnels.
2. (1) To make the raising more convenient and safer; (2) to make the raising easier.
3. Mechanical advantage is the relationship between how much load can be moved and the amount of force required to move it.
4. Theoretical mechanical advantage does not consider loss of force through factors such as friction, abrasion, and rope stretch. Actual mechanical advantage is the MA after loss of force through factors such as friction, abrasion, and rope stretch.
5. (a) 400 pounds
   (b) 200 pounds
   (c) 133.33 pounds
   (d) 100 pounds.
6. Traveling pulley
7. (1) 2:1 + 2:1 (2×2) = 4:1; (2) 2:1 + 3:1 (2×3) = 6:1.
8. They are *not* designed for the high stresses resulting from the multiplication of forces that takes place in

hauling systems. The use of personal ascenders in hauling systems can result in tearing of the rope or in structural failure of the ascender.

9. It should be positioned as far forward of the hauling system (toward the load) as possible while still being safely in reach of the rescuers.

10. There will be too much slack in the PCD's anchor sling. This will result in two problems: (1) possibly dangerous shock loading of the PCD, its sling, and its anchor can occur and (2) the hauling team will lose some of the purchase it has gained when it sets the PCD to reposition for another bite.

11. (1) The friction can increase severely, resulting in a tremendous increase in load for the haul team; (2) it can result in severe damage to the rope and other equipment.

12. Any two of the following: (1) Edge rollers; (2) directionals; (3) changing the position of the haul rope; (4) padding the rope; (5) reducing the load.

13. Tag lines.

14. (a) 1:1: One main-line rope, one anchor sling, two locking carabiners, and one rope grab (PCD), plus a separate belay system appropriate for the load being hauled.

(b) 2:1: One main-line rope, one haul rope, two anchor slings, three locking carabiners, two rope grabs (one PCD and one haul cam), and one pulley, plus a separate belay system appropriate for the load being hauled.

(c) 3:1 (Z-rig): One main-line rope, three locking carabiners, two pulleys, and two rope grabs (one PCD, one for hauling), plus a separate belay system appropriate for the load being hauled.

(d) 4:1 (piggyback): One main-line rope, one hauling rope, three locking carabiners, two pulleys, and two rope grabs (one PCD, one for hauling), plus a separate belay system appropriate for the load being hauled.

15. It creates a diminishing V, which tends to get easily snagged on brush, rock, building projections, and other objects as it advances. Also, because two strands of rope are going over the edge, additional friction is created.

Chapter 19: Tower Rescue

1. (1) Working at height; (2) EME/RF exposure; (3) electrical hazards; (4) the weather; (5) ice; (6) high winds; (7) lightning; (8) birds; (9) bees; (10) wasps.

2. *Advantages:* (1) The rescuer is securely attached to the rope at all times; (2) once the rope has been secured, additional rescuers can safely ascend with the aid of a rope grab. *Disadvantages:* (1) It requires a lot of bulky equipment, which increases the weight a rescuer must carry while ascending; (2) It requires the use of high-stretch ropes, which are not desirable for lowering operations because they have thinner sheaths, which are more susceptible to abrasion and cutting; (3) using ropes for lead climbing may create rope management concerns, such as rope entanglement or contact with electrical equipment or wires.

3. *Advantages:* (1) Lanyards limit the distance a rescuer can fall; (2) they offer more freedom of movement around and within the structure; (3) they allow a rescuer to move independently; (4) multiple rescuers can ascend or descend at the same time; (5) rescuers can proceed at their own speed; (6) rescuers can use lanyards to safety themselves off. *Disadvantages:* (1) A lanyard may not reach around a tower leg; (2) a lanyard that is not adjustable could create a greater fall hazard; (3) when lanyards are used with step bolts, there is the potential for step bolt failure; (4) lanyards generally need anchor points above the rescuer's connection on his or her harness.

4. The ability to ascend, descend, and traverse.

5. Free standing towers, guyed towers, and monopoles.

6. The operation will be either a tower-based rescue or a ground-controlled rescue.

7. The lanyard system.

Chapter 20: Highlines

1. Any four of the following: (1) To bypass an obstacle; (2) to avoid hazardous terrain; (3) to avoid difficult terrain; (4) for emergency evacuation; (5) in tactical situations.

2. (1) Potential stress and failure of equipment; (2) length of time required to set up the system; (3) getting initial personnel and rope across

3. (1) Main line; (2) near-side anchor; (3) far-side anchor; (4) load; (5) pulleys; (6) tag line; (7) haul line; (8) lowering/belay line.

4. Two, two.

5. To stabilize a load and to spread its weight out along the rope.

6. (1) To keep the two pulleys on the main line from spreading too far apart and becoming unwieldy during operations and (2) to serve as a stabilizer should one of the pulleys fail.

7. Pigtail and ascender attachments or two Prusik loops, one long and one short.

8. Head first, to minimize the subject's exposure to a head-down configuration.

9. Head first, to minimize the subject's exposure to a head-down configuration.

10. (a) A lowering/belay system is used primarily to control the speed of the load by running through a lowering device; (b) a tag line is used to maintain contact with or control of the load from either side.
11. Attached to the rigging plate above the litter.
12. A brake device.
13. Overstressing and failure of the rope, other equipment, or the anchors could result.
14. 200 pounds (91 kg); 100 feet (30 m); 10.
15. (1) the weight of the load; (2) the length of the rope span.
16. (a) 10 feet (3 m)
    (b) 20 feet (6 m)
    (c) 20 feet (6 m)
    (d) 10 feet (3 m)
17. 1 Main-line rope; 1 lowering/belay rope; 1 tag line/haul rope; 17 locking carabiners.
18. (1) As narrow a span as possible; (2) room on both sides to rig and derig the load and for personnel to get on and off; (3) suitable anchors.
19. (1) Use a line gun first to shoot over a smaller diameter rope, attach it to a main line, and pull the main line over; (2) personnel who go across to the far side trail the rope behind them; (3) lower the far-side end of the main-line rope to the ground, have someone pull the end to the base of the structure on the other side, and have the far-side team drop a haul line to the ground; the two ends are tied together, and the team then pulls up the main-line rope.
20. (1) Recheck rigging, including anchors on both sides; (2) make sure all personnel are ready.

Chapter 21: Helicopter Rescue Operations

1. (1) Is this plan in the best interest of the rescue subject and rescuer safety? (2) Is there a better way to do it? (3) If darkness or poor weather is hampering a helicopter response, will the subject be better served by an evacuation in the morning or in improved conditions?
2. *Type 1*—touchdown pad: 30 feet × 30 feet (9 m × 9 m); safety circle: 110 feet (33.5 m). *Type 2*—touchdown pad: 20 feet × 20 feet (6 m × 6 m); safety circle: 90 feet (27.4 m). *Type 3*—touchdown pad: 15 feet × 15 feet (4.6 m × 4.6 m); safety circle: 75 feet (22.9 m).
3. Any seven of the following: (1) never approach the helicopter until the pilot or crew directs you to; (2) never walk toward the tail rotor; (3) approach and depart on the down slope side of the aircraft; (4) use the door latches as instructed; (5) fasten your seat belt on boarding the helicopter and leave it secured until the pilot signals for you to disembark; (6) keep landing areas free of loose debris that rotor wash may pick up; (7) do not throw items from the helicopter; (8) provide visual wind indicators for landing and takeoff; (9) wear a helmet and use eye and hearing protection; (10) know the aircraft's layout and have a mental plan for what to do in the event of a crash or in-flight emergency.
4. Fire-resistant clothing; flight helmet; footwear and hand, eye, and ear protection; harnesses; and a personal flotation device (when flying over water).
5. Any seven of the following: noise; vibration; thermal changes; fatigue; barometric pressure; decreased humidity; decreased partial pressure of oxygen; G forces.
6. Cable breakage, entanglement, spin, static discharge.
7. Entanglement of the short haul line; hinders the pilot's ability to safely execute an autorotation; spinning of a loaded litter during a short haul operation.
8. Any seven of the following: (1) using media aircraft; (2) conducting a rescue with an unknown crew or aircraft; (3) exceeding the operating capabilities of the aircraft or crew; (4) improvising with an unpracticed or recognized technique; (5) radio incompatibility problems; (6) preoccupation with minor details (i.e., not maintaining the "big picture"); (7) inadequate leadership (e.g., failure to designate command); (8) pressing (i.e., "mission-it is" dictates operational decision making); (9) failure to delegate tasks and assign responsibilities; (10) failure to communicate intent and plans (i.e., lack of a briefing).

Chapter 22: Testing of Systems and Equipment

1. D
2. D
3. D
4. C
5. B
6. B
7. C

Glossary

A

Abrasion The damaging wear on rope and other equipment caused by rubbing against abrasive material.

Actual Mechanical Advantage (AMA) The useful mechanical advantage of a machine, such as a pulley system. It is calculated by subtracting the effects of friction from the theoretical mechanical advantage (TMA) of the system, or it can be measured by determining the actual input and output forces of the system in use.

After-Action Review See Hot Debrief.

Anchor *(n)* A secure tie-in point for attaching a line; (v) to attach a line to an anchor.

Anchor Point A single secure connection for an anchor; an anchor point is used either alone or in combination with other anchor points to create an anchor system capable of sustaining the actual or potential load on a rope rescue system.

Anchor System One or more anchor points rigged to provide a structurally sound connection for elements of a rope rescue system.

Arm Rappel (Guide's Rappel) A type of rappel in which the rope wraps around both outstretched arms and across the person's back. The technique is sometimes used in sloping terrain. It does not give enough control for vertical situations.

Artificial Anchors The use of specially designed hardware to create anchors where good natural anchors do not exist.

Ascenders Rope grab devices used by individuals to ascend a fixed rope or, with specific types of ascenders, to devise hauling systems. The two basic categories of ascenders are light-use ascenders, which normally are used for no more than one person's body weight, and general-use ascenders, which are used as personal ascenders and in hauling systems for progress capture devices and as rope grabs.

Ascending A means of moving up a fixed rope using either mechanical devices or friction hitches attached with slings to the climber's body.

Ascender Slings Attachments, usually webbing or rope, that connect a climber to the ascenders.

ASTM (formerly known as the American Society for Testing and Materials) An international organization that develops standards through a "full consensus" method. ASTM standards that apply to the rope rescue environment include those relating to search and rescue, recreational climbing equipment, and arboriculture equipment.

Automatic Belay A belay that locks off the belayed rope automatically when a sudden force is applied. Such belays do not depend on the belayer to activate the device to arrest a sudden fall, but they may require the device to be fed rope to operate correctly.

Autorotation A rotorcraft flight condition in which the lifting rotor is driven entirely by the action of the air while the rotorcraft is in motion. No engine power is supplied to the main rotor, and lift is developed from the free turning of the rotor blades, which are driven by aerodynamic forces. Rotor inertia is used as the helicopter nears the ground to control the descent.

Auxiliary Tender An optional rescuer who, in order to assist the rescue, rappels or ascends alongside the litter. This person's duties may include medical assessment and/or primary treatment of the rescue subject, as well as assisting in getting the litter over the edge, in handling the litter on the vertical face, and in loading the subject into the litter.

B

Backing Up The creation of a secondary or redundant system designed to provide added security, and the creation of one or more additional independent anchors to sustain the high angle system should the initial anchors fail. Backing up may be done at the same anchor point if it is very solid or at other anchor points.

Back Tie A connector from a primary anchor to a second, back-up anchor.

Back-Up (Safety) Knot A second knot used to secure the tail of a primary knot; also known as a safety or keeper knot.

Backyard Testing Testing performed by field-type personnel in a less than ideal or an uncontrolled environment.

Basket Litter A litter with a rigid structure that is shaped to hold a rescue subject. It is constructed of rugged materials so as to protect the subject and to resist damage when used in the rescue environment.

Bauman Bag A device for transporting rescue subjects (it is generically known as a heli-rescue bag in Europe). The Bauman bag is a hammocklike stretcher, constructed of Cordura, that has suspension straps that join to a single connection point overhead.

Belay To protect against falling by managing an unloaded rope (the belay rope) in a way that secures one or more individuals in case the main line rope or support fails.

Belay Device A braking mechanism through which a secondary line, also called the belay line, is rigged. The device must allow free run of the belay rope through it when the system is operating correctly; it must exert a slowing or stopping action on the belay line if an uncontrolled descent or fall occurs on the main line.

Belay Line A type of tag line set up to prevent an uncontrolled lowering of a load.

Belay Plate A common type of belay device; it is a simple metal plate with one or more slots for rope that is used in conjunction with a carabiner to exert friction on a belay rope.

Belayer The person who controls a safety rope connected to another person or persons to keep them from falling.

Bend A class of knot that joins two ropes or pieces of webbing.

Bight The open loop in a rope formed when the rope is doubled back on itself.

Body Rappel (Dulfersitz Rappel) A type of rappel that uses the body as friction by running the rope through the legs, across one hip, over the opposite shoulder, and to a braking hand. Because of the discomfort involved and the potential injury to body parts, this rappel has largely been supplanted by other techniques.

Bolts Metal devices used to create semipermanent anchors on a rock surface; a hole is drilled into the rock, and the device is set in the hole. A hanger usually is attached to the bolt so that the bolt can be used as an anchor point.

Bombproof Jargon for an anchor or anchor system believed to be very secure.

Brake Bar Rack A descending device consisting of a U-shaped metal bar to which several metal bars are attached that create friction on the rope. Some racks are limited to use in personal rappelling, whereas others may also be used for lowering rescue loads. Also known as a rappel rack.

Brake Hand The hand that grasps the rope to help control the speed of descent during a rappel. The dominant hand (e.g., the right hand in a right-handed individual) usually is the brake hand.

Brakeman The person who operates the braking device that controls the rate of descent of a litter in a low angle evacuation.

Break-Apart Litter A litter designed to be separated into sections so that it can be transported to the rescue site more easily and can be stored in smaller spaces.

Bridle See Spider.

C

Cams Devices used in climbing for protection or anchoring that lodge in a rock crack. Active cams with springs adjust to the width of the crack. Passive cams (nuts, stoppers, and chocks) wedge to fit the crack.

Carabiner Metal snap links used to connect elements of a high angle system.

Carabiner Wrap A rappel technique that uses several rope wraps around a seat harness carabiner to create friction and control the descent. It generally is not considered a safe and secure technique for rappelling.

Cargo Let-Down A method of lowering cargo from a hovering helicopter using a let-down line or rope controlled through a friction descent device.

CEN (European Committee for Standardization) The standards-setting authority for the European Union. CE standards cover a wide range of products, including those used for recreational climbing, protection from industrial falls, and rope access.

Center of Gravity (CG) The point in a helicopter where all forces are balanced. In a single-rotor helicopter, this is a range forward or aft beneath the rotor mast. The distribution of the weight of the fuel, the personnel, and the cargo in the helicopter affects this critical balance for safe flight.

Changeover To transfer from an ascending mode to a rappelling mode or from a rappelling mode to an ascending mode while on rope.

Chest Harness A type of harness worn around the chest for upper body support. In the high angle environment, it should never be used as the only source of support; it should always be used in conjunction with a seat harness.

Chicken Loop A safety loop that fits around the ankle to secure the ascender sling and prevent the foot from slipping out of the sling should an upper connection fail and the climber fall backward.

Clear Text Spoken communication style that avoids the use of any abbreviated codes in order to facilitate understanding by all emergency personnel.

Collective Pitch System The flight control mechanisms by which the pitch of all rotor blades is varied equally and simultaneously. The collective pitch control regulates the pitch angle of the main rotor blades. It is used as the primary power control. As the pitch of the blades is increased, lift is induced, causing the helicopter to lift off the ground, hover, or climb, as long as power is available.

Commercial Operator A person who, for compensation or hire, engages in the carriage by aircraft in air commerce of persons or property.

Component A single piece of equipment in a rope system.

Component Testing Measurement of how a single piece of equipment performs under a certain set of criteria.

Compound Pulley System Any combination of two or more simple pulley systems rigged in such a way that the first acts on the second.

Conditional Belay A belay that does not lock automatically when sudden force is applied; also known as a manual belay or brake belay. A traditional one-person belay (as discussed in Chapter 8) is considered a conditional belay, because most arrest the falling load only if properly activated by the belayer.

Counterbalance Haul System A procedure for hauling that uses a 1:1 ratio and a haul team that moves in a direction opposite to the load.

Cyclic The flight control mechanism that permits the helicopter to move forward, sideways, and backward by corresponding tilting of the rotor disc.

D

Density Altitude The actual pressure altitude corrected for temperature and humidity, which provides a measure of the air density.

Descender A rappel device that creates friction by means of a rope running through it; it is attached to a rappeller to control descent on a rope. Most descenders can also be used as a fixed brake lowering device. Also called a descent control device.

Descending See Rappelling.

Directional A technique for repositioning a rope at a more favorable angle than would exist by running the rope directly to the anchor.

Double Line Lowering The use of two ropes attached to the litter in a lowering; the ropes are rigged so that they may be operated independently to change the angle of the litter. Also called scaffold lowering.

Double Pulley A pulley with two sheaves; it can be rigged on two ropes or used to create mechanical advantage hauling systems.

Downloading A fixed weight reduction used in the load calculation process for helicopters that provides a built-in margin of safety; it is different for each make and model of helicopter.

Drop Zone The area immediately under and around the tower where objects may fall. It could extend out 30 to 50 feet (10 to 16.5 m) or farther from the base of the tower if the object that is dropped bounces off the structure or is blown by the wind.

Dulfersitz Rappel See Body Rappel.

Dynamic Relating to a moving force.

Dynamic Rollover As a helicopter lifts off from a sloping landing zone, if one skid or wheel is still on the ground, the helicopter may pivot about this skid or wheel. If this happens, the pilot can reach the "stop" on the cyclic as it runs out of cyclic travel and will not be able to stop the rollover. If a roll rate is permitted to develop, a critical angle may be reached at which the roll cannot be corrected, and the helicopter will roll over onto its side. Dynamic rollover also occurs on level surfaces, such as when a skid or wheel becomes stuck on a landing zone or is restrained by a tie-down during takeoff.

Dynamic Rope A type of rope designed for high stretch to reduce the shock on the climber and anchor system. This type of rope is usually used in rock climbing and mountaineering and is certified by the Union of International Alpine Associations (UIAA) or the European Committee for Standardization (CEN) as such.

Dynamometer Any of several instruments used to measure force. The simplest version is a type of spring scale that can measure the load on a system into which the device has been inserted.

Dulfersitz Rappel See Body Rappel.

E

Edge Rollers In-line, free-turning rollers that are anchored at the edge of a wall or cliff face to reduce rope friction.

Edge Tender The person connected to a safety attachment who works at the edge of a drop in a high angle lowering. This individual's duties include assisting in getting the litter over the edge, reducing edge abrasion to ropes, and when necessary, relaying communications between the litter tender and the brakeman.

Electronic Load Cell A force measurement device with electronic measurement capabilities.

EME or RF Exposure *EME (electromagnetic energy)* is nonionizing radiation. *RF (radio frequency)* radiation is exposure to nonionizing electromagnetic energy at radio frequencies. The major concern with RF energy is tissue heating.

Emergency Locator Transmitter (ELT) A radio transmitter attached to an aircraft that operates from it own power source on 121.5 MHz and 243 MHz. It aids location of downed aircraft by radiating a downward sweeping audiotone two to four times per second. It is designed to function without human action after an accident.

Emergency Seat Harness A temporary tied harness that is used when a manufactured, sewn seat harness is not available.

English Reeve System One of several rigging systems that can be added to a highline to control the load from either side. Controlling the system's lines from either side, rescuers can raise or lower a load from the carrier at any position along the highline.

Equipped Weight The empty weight of the helicopter plus the weight of the equipment required for the mission plus the weight of oil.

Escape Belt A device that fastens around the waist like a belt that is intended for use by the wearer only as an emergency self-rescue device. It should never be used as the sole means of suspension.

External Load A load that is carried or extends outside the aircraft's fuselage.

F

Fall Factor The distance fallen in relationship to the amount of rope used to catch the fall. The fall factor calculation is used to estimate the impact force on a rope when it is subjected to stopping a falling mass.

Figure 8 Descender A device used for rappelling and in some cases for lowering. The descender has the general shape of the numeral 8, with a large ring to create friction on the rope and a smaller ring to attach to a seat harness.

Fixed Pulley A pulley that is anchored and does not move as the load moves. Also known as a change of direction pulley. Fixed pulleys do not add mechanical advantage to a system but may make it more convenient to pull.

Flexible Litter A litter that does not have an inherent rigid structure, but rather is made of a flexible material, usually plastic, that can be wrapped closely around the subject.

Flight Crew Member A pilot, flight engineer, or flight navigator assigned to duty in an aircraft during flight time.

Flight Following The method and process by which an aircraft is tracked from departure point to destination. Flight following is the knowledge of the aircraft and condition with a reasonable degree of certainty such that, in the event of mishap, those on board may be rescued. It typically is accomplished through a position check on the radio at regular intervals.

Foundation Knot A simple knot that is tied as the first step in tying a more complex knot; examples are the overhand knot and the simple figure 8 knot.

Freestanding Tower A self-supporting structure with three or four legs. It generally is wider at the base and narrower at the top.

Full Body Harness A type of harness that offers pelvic and upper body support as one unit.

G

General-Use Ascenders A mechanical rope grab device that operates primarily by the force of a cam action wedging the rope against the inside of the device's shell. General-use ascenders are designed to slide in one direction on a rope. They are used for personal ascenders and in hauling systems for progress capture devices and rope grabs.

Ground-Controlled Rescue A rescue in which the lowering and belay lines are controlled and operated from a ground position and not on the tower.

Ground Effect When a helicopter is in a low hover, the ground interrupts the airflow under the helicopter, and the velocity of the induced airflow to the rotor system is reduced. The result is less induced drag and a more vertical lift vector. This ground cushion, or ground effect, is beneficial in flight because it increases lift capability for the helicopter, which therefore requires less power to maintain a hover. Ground effect occurs when the helicopter is at a very low altitude, usually one half the rotor diameter. Ground effect is hampered by uneven terrain, vegetation, or water beneath the rotor disc.

Guide Hand The hand that cradles the rope to help balance the rappeller. The nondominant hand (e.g., the right hand in a left-handed individual) is usually the guide hand.

Guyed Tower A narrow column that sits on a base and is stabilized by a series of guy wires attached to the tower at pre-engineered positions.

H

Harness Suspension Pathology A potentially fatal condition that can occur when a person hangs motionless in a seat harness for a long period. The position in the harness, along with harness strap compression, reduces venous blood flow from the extremities (particularly the legs) to the right side of the heart, with subsequent reduction in cardiac output. This can result in unconsciousness and possibly death in minutes.

Haul Cam A rope grabbing device that grips the rope to provide the "bite" in hauling.

Haul Line A type of tag line that the haul team uses for pulling on a load; with highlines, it is used to transport the load across the highline.

Haul System Efficiency The result of dividing the actual mechanical advantage (AMA) of a haul system by the theoretical mechanical advantage (TMA). This value is expressed as a percentage.

Haul Team The group of individuals who provide the power to raise the load.

Hazard Map A map of the operational area that identifies all the known aerial hazards, including but not limited to power lines, overhead cables, towers, and military operations areas.

Heavy Helicopter A helicopter with a certified gross weight greater than 12,500 pounds (5,670 kg). Under the ICS helicopter typing system, a heavy helicopter is a type 1 helicopter; it must have an allowable payload at 59° F (15° C) at sea level of 5000 pounds (2268 kg) and 15 or more passenger seats (unless in a restricted category).

Height-Velocity Curve A chart in the helicopter flight manual that indicates the combinations of altitude and forward airspeed required to ensure a safe autorotation.

Helibase Under the incident command system (ICS), a designated facility for conducting helicopter operations that has refueling capability. The U.S. Federal Aviation Administration (FAA) term for a permanent helicopter facility is *heliport*.

Helicopter A rotorcraft that depends principally on its engine-driven rotors for horizontal motion.

Helicopter Rappel Insertion of personnel at a site by means of rappelling on a fixed rope from a helicopter in a hover.

Helispot A temporary helicopter landing zone, which may incorporate a natural or an improved takeoff and landing area.

Helmet A head covering that protects against head injury both from falling objects and from head impact. In this book, helmet denotes head protection specifically designed for high angle work or specialized uses (e.g., flight helmet).

High Angle A very steep environment in which a person is supported primarily by the rope system. One or more ropes are necessary to keep the person from falling.

Highline (also Tyrolean or Telpher) A system of using a rope suspended between two points to move people or equipment over an area that is a barrier to a rescue operation. Also known as a Telpher or Tyrolean.

Hitch A knot that attaches to or wraps around an object or rope in such a way that when the object or rope is removed, the knot falls apart.

Hoist Rescue Insertion or extraction of personnel on a lightweight cable using an electric or hydraulic hoist that is anchored to a helicopter.

Horizontal Highline A highline in which the two suspension points are nearly on the same level.

Hot Debrief (After-Action Review) Immediate review after an emergency response operation, conducted with involved personnel, to identify operational deficiencies and planned corrective actions.

Hover A condition of flight in which the helicopter remains fairly stationary over a given point, moving neither vertically nor horizontally.

Hover Ceiling The highest altitude at which a helicopter can successfully hover while loaded to its maximum gross weight. In and out of ground effect hover ceilings are computed at maximum gross weight.

Hover in Ground Effect (HIGE) To operate at an altitude (usually equal to one half the rotor diameter above the surface) at which the positive influence of ground effect is attained.

Hover Landing A landing that does not meet the definition of toe-in, single-skid, or step-out landings. Hover landings are characterized by a need to maintain a substantial amount of hover power while the landing gear is not in contact with the surface. Hover landings normally are required because of the nature of the surface (e.g., swampy ground, tundra or muskeg, snow, or lava rock).

Hover Out of Ground Effect (HOGE) Hovering at a high enough altitude that the added benefit of ground effect is not obtained.

Hypothesis A tentative explanation for an observation, phenomenon, or scientific problem that can be tested by further investigation.

I-K

Incident Command System (ICS) A standardized emergency management system (also referred to as the incident management system [IMS]) that was developed to organize all functions needed to manage and support the response to an emergency situation.

Incident Safety Officer (ISO) The person responsible for monitoring current and projected hazards associated with dangerous conditions affecting rescuers and others.

Initial Incident Commander First emergency responder to arrive at the scene; this individual assumes the role of incident commander until he or she is relieved.

Instrument Flight Rules (IFR) FAA rules governing the operation of aircraft in weather conditions below the minimum for flight under visual flight rules; that is, conditions under which instruments are essential for flight navigation.

Kernmantle A rope design consisting of two elements: an interior core (kern), which usually supports the major portion of the load on the rope, and an outer sheath (mantle), which serves primarily to protect the core but also may support a minor portion of the load.

Kevlar The trade name for a type of Aramid fiber, manufactured by the DuPont Corp., that has high tensile strength, low elongation, and high resistance to heat.

Kilonewton (kN) A unit of measure for force equal to 1,000 newtons. It is used to test impact loads on ropes, the breaking strength of carabiners, and for other force measurements. See also Newton.

Knot A fastening made by tying together rope or webbing in a prescribed way. Knots include bights, bends, and hitches.

Kootenay Carriage A modified knot-passing pulley that is used on highlines as the main-line pulley for single and double main-line systems or as a high-strength tie off.

L

Ladder Belt A device that fastens around the waist and is intended for use as a positioning device for a person on a ladder. It should never be used as the sole means of suspension.

Laid Rope Ropes made by twisting three or more strands together with the twist direction opposite that of the strands. Plain, or hawser, laid ropes have three strands, whereas shroud laid ropes have four strands.

Landing Zone (LZ) Any improved or unimproved helicopter landing site that has an adequate touchdown pad and approach and departure paths. Under ICS, a landing zone is referred to as a helispot or helibase.

Lanyard A piece of rope or webbing that connects a rescuer's harness to a lifeline or anchorage.

Lanyard Climbing The use of one or more lanyards to ascend a structure.

Lead Climbing A two-person climbing method involving protective anchors (protection) placed by the individuals as they climb.

Light Helicopter A helicopter with a certified gross weight of less than 6,000 pounds (2,721 kg). Under the ICS helicopter typing system, a light helicopter is a type 3 helicopter; it must have an allowable payload at 59° F (15°) at sea level of 1,200 pounds (544 kg) and four to eight passenger seats.

Light-Use Ascenders Also called a personal ascender or personal ascent device, a light-use ascender is a rope grab device used to travel up (ascend) a fixed rope. Light-use ascenders normally are used for no more than one person's body weight.

Litter Attendant An individual who helps control the litter or attends to a rescue subject's medical needs during a low angle evacuation. Also known as a litter tender.

Litter Captain In low angle evacuation, the person who manages the litter team and coordinates the litter movement with other members of the rescue team.

Litter Medical Kit (LMK) A smaller version of the rescue team medical kit that is designed for the management of emergency problems that may arise while the rescue subject is on rope or restrained in a litter or when the larger rescue medical kit is unavailable.

Load The total combined objects and persons being lowered or raised by a rope in a high angle system. Some examples include a rescue subject and a rescuer, or a subject in a litter with one or two attached litter tenders.

Load Calculation Calculation of the helicopter's lifting capability for a given altitude and temperature.

Load-Distributing Anchor System (LDA) An anchor system established from two or more anchor points that (1) maintains near-equal loading on the anchor points despite direction changes on the main line rope and (2) reestablishes near-equal loading on remaining anchor points should one or more of them fail. This system is sometimes referred to as a self-equalizing anchor.

Load Ratio The ratio of the component's minimum breaking strength to the anticipated load.

Load-Releasing (LR) Hitch A type of hitch usually tied in webbing or accessory cord in such a way that it can sustain major loads and, with tension still on it, can be used as a mechanism to release the tension in the system into which it is inserted. Well-constructed load-release hitches allow the load to be let out several meters under control.

Load-Sharing Anchors An anchor system established from two or more anchor points that distributes the load among the anchor points but does not adjust to direction changes on the main line.

Locking Carabiner A carabiner with a locking sleeve on the gate side that secures the gate shut.

Locking Off The technique of jamming a rope into a descender or tying off securely so that the rappeller can stop the descent and operate hands free of the rope.

Longline A line or set of lines, typically steel cable, used for external sling load operations to deliver supplies to a site where a helicopter could not safely land.

Low Angle An environment, such as a flat or mildly sloping area, in which a rescuer is supported primarily by the surface and not by the rope system. One or more ropes may be used for safety or for lowering.

Low Angle Evacuation Movement of a rescue subject in an environment in which the load is supported primarily by itself rather than the rope rescue system (e.g., flat land or mild sloping surface). The litter is attached to a rope for safety and control. Also known as slope evacuation or scree evacuation.

Low-Stretch A quality of a type of rope designed to be used in applications such as rescue, rappelling, and ascending in which high stretch would be a disadvantage and no falls, or only very short falls, are expected before the climber is caught by the rope. The term low-stretch rope can refer to ropes with slightly more elongation than the traditional static ropes or to both types of ropes (see Static Rope).

Lowering The process and system by which a load is lowered while controlled from above. A lowering rope is weighted through its entire operation and moves consistently in a downward direction.

Lowering/Belay Line The line attached to a load on a highline that is used to control the load from the near-side point.

M

Main Line The line (or lines) that provide the support of the load.

Main Rotor The rotor that supplies the principal lift to a rotorcraft.

Manifest A written list of personnel and/or cargo to be transported and their weights.

Manner of Function The method in which a particular piece of equipment was designed to be used.

Master Attachment Point The point where rigging comes together for maximum strength.

Maximum Gross Weight The certified maximum allowable weight of an aircraft, as determined by the manufacturer and approved by the FAA, at which that particular aircraft can safely fly. This weight is the equipped weight of the aircraft plus that of the useful load (i.e., pilot, passengers, cargo, and fuel).

Maximum Performance Takeoff A steep ascent upon takeoff, done to clear obstacles, that involves limited forward airspeed and that approaches the flight limitations of the helicopter.

Mechanical Advantage (MA) The ratio of the output force produced by a machine to the applied input.

Medical Preplanning The prediction of conflicts that may arise between subject care and rescue operations as well as the prognostic adaptation of medical and rescue systems.

Medium Helicopter A helicopter with a certified gross weight between 6,000 pounds (2,721 kg) and 12,500 pounds (5,669 kg). Under the ICS helicopter typing system, a medium helicopter is a type 2 helicopter; it must have an allowable payload at 59° F (15° C) at sea level of 2,500 pounds (1,134 kg) and nine to 14 passenger seats (unless it is in a restricted category).

Monopole A cylindrical, self-supporting column that is larger at the base and narrower at the top. Monopoles usually are associated with PCS (personal communication systems [e.g., cell phones, pagers]) antennas.

Mountaineering The use of combined skills, such as climbing and snow and ice travel, to ascend a mountain.

Multipoint Anchor Anchors involving two or more anchor points.

Münter Hitch A type of running knot commonly used in belaying that slips around a carabiner to create friction against itself. It is also known as the Italian hitch or half ring bend.

Münter Hitch Rappel A limited-use rappel technique involving a Münter hitch attached to the seat harness carabiner.

N-O

National Fire Protection Association (NFPA) A U.S. organization that sets standards and fire service guidelines for rope and related equipment, along with performance standards for rope rescuers in the fire service.

Newton (N) The unit of force required to accelerate a mass of 1 kilogram 1 meter per second per second. The impact loads on rope and the breaking strength of equipment usually is expressed in kilonewtons (kN); a kilonewton is 1,000 newtons. If the English system is used, this is expressed in pounds/force (lbf). One newton equals 0.225 lbf. See also Kilonewton.

Nomex A fire-resistant aramid fiber manufactured by the DuPont Corp. It is used in the manufacture of protective clothing.

Nonlocking Carabiner A carabiner without a means to secure the gate shut.

Null Hypothesis A statistical hypothesis formed to determine whether obtained results are significant.

Nylon 6 A type of nylon used in rope manufacturing. Because of its shock-absorbing qualities, nylon type 6 is found in most climbing ropes. See Perlon.

Nylon 6,6 A type of nylon used in rope manufacturing. With its resistance to wear and reduced elongation under load, most static ropes are constructed of type 6,6. In North America it is manufactured by DuPont and the Monsanto Corporation.

One-Skid Landing The maneuver of placing one skid of the helicopter on the ground while the other remains above the ground, typically performed in steep terrain. When the skid is in contact with the ground, the center of gravity can shift laterally.

P

Packaging Proper placement of a rescue subject in a litter for transport; it takes into consideration the subject's **primary medical problems and physical stabilization of the individual in the litter.**

PBI (Polybenzimidazole) A synthetic fiber produced by Celanese AG. It has no melting point, will not ignite, and retains fiber integrity and suppleness when exposed to a flame.

Pendulum (v) To swing on a rope.

Perlon A trade name for a version of nylon type 6.

Pickoff Rescue A rescue in the high angle environment involving an uninjured or slightly injured subject in which a single rescuer usually has direct physical contact with the subject and in which a litter is not initially used in the rescue operation.

Piggyback System (Pig-Rig) A compound pulley system in which one hauling system pulls (or piggybacks) on another hauling system. The term is often used for a specific type of 4:1 hauling system in which one 2:1 system is attached to (piggybacked onto) another 2:1 system to create a 4:1 system.

Pigtail A short piece of rope with which the litter tender attaches to the litter system.

Pilot in Command (PIC) The person who (1) has final authority and responsibility for the operation and safety of the flight; (2) has been designated as pilot in command before or during the flight; and (3) holds the appropriate category, class, and type rating, if appropriate, for the conduct of the flight.

Piton A slender metal wedge, with an eye for attachment, that is driven into a rock crack for climbing protection or for anchoring.

Pitot Tube A projecting tube on the front of the helicopter fuselage that measures ram air pressure and delivers that pressure to the airspeed indicator.

Polyester A type of fiber used in some rope manufacturing. Also known by the trade name Dacron.

Polyolefins A group of fiber types (e.g., polypropylene, polyethylene) used in the manufacture of ropes often used in water applications.

Pounds/force (lbf) In the English system, a unit of measure for force; it is used to test impact loads on ropes, the breaking strength of carabiners, and for other force measurements. The impact loads on rope and the breaking strength of equipment usually are expressed in kilonewtons (kN), a measurement in the SI system. To convert lbf to kN, multiply by 0.004448.

Power-On Landing A landing maneuver in which both skids are in full contact with the ground while full power is maintained; this maneuver is performed to maintain the position of the aircraft on a marginal touchdown pad.

Precautionary Landing A landing conducted by the pilot because of an apparent failure of the helicopter flight systems, which would make continued flight unsafe.

Preplan Written or mental contingency preparation for possible emergency operations.

Progress Capture Device (PCD) A rope grab device, general-use ascender, or hitch placed on the rope in a hauling system to prevent the rope (and the load) from slipping back down as the haul system is reset. Also commonly referred to as the ratchet.

Prusik A type of friction hitch used in ascending and belaying. Some individuals use the term **Prusik** synonymously with ascending (e.g., to Prusik), even when mechanical devices are used.

Prusik Loop A continuous loop of rope in which a Prusik hitch is tied.

Prusik Minding Pulley (PMP) A pulley with specially shaped side plates that help manage Prusik hitches.

Public Aircraft A government-owned, leased, or hired aircraft that is performing work "exclusively in the service" of any federal, state, or local government agency.

Pulley A device with a free-turning, grooved metal wheel (sheave) that is used to reduce rope friction; it also has side plates to which a carabiner may be attached.

R

Rappel Rack See Brake Bar Rack.

Rappelling Controlled descent of a rope using friction to obtain the control. Normally the friction is created by rope running through a descender.

Rock Climbing Ascending while making direct contact with the rock. Rope and other equipment may be used for safety in the event of a fall.

Rope Access The commercial use of mountaineering and caving rope techniques to access work sites. To ensure safe operation, the systems usually involve at least main and belay (safety) lines.

Rope Grab A device that grips the rope. The two types are mechanical rope grabs, which usually are made of metal and which grip the rope with a camming action, and rope or webbing rope grabs, which use a hitch to grip the rope.

Rope Handler The person in a lowering operation who assists the brakeman with rope management.

Rope History Log A document that tracks the history of a particular rope. The log contains entries that indicate the manufacturer, diameter, design, tensile strength, date of purchase, when the rope was used, how it was used, and any abuse that could affect its performance or safety.

Rope Rescue Rescue in a high angle, steep, or extreme environment where the use of rope and related equipment is necessary.

Rope Tag Identification placed on a rope that distinguishes it from other ropes.

Rotorcraft-Load Combination The combination of a rotorcraft and an external load, including the means of attaching the external load. Rotorcraft-load combinations are designated by the FAA as Class A, Class B, Class C, or Class D. In Class A rotorcraft-load combinations, the external load cannot move freely, cannot be jettisoned, and does not extend below the landing gear. In Class B rotorcraft-load combinations, the external load can be jettisoned and is lifted free of land or water during the rotorcraft operation. In Class C rotorcraft-load combinations, the external load can be jettisoned and remains in contact with land or water during the rotorcraft operation. In Class D rotorcraft-load combinations, the external load is other than a Class A, B, or C and has been specifically approved by the administrator for that operation.

Rotor Disc The circular area swept by the rotating blades in one revolution.

S

Safety Circle An obstruction-free area on all sides of the helicopter touchdown pad that allows a safe approach to and departure from the touchdown pad.

Safety Knot See Back-Up Knot.

Seat Harness A system of nylon or polyester webbing that wraps and supports the pelvic region to attach the wearer to the rope or other protection in the high angle environment. The three NFPA classes of harnesses are Class I (a light duty seat harness meant for emergency escape and work by one person), Class II (a seat harness meant for heavy duty work by one person or for use in rescue situations in which another person's weight may be added in the course of the rescue), and Class III (a full-body harness meant for fall protection and rescue activities in which inversion might occur).

Short Haul The transport of one or more people externally suspended below a helicopter. Also, the use of a helicopter and an externally attached line to insert or extract personnel in areas that preclude a normal landing.

Simple Pulley System A simple machine consisting of a pulley and rope that provides a mechanical advantage.

Single Line Lowering The use of one main lowering rope with a belay to lower a litter.

Single Rope Technique (SRT) Ascending and descending directly on the rope without direct aid from contact with the rock, walls, or structures.

Situational Awareness The ability of an individual to know what is going on around himself or herself at all times. Situational awareness is maintained by obtaining updated information about the external environment and about all operational conditions in order to form an accurate mental image of a mission.

Size Up Continuous evaluation of information, resulting in the development of a rescue plan.

Sling Load An external load supported by a sling, net, bag, or some combination of these that is attached with a longline to the helicopter by means of a cargo hook.

Software A category of high angle equipment that is not hardware (e.g., rope and webbing).

Span of Control The ratio of subordinate personnel to one supervisor during an emergency incident. The optimum span of control is considered to be 5:1; this may be increased to a maximum of 7:1.

Spectra Trade name for a high modulus polyethylene fiber with high tensile strength.

Spider The system of attaching a lowering rope to a litter. A spider usually has four or more legs that connect to various points of a litter to equalize loading. Sometimes called a bridle or harness.

Spotter The flight crew member positioned in a helicopter to direct activities during helicopter rappel and short haul missions.

Static Rope A type of rope designed to be used in applications such as rescue, rappelling, and ascending in which high stretch would be a disadvantage and in which no falls, or only very short falls, are expected before the person is caught by the rope. Static ropes have slightly less elongation than low-stretch ropes built to the same standard. Less elongation prevents loss of system efficiency to rope stretch (see Low-Stretch Rope).

Static Testing For the purposes of this chapter, the term refers to testing performed with the subject at rest and without motion or momentum created in the system; the opposite of dynamic testing.

Step-Out Landing A landing used for dropping off or picking up passengers and cargo (other than the rappel/short haul method) while the helicopter is held in a hover. The helicopter is not in contact with the ground, and the center of gravity can shift laterally and longitudinally.

Steep Angle Highline A highline in which one of the suspension points is considerably higher than the other.

Stopper Knot A knot tied in a rope to help provide bulk. For example, a simple figure 8 knot may be tied in the bottom end of a rope to prevent a person from rappelling off the end, or it may be tied in the top of the rope to prevent the rope from accidentally slipping through equipment.

Subject The person being rescued, or one who is in harm's way; also called the victim.

Supplemental Type Certificate (STC) The airworthiness approval required by the FAA (FAR* Part 21.113) when a design modification involves a change in materials, parts, and appliances on the aircraft. Rescue equipment, which is attached to a helicopter, is affected by the scope of this requirement.

System The combination of various components used in the high angle environment to construct a functioning unit. Two examples would be a lowering system or an anchor system.

System Safety Factor The ratio between the maximum load expected on a high angle system and its breaking strength. The larger the ratio, the greater the safety factor.

Systems Testing Assembly of all the components of a rescue system in the manner in which they are to be used and then testing the system to see if actual performance meets expectations.

T

Tag Line A line attached to the load on a highline that is used to maintain contact or control of the load from either side.

Tail Rotor The rotor on the end of the tail boom that produces thrust in the opposite direction to the torque reaction of the main rotor.

Tall Tower As a rule of thumb, some instructors consider anything over 200 feet (61 m) to be a tall tower.

Tandem Prusik Belay System Two triple-wrap Prusik hitches of differing lengths set a few inches apart in a series on a belay rope, used to grab the rope in case of main-line failure or to hold the load while the lowering and raising systems are adjusted.

Tandem Pulleys Two in-line pulleys on the same rope. Tandem pulleys are used in highlines to stabilize a load and to distribute its weight along the rope.

Tensile Strength A measurement of the greatest lengthwise stress under slow pull conditions that a rope can resist without failing.

Telpher Another name for a highline.

Theoretical Mechanical Advantage (TMA) Calculated mechanical advantage without allowance for friction and other losses of advantage.

Touchdown Pad A designated area, which may have a prepared or improved surface, where the helicopter skids are placed.

Toe-In Landing A landing maneuver in which the helicopter rests on the toes of the skids; toe-in landings are used to drop off or pick up passengers or cargo. To execute the maneuver, a significant amount of hover power (within 15% of hover power) must be held to keep the helicopter from falling backward. When the helicopter is operated in this manner, the potential exists for a

---

*See the section, Applicable U.S. Federal Regulations, p. 000.

significant lateral and longitudinal shift in the center of gravity during loading and offloading. In addition, when the helicopter is balanced on the forward one third or less of the skid tube, main rotor blade clearance is another significant concern.

Torque A twisting force that causes a counter-rotating motion. In a helicopter with a main rotor that rotates counterclockwise, the fuselage rotates clockwise. The tail rotor produces anti-torque to counteract this force. The maximum continuous upper torque limit is 100%; however, a transient over-torque may be tolerable to the helicopter power plant.

Tower-Based Rescue A rescue in which the lowering and belay lines are controlled and operated from a position on the tower.

Translational Lift The additional lift generated as the helicopter transitions from a hover to horizontal flight. Transitional lift is due to the increased efficiency of the rotor system as it generates more lift in forward flight with a higher inflow velocity of air mass comparison with a hover.

Traveling Pulley A moving pulley that is attached to a load or to a haul cam, which adds to the mechanical advantage.

Tree Wrap A technique for running a rope around a tree trunk to create friction for a braking effect in litter lowering.

Tying Off Short A safety technique that creates an extra point of attachment during ascending by tying the person directly into the main-line rope.

Tyrolean Another name for a highline.

U-Z

UIAA (Union of International Alpine Associations) An organization that sets performance standards for ropes, harnesses, ice axes, helmets, and carabiners to be used by climbers and mountaineers.

Unified Command Management of an emergency incident through the incident command system in which multiple agencies or jurisdictions are involved, each one having an incident commander assigned to the operation.

Vertical Caving Traveling through caves with vertical or near vertical sections that require the use of rope and ascending and descending equipment.

Vertical Reference A technique used by the helicopter pilot and flight crew, while operating above the ground, to determine the height of the aircraft and any associated external load through visual clues. Surface landmarks and references are used during approaches, departures, and external-load positioning maneuvers at landing or work areas.

Visual Flight Rules (VFR) The rules for conducting flight operations under visual meteorological conditions (VMC). Aircraft flying under VFR are not required to be in contact with air traffic controllers and are responsible for their own separation from other aircraft. The term also is used in the United States to indicate weather conditions that meet or exceed minimum VFR requirements.

Wire Strike Protection System (WSPS) A device designed to protect a helicopter in the event of a collision with a power line or other wire obstacle. If a helicopter suffers a wire strike, the wire could become entangled in the rotor system and lead to destruction of the aircraft. The WSPS has cutting blades set at the top and bottom at the front area of the aircraft. This allows the device to sever a wire on contact.

Z-Rig Common name given to a specific type of 3:1 hauling system. The name is taken from the general shape that the rope makes as it runs through the system.

Illustration Credits

Fig 11-2, 11-5, 11-6. Paul Ross, photographer.

Fig 20-10. Wren Industries, Grand Junction, Colorado.

Fig 20-11. Rescue Technology, Carrollton, Georgia.

Fig 21-1. A, Kingman Daily Miner. B, Carmen L. Burgess.

Fig 21-2. REGA, Swiss-Air Rescue.

Fig 21-5. Glenn Grossman, photographer.

Fig 21-6. Los Angeles County Sheriff's Department Aero Bureau.

Fig 21-10. NPS.

Fig 21-11, 21-16. Images Courtesy of Dominik Hunziker, Saedan, Switzerland.

Fig 21-17. NPS, Yosemite Search and Rescue.

Fig 21-19. Paul Ross, photographer.

Fig 21-20. Image Courtesy United States Coast Guard. Jacquelyn Zettles, photographer.

Fig 21-21. Dominik Hunziker, Saedan, Switzerland.

Fig 21-22. Austin/Travis County EMS.

Fig 21-23. Sikorsky Aircraft Corp.

Fig 21-24. Heli-Rescue Consult.

Fig 21-26. USFS.

Fig 21-27. REGA, Swiss-Air Rescue.

Fig 21-29. Heli-Rescue Consult.

Fig 21-30. Department of Defense.

Fig 21-31. Barry Smith, photographer.

Fig 21-32. Paul Ross, photographer.

Figs 22-2 to 22-4. Seattle Mountain Corporation (SMC), Ferndale, Washington.

Index

A

Abrasions, 21
  damaging ropes, 37
  definition of, 20
  prevention of, 37
  weld, 178
Accessory code, 29
Actual mechanical advantage (AMA), 280
  definition of, 278
Adjustable spiders, 265f
  creating from rope, 264
Adjustable tie-ins for low angle evacuation, 235f
Adrenaline rush, 5
Advanced life support, 188, 189
After-action review (hot debrief), 176
Agency representative, 172
Air ambulances, 321–322. *See also* Helicopters
Aircraft
  military, 322
  public, 321, 334–335
    definition of, 319
Aircrew. *See* Crew
Air Traffic Controller (ATC), 63
  rigging, belaying, 106–109
Airway
  assessment of, 187–188, 206b
  interventions for, 188
  management of, 218
Albuterol, 187t
Alcohol, 5
Altitude, density
  definition of, 318
  of helicopters, 330–331, 332f
Aluminum carabiners *vs.* steel carabiners, 52
AMA. *See* Actual mechanical advantage (AMA)
Ambu bags, 186t
Ambulances, air, 321–322
American National Standards Institute (ANSI), 14
  standards of, 16, 359
American Society for Testing and Materials (ASTM), 14
  carabiner labeling, 53
  definition of, 10
  standards of, 359
Amplitude modulation (AM) radio tower, 297
Anchor plates, 87–88, 88f
Anchor points, 80, 83
  backing up single, 89f
  definition of, 80f
  direction of pull on, 81

Anchor points *(Continued)*
  multiple slings on, 89–90
  webbing placed around, 86
Anchors, 28, 79–94. *See also* Artificial anchors
  backing up of, 83–84, 84f, 90
  definition of, 80f
  on elevator housing, 81
  extending, 88
  far-side, 305–306
  with figure 8 follow-through knots, 85
  of hauling system, 241f
  load-distributing, 91
  load-sharing, 90–91, 91f
    definition of, 80f
    forces on, 93f
  to machine housing, 81
  materials for rigging highlines, 312
  multipoint, 83, 89
    definition of, 80f
  natural, 80
  near-side, 305
  placement of, 81
  portable, 89
  positioning of, 81–82
  presewn slings for, 85–86, 86f
  rigging, 7
  rock, 61
  rope for, 84
  to scuppers, 81
  self-equalizing, 91, 93f, 94f
  skills checklist for, 362
  to stairwell beams, 81
  straps for, 86, 86f
  strength of, 81
  on structures, 80
  using vehicles for, 88–89
  to wall sections between windows and doors, 81
  webbing for, 85, 87f
Anchor system, 80, 244–245
  definition of, 80f
  load-distributing, definition of, 80f
  for low angle evacuation, 231
  for low angle lowering, 236
  two-point load distributing, 91–92
Anderson, Russ, 3
ANSI. *See* American National Standards Institute (ANSI)
Antiemetics for helicopter operations, 337
Anti-torque, 328
Aramids, 24, 141

Arizona DPS aircrew, 322f
Arm rappel (guide's rappel), 116, 117, 117f
Artificial anchors, 61, 80, 81
    definition of, 80f
Ascenders, 60
    attaching to rope, 150–151
    attachments on highline, 309
    backing down rope, 151
    definition of, 48, 144
    general-use, 61, 61f, 144
        definition of, 144
        in rescue hauling systems, 284–285
    left-handed, 148
    light-use, 60, 144–145, 148
        definition of, 144
        in rescue hauling systems, 284
        using, 149, 150f–151f
    mechanical, 144
        for personal use, 148, 148f
    right-handed, 148
    types of, 144–145
Ascender slings, 148
    attaching to ascender, 148–149
    definition of, 144
Ascending, 3, 7
    definition of, 2, 144
    over edge, 157–158
    purpose of, 144
    ropes for, 21
    skills checklist for, 365
    techniques for, 143–164
Ascending system
    creation of, 151–152
    examples of, 154–157
    practice, 154–155, 154f
Assistance, failure to ask for, 5
ASTM. *See* American Society for Testing and Materials (ASTM)
ATC. *See* Air Traffic Controller (ATC)
Ativan. *See* Lorazepam (Ativan)
Autolock, 50–51
Automatic belay, definition of, 192
Autorotation, 329
    definition of, 318
Auxiliary tender
    definition of, 250
    with litters, 270, 270f
Axles of pulleys, 64

B

Backing up
    of anchors, 83–84, 84f
    definition of, 80f
Back ties
    definition of, 80f
    pretensioned, 90
Back-up (safety) knot, definition of, 68f
Backup of other rescuers, 6
Backyard testing, 350
    definition of, 348
Bagged ropes, 35, 35f, 43, 139f
Bag mask, 186t
Bag-valve-mask (BVM), 188
Ball bearings, 64–65
Basic life support, 189

Basket litter, definition of, 214
Bathing, ropes, 40–42
Bauman bag, 342, 343f
Beam clamp, 89f
Bearings, 64
Belay, 62–63
    Air Traffic Controller (ATC) rigging, 106–109
    arranging direction of, 112
    automatic, definition of, 192
    body, 63, 113–114
    bottom, 113, 113f
    brake, 192
    communications, 102
    conditional, 192
    decisions about, 99
    definition of, 98
    failure of, 99–100
    on level ground, 103f
    in low angle evacuation, 237
    lowering, 100b
        feeding out in, 195–197, 196f
        with single line *vs.* double line, 264b
    one-person *vs.* rescue, 98
    pickoff rescue, 205
    practicing with one-person weight or dummy, 105
    rescue, 191–201
        skills checklist for, 366
    rope grab devices for, 61
    ropes for, 113
    self, 137
    signals for, 101–102
    situations requiring, 98–99
    taking in slack, 197
    techniques, 102
    TRE rigging, 109–112
Belay devices, 63, 98, 106f. *See also* individual devices
    assisted catch, 109
    definition of, 98
    free running, 106
    personal, 63f
Belayers, 2, 98
    definition of, 2, 98
    for high angle lowering system, 252
    securing, 113
Belay line, 98
    definition of, 98, 304
Belay plates, 106
    definition of, 98
    in figure 8 descenders, 109
    on level ground, 108f
Belay rope, locked, releasing, 201
Belay system, 98
    elements of, 99f
    for high angle lowering system, 252
    for litter lowering, 266–267, 266f
    practice, 100–101, 100f
Belts
    escape, 10, 142f
    gunner's, 337
    ladder, 10, 13
    life, 13
    pompier, 13
    safety, standards for, 359

Bend
definition of, 68f
figure 8, 73, 73f
overhand, 86
ring, 74, 86
Bight
definition of, 68f
knots on, 71, 71f
Biners, 48
Black Diamond. *See* Air Traffic Controller (ATC)
Blanket
across litter, 218f
wrapped around patient, 219f
Body belays, 63, 113–114
Body rappel (Dulfersitz rappel), 116
Bolts, 62, 62f
definition of, 48
Bombproof, 81
definition of, 80f
Boots, 12
Boredom, 178
Bottom belays, 113, 113f
Bowline knots, 71, 85
on coil, 75, 76f
interlocking long-tail, 75, 77f
for loop, 234b
with overhand backup, 72f
Bowlines, 68–69
Braided rope, 25–26, 25f
Brake and anchor systems for low angle lowering, 236
Brake bar rack, 58–59, 58f, 130–137
attaching to harness, 130, 130f
attaching to rope, 131, 132f–133f
characteristics of, 59b
clearing from edge, 138f
definition of, 48, 116
down vertical face, 134–137
getting off rope, 133
with hyper-bar, 58, 59f
incorrect lacing of, 133f
on level ground, 130–133
locking off, 260, 260f
for low angle evacuation, 236
to lower, 259–260
practice rescuer down vertical drop, 261
practice rescuer on slope, 258–260, 259f
on slope, 133–134, 135f, 136f
on vertical, 262f
operating, 131
personal *vs.* rescue versions of, 59
tie-off bar, 58
tying off, 131–133, 134f
unlocking, 133, 260
Brake belays, 192
Brake device for high angle lowering system, 252
Brake hand, 117
definition of, 116
Brakeman, 231
definition of, 230
for high angle lowering system, 252
stance for lowering, 255f
Brake systems for double line lowering, 271
Brake tube, 237b, 271, 272f

Break-apart litter, 214, 216, 216f
Breathing
assessment of, 187–188, 206b
interventions for, 188
Bridle, 250
Briefing. *See also* Hot debrief (after-action review)
emergency, 328b
Broken ground evacuation, 230
Budget for medical care, 184
Built-in fall protection in tower rescue, 297–298
Bushings, bronze, 64
Butterfly coil, 36f
Butt thrust, 129, 129f
BVM. *See* Bag-valve-mask (BVM)

C
Calls, 101
Call when needed (CWN) for-hire commercial operators, 322
Cams
definition of, 48
hard, 60
haul, 283
definition of, 278
ratchet, 242b
safety, 242b
soft, 60
spring-loaded, 63f
tender, 285
Canvas pads, 37, 37f
Carabiners, 2, 48–55
aluminum *vs.* steel, 52
brake bars, 53–55, 54f
buying, 53
care and inspection of, 56
clipping across ascender and rope, 149f
cross-gate forces on, 178
definition of, 2
designs of, 49f
D-shaped, 49, 49f
gate opening, 50, 50f, 51f
hard linking, 53
HMS, 50, 102
labeling of, 53
latches for, 48, 49f
loading, 54f
locking, 50–51, 52, 52f
definition of, 48
long-axis testing of, 349f
nonlocking, 50
definition of, 48
overloading of, 349f
parts of, 48f
reversed and opposed, 51f
screw links, 55–56, 55f
shapes of, 49–50
sizes and strengths, 50
standard labeling, 53
steel *vs.* aluminum carabiners, 52
strength of, 51
testing of, 348–350
three-way loading, 55
troubleshooting problems with, 56b
unlocked gates, 178

Carabiner wrap, 137
  definition of, 116
Cargo lowering in helicopter rescues, 343, 345f
CAT, 60
Caver's coil, 36f
CE. *See* European Committee for Standardization (CE)
Center of gravity
  definition of, 318
  of helicopters, 332
Cervical spine
  devices, 186
  immobilization equipment for, 186
  with litters, 218–219
Chain coil, 42f
Change of direction pulley, 280
Changeover, 144, 158–163, 158f–159f, 161f–163f
  definition of, 144
  procedures for, 158–163
Chest harnesses, 15
  definition of, 10
Chicken loops, 154, 154f
  definition of, 144
Circulation, assessment of, 188–189
CISM. *See* Critical incident stress management (CISM)
Clear text, 169
  definition of, 166
Climbing, 2–3
  boots for, 12
  recreational, 359
  technical, 20
  tower rescue, 297–298
Climbing gym, indoor, 3
Climbing helmet certification, Union of International Alpine
    Associations (UIAA), 11
Clog, 60
Closed loops
  tying directly to head of litter for low angle evacuation, 232–233
  webbing for, 234b
Clothing, 12
  fire-resistant for helicopters, 333–334
Clove hitches, 75, 75f
CLR. *See* Component load ratio (CLR)
CMI, 60
Coanda effect, 328
Code of Federal Regulations (CFR)
  Title 14, 335
Coils, 35, 36f, 75, 76f
Cold, protection from, 10–11, 217–218
Cole rack. *See* Brake bar rack
Collective pitch system, 328
  definition of, 318
Combination seat/chest harnesses, 15f
Combi-Tube, 188
Commands, 101, 242b
Commercial rope protector, 38–39, 38f
Commercial tie-in system, 221–222, 224f
Communications, 173–174
  belay, 102
  digital, 174
  for hauling in low angle evacuation, 241
  for hauling systems, 288
  helicopter, 324
  in high angle lowering system, 252–253

Communications *(Continued)*
  human side of, 174
  ineffective, 178
  for low angle evacuation, 237–238, 239b
  for pickoff rescue, 203
  with rescue subject, 208b
  for safety, 176–177
  simplex, 173–174
  skills for, 7
Complex pulley systems, 282b
Component load ratio (CLR), 28
Component testing, 348
Compound mechanical advantage, 280–282
Compound pulley system, 280
  definition of, 278
Concentration, inability to, 5
Conditional belay, 192
Conduction, 11
Confined space
  hauling from, 289, 289f
  rescue from, 3
Conforming backboard, 189
Continuous sequence for double line lowering, 272
Convection, 11
Copilot, 326
Cordage, standards for, 359
Cordage Institute, standards of, 359
Cotton, 12
Counterbalance haul system, 244
  definition of, 230
  elements of, 245f
Creep, 22
Crew
  approach and departure around a helicopter, 333f
  Arizona DPS, 322f
  briefing of, 328f
  helicopter rescue, 326–328
  in PPE, 333f
Crew chief, 326
Critical incident stress management (CISM), 173
Crush syndrome, 14
Cycle limits, 338
Cyclic, 328
  definition of, 318

D

Danger signs for high angle rope technicians, 5
Decadron injectable, 187t
Dehydration, 11
Denier, 23
Density altitude
  definition of, 318
  of helicopters, 330–331, 332f
Descenders, 56, 59, 116. *See also* Figure 8 descenders
  clearing, 129
  definition of, 48, 116
  personal escape, 142, 142f
  types of, 56–58
Descent control devices, 116
Detail, attention to, 6
Dextrose, 187t
Diazepam, 187t
Digital communication, 174

Directional, 82–83, 82f
    definition of, 80f
    in hauling system, 285–286
    location of, 83
Dirt on ropes, 40
Disc area, 328
Discoloration of ropes, 40
Distraction, 178
Double braided rope, 25–26, 26f
Double line lowering
    changing litter angle during, 273f
    definition of, 250
    litter tie-ins for, 271
    spiders, 271f
    systems, 270
Double line to single point spiders, 270
Double line to two point spiders, 270–271
Double overhand knot, 74, 74f
Drop lines, standards for, 359
Drop zone, definition of, 296
Drugs. *See* Medications
D-shaped carabiners, 49, 49f
Dual brake litter lowering, requirements for, 274
Dulfersitz rappel, 116
Dust abatement with helicopters, 324
Dynamic, definition of, 348
Dynamic kernmantle, 26, 26f
Dynamic measurement, 355
Dynamic rollover, 324
Dynamic rope, 21
    core of, 21f
    definition of, 20
    for litters, 22
    vs. static ropes, 27
Dynamic short haul, 343, 344f
Dynamometer, 355–356, 355f
    definition of, 348

E

Ear protection for helicopters, 334
ECAC. *See* European Civil Aviation Conference (ECAC)
Edge
    ascending over, 157–158
    clearing brake bar rack from, 138f
    getting over, 129–130, 258
        in hauling systems, 288
        in litter lowering, 268
    rollover, ascending over, 157
    undercut, 130
        ascending over, 158
        getting over in litter lowering, 268
Edge rollers, 38f
    definition of, 34
    in hauling system, 285
Edge safety line, 177f
Edge-stitched (shuttle loom) webbing, 30f
Edge tender
    definition of, 250
    for high angle lowering system, 252
Efficiency (of a haul system), 280
    definition of, 278
Electromagnetic energy (EME), 296, 297
Electronic load cell, 348, 355, 356

Elevator housing, anchoring to, 81
EME. *See* Electromagnetic energy (EME)
Emergency briefing, 328b
Emergency cable cutters, 339
Emergency descent, 59
    systems for, 137
Emergency medical skills, 7
Emergency medical technicians, basic level interventions, 188
Emergency seat harnesses, 10, 13
Energized power lines, 297t
English reeve system, 304, 315, 315f
Entanglements in helicopter short haul operations, 343
Environmental forces, 179
    protecting litter patient from, 217–218
Epinephrine, 187t
Equipment
    care of, 6
    fire service rescue, 3
    immobilization for cervical spine, 186
    location and mobility of, 168–169
    medical care, 184, 185t, 186t
    personal protection, 5, 333–335, 359
    for person wearing a seat harness, 206b
    for pickoff rescue, 203–204
    for rigging highlines, 312
    standards for, 359
    testing of, 347–357
    for tower rescue, 297, 302
Escape belts, 10, 142f
ET intubation, 188
Etrier, 310
European Civil Aviation Conference (ECAC), 335b
European Committee for Standardization (CE)
    climbing helmet certification, 11
    definition of, 10
    standards of, 359
European Committee for Standardization/Union of International
        Alpine Association (CE/UIAA) carabiner labeling, 53, 53f
European Joint Aviation Authorities (JAA), 335b
Extended attack, 173
Extremities, splints for, 186t
Extrication device
    Kendrick, 220
    spinal, 189
Eyes, protection of, 218
    in helicopters, 334

F

Fabrics
    for clothing, 12
    softeners for, 42–43
Face, protection of, 218
Fall factor, 22
    definition of, 20
    of ropes, 22–23
Falling objects damaging ropes, 37
FAR. *See* Federal Aviation Regulations (FAR)
Far-side anchor, 305–306
Fast roping, 341b
Fatigue, 178
    physical, 5

Federal Aviation Regulations (FAR), 335
Fibers for ropes, 23–24
Figure 8
    attaching, 119–121
    with ears, 58f
        to lower down vertical face, 257–258, 257f
        lowering on steep slope, 253–257, 254f
    laced for lowering, 255f
    problems with, 205
Figure 8 bend, 73, 73f
Figure 8 brakes, locking off, 256f
Figure 8 descenders, 56, 57f, 118, 118f, 119f
    belay plates in, 109
    definition of, 48, 116
    double wrapping, 125–127, 127f
        hand position with, 128f
    down vertical face, 122–128, 124f
    with ears, 3, 57, 119–128, 119f
    with girth hitch, 57f, 118–119, 118f
    on level ground, 120f
    locking off, 121–122, 121f, 125, 126f
    for low angle evacuation, 236
    on slope, 122, 123f
Figure 8 knots, 69–71, 70f, 72, 85
    on a bight, 71, 71f
Financial resources for medical care, 184
Fire captain giving instructions, 175f
Fire hose rope pads, 37, 37f
Fire Rescue Escape Device, 142, 142f
Fire-resistant clothing for helicopters, 334–335
Fire service rescue, 3
    standards for, 359
Fisherman's knot, 73, 73f
540 degrees Rescue Belay, 63, 198–201, 198f, 199f, 200f
    locking off and releasing with, 201f
    manually locking off belay rope, 200–201, 201f
Fixed pulley, 280
    definition of, 278
Flanges, 299
Flash rappels damaging rope, 39
Flat webbing, 30
Flexible litter, 216–217
    definition of, 214
Flicker seizures, 337
Flight
    helmets for, 334
    stressors of, 337, 337b
Flight following, 323
    definition of, 318
Flotation devices for helicopters, 335
Flow-restricted oxygen powered (FROP), 188
Flumazenil, 187t
Foot supports, 14
Footwear, 12
    for helicopters, 334
Foundation knot, 68f
4:1 rule, 40
Fractures, litter packaging, 220
Frame of light-use ascenders, 148
Free climbing, 2
    in tower rescue, 297
Free solo climbing, 2

Freestanding tower, 299, 300f
    definition of, 296
Friction
    brake bar rack for lowering, 259–260
    gaining extra, 125, 127–128, 128f
Friction hitches, 144
    in rescue hauling systems, 283–284
FRIES. See Fast rope insertion/extraction system (FRIES)
FROP. See Flow-restricted oxygen powered (FROP)
Full body harnesses, 15, 15f
    definition of, 10
Full spine splints, 186

G
Gate opening carabiners, 50, 50f, 51f
General-use ascenders, 61, 61f, 144
    definition of, 144
    in rescue hauling systems, 284–285
General-use rope grab, free running in rescue hauling systems, 285
Gentex SPH-5 helmet, 334
Gibbs, 61
Girth hitches
    figure 8 descenders, 57f, 118–119, 118f
    webbing, 88f
Glossy marks on ropes, 40
Gloves for helicopters, 334
Gore-Tex, 12
Grapevine knot, 73, 73f
Gravity, center of
    definition of, 318
    of helicopters, 332
Grease, removal of, 43
GriGri, 63
Ground-controlled rescue, 296
Ground effect, 328
    aerodynamics, 330f
    definition of, 318
Guide hand, 116, 117
Guidelines and procedures, 167–168
Guide's rappel. See Arm rappel (guide's rappel)
Gunner's belts, 338
Guyed tower, 296, 299, 301f

H
Half boards, 220
Half hitches, 70f
Half spine splints, 186
Halogen bulbs, 16
Haloperidol, 187t
Hand, 21
    guide, 116, 117
    protection for helicopters, 334
Hand signals, 325f
Hangers, 62
Hard cams, 60
Hard linking carabiners, 53
Hardware, 47–65
    securing, 16
    standards for, 359
Harnesses. See also Seat harnesses
    attaching brake bar rack to, 130, 130f
    chest, 15
        definition of, 10

Harnesses *(Continued)*
  emergency seat, 13
    definition of, 10
  full body, 15, 15f
    definition of, 10
  for helicopters, 334
  radio chest, 174, 174f, 253f
  rescue, 14
  seat/chest, 15, 15f
  standards for, 15–16, 359
Harness suspension pathology, 13–14
  definition of, 10
Hasty packs, 168
Haul cams, 284
definition of, 278
Hauling
  belay practice system, 101f
  commands for, 242b
  rope grab devices for, 61
Hauling systems, 277–293
  anchors, forces on, 241f
  communications, 288
  counterbalance, 244
    definition of, 230
    elements of, 245f
  elements of, 284–285
  multiforce, 246
  4:1 piggyback, 292–293, 293f
  preventing edge friction in, 287–288
  purpose of, 278–279
  skills checklist for, 371
  1:1 TMA, 289, 289f
  2:1 without the diminishing V, 290, 291f
  3:1 Z-rig, 291–292, 292f
Haul line, 306
  definition of, 304
Haul rope changing position of, 287
Haul team, 231
  definition of, 230
  for low angle evacuation, 241
Hazards, 178
  of helicopter short haul operations, 341–342
  of tower-based rescue, 296–297
Head, 189
  immobilization, 224
Headgear, 10–11
Headlamps, 16, 16f
Heat, protection from, 10–11
Heat fusion, 39
Heavy helicopter, 322, 323f
Heights, fear of, 4
Height-velocity curve, 330
  definition of, 318
  of helicopters, 331f
Helibase, 324
  definition of, 318
Helicopter manager, 326
Helicopter rappel, 340–341
Helicopter rescue crews, 326, 328
Helicopter rescue hoist, 339f
Helicopter rescue operations, 317–345
  outside assets, 321–322

Helicopter rescue training, 335b
Helicopters
  aerodynamics of, 328
  communications, 324
  controls of, 329f
  decision making, 320b
  definition of, 318
  federal regulations for, 335
  flight characteristics and limitations, 328–330
  flying in mountainous terrain, 321f
  heavy, 322, 323f
  hoist rescue, 338–339
  landings, 330
  landing zones, 324
  mission management of, 323
  night rescue operations by, 321
  nighttime limitations of, 321
  performance of, 332–333
  personal protective equipment (PPE) for, 334–335
  rescue, 320
    decision making, 320
    mission planning and preplanning, 321
    situational awareness, 320
    techniques of, 337–344
  rescue scene, taking off from, 320f
  rescue subjects, care of, 336
  rescue subjects in interior, 337f
  resource categories of, 322–323
  safety of, 333
  short haul operations, 341–342, 342f
    hazards of, 342
    procedures for, 342
  types of, 323t
  weather limitations of, 320–321
  when to use, 320
Heli-rappelling, 340, 340f
Helirescue bag, 341
Helispot, 321, 326f, 327f
  definition of, 318
  manager, 333f
Helmets, 5, 10–11
  chin strap, 10–11
  climbing, 11
  definition of, 10
  flight, 334
  for patients on litters, 224
  removal of, 225b
  standards for, 359
Hexcentrics, 62f
HIGE. *See* Hover in ground effect (HIGE)
High angle, definition of, 2
High angle environment, 1–8
  climbing, 2–3
  mountaineering, 2
  vertical caving, 3
High angle lowering
  medical considerations for rescue subjects in, 269–270
  skills checklist for, 370
High angle lowering system, 249–276
  belays for, 252
  braking systems for, 252
  communication in, 252–253

High angle lowering system *(Continued)*
  elements of, 251–252, 251f
    load attachments to main-line rope, 251
  principles of, 253
High angle rescue, 3–4
  industrial rescue, 3
  rope access, 3–4
  tactical operations, 3
  tower rescue, 4
High angle rope technician, 4–5
High directionals for rigging highlines, 312
Highlines, 303–315
  definition of, 304
  determining amount of sag in, 310
  elements of, 305–306
  forces on, 311f
  loads, 306–307
  problems with, 305
  rigging of, 312–315
  skills checklist for, 372
  use of, 304–305
High-modulus polyethylene (HMPE) extended chain, 24
High-strength tie-off, 84, 84b
High-stretch rope, 21
Hitches. *See also* Münter hitches; Prusik hitches
  clove, 75, 75f
  definition of, 68f, 144
  friction, 144
    in rescue hauling systems, 285
  girth
    figure 8 descenders, 57f, 118–119, 118f
    webbing, 88f
  half, 70f
  Italian, 63
  load-releasing (LR), 193
    definition of, 192
  radium releasing, 193–195, 194f, 195f
  tensionless, tying, 84, 84b, 85f
HMS carabiner, 50, 102
HOGE. *See* Hover out of ground effect (HOGE)
Hoist operator, 338, 339f
Hoist rescue, 338–339
  definition of, 318
  helicopters, 337–338
Hollow braided rope, 25
Horizontal highline, 304, 305f
  definition of, 304
  load on, 308f
Hot cutter, 43f
Hot debrief. *See* After-action review (hot debrief)
Hot debrief (after-action review), 166, 175f, 176
Hot loading, 324
Hot off-loading, 324
Hover, 328
  definition of, 318
Hover ceiling
  definition of, 318
  of helicopters, 332
Hovering over water, 329
Hover in ground effect (HIGE), 329
  definition of, 318
Hover landing, 331
  definition of, 318

Hover out of ground effect (HOGE), 329
  definition of, 318
Hydration, 11
Hyper-bar, brake bar rack with, 58, 59f
Hypotension, 188
Hypothesis, definition of, 348
Hypovolemic shock, 188

I

IAFF. *See* International Association of Fire Fighters (IAFF)
ICS. *See* Incident command system (ICS)
IFR. *See* Instrument flight rules (IFR)
Immobilization equipment for cervical spine, 186
Incident assignment, 178–179
Incident command system (ICS), 169
  definition of, 166
    example of, 170f–171f
Incident personnel, 179
Incident review, 176
Incident risk management process, 177–178
Incident safety officer (ISO), 172
  definition of, 166
Indoor climbing gym, 3
Industrial rescue, 3
In-flight emergency, 335
Initial attack, 173
Initial incident commander, 169
  definition of, 166
Injectable medications, 187t
Instrument flight rules (IFR), 323
  definition of, 318
Insulation, 12
Interlocking long-tail bowlines, 266
International Association of Fire Fighters (IAFF), 3
International Society of Fire Service Instructors (ISFSI), 3
International system of units (SI), 1
Intravenous fluids, 186t
Investigation, 172–173
ISFSI. *See* International Society of Fire Service Instructors (ISFSI)
ISO. *See* Incident safety officer (ISO)
Italian hitches, 63

J

JAA. *See* European Joint Aviation Authorities (JAA)
Jammed devices
  extricating, 140
  extricating an obstruction from, 160
Jenny bag, 341–342
Jumar, 60

K

Kendrick extrication device, 220
Kernmantle, 26
  definition of, 20
  dynamic, 26, 26f
  static, 26–27, 26f
Ketorolac tromethamine, 187t
Kevlar, 24
  definition of, 20
Knees over edge rappel, 129, 129f
Knives, 17

Knots
    affect on ropes, 68–69
    backing up, 69
    back-up (safety), 68f
    on bight, 71
    bowline, 71, 85
        on coil, 75, 76f
        interlocking long-tail, 75, 77f
        for loop, 234b
        with overhand backup, 72f
    double overhand, 74, 74f
    dressing, 69
    figure 8, 69–71, 70f
    figure 8 follow-through, 72f, 85
    fisherman's, 73, 73f
    foundation, 68f
    grapevine, 73, 73f
    overhand, 69, 70f, 71f
    passing for litter lowering, 274–277, 275f
    passing for pulleys, 65, 65f
    Prusik, 17
    qualities of, 68
    safety, 68f
    skills checklist for, 361
    stopper, 68f
    strength loss through, 39
    tape, 86
    water, 74, 86
Kootenay Carriage, 65, 306
    definition of, 304
Krabs, 48

L

Ladder belts, 13
    definition of, 10
Ladder splints for extremities, 186t
Laid rope, 25, 25f
    definition of, 20
Landing
    hover, 331
        definition of, 318
    one-skid, 331, 332f
        definition of, 319
    power-on, 331
        definition of, 319
    precautionary, definition of, 319
    snow, helicopters, 324
    step-out, 331
        definition of, 319
    toe-in, 331
        definition of, 319
Landing zone, 318
Lanyard
    definition of, 296
    standards for, 359
Lanyard climbing, definition of, 296
Lanyard systems, 298–299, 299f
Large-diameter rope, 27
LDA. *See* Load-distributing anchor system (LDA)
Lead climbing, 2
    definition of, 296
    in tower rescue, 298
Leadership, 173

Leapfrogging, 236
Leather, 12
LED. *See* Light-emitting diode (LED)
Left-handed ascenders, 148
Liaison officer, 172
Life belts, 13
Lifelines, standards for, 359
Life safety rope
    establishing responsibility for, 40
    National Fire Protection Association (NFPA) guidelines for, 28–29
Light, sources of, 16
Light-emitting diode (LED), 17
Light helicopter, 322, 322f
    definition of, 318
Light-use ascenders, 60, 144–145, 148, 148f
Litter attendant
    definition of, 230
    on hoist or short haul, 336f
Litter captain, definition of, 230
Litter lowering
    of live subjects, 266–267
    passing knots for, 274–277, 275f
Litter lowering systems, 261–266
Litter medical kit (LMK), 185–187
Litters, 186, 213–227
    belay system for lowering, 266–267, 266f
    blanket across, 218f
    carrying of, 225–226
    changing angle for double line lowering, 271–272
    functions of, 214
    in high angle rescue, skills checklist for, 368
    loading subject into, 269–270
    loads on highlines, 307, 309f
    for low angle evacuation, 231
    metal basket, 214, 214f
    packaging patient in, 217, 221
        materials for, 221
        for rope rescue, 220–221
    packaging spinal injuries, 219
    patient tie-ins, 221–224
        completed, 224f
        lower torso, 223f
        upper torso, 222f
        webbing placement for, 221f
    plastic basket, 215, 215f
    with plastic-covered head and end rails, tying main-line rope to for low angle evacuation, 233f
    position for lowering, 261
    protecting patient in, 217
    rigging of, 264f
        highlines, 312–313
        for low angle evacuation, 232–233, 232f
        for single line lowering, 261–262, 267–268, 267f
    rigid, for low angle evacuation, 231
    ropes for, 21–22
    selection of, 216
    shield on, 219f
    soft, 186
    spinning of in helicopter short haul operations, 342
    stabilizing subject in, 221
    tie-ins
        for double line lowering, 271
        for low angle evacuation, 232

Litters *(Continued)*
with two-point Yosemite system, 183f
tying a loop onto, 233f
tying closed loop directly to head of
for low angle evacuation, 232–233
tying main-line rope directly to head of
for low angle evacuation, 232
types of, 214–217
vapor barrier across, 218f
Litter slings, 225–226, 226f
Litter system, 244
Litter team for low angle evacuation, 234
Litter tenders
attachments, 274, 307
body positions for low angle evacuation, 234
definition of, 250
in high angle lowering system, 251
in low angle evacuation, 232
position of, 269, 269f
on highlines, 310
strategy for low angle evacuation, 235
tie-ins, 265, 266f
for low angle evacuation, 235–236, 235f
Litter wheels, 226, 226f
LMK. *See* Litter medical kit (LMK)
Load, 306
beginning movement in highlines, 313–314
calculation for helicopters, 324–326
completing transfer in highlines, 314
definition of, 250
in high angle lowering system, 251
highlines, 306–307
horizontal highline, 308f
one-person belaying, 97–114
Münter hitch, 103
skills checklist for, 363
one-person in highlines, 306–307, 309f
reducing weight of in hauling systems, 288
sling, 343
definition of, 319
two-person in highlines, 307
Load calculation, definition of, 318
Load-distributing anchor system (LDA), 91–92
definition of, 80f
Loading
carabiners, 54f
hot, 325
pins for, 349
shock, 28
Load ratio, 28
component, 28
definition of, 20
system, 28
Load-releasing (LR) hitches, 193
definition of, 192
Load-sharing anchors, definition of, 80f
Local rescue needs, 166–167
Locked belay rope, releasing, 201
Locking carabiner, 50–51, 52, 52f
definition of, 48
Locking off, 119
brake bar rack, 260, 260f
definition of, 116

Locking off *(Continued)*
figure 8 descenders, 121–122, 121f, 125
in lowering, 255–256
Long bone fractures, litter packaging, 220
Longline, 343
definition of, 318
Lookout, 174
Loops
bowline knots, 234b
equipment for seat harnesses, 16f
tying onto litter, 232–233, 233f
Lorazepam (Ativan), 187
Low angle, definition of, 2
Low angle evacuation, 229–247
braking systems for, 236–237
definition of, 230
elements of, 230–231, 231f
examples of, 230, 230b
hauling, 240–246
2:1 hauling system for, 245, 245f, 246f
vs. high angle evacuation, 230b
1:1 mechanical advantage hauling system, 240–241, 240f
mechanical *vs.* human power, 240
of more than one rope length, 239–240
need for, 230
rescue subject tie-ins, 264–265
safe movement of personnel in, 246
skills checklist for, 369
standard requirements for, 232–234
Low angle lowering
brake and anchor systems for, 236
typical, 238–239
Lowering. *See also* Double line lowering; Litter lowering
vs. belay, 100b
with brake bar rack, 259–260
practice rescuer down vertical drop, 261
practice rescuer on slope, 258–260, 259f
on vertical, 262f
commands for, 254b
definition of, 98
feeding out belay in, 195–197, 196f
single line *vs.* double line, 261
with belay, 264b
using figure 8 with ears on steep slope, 253–257
Lowering/belay line, 306
attachments on highlines, 310
definition of, 304
Lowering/raising pickoff, 211–212
Lowering system, main-line, 266
Low-risk methods, 5–6
Low-stretch, definition of, 20
Lug soles, 12

M

MA. *See* Mechanical advantage (MA)
Machine housing, anchoring to, 81
Main line, 305
definition of, 304
Management. *See* Organization and management
Manner of function, definition of, 48
Master attachment point, 90–91
definition of, 80f

Maximum gross weight
definition of, 318
of helicopters, 332–333
Maximum performance takeoff, 324
definition of, 319
Maximum working temperature, 141
MBS. *See* Minimum breaking strength (MBS)
Mechanical advantage (MA)
calculating, 279f, 280, 282–283
definition of, 278
incremental addition of, 282
multiplying, 280–282
ways to add, 282
Mechanical ascenders, 144
Mechanical rappel devices, 118–119
Mechanical rope protection devices, 38–39
Medical attendant for low angle evacuation, 232, 234
Medical care, 182–187
assessment and interventions, 187–189
control, 183–184
equipment, 184, 185t, 186t
financial resources, 184
integrating with rescue, 190
litter medical kit (LMK), 185–187
medical personnel, 182–183
patient benefits, 184–185
preplanning, 182, 182t
skill level, 183
special cases, 183
Medical considerations, 181–196
pickoff rescue, 205
Medical (trauma) patients, 189
Medications, 5
injectable, 187t
for litter medical kit (LMK), 186–187
Medics on helicopters, 327
Medium helicopter, 322, 323f
definition of, 319
Melted rope end, 43f
Mental impairment, 5
Metal basket litters, 214, 214f
Metal rope protection devices, 38
Mildew, removal of, 43
Military aircraft, 322
Military extraction techniques, 341b
Minimum breaking strength (MBS), 28
Mission, 178–179
Monopole, definition of, 296
Morphine sulfate, 187t
Mountaineer coil, 36f
Mountaineering, 2
ropes for, 20
Multiforce haul systems, drawbacks to, 246
Multiplying rule, exception to, 282b
Multipoint anchors, 83
definition of, 80f
Münter hitches, 63, 100b, 102
definition of, 98
on level ground, 105f
one-person load belaying, 103
practicing with, 105
tying, 104f
Münter hitch rappel, 137, 139f
definition of, 116

N
Naloxone, 187t
National Fire Protection Association (NFPA), 3
carabiner labeling, 53, 53f
climbing helmet certification, 11
definition of, 10, 166
harness standards, 16
life safety rope guidelines, 28–29
standards of, 167, 359
Natural fiber rope, 3, 23
Near-side anchors, 305
Near-side rigging with pretensioned back-ties, 313f–314f
Needle loom webbing, 30
NFPA. *See* National Fire Protection Association (NFPA)
Noise on helicopters, 337
Nomex, 333–334
Nonlocking carabiner, 50
definition of, 48
Nonmedical patients, 189
Nose of light-use ascenders, 148
Notification, 172
Null hypothesis, 351–354
definition of, 348
Nylon, 24, 29, 141
substances damaging, 36
Nylon 6,6, 24
definition of, 20
Nylon 6 (Perlon), 24
definition of, 20
Nylon fiber rope, 23

O
Occupational Safety and Health Administration (OSHA), 3
secondary safety systems, 137
standards of, 359
Oil, removal of, 43
One-person belay device, rigging, 107f
One-person load belaying, 97–114
Münter hitch, 103
skills checklist for, 363
One-person loads on highlines, 306–307, 309f
One-skid landing, 331, 332f
definition of, 319
Operations chief, 173, 327
Oregon spine splint (OSSII), 220
Organization and management, 166–174
command staff, 172
communications, 173–174
critical incident stress management (CISM), 173
goals and direction, 173
guidelines and procedures, 167–168
incident command system (ICS), 169
incident safety officer (ISO), 172
investigation, 172–173
leadership, 173
maintaining, 175
multijurisdictional/multiagency operations, 169–172
notification, 172
resource allocation, 173
response, 172
span of control, 169
Organizations setting standards, 359
OSHA. *See* Occupational Safety and Health Administration (OSHA)
OSSII. *See* Oregon spine splint (OSSII)

Outside helicopter rescue assets, 321–322
Overconfidence, 5
Overexcitement, 5
Overhand bend, 86
Overhand knot, 69, 70f, 71f
Overloading
  of carabiners, 349f
  of rope, 36–37
Oxygen, 186t
  for helicopter operations, 337

P

Packaging
  definition of, 230
  for litter
    fractures, 220
    spinal injuries, 219
  for low angle evacuation, 234
Padding for patients on litters, 225
Parapets, getting over in litter lowering, 268
Pararescuers on helicopters, 326
Patients. *See also* Rescue subjects
  on litters
    helmets for, 224
    padding for, 225
    protecting from environmental forces, 217–218
    tie-ins for, 221–224
  medical (trauma), 189
  medical care of, 184–185
  nonmedical, 189
  vapor barrier wrapped around, 219f
PBI, 334–335
PCD. *See* Progress capture device (PCD)
PEAD. *See* Pharyngeal/esophageal airway device (PEAD)
Peak force indicator, 355
Pendulum, definition of, 80f
Perlon. *See* Nylon 6 (Perlon)
Personal ascent devices, 60, 60f
Personal belay device, 63f
Personal equipment and protection, 9–18
Personal escape
  descenders, 142, 142f
  devices and kits, 141
  rope, 24, 141
Personal flotation devices for helicopters, 335
Personal protective equipment (PPE), 5
  for helicopters, 334–335
  standards for, 359
Personnel safety lines, 246f
Petzl, 60, 61
Pharyngeal/esophageal airway device (PEAD), 188
Physical fatigue, 5
Physical impairment, 5
Physical safety, 5
PIC. *See* Pilot in command (PIC)
Pickets, 89, 89f
Pickoff rescue
  belay, 205
  definition of, 204
  medical assessment of, 206b
  medical considerations, 205
  procedure for, 207f
  situations involving, 203

Pickoff rescue *(Continued)*
  sizing up situation, 208b
  skills and equipment for, 203–204
  skills checklist for, 367
  teamwork and communication in, 203
  techniques for, 203–212
Piggyback system, 280. *See also* Hauling systems
  definition of, 278
Pig-Rig. *See* Piggyback system
Pigtail
  definition of, 250
  highlines, 307–309
Pilot in command (PIC), 326
  definition of, 319
Pitons, 61
  definition of, 48
Plaited rope, 25, 25f
Plans chief, 173
Plastic basket litters, 215, 215f
PMI, 60, 61
PMI Hasty Harness, 209f
PMI PED descenders, 142, 142f
PMP. *See* Prusik Minding Pulley (PMP)
Police line barricade, 167f
Polyester, 24, 29, 141
  definition of, 20
  substances damaging, 36
Polyester fiber rope, 23
Polyester pile, 12
Polyethylene, 23
Polyolefins, 23
  definition of, 20
Polypropylene, 12, 23
Pompier belts, 13
Power lines, energized, 297t
Power-on landing, 331
  definition of, 319
PPE. *See* Personal protective equipment (PPE)
Preboarding helicopters, 332
Precautionary landing, definition of, 319
Preparation and training, 190t
Preplanning, 165–179
Prerigging, 236
Presewn slings for anchors, 85–86, 86f
Pretensioned back tie, 91f
Procedures, 167–168
Prochlorperazine, 187t
Progress capture device (PCD), 231, 242–244, 243f, 244f, 283
  definition of, 230
  free running, 243–244
  Prusik-type, 244
  in rescue hauling systems, 283–284, 284f
    alignment of, 286f
    setting on automatic, 286f
  spring-loaded, 244
Protection, 2
Protective gear, 6
Prusik, 265
  definition of, 48, 144
Prusik hitches, 29, 60, 144, 145
  rope selection for, 145
  three-wrap, 147, 147f
  weighting, 145

Prusik knot, 17
Prusik loops
    attaching to rope, 145, 146f–147f
    creation of, 145
    definition of, 144
Prusik Minding Pulley (PMP), 65, 197, 197f, 198f
    definition of, 192
Public aircraft, 322, 334–335
    definition of, 319
Pulley and anchor system, 244–245
Pulleys, 64, 64f, 306
    change of direction, 280
    definition of, 48, 279
    fixed, 280
        definition of, 278
    knot-passing, 65, 65f
    low angle evacuation
        1:1 mechanical advantage hauling system, 240–241
    tandem, 65, 306
        definition of, 304
    traveling, definition of, 278
Pulley system
    complex, 282b
    compound, 280
        definition of, 278
    simple, 280
        definition of, 278

R

Radiation, 11
Radio
    channels, 174
    for high angle lowering system, 253
Radio chest harnesses, 174, 174f, 253f
Radio frequency (RF) exposure, 297
    definition of, 296
Radio tower amplitude modulation (AM), 297
Radium releasing hitches, 193–195, 194f, 195f
Rain, protecting litter patient from, 217–218
Raising operation, taking in slack in, 197
Rappelling, 115–142, 340, 340f
    arm, 116, 117, 117f
    body, 116, 117–118, 117f
    control of, 116
    definition of, 2, 116
    flash, 39
    getting over edge, 129–130
    helicopter, 338–340
        definition of, 318
    knees over edge, 129, 129f
    Münter hitch, 137, 139f
        definition of, 116
    ropes for, 21
    safely, 7
    skills checklist for, 364
    stance for, 128
    training for rope rotation in, 39
    using body friction, 117–118
Rappelling devices, 56, 116
    mechanical, 118–119
Rappel rack. *See also* Brake bar rack
    definition of, 48
Ratchet cams, 242b

Recreational climbing, standards for, 359
Redundant systems, 5, 175
REGA knotted rope technique, 341f
Repeater channels, 173
Requirements for Rope Access Work, 4
Rescue
    cache preplanning, 168–169
    integrating with medical care, 190
    review of tactics, 167
    ropes for, 21–22
Rescue 8, 3, 57
Rescue Belay, 540 degrees. *See* 540 degrees Rescue Belay
Rescue belaying, 191–201
    skills checklist for, 366
Rescue chest harnesses, 210–211, 211f
Rescue harnesses, 14
Rescue hauling systems, 278
    4:1 (piggyback) hauling system, 292–293, 293f
    2:1 hauling system without the diminishing V, 291f
    rigging and using, 287–292
    1:1 TMA, 287–289, 290f
    3:1 Z-rig hauling system, 291–292, 292f
Rescue highlines, 304
Rescuer
    characteristics of effective, 5
    on helicopters, 328
        let-down/lowering, 343
    standards for, 359
Rescue rope, 33–45
    material for, 23
Rescue ruck apparatus, 168f
Rescue sling, arrangement of, 208f
Rescue subjects. *See also* Patients
    in helicopters, 336, 337f
    loading into litters, 269–270
    lowering live in litters, 266–267
    medical considerations for high angle lowering, 269–270
    removing weight on rope, 209
    seat harnesses placed on, 209–210
    stabilizing in litters, 221
    tie-ins for low angle evacuation, 264–265
    unconscious, 212
Rescue team leader for high angle lowering system, 252
Research coordinator, 350–351
Respiration, 11–12
Response, 172
Rigging
    Air Traffic Controller (ATC), 106–109
    anchors, 7, 312
    highlines, 312–315
    litters, 264f, 267–268, 267f
        for low angle evacuation, 232–233, 232f
        for single line lowering, 261–262
    near-side with pretensioned back-ties, 313f–314f
    one-person belay device, 107f
    rescue hauling systems, 287–292
    TRE, 109–112
Rigging plate, 265f
    as master attachment point, 264
Right-handed ascenders, 148
Rigid litters for low angle evacuation, 231
Ring bend (water knot), 74, 86
Rock anchors, 61

Rock climbing, definition of, 2
Roll module, 39
Rollover edge, ascending over, 157
Roof drain holes between windows and doors, 81
Roof roller, 39, 39f
Rope, 19–31. *See also* Dynamic rope; Static rope
  for anchors, 84
  angle of, 130, 130f
  attaching ascenders to, 150–151
  attaching brake bar rack to, 131, 132f–133f
  attaching Prusik loop to, 145
  backing ascenders down, 151
  bagged, 35, 35f, 43, 139f
  belaying, slack in, 113
  bending, 40, 40f, 69f
  braided, 25–26, 25f
  breaking strength of, 29
  care of, 6, 34
  coils, 35, 36f, 75, 76f
  colors of, 29
  commercial protectors of, 38–39, 38f
  construction of, 24–27
  creating spiders from, 262
  damaged, 36–40
  determining for task, 20
  double braided, 25–26, 26f
  dressing ends of, 43
  fall factor of, 22–23
  fibers made from, 23–24
  getting off of, 257, 260
  haul, 286
  high angle lowering system, 251–252
  high-stretch, 21
  hollow braided, 25
  inspection of, 40, 41f
  laid, 25, 25f
    definition of, 20
  large-diameter, 27
  life safety
    establishing responsibility for, 40
    National Fire Protection Association (NFPA) guidelines for, 28–29
  for low angle evacuation, 231, 237
  maximum working temperature, 141
  mechanical protection devices, 38–39
  melted end of, 43f
  metal protection devices, 38
  natural fiber, 23
  nylon fiber, 23
  overhand knot for, 69
  overloading, 36–37
  personal escape, 24, 141
  plaited, 25, 25f
  polyester fiber, 23
  preventing rappelling off end of, 140
  protecting below you, 139–140
  for rappelling and ascending, 21
  removing subject's weight on, 209
  rescue, 21–22, 33–45
    material for, 23
  retiring, 40, 41b
  rotation in rappelling training, 39
  selection of, 27
    for Prusik hitch, 145

Rope *(Continued)*
  size of, 27
  special cleaning problems, 43
  stacking of, 43, 44f
  standards for, 359
  storing, 34–35
  strength of, 27
  synthetic fiber, 23
  tagging, 34
  for technical climbing and mountaineering, 20
  tensile test standards of, 29
  throwing of, 45f
  trapping, avoidance of, 163f
  washing, 40–42
Rope access, 3–4, 21
  definition of, 2
Rope grabs, 50
  for belaying and hauling, 61
  definition of, 48
  in hauling systems, 284
  nature of, 284
Rope handlers
  definition of, 230
  for high angle lowering system, 252
  hints for, 43–45
  in low angle evacuation, 237
Rope history log, 34, 34f
  definition of, 34
Rope pads, 37
  fire hose, 37, 37f
  in hauling systems, 288
  improvised, 37–38
Rope rescue, 3
  compartmental storage of equipment, 168f
  definition of, 2, 166
  technician skills, 7
Rope system, 244
Rope tag, 34
  definition of, 34
  example of, 34f
Rope washers, 42f
Rotor blades, 328

S

Safety, 175–176
  communications for, 176–177
  of helicopters, 333–334
  high angle rope technician, 4
  in litter lowering systems, 261
  physical, 5
  Prusik, 137–138
  rappelling, 7
  tower-based rescue, 299–300
  tying off short, 154
Safety belts, standards for, 359
Safety cams, 242b
Safety circle, 324
  definition of, 319
Safety knot, definition of, 68f
Safety lever of light-use ascenders, 148
Safety lines, 5, 6
  edge, 177f
  personnel, 246f

Safety officer, 6
　for high angle lowering system, 252
Safety person, 2
Safety systems, secondary, Occupational Safety and Health
　　Administration (OSHA), 137
Safety tether strap, 338
Safety tie-in on highlines, 310
SAS. *See* Special Air Services (SAS)
Scouts for low angle evacuation, 234
Scuppers, anchoring to, 81
Search and rescue, precision in, 178–179
Seat/chest harnesses, 15
Seat harnesses, 13
　definition of, 10
　emergency, 10, 13
　equipment loops, 16f
　manufactured, placed on subject, 209
　manufactured sewn, 13f
　qualities of, 14
　rescue of person not wearing, 209–211
　rescue of person wearing, 205–209
　tied, placed on subject, 210
　tied hasty, placed on subject, 210, 210f
Seattle Manufacturing Co. (SMC), 349
　Escape 8 descenders, 142, 142f
Seizures, flicker, 337
Self-belay, techniques for, 137
Self-rescue, preparation for, 6
Sheave of pulleys, 64
Shell (clothing), 12
Shock, signs of, 188
Shock absorption, 28
Shock loading, 28
Shoes for helicopters, 334
Short haul
　definition of, 319
　dynamic, 342, 343f
Short haul operations
　helicopters, 341–342, 342f
　　hazards of, 341–342
　　procedures for, 342
Short rope, fall factor of, 22–23
Shoulder slings, 16
Shuttle loom webbing, 30
Side plates of pulleys, 64
Signals
　for belay, 101–102
　hand, 325f
　yes-or-no, 174
Sikorsky hoist rescue, 338f
Simple mechanical advantage, 280, 281f
Simple pulley systems, 280
　definition of, 278
Simplex communication, 173–174
Single line lowering
　definition of, 250
　litter rigging for, 261–262
Single rope technique (SRT), 1, 3, 21, 60
　definition of, 2
Single unit roller, 38, 38f
Situational awareness, 176, 177b, 327
　definition of, 166, 319
　loss of, 5

Size up, definition of, 296
Sked litter, 216, 217f
Sling load, 343
　definition of, 319
Slings, creating from webbing, 86
Slip clutch, 339
Slopes
　brake bar rack lowering on, 133–134, 135f, 136f, 258–260, 259f
　figure 8 descenders on, 122, 123f
　in helicopter landings, 324
　steep
　　evacuation with progress capture devices (PCD) in, 242–243
　　lowering with figure 8 with ears, 253–257, 254f
SLR. *See* System load ratio (SLR)
SMC. *See* Seattle Manufacturing Co. (SMC)
Snap links, 48
Snow landing by helicopters, 324
Society of Professional Rope Access Techniques (SPRAT), 4
Socks, 12
Soft cams, 60
Soft litters, 186
Solid braided rope, 25
Solution dying of ropes, 29
Span of control, 169
　definition of, 166
Special Air Services (SAS), 3
Special procedure insertion and extraction system (SPIES), 340b
Spectra, 29
　definition of, 20
Spiders, 261–264
　adjustable, 265f
　　creating from rope, 264
　anchor strip for, 262
　attaching to main-line lowering rope, 263
　construction of, 261–262
　creating from rope, 262
　definition of, 250
　for double line lowering systems, 270, 271f
　double line to single point, 270
　double line to two point, 270–271
　highlines, 307
　sizing for dual brake litter lowering, 274
　webbing sling for, 262
SPIES. *See* Special procedure insertion and extraction system (SPIES)
Spinal extrication device, 189
Spinal immobilization
　commercial devices for, 219–229
　equipment for, 186
Spinal injuries
　packaging for litter, 219
　protection in flexible litter, 217
Spine, 189
　boards, 219, 220f
　cervical
　　devices, 186
　　immobilization equipment for, 186
　　with litters, 218–219
　splints, 186
Spiral weave (needle loom) webbing, 30f
Spotter, 326
SPRAT. *See* Society of Professional Rope Access Techniques
　　(SPRAT)
Spreader on highlines, 310

SRT. *See* Single rope technique (SRT)
Stairwell beams anchoring to, 81
Standards, 359
Static kernmantle, 26–27, 26f
Static measurement, 355
Static rope, 3
 core of, 21f
 definition of, 20
 vs. dynamic ropes, 27
 for litters, 22
Static testing, definition of, 348
STC. *See* Supplemental type certificate (STC)
Steel carabiners *vs.* aluminum carabiners, 52
Steep angle highline, 304, 305f
 definition of, 304
Steep slopes
 evacuation with progress capture devices, 242–243
 lowering with figure 8 with ears, 253–257, 254f
Step-out landing, 331
 definition of, 319
Sticht plate, 63
Stokes-style litter, 342
Stopper knot, 68f
Stoppers, 62f
Study objective, 351
Subjects. *See also* Rescue subjects
 definition of, 166
Suction, equipment for, 186
SUDOT, 174
Sunglasses for helicopters, 334
Supplemental type certificate (STC), 335
 definition of, 319
Surface-applied dying of ropes, 29
Survival plan checklist, 335
Synthetic fiber rope, 23
System
 definition of, 2
 testing of, 347–357
System efficiencies, calculating, 283, 283f
System load ratio (SLR), 28
System safety factor
 definition of, 20
 determining, 27–29
Systems testing, 350
 definition of, 348

T

Tactical operations, high angle rescue, 3
Tag line, 306
 attachments for on highlines, 310
 definition of, 278, 304
 in hauling systems, 288, 288f
Tall tower, 296
Tandem Prusik belay, 64, 193
Tandem Prusik belay system, 192–193, 192f
 construction of, 193
 definition of, 192
 operating, 195
Tandem Prusik system, 285f
Tandem pulleys, 65, 306
 definition of, 304
Tangles, prevention of, 43–44
Tape knot, 86
Team concepts, 6

Team skills, 7
Teamwork and communication in pickoff rescue, 203
Technical climbing, ropes for, 20
Technical rescue, 3
Telpher, definition of, 304
Temperature. *See also* Cold; Heat
 on helicopters, 336
 maximum working, 141
10% rule for highlines, 310
Tensile strength, 27, 34
 definition of, 20
Testing, 347–357
 crunching results of, 356
 methods of, 354–355
 performance of, 350
 planning of, 350–351
 results of, 355
 sample project planning sheet, 352f–354f
 variance in, 351f
Theoretical mechanical advantage (TMA), 280
 definition of, 278
Think systems, 5
Third man with litters, 270
Three-ascender system, 155–157, 155f
Three-point suspension of helmets, 10–11
Three-way loading carabiners, 55
Three-wrap Prusik hitches, 147, 147f
Tie-ins
 commercial, 221–222, 224f
 of light-use ascenders, 148
 for litters
  for double line lowering, 271
  for low angle evacuation, 232
  webbing of, 221f
 for low angle evacuation, 231
  adjustable, 235f
  litter tender, 235–236, 235f, 265, 266f
  rescue subject, 264–265
 for rescue subject, 221–224
 safety on highlines, 310
Tie-in system, commercial, 221–222, 224f
Titanium tubing litter, 215
TMA. *See* Theoretical mechanical advantage (TMA)
1:1 TMA hauling system, 287–289, 288f
Toe-in landing, 331
 definition of, 319
Top roping, 2
Torque, 328
 definition of, 319
Touchdown pad, 324
 definition of, 319
Tower
 amplitude modulation (AM) radio, 297
 freestanding, 299, 300f
  definition of, 296
 guyed, 299, 301f
  definition of, 296
 tall, 296
Tower-based rescue, 4, 295–302
 climber exhaustion, 299
 climbing, 297–298
 completing, 302
 contacts and resources, 302
 definition of, 296

Tower-based rescue *(Continued)*
  equipment and personnel, 302
  hazards of, 296–297
  need for, 296
  personal rescue equipment, 297
  preplanning, 302
  rescue gear, 297
  rescuer safety, 299–300
  size up, 301–302
  training, 302
Training, 190t
Training deficiencies, identification of, 167
Translational lift, 330
  definition of, 319
Traveling pulley, definition of, 278
TRE belay device, 63
  level ground, 110f–111f
  rigging, 110f
TRE rigging, belaying, 109–112
Tree wrap, 230
  for low angle evacuation, 236–237, 238f
Trigger, belay practice system, 101f
Tripods used as directionals, 287f
T system, 283–284
Tubular webbing, 30
Tunnel vision, 5
Two brake lowering system, 272–274
Two-person loads, highlines, 307
Two-point Yosemite system on litter, 183f
Tying off short, 152–154, 152f–153f
  definition of, 144
  maintaining safety, 154
Type 1 rescue, 189
Type 2 rescue, 189
Tyrolean, definition of, 304

U
UHMWPE. *See* Ultra-high molecular weight polyethylene (UHMWPE)
UIAA. *See* Union of International Alpine Associations (UIAA)
Ultra-high molecular weight polyethylene (UHMWPE), 141
Unconscious subject, 212
Undercut edge, 130
  ascending over, 158
  getting over in litter lowering, 268
Underwear, 12
Unified command, 169
  definition of, 166
Union of International Alpine Associations (UIAA)
  climbing helmet certification, 11
  definition of, 10
  standards of, 359
Unlocking in lowering, 256–257
Urination, 11

V
Vacuum mattress, 189
Vacuum splints, 186, 220

Vapor barrier
  across litter, 218f
  wrapped around patient, 219f
Vehicles used for anchors, 88–89
Vertical caving, 3
  definition of, 2
Vertical face
  brake bar rack down, 134–137
  figure 8 with ears to lower down, 257–258, 257f
Vertical lowering, 250
  with brake bar rack, 261, 262f
Vertical reference, definition of, 319
Vertical rescue, 3
Vertical sports, ropes for, 23
VFR. *See* Visual flight rules (VFR)
Vibram, 12
Vibration on helicopters, 336
Visual flight rules (VFR), 323
  definition of, 319
VOX (voice operated exchange) headset, 174

W
Warning call, 7
Washing ropes, 40–42
Water, hovering over, 329
Water ditching survival training, 336
Webbing, 29–30
  for anchors, 85, 87f
  care of, 43
  for closed loop, 234b
  clove hitch for, 75
  construction of, 30
  creating slings from, 86
  for litter tie-ins, 221f
  overhand knot for, 69
  placement around anchor points, 86
  size of, 30
  sling for spiders, 262
  strength of, 30–31
Weld abrasion, 178
Wetness, protection from, 12
Whistle command system, 174
Wind
  indicators for helicopter landings, 324
  protecting litter patient from, 217–218
Wire baskets, 186
Wool, 12
Workplace, standards for, 359

Y
Yes-or-no signal, 174

Z
Z-rig, 282
  definition of, 278
  3:1 hauling system, 291–292, 292f